# BONE AND MINERAL RESEARCH/7

The cover illustration is a phase-contrast micrograph of an osteoclast. It was reproduced from the paper by T.J. Chambers and C.J. Dunn: 'Prostacyclin inhibits the cytoplasmic activity of isolated osteoclasts' which appeared in *Current Advances in Skeletogenesis* (Fig. 1a, p. 151; Editors: M. Silbermann and H.C. Slavkin; Excerpta Medica, 1982), by courtesy of the authors.

# BONE AND MINERAL RESEARCH/7

## A regular survey of developments in the field of bone and mineral metabolism

*Edited by*

**JOHAN N.M. HEERSCHE**
*MRC Group in Periodontal Physiology*
*University of Toronto*
*Toronto, Canada*

**JOHN A. KANIS**
*Department of Human Metabolism and Clinical Biochemistry*
*The University of Sheffield Medical School*
*Sheffield, S. Yorkshire, U.K.*

**1990**
**ELSEVIER**
**Amsterdam – New York – Oxford**

ISBN 0-444-81371-3 (volume)
ISBN 0-444-90409-3 (series)

*Published by:*
Elsevier Science Publishers B.V. (Biomedical Division)
P.O. Box 211
1000 AE Amsterdam
The Netherlands

*Sole distributors for the USA and Canada:*
Elsevier Science Publishing Company, Inc.
655 Avenue of the Americas
New York, NY 10010
USA

**Printed in The Netherlands**

This volume was produced under the auspices of the International Conferences on Calcium-Regulating Hormones, Inc.

# List of Contributors

**E. F. Eriksen**
*Medical Department III, Division of Endocrinology and Metabolism, Aarhus Amtssygehus, 8000 Aarhus C, Denmark*

**A.J. Friedenstein**
*Immunopharmacological Laboratory, The Gamaleya Institute for Epidemiology and Microbiology, Academy of Medical Sciences of the USSR, Gamaleya Str. 18, Moscow D-98, USSR*

**M.F. Holick**
*Boston University School of Medicine, 80 East Concord St., M-1013 Boston, MA 02118, USA*

**D.A. McCarron**
*Division of Nephrology and Hypertension, Institute for Nutrition and Cardiovascular Research, Department of Medicine, Oregon Health Sciences University, 3181 S.W. Sam Jackson Park Road, Portland, OR 97201, USA*

**G. Milhaud**
*VA 163 CNRS, Faculté St. Antoine, 27 rue Chaligny, Paris, France*

**L. Mosekilde**
*Medical Department III, Division of Endocrinology and Metabolism, Aarhus Amtssygehus, 8000 Aarhus C, Denmark*

**J.M. Moseley**
*Department of Medicine, University of Melbourne, and St. Vincent's Institute of Medical Research, St. Vincent's Hospital, Fitzroy, Victoria 3065, Australia*

**A.M. Perault-Staub**
*UA 163 CNRS, Faculté St. Antoine, 27 rue Chaligny, Paris, France*

**S.H. Ralston**

*University Department of Orthopaedic Surgery, Western Infirmary, Glasgow G11 6NT, UK*

**D.W. Rowe**

*Department of Pediatrics, University of Connecticut Health Center, Farmington, CT 06032, USA*

**J.F. Staub**

*UA 163 CNRS, Faculté St. Antoine, 27 rue Chaligny, Paris, France*

**L.J. Suva**

*Department of Medicine, University of Melbourne, and St. Vincent's Institute of Medical Research, St. Vincent's Hospital, Fitzroy, Victoria 3065, Australia*

# Contents

# Editors' Foreword

JOHAN N.M. HEERSCHE and JOHN A. KANIS

Our aim in putting together this 7th volume of the *Bone and Mineral Research* series has been to present high quality up-to-date reviews and in-depth analyses in areas where developments are, or potentially could be, of great interest to the Bone and Mineral research community. It is self evident that we hope to have been able to maintain the high standards established in this series under the stimulating direction of Dr. William A. Peck, the Editor of the first six volumes.

Within the wide field of bone and mineral research, progress has been astounding in some areas, whereas in other areas slow and gradual accummulation of knowledge has resulted in an increased insight, which make a review appropriate. We have attempted to include reviews in both areas and, in addition, to include chapters which emphasize the development of new concepts.

In the first chapter, by Perault-Staub and her co-workers, calcium homeostasis is re-visited. In it, the importance of oscillatory behaviour associated with the dynamics of calcium regulation is emphasized, and new models are proposed related to the importance of self-regulation of plasma calcium homeostasis within a framework of the dynamic organization of all biological systems.

Next is a discussion of current views on calcium and hypertension. Controversial as this issue may be, we felt that a critical evaluation of the evidence relating increased serum total calcium or ionized calcium to hypertension would be of interest and would help focus thought and experimentation in this area.

Cancer-associated hypercalcaemia is one of the areas that has seen remarkable progress in recent years. A classic overview of the complexity of the issue and the variety of factors involved in the various forms of this syndrome is given in Chapter 3, and is followed by an in-depth review in Chapter 4 of our current knowledge of the parathyroid hormone-related peptide (PTHrP), the recently discovered major mediator of humorally mediated cancer-associated hypercalcaemia.

The emerging importance of molecular biology as a tool to resolve basic issues related to diseases of bone and mineral metabolism, evident from this chapter, is further emphasized in the following chapter on oesteogenesis imperfecta, in which the genetic abnormalities resulting in many forms of osteogenesis imperfecta are discussed. The concepts and approaches developed in studying this disease will likely serve as a model for future forays into resolving other genetic matrix-based bone diseases.

With regard to the origin and lineage of the cells actually forming the bone matrix, knowledge remains fragmentary. However, without the highly original and pioneering investigations of Friedenstein, this field would be lagging even further than it does now. Reading how these new concepts were developed and how interaction between the haemopoietic and stromal systems may be crucial for generating new supplies of bone-forming cells is fascinating. In addition, the approach may prove to be of great importance to solve the greatest current riddle in bone metabolism: discovering the cause and a cure for osteoporosis. Some aspects of this latter problem are highlighted in Chapter 7, where estrogen's actions on bone are being discussed. Despite the long-standing recognition that estrogen-deficiency is one of the most important causes of osteoporosis, and despite an enormous scientific effort, this area is still a clear example of one where more insight is acquired continuously, where insight into the cellular aspects of estrogen action and the mechanisms of its clinical effects is now greater than ever before, but where the great breakthrough is still to come.

Last but not least, an entirely 'non-bone' target organ of the 'bone hormones' of the vitamin D family is discussed in Chapter 8. In this chapter, an extensive discussion of the physiology and photobiology of vitamin D can be found, together with a new and exciting possible use of $1,25(OH)_2D_3$ and its analogs for treatment of psoriasis.

We hope this book may provide enjoyable reading over the Christmas holidays, during weekends in the sun, in front of the fireplace, or just simply while at work, and thus provide the seeds for new thoughts and experiments.

*Bone and Mineral Research/7*
*Johan N.M. Heersche and John A. Kanis, editors*



# Extracellular calcium homeostasis

A.M. PERAULT-STAUB, J.F. STAUB AND G. MILHAUD

*UA 163 CNRS, Faculté St. Antoine, 27 rue Chaligny, Paris, France*

'Bien loin (. . .) que l'animal (. . .) soit indifférent au monde extérieur, il est au contraire dans une étroite et savante relation avec lui, de telle façon que son équilibre résulte d'une continuelle et délicate compensation établie comme par la plus sensible des balances.'

(Claude Bernard. Leçons sur les phénomènes de la vie communs aux animaux et aux végétaux)

## Introduction

The aim of this review is to propose a reappraisal of the concepts of calcium homeostasis in the light of recent advances not only in the calcium field, but also in many other domains. The decisive events underlying this reappraisal are the manifestations of periodic behaviour by numerous parameters, all more or less directly related to calcium metabolism, and especially the documented circadian behaviour of total as well as ionized plasma calcium concentration in rat (Milhaud et al., 1972; Hunt and Perris, 1974; Talmage et al., 1975a; Staub et al., 1979) and in man (Jubiz et al., 1972; Kanabrocki et al., 1977; Markowitz et al., 1981; Perry et al., 1986). The thesis we will develop states that (1) the stability of calcium metabolism (plasma calcium concentration included) being viewed as the property of a self-organized system, maintained out of its thermodynamic equilibrium and the relative constancy of the plasma calcium concentration around a small amplitude circadian variation (central aspect for calcium homeostasis) as the property of a particular sector of this global system, (ii) plasma calcium behaviour resulting to a large extent from the complementarity, at the plasma level, of the self-oscillating behaviours of the main metabolic functions, intestine, kidney and bone, (iii) special attention being paid to the self-oscillating nature of calcium bone efflux. In our opinion, it results from the dynamic organization of bone as an organ and, especially, of nonlinear mineral reactions, highly constrained by the organic constituents of bone matrix and occurring at mature bone surface, under the cellular osteoblast-lining cell-osteocyte complex.

As for any biological system, the independence of calcium metabolism evolves largely from adapting its mineral spatio-temporal organization and its endocrine system to the sequential events which characterize the *milieu extérieur* (e.g. day/light schedule). We suggest that small daily plasma calcium variation stems from self-regulation processes, including specific interactions between bone as self-oscillating organ and calcium-regulating hormones, with their inherent circadian features. Of course, the flexibility and diversity of such a mode of regulation differ in many respects from the control foreseen by the classical homeostasis schemas. Nevertheless, even if the prevalence of hormonal control through negative feedback mechanisms is questionable, interdependence between metabolic system and hormonal metabolism (production, secretion, degradation, for instance) is obviously considered in this new schema. The requirement for a reappraisal of the traditional concepts of homeostasis has already been discussed in the literature, pertaining to the calcium (Neuman, 1969; Parfitt, 1979; Perault-Staub et al., 1974), and, more generally, to physiological and theoretical studies of the spatio-temporal organization of living system and its stability (Yates, 1982a; Moore-Ede, 1986; Waddington, 1968; Thom, 1968; Nicolis and Prigogine, 1977).

This chapter will review (i) generalities about homeostasis versus oscillatory behaviour and about contemporary advances in spatio-temporal organization, regulation and control of biological system (Section 1); (ii) current knowledge and understanding the dynamic organization and regulation of calcium metabolism (Sections 2 and 3); (iii) oscillatory behaviours associated with calcium dynamics and regulation (Section 4). Proposition of a temporal self-organized model for calcium metabolism in the rat will be presented in Section 5 and its implication for a self-regulation schema of plasma calcium homeostasis will be discussed in Section 6.

## 1. General considerations

Any living system can be defined as a dynamic system, involving a set of numerous physico-chemical reactions coordinated both in space and time. This system is open to its natural environment, with which it interfaces for energy, matter and information transfers. From a thermodynamic point of view, a living system is maintained in a state of non-equilibrium and its integrity rests on the nature of its relationships with its environment. Note that the modernity of this definition has less to do with the terms themselves, than with the meaning that these terms and their underlying relationships have today, as a result of recent progress in thermodynamics, physics and biology.

The same is true for more specific concepts such as homeostasis, introduced by Cannon (1929) and based on one century-old idea of *'fixité du milieu intérieur'* proposed by Claude Bernard (1878). Let us ask a primary question: Was the initial concept of homeostasis so acute that it might still be valid, even in the light of the recent spectacular developments in biological science? The proposition of other terms such as homeorhesis (Thom, 1968) and chreod (Waddington, 1968) or homeokinesis (Soodak and Iberall, 1978; Yates, 1982a) seems, in contrast, to indicate the need for a reappraisal of this field. We may also ask: Does homeostasis, as such, still possess its original meaning? These fundamental questions need to be raised and explored in detail, before embarking on a study of the specific question of calcium homeostasis.

Considering the strong interaction of a living system with its environment, the definition of a living system requires the determination of some organizational properties different from those of its *milieu extérieur,* endowing it with spatial and temporal specificities. An important part of the scientific approach to this problem is descriptive and concerns the study of 'states'. Hence, peculiarities of the spatial organization of living system with its high degree of complexity have been largely studied from the anatomical to molecular level, via intercellular, cellular and subcellular levels. Nevertheless, beyond description of these peculiarities, physico-chemical explanations have been suggested for the genesis and the development of such a spatial complexity (e.g. models for morphogenesis: Meinhardt, 1982; Harrison, 1987). Even though they may be still incomplete, these explanations emphasize the importance of the physical properties of the biological constituents and the pertinence of physical notions of a more general nature, such as notions of diffusion (Turing, 1952) and convection, phase transition (Yates, 1982a) (with the associated problems of interface, surface phenomena, maintenance of metastable forms, clustering, fusion, aggregation, polymerization: Aloia, 1983), i.e. many physico-chemical situations maintained in dynamic nonequilibrium conditions.

Surprisingly, there appears to have been no parallel or connection proposed between the temporal organization of a living system and the complexity of its spatial organization. In contrast, it is the constant behaviour, i.e. the simplest temporal organization, which is viewed as the most significant temporal expression of a living system. Thus, in spite of its evident spatio-temporal organization, a living system is considered as a system homogeneous in time which, of course, strengthens the descriptive power of the spatial studies. However, this constant behaviour does not describe a state of thermodynamic equilibrium, but a state of dynamic equilibrium, or steady-state (a distinction introduced in biological systems by Burton, 1939) i.e. under its formal definition, the state of an open system in which the quantities of components remain fixed in time in the face of constant fluxes through the system.

It is today well-established that the steady-state is only one of several temporal stable behaviours that a complex dynamic system is *a priori* able to exist in. Oscillatory behaviours (self-sustained periodic or aperiodic behaviours: Nicolis and Prigogine, 1977; Segel, 1984), which are known as stable behaviours for dynamic systems maintained far from their thermodynamic equilibrium, can be expected. There has been, for many years, evidence for oscillatory behaviours in living systems, and a conceptual framework for the temporal and spatio-temporal organization of biological system has been developed (Rapp, 1980; Moore-Ede et al., 1982; Winfree, 1987; Edmunds, 1988) around the idea that oscillatory behaviour is a fundamental property of living system. Thus, for instance, Goodwin (1970), in his paper on biological stability, concludes that: 'oscillatory behaviour is the fundamental dynamic mode of living, self-reproducing systems, as we know them at and above the cellular level. The oscillation is not imposed by the environment; nor is it incidental to the living process. It is central to its organization'.

Thus, from a temporal point of view, the two concepts of the organization of living system seem to be in opposition. But what does this apparent paradox really mean?

## 1.1. Two concepts of temporal organization in biological systems

### *1.1.1. Homeostasis*

The apparent contradiction between the two concepts of temporal biological organization, namely constancy and oscillatory behaviour, questions the current understanding of the notion of homeostasis, which, everyone agrees, is of prime importance for the development of physiological sciences. It is not an easy question to answer, due to the ubiquitous use of this term, from intracellular to sociological or ecological levels of organization. Nevertheless, two ideas could clarify our thoughts on homeostasis. (1) The concept is centred on the steady-state: the normal temporal expression of a biological system is considered to be a constant behaviour. Claude Bernard wrote that this kind of behaviour is 'a primary condition for the freedom and independence of living bodies in relation to the environment surrounding them', environment, which is, in contrast, highly variable and undergoes unpredictable fluctuations. (ii) The steady-state is maintained by appropriate means: when, by extension of Bernard's writings on the 'fixité du *milieu intérieur*', Cannon (1929) introduced the concept of homeostasis, he described how this state might be obtained: 'Changes in the surrounding (*milieu extérieur* for Claude Bernard) excite reactions in this system, or affect it directly, so that internal disturbances of the system are produced. Such disturbances are normally kept within narrow limits, because automatic adjustments within the system are brought into action, and thereby wide oscillations are prevented and internal conditions are held fairly constant. . . 'If a state remains steady it does so because any tendency towards change is automatically met by increased effectiveness of the factor or factors which resist the change'.

Let us recall that Claude Bernard wrote before endocrinology was established and that Cannon drew attention to the role of the autonomic nervous system. It is only in 1954 that Selye and Rosch (1954) pointed out that the ability of living system to adapt successfully to its environment depends, also, on endocrine systems. The engineering discipline called cybernetics (Wiener, 1948) found, in the sixties, a new domain of application (Goldman, 1960) within the conceptual framework proposed by Cannon and the integrative action of the nervous and endocrine systems. It led to the successful development of heuristic models to explain homeostasis. The specific cybernetic concepts of control and information theory introduced the notions of errors or stimuli, corrective response, negative feedback and so on, into diagrams of biological control. Since then, a biological control system and a cybernetic system — defined as: a set of variables whose constancy, controlled over time, is regulated by an error sensing device which, through feedback mechanisms activated by the error, damps any perturbation in order to maintain the constancy of the inherent set-value — have been considered to be analogous. Even if serious criticisms are now made against the extensive use of this engineering theory (Yates, 1982b), cybernetics have greatly influenced the thinking about homeostasis. It helped to clarify a certain view of the hierarchical organization of biological systems (dividing the organism into controlled and controlling systems) and to specify the role of regulatory factors such as endocrine or neuro-endocrine agents. D.S. Riggs (1970), in his book on *'Control Theory and Physiological Feedback Mechanisms'* proposed a variety of powerful mathematical methods, which are extensively used in the life sciences. Application of cybernetics to homeostasis has even been so successful that, in the mind of most biologists, homeostasis is now directly associated with cybernetics concepts. Nevertheless, D.S. Riggs emphasized, in his introduction, that 'the most fully developed and most easily comprehended methods of control theory deal with linear systems while most biological systems are nonlinear. This hindrance is intrinsic, and it is no good trying to sneak around it by applying inappropriate linear methods to grossly nonlinear systems, simply because the linear methods are easy to use'. He also states, in Chapter 7 on the Analysis of nonlinear feedback systems in a steady-state and the limitations inherent to exclusive steady-state considerations, that: 'First, we must restrict our attention to step inputs applied at time zero and maintained constant therafter, . . . Second, we must exclude from consideration systems which exhibit a limit cycle (i.e. periodic behaviour) in response to a constant input.' In spite of these warnings and, in fact, due to the numerous positive aspects of the cybernetic approach, there is a tendency to overemphasize the use of the steady-state as a representation of the temporal organization in biological systems. This may be responsible for the use of the term 'homeostasis' as soon as a regulated system can be approximated in a steady-state, or for the extension of homeostasis to any organizational level, for instance, in biochemical pathways where the oscillatory behaviours were, until recently, considered by some scientists (Hermann, 1980) as 'the less commonly recognized expressions of control'.

### *1.1.2. Oscillatory behaviour*

Although oscillatory (mainly periodic) behaviours in living systems have been observed since the early development of biology, it is significant that this type of temporal expression has only recently contributed to laying the foundations of fascinating theory(ies) on organization and regulation of living systems (Pittendrigh, 1961; Goodwin, 1970; Pavlidis, 1973; Nicolis and Prigogine, 1977; Winfree, 1987). Such a delay in proposing valuable theories has its corollary in the widespread prevalence of behavioural schemas associated with the use of steady-states (see just above) to describe biological systems. It originates in part from the scattered numbers of purely physico-chemical examples displaying such an oscillatory behaviour, and from the difficulty of developing a physical theory able to provide a rational and scientific explanation for the emergence of such oscillatory phenomena. It is now recognized that self-sustained oscillations do occur in a broad spectrum of chemical systems so long as reactions take place in situations involving fluxes of energy and/or matter (open system), in contrast to classical situations in which reactions spontaneously evolve towards thermodynamic equilibrium (Field, 1985). The importance of open systems in biology was recognized by Schrödinger (1945).

The theoretical researches of Prigogine and Balescu (1956) have examined the thermodynamic feasibility of periodic chemical reactions. Simple theoretical nonlinear models (Brusselator: Nicolis and Prigogine, 1977; Oregonator: Field and Noyes, 1974), hypothetical schemas of chemical reactions including autocatalytic processes, were studied. These described the fundamental property required to generate oscillatory behaviours; the set of the more or less complex behaviours foreseen by these theoretical models have been successfully compared with experimental oscillatory results, the most famous of them being the Belousov-Zhabotinskii reaction (Belousov, 1951). Then, as stated by Rapp (1987), 'the scientific community was receptive to the idea of spontaneous periodicity'. These discoveries gave rise to a renewal of interest for periodic manifestations in biological systems as oscillations were found in biochemical reactions. The classic example is the glycolytic pathway (Chance et al., 1967; Hess and Boiteux, 1971) for which, under suitable experimental conditions, autonomous oscillations (order of minutes) have been observed when glucose enters the system at a constant rate. Since this first example in cell-free system, numerous periodic phenomena have been described in a wide range of organisms (from single-cell to human), covering a large frequency range (from fractions of a second to years) and involving a whole spectrum of processes (from protein synthesis to neural activity). A first, simple autocatalytic model was proposed by Sel'kov (1968) which accounts for the various experimental results of the glycolytic system. Later, Goldbeter and Nicolis (1976) described an allosteric model which established a link between the cooperative properties of an enzyme (positive feedback) and the coherent spatio-temporal behaviour of the system as a whole. Models based on autocatalytic processes have also been proposed for the cell division cycle (Tyson and Kauffman, 1975). Nonlinear models including both an inhibitor feedback loop and a source of delay in this negative feedback have been suggested for other biological oscillators such as oscillations in calcium-cyclic AMP (Rapp and Berridge, 1977) or for cell division cycle

(Tyson and Othmer, 1978). Thus, while it is clear that there is no single mechanism for generating all biological oscillations, relevant physico-chemical mechanisms are now available which are suitable for modelling biological oscillations.

Besides their stability, nonlinear oscillators have the remarkable property of being able to react specifically towards other extrinsic periodic phenomena, for instance, by phase entrainment and period synchronization. This type of peculiarity is clearly of great interest to physiologists when the endogenous periodicity (circadian or seasonal) is similar to the natural periodicity of the *milieu extérieur* from which the living system has evolved and in which it expresses itself (Moore-Ede et al., 1982; Edmunds, 1988). It has been suggested that a major factor in the evolutionary development of a living system's identity lies in the fact that the living system succeeds, through selection, in integrating some repetitive temporal features of its environment into its own structure. By doing so, a living system performs better in its particular environment, because these endogenous oscillations remain very sensitive to the influence of the native environmental periodic events, with which they are able to harmonize in frequency and phase. Rhythmic expressions provide beautiful examples of the mode of temporal organization in living system. In this context, hormonal and central nervous systems (suprachiasmatic nuclei for instance), with their prominent rhythmic profile, are prime candidates for intermediary factors between the environment and the target metabolic system, acting as circadian pacemakers. Another consequence of the dynamic reactivity of nonlinear oscillators is that, through coupling together, they can generate complex oscillatory behaviours (Golbeter and Decroly, 1983) and rhythmic patterns whose periodicity is a combination of the initial frequencies. For instance, Winfree (1967) and Pavlidis (1969) suggested that a low-frequency behaviour as circadian rhythmicity may originate from the coupling of a number of biochemical oscillators whose period is of the order of minutes.

In summary, the foundation for a new view of the temporal organization of living systems lay both in experimental evidence for large number of oscillatory phenomena and in recent development of a conceptual framework able to explain their generation and their self-regulation ability. This view is all the more fascinating since, on the basis of purely physico-chemical principles, it encompasses spatial and temporal organization, the key principle being the ability of complex systems to produce stable heterogeneities in both space and time. This property is directly dependent upon the expression of nonlinear processes within a system which, mathematically, has rarely analytical solutions. However, the dynamics of such formal systems may now be studied by numerical and computational methods. Thus, promising advances in this concept of biological organization are linked to developments in the mathematical theory of nonlinear systems. They also involve the elaboration of theory(ies) applicable to biology: e.g. the kinetic theory as presented by Harrison (1987) which 'envisages pattern and form (in space and time) as being generated by movement away from equilibrium, explicable therefore only in terms of rates of chemical reactions and transport processes', or homeokinetics, introduced by Soodak and Iberall (1978) and

Yates (1982a), which is a 'physical theory for complex systems based upon statistical mechanics, nonlinear dynamics and irreversible thermodynamics' and in which 'nonlinear oscillators are used as dynamic regulators'.

## 1.2. Pertinence of the homeostasis concept to oscillatory behaviour

The circadian rhythm because of its periodicity close to 24 h is one of the periodic behaviours best known to physiologists. Surprisingly, some biological variables as 'vital' as body temperature or plasma concentration of numerous minerals, including calcium, usually described as examples of homeostasis, show circadian variations (Palmer, 1976). This prompted biologists to analyse these periodic phenomena as resulting, more or less directly, from periodic perturbations arising from variations in the *milieu extérieur*. It is now shown experimentally that these oscillations are intrinsic properties of living systems: they persist generally, but not necessarily with the same characteristics (different period and amplitude values, free-running), in the absence of external oscillatory phenomena (Moore-Ede et al., 1982). It is understandable that the problem of the compatibility between homeostasis and oscillatory behaviours has been questioned if there are real discrepancies between the regulation and control mechanisms for these two concepts of temporal organization. The biologist's stand-point towards this problem arises from both phenomenological and conceptual considerations. Scientists interested in the foundations of theoretical biology, such as Waddington (1968), Thom (1975), Nicolis and Prigogine (1977), Yates (1982b), Pattee (1970) and others, with their conceptual and formal researches about thermodynamics and life, evolution, development, self-organization, morphogenesis, etc. have made major contributions.

### 1.2.1. *The physiologists' stand-point*

#### 1.2.1.1. *Exclusion*

We will devote little space to the once-current approach in which the two aspects of the temporal organization of biological systems were studied separately. Two decades ago, scientists interested in homeostasis used the formal schema suggested by control system theory to examine maintenance of a system in a steady-state through feedback mechanisms. It would be unfair to underestimate the important advances provided by cybernetic models of homeostasis, and to be unaware that Jones (1973), in his text devoted to homeostatic regulation, pointed out that classical application of feedback systems in biological field may be too limited a view. Nevertheless, it appears that authors, too convinced by the explanatory power of relatively simple comprehensive models built around this basic schema, had a tendency to consider real rhythmic expression as an 'error' resulting from periodic exogenous perturbation. Amplitude of the periodic event was even interpreted as the coefficient of variation of the set value (here the mean periodic value has no actual meaning for the system itself) i.e. as an index of the precision with which the (theoretically expected) set value was maintained (Bronner, 1982). Thus, in order to avoid the complexities due to periodic manifestations (judged devoid of significance), experimentation was performed over a relatively short time-lapse compared to the (known or expected) periodicity of the studied parameter or at the same phase of the rhythm.

Conversely, chronobiology (Halberg, 1969), a scientific discipline mainly interested in rhythmic events, was born. Chronobiologists started with a serious handicap because they had only empirical model to fund their thinking and, even now, although great progress has been made in understanding the genesis of rhythmic feature, these formal models are so complex that they are not easily handled by the biologist. Hence, chronobiology is more descriptive than explanatory. Its main contribution concerns the study of the connections and relationships that exist between the various periodic events in an organism, not only under physiological conditions, but also in pathology and therapeutics (Reinberg and Halberg, 1979).

#### *1.2.1.2. Association*

The stand-point of physiologists, skilled in biological rhythmicity, who devoted themselves to reach a compromise between homeostasis and rhythmicity, was more fruitful for the thesis we develop here. Aschoff (1979) noticed, 'the rhythmic structure of biological systems can be considered a principle, complementary to that of homeostasis'. Moore-Ede also argued the prefix 'homeo' was coined by Cannon as implying some variation around a constant value. Within the framework of such an association, Moore-Ede (1986) proposed 'a mature understanding of homeostasis which should encompass both reactive and predictive homeostasis'. He suggests an extension of the classical schema of homeostasis in which controlling agents only react to a change which has already occurred. Moore-Ede introduces the peculiarities of the physiology and behaviour of most living organisms in the endeavour to adapt to their natural environment (the seasons of the year and the day-night cycle).

Following this schema, the organism should have developed some intrinsic type of time-measuring device which enables the prediction of a repetitive (mainly circadian) event. Thus, before the time at which this foreseeable event will take place, the organism activates special mechanisms (e.g. protein synthesis). The internal repercussion of the rhythmic event is then efficiently counterbalanced and homeostatic conditions are maintained. Explicit consideration of the oscillatory nature of the living system and of its relationships to adaptation and anticipation within a homeostatic schema is obviously important. Apparently relieved of the necessity of constancy, Moore-Ede supports his argument with examples as different as food availability, potassium balance, sleep-wake cycle or thermoregulation, i.e. he illustrates his homeostasis schema by studying both variables which have a nearly constant behaviour and belong to plasma and extracellular fluids (i.e. to the *milieu intérieur* defined by Claude Bernard), and behavioural variables, with highly circadian pattern. A careful analysis of this schema reveals that the association of oscillatory behaviour with homeostasis implies the use of the cybernetic key-words, i.e. corrective response and more or less implicitly, error and set-value concepts.

However, the author further suggests modulating them by using a temporal qualification such as 'corrective response initiated in anticipation', 'cyclic variation in physiological set-point'. Therefore, and without minimizing the interest of this study, one may question the validity of the integration of oscillatory behaviours by extension of a conceptual framework, intially designed for a basically constant system (i.e. approximated to a linear system). The real impact of oscillatory events with their nonlinear nature and their reactional specificities (self-regulation) may be underestimated in favour of homeostasis.

### *1.2.2. Stability and constancy*

As previously mentioned, one of the theories of temporal organization in living systems, homeostasis, may benefit from a series of successive developments, improvements and 'complexifications', while the other, oscillatory behaviour, is topical and expanding rapidly. So, what undoubtedly distinguishes the two theories is the background system theory that has developed a great deal since the publication of homeostasis statements, a century or even 50 years ago. Let us revisit Claude Bernard's and Cannon's papers with a dual approach. Let us replace the propositions in their initial cultural context and re-evaluate these authors' intuitive power in analyzing their idea in the light of the contemporary knowledge on system regulation and organization.

#### *1.2.2.1. Stability*

The writings of Claude Bernard and Cannon may be re-read bearing in mind one of the central problems in biology, i.e. the stability of biological systems. Indeed, although Claude Bernard and Cannon emphasized words such as constancy, 'fixité', uniform, rigid, steady-state, these words were by themselves less important than the impression gave by them of the high degree of permanence and of stability shown by the living system, especially if compared to the inconstancy offered by the *milieu extérieur.* This is illustrated in the following quotation 'All the vital mechanisms, however varied they may be, have only one object, that of preserving the conditions of life in the internal environment' (translated by Cannon from Claude Bernard). It is the very reason for which Yates (1982a) translated 'fixité' by 'stability' rather than fixity. The notion of stability was for Claude Bernard, by necessity linked in his mind to the notion of constancy: the stability of oscillatory regimes in autonomous systems (Poincaré, 1890) was too contemporary to have significant influence on his thought. Furthermore, Claude Bernard and Cannon ignored temporal expressions such as chaotic behaviours which are today thought to be interesting features of biological systems (Goldberger and West, 1987), and the strong relationship which exists between spatial and temporal organization in complex nonlinear systems? Thus, intuitive though they might have been, they could obviously not suspect such a behavioural diversity hidden behind the stability concept: 'a system is stable if its form (in space and time) persists and continues to carry out characteristic behaviours in spite of random or systematic, time-varying inputs that tend to perturb its behaviour. Stable systems persist' around only rest (using Yates, 1982a terminology, i.e. constant) states if linear systems, and around either rest or motional (oscillatory for instance) states if nonlinear systems. It is also in this context that Waddington (1968) and Thom (1968) discussed the term of homeostasis, introducing homeorhesis, i.e. stabilized flow (or trajectory) rather than stabilized state. So far, unfortunately, these definitions have not become firmly enough fixed in minds of numerous biologists who, in 1990, persist in confusing stability and constancy.

Scarcely developed by Claude Bernard, the capacity for adaptation and evolution of living systems, i.e. for modification of some behavioural characteristics, is today associated with the notion of resilience. This notion is defined as the 'measure of the ability of the system to absorb changes of state variables, driving variables, and parameters, and still persists. In this definition, resilience is a property of the system' (Holling, 1976). In first analysis, this concept seems *a priori* antinomic to that of stability. It is well-known today that some quantitative modification of parameter values, in nonlinear systems, can lead through bifurcations, to qualitative changes in the stable dynamic behaviours (change from constant to oscillatory behaviour, for instance). Thus nonlinear systems are substantially analogous to the essential characteristics of the biological systems and could thus bridge the gap between homeostasis, adaptation and evolution.

*1.2.2.2. Constancy*

*1.2.2.2.1. Where.* Since, for Claude Bernard and Cannon, constancy and stability were closely linked, one understands today why these authors chose to illustrate the stability of biological systems by factors which, at a first approximation, exhibit a constant behaviour. Nevertheless, it is significant that the milieu chosen by Claude Bernard was 'blood plasma, together with all interstitial liquids', i.e. the fluid shared by all the organs and their constitutive cells of the body. Similarly, Cannon defined homeostasis as the 'relatively uniform condition of the fluid matrix in which the living cells of the organism exist'. These authors have exemplified the constancy in biological systems by the behaviour of variables involved in a high-order of organization. The order is even higher for blood plasma than for interstitial liquids, as compositions of the blood plasma and the extracellular fluid of numerous specific organs differ, due to their own metabolic activity, microcirculation, perfusion rate (Neuman, 1969).

*1.2.2.2.2. Why.* Claude Bernard explained the increase in complexity of living systems by the initial emergence and subsequent maintenance during evolution, of a *milieu intérieur* which is 'the source and confluent of all the elementary exchanges'. Its 'fixed' composition, if expressed in modern terms, is neither that of the intracellular milieu, nor that of the *milieu extérieur.* Thus, he established (at least for some 'vital' variables) the necessary conditions for the expression of the elementary constituents of life, the cells. By differentiation and specialization, they are in charge of the metabolic functions of organs and, at a higher level, of the properties of the organism as a whole. This fundamental proposition appears even more pertinent if we examine it in modern language. Let us, for instance, interpret some variations observed in the concentration of plasma constituents in term of information (as is done in cybernetics). Unlike the nervous system which is highly organized in space, plasma is homogeneous in space, as a consequence of its rapid mixing. Then, blood plasma may be viewed as a crude system used as an information vehicle for the coordination, in time, of various physiological functions. Two cases may be predicted. Either, the information conveyed by the plasma — namely the temporal variation of a given constituent — is deciphered by specific cells (e.g. target cells for a hormone) so that, large variations in the plasma concentration of this constituent (nonhomeostatic variable) can be expected, contributing to temporal variations in some specific cellular function. Or, the information is ubiquitous and every cell is more or less sensitive to the concentration variation of this plasma constituent (essential constituent such as calcium for instance). In the latter case, there may be at least one reason for which the concentration of this kind of plasma constituent needs to be kept constant (homeostatic variable), i.e. devoid of temporal information. Indeed, plasma variation in concentration of this 'essential' constituent should induce a synchronization in time with the whole organism. But, it is not at all evident that, within an organism, the principles for optimal integration of the physiological functions rest on such a simultaneity in time (one rather observes a diversity in time-schedule associated to a diversity in functions). In summary, under physiological conditions, the 'homeostatic' variables should not be informative, for the system itself, according to the term presently used.

*1.2.2.2.3. How.* We can now examine how, within the modern framework of dynamic organization of biological systems, 'constant' behaviour of some variables in blood plasma can be realized. But, first, can a real phenomenon be shown to have or not have a constant behaviour? In a formal manner, an oscillatory (periodic or aperiodic) behaviour can be considered as constant behaviour either when the amplitude of the oscillations tends towards zero, or, if periodic, when its period tends to a null or infinite value. This remark illustrates how, in practice, constancy is always a hypothetical behaviour since only retained by default: Constancy may be assumed as long as a phenomenon does not differ significantly from a constant one. In reality, there is no simple criterion for deciding whether a biological parameter is basically constant and whether, more generally, the system to which it belongs operates in the steady-state. We use approximations suffering from several potential artefacts: sampling frequency, experimental duration, accuracy of measurements, premature conclusion that the system is in a steady-state from the approximation of kinetic data (tracers or perturbation studies) to a sum of exponential terms, etc. Conversely, a system is not in a steady-state, if one of the system variables significantly fits an oscillatory pattern, the reason being intrinsic or extrinsic. But, and this is fundamental for homeostasis, this situation does not exclude some other variables within the system oscillating with such a small amplitude that their behaviour could be approximated to a 'constancy' lying on the borderline of an oscillatory behaviour. Consequently, oscillating and constant behaviour may coexist within the same complex system. The quasi-constant behaviour of some variables inside a pool can result from the counterbalancing of oscillatory influxes and effluxes, having quite large amplitudes. In this sense, the time exclusion contained in the homeostasis concept rests on a very subtle use of nonlinear oscillatory manifestations, perfectly expressed by the living system, but whose basic features may be reasonably expected today accessible for analysis.

## 1.3. Circadian time keeping and homeostasis

We can now set up a conceptual framework for the category of metabolic systems which includes calcium metabolism. Homeostasis should be viewed as the ultimate achievement, at a high organizational level, of a homogeneity (constancy) which is stable in space and time. This homogeneity arises from the harmonious composition of dynamic oscillatory processes originating from both the spatio-temporal heterogeneity of each organ and the behavioural relationships that the system, as a whole, maintains with its *milieu extérieur*. With the peculiarities of its own metabolism and its specific actions on target cells, the regulatory (endocrine and nervous) system will actively participate to optimize this integrative dynamic organization from which some fundamental principles of self-regulation emerge.

### *1.3.1. General*

The homeostasis of an exogenous metabolite is directly related to its ingestion by feeding. In most animals, feeding is a circadian event associated with the major behavioural events (sleep-wake and rest-activity cycles) which govern the temporal relationships of the system with its *milieu extérieur*. According to our proposed conceptual framework, any study of the organization of this metabolism and its normal temporal regulation requires consideration of circadian time-keeping, i.e. of intrinsic nonlinear oscillators having a periodicity of circa 24 h. Circadian feeding is probably only one of several circadian features inherent in the metabolite's physiology. So that other circadian manifestations either of the 'homeostatic' parameter (variation of small amplitude), or of some specific metabolic functions and regulatory mechanisms should be observed. Such kinetic data raises specific problems related to (i) the intrinsic nature of periodic behaviours and their dependence upon the known zeitgebers or other internal synchronizers; (ii) once the intrinsic nature of the periodic event is recognized, the kind of the nonlinear processes involved in generating the oscillatory behaviour and the role of the environmental constraints imposed by the biological milieu; (iii) their integration into a comprehensive schema including both the overall dynamic organization and the principles of self-regulation.

### *1.3.2. Plasma calcium homeostasis*

Ever since McLean and Hastings (1935) first described the concentration of calcium in the blood as 'one of nature's physiological constants', conventional reports on plasma calcium homeostasis have focussed on the 'steady-state' level of plasma calcium concentration and its 'minute-to-minute' achievement by equilibration of irreversible calcium fluxes coming from and going to the main metabolic functions, i.e. bone, kidney and intestine (Bronner, 1975, 1982; Stewart and Broadus, 1987). Classical kinetics studies of calcium metabolism *in vivo* have all contributed to extending this notion of steady-state to the so-called exchangeable part of calcium metabolism and, from this, to quantifying the constant calcium fluxes related to bone, kidney and intestines (Aubert and Milhaud, 1960). As a result, calcium metabolism under physiological conditions is currently described as being in a dynamic state devoid of any temporal information. Hence, the prevalence of (i) experimental designs based on the study of the effects of acute or long-term perturbations, e.g. calcium challenge, changes in dietary or hormonal conditions; (ii) cybernetic interpretation of the results, largely based on hormonal control mechanisms that the organism is able to develop in order to preserve the 'steady-state' of plasma calcium concentration (Aurbach et al., 1985).

Our conceptual framework for plasma calcium homeostasis is unconventional, free from any systemic notion of 'steady-state'; we focus on the major role played by the intrinsically periodic events (mainly circadian ones) which are more or less directly related to calcium metabolism. The central idea is that, under normal conditions, the circadian behaviour carries temporal information of the highest significance for both the establishment and the maintenance of plasma calcium homeostasis. The existence of such internal dynamics in both metabolic (bone, kidney, intestines) and hormonal (parathyroid hormone, PTH; calcitonin, CT, and vitamin D) systems in the physiological state, prompted us to approach the problem of plasma calcium homeostasis by direct observation of spontaneous variations under normal conditions. As previously noted, further development of this concept requires explicit consideration of a pluridisciplinary knowledge of the internal organization (nonlinear dynamics) of metabolic functions and hormonal systems (Staub et al., 1988).

Before we present our results obtained for calcium metabolism in such a new conceptual framework, we will summarize the most significant dynamic aspects of calcium metabolism and its organization, with special emphasis on mineral hard tissue metabolism, and survey the classic, but still developing, theories of extracellular calcium homeostasis.

## 2. Current knowledge of the dynamic organization and regulation of calcium metabolism

**Warning:** The reader expert in calcium metabolism may find this survey, despite our efforts, as relating a simple list of 'facts', more or less evident, either vague or very precise and containing details which are not directly related to our purpose. We agree with and support the evidence that calcium metabolism, like any biological system, must not be only thought of, but also treated as, more than a compilation of mechanisms at various levels of organization. Nevertheless, we have retained this form of presentation which points to the distinction between knowledge and understanding. From these 'facts' (although they must be not weakened by some implicit current understanding), the hidden properties governing spatio-temporal expressions of both calcium metabolism and its regulatory processes must be distilled. A modeling approach offers a suitable rational framework, within which current pertinent data may be used to reveal these buried properties which are intimately associated with the overall physiological behaviour of a given metabolism. But, even with a model which provides good qualitative or quantitative approximations of the physiological behaviours, it is also necessary to use iterative procedures to realize its heuristic potential integrating other relevant data available in the vast store of current knowledge.

### 2.1. General

The biological importance of calcium, the most common mineral ion, has been known for a century (Ringer, 1883). The role of calcium in biological systems is diverse, multifaceted and fundamental. It is widely involved in many physiological processes, including skeleton growth and modelling, the maintenance of the integrity and permeability of cell membranes, the coupling of muscle excitation and contraction, the control of many enzymes and blood coagulation, the regulation of nerve excitability and the action of many hormones. Its ubiquitous function depends on the maintenance of plasma ionized calcium concentration at a certain level, the concept of plasma calcium homeostasis: below this level, the neuromuscular and skeletal systems cease to function normally; above this level, toxicity of many enzyme systems occurs.

Whereas organic metabolism deals with the formation, by covalent interactions, of a series of organic substrate molecules (metabolite cycles) catalyzed by enzymes and cofactors, that of calcium like any mineral metabolite, mainly involves electrostatic (noncovalent) interactions with other molecules or ions, i.e. calcium remains intact. This applies to calcium in solution, e.g. for $Ca^{2+}$ complexing with organic ligands or with other mineral (anions) constituents, and to the crystal structure of the solid calcium-phosphate (Ca-P) mineral phase in hard tissues. A common step in all these reactions is the replacement of the water molecules coordinating $Ca^{2+}$ with specific binding ligands (organic: Seamon and Kretsinger, 1983, or mineral: Posner and Betts, 1981) and free energy, also called Gibbs activation energy, is here the most important of the thermodynamic functions to take into account. Water exclusion ultimately leads to the precipitation of a solid phase in hard tissues. So, a major dynamic event for calcium metabolism is not a problem of chemical reaction strictly speaking, but a problem of phase transformation (solute ions/solid phase and vice versa). The dynamic organization of calcium metabolism has then to be considered as partly related to problems of nucleation, of solubility product, of interfacial tension, of crystal surface, size, geometry, of interfacial phases, etc., as foreseen by Best and Hearon (1960). It is a question of a series of phenomena belonging to the domain of physics rather than to that of chemistry and their reactional characteristics (rate, nonlinearity) being intrinsic properties of mineral materials, even if these mineral reactions are catalyzed by organic materials. The other dynamic aspect of calcium metabolism, and not the least, concerns calcium in aqueous solution with its central role as pivotal intracellular messenger. The natural selection of calcium as messenger rather than sodium, potassium or magnesium has been attributed (Williams, 1970; Carafoli, 1987) to its physical properties (radius, 6 – 8 coordination number) in respect to tightly and specifically binding the messenger to various biological ligands (cooperatively activated, buffering and storage structures). Rapid $Ca^{2+}$ movements in soft tissues involve membrane transport, monitored by diffusion gradients, electrophoretic, selective channels and energy-dependent mechanisms. The dynamic characteristics of these rapid and irreversible fluxes of calcium in soft tissues are largely dictated by the specificity of the biological material which controls them.

The nature and location of any calcium transformation and transfers occurring *in vivo* are dependent upon the cellular or organic milieu in which they operate, be it buffering of cytosolic $Ca^{2+}$ by specific calcium-binding protein or catalysis of primary nucleation of Ca-P salts by specific bone components. It is nevertheless very likely that the peculiarities of the reaction processes of calcium as a reactive mineral material strongly influence the overall dynamics of calcium metabolism *in vivo,* and consequently, plasma calcium homeostasis.

### *2.1.1. In vivo calcium metabolism*

Mammals obtain their calcium from food (exogenous source). 98 – 99% of this endogenous calcium is associated with the bone crystals in the skeleton (Ca-P salts) and the remaining 1 – 2% is subjected to a variety of calcium movements occurring rapidly inside the cell and between the inside and outside of the cell, taking into account the large concentration difference between intracellular (sub $\mu$M) and extracellular (mM) concentrations of free $Ca^{2+}$. Thus, the dynamic organization of calcium metabolism can be summarized by three types of movements: (i) between the organism and the outside world; the fluxes of calcium across the epithelial cells (ion-transporting cells) in the kidney and intestine, with a strong behavioural component for this latter process (food intake and activity habits); (ii) between the ECF and soft tissues, with a diversity of intracellular buffering structures and cellular functions in which $Ca^{2+}$ is implicated; (iii) between the endoskeleton and ECF, the phase transformation mediated both by specialized (lineage osteoblast and osteoclast) cells at the interface between hard tissues and ECF and by properties arising from the physico-chemical organization of the mineral constituents in bone.

Plasma integrates all these calcium movements. Plasma calcium homeostasis in vertebrates results from the quasi-counterbalancing of these various calcium fluxes, leading to achievement of a quasi-constant level of plasma ionized calcium concentration, with a slight age-dependent drop. To be more precise, plasma calcium concentration shows a circadian rhythm of small amplitude and such a rhythmic manifestation also qualifies a large number of biological functions implicated, more or less directly, in plasma calcium homeostasis. However, since they have, till now, been nearly always ignored in classical homeostasis schema, they shall be especially surveyed in Section 4 to be further explicitly considered inside the new schema of calcium metabolism and plasma calcium homeostasis proposed in Sections 5 and 6.

### *2.1.2. The associated hormonal systems*

Many systemic (hormones) and local (e.g. bone growth factors), may influence the dynamic characteristics of calcium metabolism. Nevertheless, as for other mineral metabolisms, some peculiar regulatory factors are specific to regulation of calcium metabolism. They are the principal calcium-regulating hormones: PTH, vitamin D, and CT. These hormones actively contribute to ensure the spatio-temporal organization of calcium metabolism, plasma calcium homeostasis included, through a complex interplay of processes concerning their own metabolism, their interaction with extracellular (mainly $Ca^{2+}$) constituents, their mutual interaction and their effect on target cells.

Recent progress in molecular and cellular biology has led to the elucidation of the major metabolic pathways of these hormones. For detailed reviews, see e.g. Cohn and Etling (1983) and Habener et al. (1984) for PTH, Jacobs (1985) for CT and DeLuca (1983) and Bell (1985) for vitamin D. We will only deal with the metabolic pathways of these calcium-regulating hormones, without considering their action on calcium metabolism which will be treated separately, when discussing their target tissue (Section 2.2).

#### *2.1.2.1. Parathyroid hormone*

*2.1.2.1.1. Biosynthesis and secretion.* *(a) Processes:* PTH is synthesized in the parathyroid chief cells from larger precursor molecules. Translation of mature mRNA yields prepro-PTH (Kemper et al., 1974), which is cleaved into pro-PTH and further converted to PTH. PTH is incorporated in secretory vesicles to be either secreted by exocytosis, stored or degraded intracellularly. There are probably two kinds of secretory granules associated with two pathways for PTH release: one involving stored (or 'mature') hormone and the other for newly synthesized PTH which is transported directly to the periphery of the cell to be secreted (Morrissey and Cohn, 1979). Parathyroid tissue and cells contain intact PTH and various fragments of PTH produced by protease degradation (Di Bella et al., 1978; biologically inactive C-terminal, mid region fragments of the molecule). PTH fragments can be substantially secreted, together with intact PTH (Hanley et al., 1978).

(b) *Regulation:* The parathyroid glands are unusual among secretory systems as PTH release is repressed and not stimulated, by high extracellular $Ca^{2+}$ concentration. This was demonstrated both *in vivo* (Care et al., 1966) and *in vitro* (Habener and Potts, 1976). It is now known that the relationship between $Ca^{2+}$ and PTH is much more complex than a simple inverse linear relationship. Direct measurement of immunoreactive hormone concentration in the parathyroid effluent blood of calves (Mayer and Hurst, 1978) and other analysis (Jung, 1982), have shown that there is an inverse sigmoidal relationship between these parameters. *In vivo* studies on calves showed that PTH secretion rate and plasma calcium are related as follows: there is a linear proportional control system over a range between 7 and 8 mg · 100 $ml^{-1}$ and up to supraphysiologic $Ca^{2+}$ concentrations, while a constant high rate of secretion is observed below this threshold of hypocalcaemia (no further rise in secretion) and a persistent basal secretion in the presence of elevated calcium concentration. The reciprocal causality between extracellular-free calcium and PTH *in vivo* has led to define the intersection point of both curves as the set-point (equilibrium operating point: Parfitt, 1969). With improved assay methodology and using *in vitro* systems, an inverse sigmoidal function relating ionized $Ca^{2+}$ and PTH release has also been described (Brown et al., 1987). Moreover, the molecular form of secreted hormone depends upon the calcium concentration; more intraglandular PTH degradation occurs at higher $Ca^{2+}$ levels (Habener et al., 1974).

Neither the biosynthesis of pro-PTH nor its conversion to PTH seem to be sensitive to the extracellular calcium concentration (Morrissey and Cohn, 1979). Thus, calcium has to regulate the activity of the secretory mechanism itself, i.e. the exocytosis and/or the rate of vesicle degradation. The changes in the molecular composition of the hormone secreted under high $Ca^{2+}$ concentration *in vitro* are in agreement with an effect of calcium on PTH degradation, decreasing the amount of intact PTH available for secretion (MacGregor et al., 1986). Adenylate cyclase and cAMP are intermediates in the control by $Ca^{2+}$ of PTH secretion (Brown et al., 1978), but the biochemical nature of the reactions elicited by cAMP is unknown. Recent data indicate that the first event in the regulation of PTH secretion by extracellular $Ca^{2+}$ is the binding of $Ca^{2+}$ to a low affinity, high capacity 'receptor' on the surface of parathyroid cells. Calcium occupancy of these sites is required to initiate intracellular signals (Wolf and Scarpa, 1987). The extracellular receptor might produce some of its effect on PTH secretion by mobilizing intracellular $Ca^{2+}$, possibly via inositol triphosphate pathway (Epstein et al., 1985; Chen et al., 1987; Shoback et al., 1988).

1,25-Dihydroxy-vitamin D (1,25-$(OH)_2$D) has a direct effect on PTH synthesis. Parathyroid cells have high-affinity receptors for 1,25-$(OH)_2$D similar to those found in the main target sites for the hormone, namely, intestine and bone (Hughes and Maussler, 1978). 1.25-$(OH)_2$D has no immediate effect on the PTH synthesis of isolated parathyroid cells, but reduces preproPTH-mRNA level by 50% at 48 h (Cantley et al., 1985; Silver et al., 1985), which suggests an action on DNA transcription. Recent reports indicate that, in the normal rat, physiological amount of $1,25(OH)_2D$ decreased parathyroid gland preproPTH-mRNA over 3 – 48 h with no change in serum calcium, confirming that $1,25\text{-}(OH)_2D$ regulates PTH gene transcription (Silver et al., 1986).

A number of other regulatory factors of PTH metabolism have been described, such as magnesium (from 1/3 to equipotent as $Ca^{2+}$) which is required at a finite concentration for normal PTH secretion (Habener and Potts, 1976), or CT (but with very high doses: Fischer et al., 1971), catecholamine, cortisol, somatostatin, secretin, etc. The physiological contribution of these factors is unclear.

*2.1.2.1.2. Extraglandular metabolism.* Secreted, PTH is taken up by tissues and intact PTH is cleared rapidly from the circulation with an apparent half-life of 2 to 5 min, by peripheral degradation (cleavage into N and C-terminal fragments) and glomerular filtration (Papapoulos et al., 1980). Kidney (Hruska et al., 1975) and liver (Neuman et al., 1975) are the main organs for peripheral catabolism of intact PTH. The half-lifes of C-terminal and mid-region fragments are longer than those of intact PTH and the biologically active N-terminal fragments (Manning et al., 1981). Thus, circulating PTH is heterogeneous, consisting of multiple fragments and this heterogeneity has to be taken in account for interpretation of radio-immunoassays.

### *2.1.2.2. Vitamin D*

Vitamin D is available in foodstuffs either from plant (ergocalciferol, vitamin $D_2$) or from animal (cholecalciferol, vitamin $D_3$) sources and is absorbed from the intestinal tract, by the fat-soluble sterol absorption mechanisms; in normal conditions, exposure of the skin to sunlight (process of photobiogenesis) leads to the formation vitamin $D_3$ from its precursor, 7-dehydrocholesterol (Holick et al., 1981). The metabolic pathways of vitamin $D_2$ and vitamin $D_3$ are identical: the term vitamin D will be used as a generic term for vitamin $D_2$, vitamin $D_3$ and their metabolites.

*2.1.2.2.1. Metabolic sequence of activation.* Vitamin D is a prohormone essentially devoid of metabolic activity. It is stored in muscle and adipose tissue and its distribution in the plasma (concentration of about $5 \cdot 10^{-9}$ M) involves carrier-proteins, albumin and a vitamin D-binding protein (DBP). This latter protein is synthesized in the liver and has a plasma concentration of about $5 \cdot 10^{-6}$ M (Haddad, 1987). DBP is the only transport protein for all vitamin D sterols, with preferential affinity for the 25-hydroxylated forms. Only 2% of the available DBP binding sites are normally occupied. The first stage of vitamin D metabolism is a 25-hydroxylation. It is believed that carrier-proteins facilitate entry of vitamin D into the liver cells where 25-hydroxylation takes place (Ponchon et al., 1969) via 25-hydroxylase (25-OHase) enzymatic activities. Circulating 25-hydroxy-vitamin D (25-OHD) is bound to DBP and is the major circulating form, with a plasma concentration 10 times greater than vitamin D. The circulating pool of the metabolite is presumably in equilibrium with a storage pool inside muscle and fat cells and includes a small fraction of free 25-OHD capable of diffusing into cells. 25-OHD has only modest biological effects. The critical second hydroxylation step takes place in the kidney (Fraser and Kodicek, 1970) with the introduction of a hydroxyl in position 1 to form 1,25-$(OH)_2$D, the most potent bioactive metabolite. The 1$\alpha$-hydroxylase (1-OHase) is located in the kidney proximal convoluted tubule (Yoon and DeLuca, 1980). Most plasma 1,25-$(OH)_2$D is bound to DBP (less affinity than for 25-OHD) and albumin with the normal concentration in the order of $10^{-10}$ M; the small unbound fraction of 1,25-$(OH)_2$D is thought to be available for distribution to tissues. Most tissues (Norman et al., 1982) contain varying amounts of cellular binding proteins and nuclear receptors for this sterol.

The kidney proximal convoluted tubule contains another mitochondrial OHase (Knutson and DeLuca, 1974), 24-OHase which produces 24,25-dihydroxy-vitamin D (24,25-$(OH)_2$D). The biological significance of this metabolite is unclear, but it is the major circulating dihydroxy-vitamin D product in mammals, with plasma concentrations approximately 100 times higher than 1,25-$(OH)_2$D.

*2.1.2.2.2. Regulation.* The formation of vitamin D does not seem to be controlled and is only a function of the vitamin D status of the organism. Recent data suggest a down-regulation of 25-OHD by 1,25-$(OH)_2$D either by inhibition of its production (Bell et al., 1984; Corlett et al., 1987) or by increasing its metabolic clearance (Halloran et al., 1986). Although 1,25-$(OH)_2$D receptors have not yet been demonstrated in hepatocytes, 1,25-$(OH)_2$D has been reported to increase hepatocyte cytosolic calcium levels (Baran and Milne, 1986) which could contribute to this control mechanism. The renal hydroxylase (OHase) is the major site of regulation of vitamin D metabolism. The serum 1,25-$(OH)_2$D is normally tightly regulated and changes very little in response to vitamin D challenge. The regulation mechanisms are thought to involve calcium, phosphorus, PTH, CT and 1,25-$(OH)_2$D itself.

Manipulation of dietary calcium has a pronounced influence on the circulating 1,25-$(OH)_2$D concentration: calcium restriction causes a rise in plasma 1,25-$(OH)_2$D and calcium load causes this parameter to fall (Boyle et al., 1971; Hughes et al., 1975). The induced changes in 1,25-$(OH)_2$D are strongly correlated with changes in PTH secretion, due to the feedback regulation of circulating PTH by the plasma ionized calcium concentration and the stimulation of renal 1-OHase by PTH. The leadership of PTH in regulating 1,25-$(OH)_2$D synthesis is well-documented (Garabedian et al., 1972). PTH action on renal 1-OHase is mediated by cAMP (Horiuchi et al., 1977) and is closely linked to the renal tubular transport of phosphate. It requires physiological concentration of extracellular calcium. Nevertheless, recent studies suggest that $Ca^{2+}$ may directly control 1,25-$(OH)_2$D biosynthesis. Medium $Ca^{2+}$ seems to be a direct regulator of 1,25-$(OH)_2$D production by kidney *in vitro* (Favus and Langman, 1986). Similarly, a direct feedback control of 1,25-$(OH)_2$D production by its regulated ion, $Ca^{2+}$ (Bushinsky et al., 1985) can be seriously proposed *in vivo*.

Renal synthesis of 1,25-$(OH)_2D$ seems to depend on the amount of 1,25-$(OH)_2D$ as example of self-regulation by complex feedback mechanism (Colston et al., 1977), because it depends on the calcium and phosphorus status (Tanaka and DeLuca, 1983). 1,25-$(OH)_2D$ modulates both its own basal synthesis and PTH-stimulated synthesis (Booth et al., 1985). PTH inhibits the renal synthesis of 24,25-$(OH)_2D$ while 25-OHD-24-OHase is enhanced by 1,25-$(OH)_2D$ (Henry et al., 1974).

Plasma inorganic phosphate is another regulator of plasma level of 1,25-$(OH)_2D$. It acts via a cyclic nucleotide-independent mechanism (Tanaka and DeLuca, 1973). Plasma phosphate concentration is inversely related to the rate of conversion of 25-OHD to 1,25-$(OH)_2D$ by mechanisms which are independent of the calcium-PTH-1,25-$(OH)_2D$ loop. It is not known whether this mechanism is linked to changes in renal OHase activity or to the ultimate metabolism of 1,25-$(OH)_2D$.

CT stimulates 1-OHase in the proximal tubule of rat kidney (Kawashima et al., 1981) *in vitro*. CT also directly stimulates 1,25-$(OH)_2D$ production *in vivo*, independently of PTH, vitamin D status and changes in plasma calcium and phosphate levels (Jaeger et al., 1986).

*2.1.2.2.3. Degradation and excretion.* The plasma half-life of vitamin D in normal humans is approximately one day, that of 25-OHD is 2 weeks, that of 1,25-$(OH)_2D$ is 12 – 15 h, while that of 24,25-$(OH)_2D$ is 6 h. The main excretory route for the major metabolites of vitamin D is the bile (Bell and Kodicek, 1969). Each 25-hydroxylated vitamin D metabolite undergoes an enterohepatic circulation (Kumar et al., 1980). They are further hydroxylated (24-OHase) in the kidney, and this initiates a catabolic cascade (Esvelt et al., 1979). Vitamin D metabolites are finally excreted in the urine and feces. It has been shown that calcium deprivation in man increases (and not decreases, as expected for a vitamin D calcium homeostatic function) hepatic inactivation of 25-OHD (decline in half-life) and that this is mediated by 1,25-$(OH)_2D$ (Clements et al., 1987).

*2.1.2.3. Calcitonin*

*2.1.2.3.1. Biosynthesis and secretion.* *(a) Processes:* CT was initially supposed to be produced by the parathyroid glands, by Copp et al. (1962). Hirsch et al. (1963) discovered it in the thyroid gland of the rat, Milhaud et al. (1965a), in human thyroid gland. The prevailing opinion at this time considered CT as a vestigial hormone in mammals. We did not agree and decided to investigate the role of this hormone in human physiology, pathology and therapeutics. CT is produced by the parafollicular C-cells. CT biosynthesis has been studied in many species, e.g. human and rat (Jacobs et al., 1979; Desplan et al., 1980), chicken (Lasmoles et al., 1983). The CT genes generate two discrete mRNAs which encode the precursor peptide for CT and another peptide, CT gene-related peptide, CGRP (Amara et al., 1982; Rosenfeld et al., 1983). The choice between these mRNAs, made by post-transcriptional events, leads to predominance of the CGRP pathway in the nervous system (CGRP is regarded as a neuropeptide) and of the CT pathway in the C-cells. In rat (Amara et al., 1984), as in human (Jonas et al., 1985), the CT-CGRP gene contains six exons and the organization of the gene is identical in both species. In the C-cells, the first four exons are spliced to generate the mature CT-mRNA. This mature mRNA encodes preproCT (in the rat: Amara et al., 1982 and human: Lemoullec et al., 1984) and is cleaved by endopeptidases to yield proCT (Birnbaum et al., 1984). CT formation involves two proteolytic cleavages with generation of three different peptides (Roos et al., 1984) among which CT and C-terminal peptide, called katacalcin (Hillyard et al., 1983), both stored and circulating (Ali-Rachedi et al., 1983) in equimolar quantity. The CT secretion rate in man has been reported to be around 15 $\mu$g/day or 1.5 I.U./day (Cecchetin et al., 1985).

*(b) Regulation:* The principal secretagogue for CT is calcium. Classical schemas postulate existence of (i) a simple relationship between CT secretion and the extracellular calcium concentration: *in vivo* as *in vitro,* high calcium concentrations stimulate CT release and low calcium levels inhibit it (Care et al., 1986; Roos et al., 1975; Parthemore and Deftos, 1978) and (ii) an influence of the extracellular calcium concentration on the thyroid gland CT content: hypocalcaemia in parathyroidectomized (PTX) rat is associated with increased thyroid CT content, whereas hypercalcaemia causes depletion in C-cells secretory granules and reduced glandular CT content (Gittes et al., 1968). Thus, a proportional control of blood calcium on CT secretion has been suggested. However, the effect of acute hypercalcaemia on glandular production of rat CT-mRNA has been examined *in vitro* (Jacobs et al., 1983) and *in vivo* (Segond et al., 1984). Injection of calcium leads to a rise in the level of translatable CT-mRNA together with a rapid secretion of CT; this suggests that there is a relationship *in vivo* between CT biosynthesis and calcium-mediated CT secretion and that calcium could act at the post-transcriptional level, presumably by activating inert CT-mRNA pools. A rise in cytosolic-free calcium concentration elicited by the rise of extracellular calcium concentration could stimulate the calcium-induced secretion of CT (Fried and Tashjian, 1986; Haller-Brem et al., 1987). CT secretion *in vitro* can be stimulated by theophylline or dibutyryl cAMP, suggesting that cAMP may be involved in the $Ca^{2+}$-mediated control of CT secretion (Care et al., 1970).

C-cells might be a target site for 1,25-$(OH)_2$D as 1,25-$(OH)_2$D-binding protein has been found in cytosol from human medullary thyroid carcinoma (Freake and McIntyre, 1982). Moreover, the steroid seems to act, in a dose-dependent manner, on CT gene transcription level in the normal rat (Segond et al., 1985; Naveh-Many and Silver, 1988).

A variety of endocrine factors may influence CT secretion (gastrin, cholecystokinin, glucagon, somatostatin: Munson, 1976). Gastrin produces an acute increase in plasma CT in patients with medullary carcinomas (Hennesy et al., 1973), in pig (Cooper et al., 1974) and is at best a rather weak CT-releasing factor in the rat, mediating postprandial calcium homeostasis (Talmage et al., 1983).

*2.1.2.3.2. Extraglandular metabolism.* The half-life of exogenous human CT is about 10 minutes (Huwyler et al., 1979). The kidney seems to be the most important clearance organ in man (Ardaillou et al., 1970) and in the rat (Milhaud and Hankiss, 1969; Onishi and Deftos, 1988). CT is bound to specific proteins in human blood (Milhaud and Szlamska, 1971). There are circulating immunoreactive species which may represent CT-fragments or dimers formed from the native hormone (Jullienne et al., 1978).

## 2.2. The main metabolic pathways and their regulation

### *2.2.1. Interface with the milieu extérieur*

#### *2.2.1.1. Intestine*

Unlike other minerals in the diet such as sodium and potassium, which are almost entirely absorbed, only a fraction of exogenous dietary calcium is absorbed by the intestine. The net absorption of calcium (ingesta minus feces) is the net balance between two processes, the transfer of calcium from the intestinal lumen to the plasma (exogenous calcium absorption) and the transfer of calcium from the plasma to the intestinal lumen (endogenous calcium secretion). These calcium movements are controlled by the epithelial cells of the duodenum, jejunum and ileum, which form a cellular interface between the ingesta and the plasma. Thus, the absorption of calcium is a function of two intestinal intrinsic factors (i) the capacity of net absorption in different intestinal segments and (ii) the residence time of the ingesta in each segment, which depends upon the peristaltic movements of ingesta moving through the intestine.

*2.2.1.1.1. Absorption.* There is strong evidence that some calcium is transported from the intestinal lumen to plasma via simple passive diffusion while another portion proceeds by active transport and facilitated diffusion. The flux of calcium from intestinal lumen to blood involves (i) a saturable component that may be defined by Michaelis-Menten kinetics (Wasserman and Taylor, 1969) which corresponds mostly to a transcellular transport and involves three steps: first, entry across the brush-border membrane which is partly carrier-mediated (Rasmussen et al., 1979). Secondly, interaction with cellular organelles. Calcium in intracellular transit is not free but complexed and may be sequestered by an intracellular organelle. Considerable evidence indicates a relationship between the quantity of various calcium-binding proteins and the intestinal transport of calcium (Wasserman and Chandler, 1985). Thirdly, extrusion across the basolateral membrane. This extrusion could be mediated by a sodium-calcium exhanger (Ghijsen et al., 1983) and a $Ca^{2+}$-ATPase (Ghijsen et al., 1982). (ii) A nonsaturable component (Wasserman et al., 1966) which directly depends upon diffusible calcium concentration in intestinal lumen and becomes increasingly significant as the lumenal $Ca^{2+}$ concentration exceeds the saturating concentration of the active transport system. It may correspond to both paracellular or intercellular transport and transcellular transport via simple diffusion. In the rat, the saturable component is mainly present in the proximal intestine, less in jejunum than in duodenum (Bronner et al., 1983) and seems absent from the ileum (Walling and Kimberg, 1974). Calcium appears to be no longer in an absorbable form in the colon (Ammann et al., 1986).

1,25-$(OH)_2$D is now recognized as the most potent agent with which organisms adapt to changes in dietary calcium. 1,25-$(OH)_2$D modifies the saturable component of calcium absorption, which varies inversely with calcium intake (Pansu et al., 1981). Vitamin D stimulates active calcium absorption to the greatest degree in the duodenum and much less in the jejunum (Harrison and Harrison, 1965). 1,25-$(OH)_2$D binds to a specific, high affinity intracellular receptor in intestinal cells (Kream et al., 1977; Wecksler et al., 1979); its nuclear localization has been demonstrated (Brumbaugh and Haussler, 1975), and its action to increase the transport of calcium across epithelial cells appears to depend on RNA and protein synthesis, leading to production of vitamin D-dependent calcium-binding protein (CaBP) (Taylor and Wasserman, 1967). 1,25-$(OH)_2$D receptor occupancy has been correlated with CaBP induction (Theofan et al., 1986) and CaBP levels correlate with intestinal calcium absorption (Roche et al., 1986). However, a clear dissociation in time exists between changes in CaBP content and transcellular $Ca^{2+}$ transport (Spencer et al., 1976) and inhibitors of protein and RNA synthesis do not block the ability of 1,25-$(OH)_2$D to stimulate calcium transport (Bikle et al., 1978). 1,25-$(OH)_2$D could also act by directly effecting the brush-border membrane to enhance permeability (Matsumoto et al., 1981). This is the 'liponomic' model in which 1,25-$(OH)_2$D induces specific alterations in brush-border membrane lipid content, leading to increased membrane fluidity which, in turn, increases calcium transport. The fluidity changes occur within 1 – 2 h, preceding the earliest detectable increase in calcium transport (Brasitus et al., 1986).

A progressive decline in receptor content from duodenum to ileum has been observed in vitamin D-deficient rats (Feldman et al., 1979). Studies *in vivo* indicate that, under physiological conditions as well as during chronic dietary restriction, increased intestinal vitamin D receptor content accompanies increased $Ca^{2+}$ active transport (Favus et al., 1988). Thus, 1,25-$(OH)_2$D could increase $Ca^{2+}$ intestinal absorption by increasing the number of intracellular receptors. Such an up-regulation of the vitamin D receptor by 1,25-$(OH)_2$D may be controlled at several steps, including a major effect on post-translational events to depress the rate of receptor degradation. Calcium absorption increases after administration of PTH, but it seems that this effect is an indirect action of PTH, via 1,25-$(OH)_2$D. In the same way, CT directly stimulates renal 1,25-$(OH)_2$D production which, in turn, increases intestinal absorption of calcium (Jaeger et al., 1986). Finally, although the intestinal transports of calcium and phosphate occur via different mechanisms, phosphate transport is stimulated by vitamin D metabolites. Thus, there may be effects on calcium absorption that are due to changes in vitamin D metabolism secondary to phosphate depletion (Lee et al., 1981).

*2.2.1.1.2. Secretion.* The mechanism by which endogenous calcium is secreted into the intestinal lumen is not entirely clear. Some results indicate that this serosa-mucosa calcium flux fulfils all the criteria for active secretion (Walling and Kimberg, 1973) while others are more consistent with movement by bulk flow and intercellular water movement (Nellans and Kimberg, 1979).

*2.2.1.2. Kidney*

The kidney, like the intestine, forms an interface between the *milieu intérieur* and the *milieu extérieur,* and calcium (as other electrolyte) movements between the renal lumen and the blood are controlled via the transport and permeability characteristics of the epithelial cells which are the determining factors of the temporal and quantitative properties of urinary calcium excretion.

*2.2.1.2.1. Excretion.* The amount of calcium filtered through the glomerular membrane is directly proportional to the ultrafiltrate plasma calcium concentration. A number of specific tubular reabsorption processes then progressively alter the volume and composition of tubular fluid as it flows through the nephron. The proximal tubule reabsorbs 50 – 60% of filtered calcium. The ratio between calcium concentration in tubular fluid and plasma ultrafiltrate (TF/UF Ca) in this part of the nephron, is between 1.0 and 1.2 (Le Grimellec et al., 1975). Although this is consistent with passive reabsorption of calcium secondary to transport of sodium and water, some authors (Ullrich et al., 1976) believe that, in the rat, 20% of total calcium transport in the proximal tubule is active, coupled to that of sodium through a process of counter-transport. About 10% of calcium reabsorption takes place in pars recta of the loop of Henle by an energy-producing metabolic process. There is no evidence for calcium transport in the ascending limb of the thin segment (Massry, 1982). In contrast, 20% of the filtered calcium is reabsorbed by the thick ascending limb and TF/UF Ca and TF/UF Na ratios in the early distal convoluted tubule are both reduced to values of 0.5 or less (Goldberg et al., 1976), indicating that most of the calcium transport takes place in the medullary and cortical segments of the thick ascending limb of the loop of Henle. Calcium transport occurs here by an active process. Finally, about 10% of filtered calcium is reabsorbed between the early distal tubule and the terminal part of the nephron (Shareghi and Stoner, 1978). In man, less than about 2% of filtered calcium load is irreversibly excreted in the urine with a mean calcium concentration ranging between 2 and 7 mM.

*2.2.1.2.2. Hormonal control.* Kidney is a target organ for both PTH (Chase and Aurbach, 1967) and CT (Marx et al., 1973; Bouizar et al., 1986). PTH and CT, like several other peptide hormones, act by stimulating intracellular cAMP generation (Morel, 1983). Until recently, there had been conflicting reports on the effects of PTH, and especially CT, on renal calcium excretion. In fact, renal effect of CT is dose-dependent in man (Milhaud et al., 1975), and recent experiments with animals acutely deprived of several hormones and infused with physiological dose of a single hormone have clearly established that, *in vivo,* both CT and PTH sharply reduce urinary calcium excretion in rat (Elalouf et al., 1983; De Rouffignac et al., 1984). CT stimulates electrolyte reabsorption by the thick ascending limb of Henle's loop and along the distal tubule. PTH also produces a significant reduction in calcium excretion by stimulating calcium transport in the cortical thick ascending limbs of the loop of Henle (Bourdeau and Burg, 1979).

Long-term administration of small amounts of 1,25-$(OH)_2D$ to PTX rats increased urinary calcium excretion (Rizzoli et al., 1977). On the other hand, there is evidence that vitamin D enhances the reabsorption of calcium in the distal renal tubule (Sutton and Dirks, 1978). Receptors for 1,25-$(OH)_2D$ have been found in kidney cells (Chandler et al., 1979), but the action of vitamin D on renal calcium excretion is not clear.

### 2.2.2. *Soft tissues*

#### 2.2.2.1. *Extracellular fluids*

Extracellular fluids are complex solutions in which only ionized calcium participates directly in most biological reactions. This ionized portion is thought to be in equilibrium with protein-bound fraction and complexed forms of calcium with anions (Robertson and Marshall, 1981). Calcium distribution among these forms varies from one fluid to another. Plasma has two main calcium fractions which are characterized as diffusible or free (ionized plus complexed forms with bicarbonate, $PO_4^{3-}$, citrate) and nondiffusible (bound to albumin and globulin). The active form, ionized $Ca^{2+}$, amounts to about 45% of the total plasma calcium concentration and is maintained, in most vertebrates, at a level of about 1.20 mM. Plasma calcium exchanges with the calcium pool of other extracellular fluids. Except for some specialized compartments with strong barriers to diffusion, such as the cerebrospinal fluid (Goldstein et al., 1979), the free $Ca^{2+}$ concentration in extracellular fluids is assumed to be equivalent to that of serum.

#### 2.2.2.2. *Intracellular calcium*

Contrasting with the function of $Ca^{2+}$ in extracellular fluids (the locus of calcium homeostasis, i.e. of spatio-temporal homogeneity in $Ca^{2+}$ concentration, see Section 1.2.2.2), the function of intracellular calcium is to carry signals to a large number of biochemical activities in the various subcellular compartments (Rasmussen and Barrett, 1984). In other words, $Ca^{2+}$ acts as an informative intracellular constituent via the cytosolic spatio-temporal variations of its concentration (Harary and Brown, 1984; Meyer and Stryer, 1988). The very low value of cytosolic calcium concentration is the main way by which calcium functions: although the total intracellular calcium concentration approaches or surpasses the mM level (same order of magnitude as the extracellular concentration), only 0.1% or less is in its ionized form (Carafoli, 1987). There is thus a very large concentration gradient between the cytosol and both extracellular fluids and intracellular organelles: mitochondria and endoplasmic (ER) or sarcoplasmic (SR) reticulum. Consequently, very small perturbations, e.g. minor changes in the physical properties of plasma membrane (which are also highly dependent on calcium concentration (Düzgünes and Papahadjopoulos, 1983)), lead to large variations in cytosolic $Ca^{2+}$ concentration (excitability properties), while only small displacements of amounts of calcium mass are involved. This illustrates the departure of intracellular calcium organization from the concept of homeostasis (see Section 1.2.2).

A very specialized regulatory machinery operates at various levels of cellular organization to determine the properties of intracellular calcium metabolism, in particular the cytosolic resting concentration (0.1 – 0.2 μM): (i) the first level is the plasma membrane, i.e. the interface with the extracellular fluids, with its poor permeability to calcium. Calcium enters the cell through the plasma membrane passively, down its electrochemical potential via either nonspecific leak or specific $Ca^{2+}$ channels. Calcium is actively extruded from the cell against the concentration gradient via $Na^+/Ca^{2+}$ exchanger, and through a specific ATPase. Another less understood membrane function is the calcium-binding capacity of membranous constituents (Levine and Williams, 1982: protein, phospholipids, or glycocalyx at the external surface of the plasma membrane). (ii) Since cells greatly limit the exchange of calcium with the extracellular milieu, a large part of intracellular calcium is self-regulated. This process involves ER or SR which is the major organelle regulating cytosolic $Ca^{2+}$ within the physiological range, and mitochondria, which has an impressive total capacity for $Ca^{2+}$ accumulation in association with phosphate. The processes implicated in calcium movements between organelles and cytosol are multiple and involve, depending on the organelle, reversible ATPase processes, specific channels, $Ca^{2+}$-induced $Ca^{2+}$ release, $Ca^{2+}$ release dependent upon inositol 1,4,5-trisphosphate (Berridge and Irvine, 1984) and $Ca^{2+}/2H^+$ or $Ca^{2+}/2Na^+$ antiport carriers. (iii) High affinity $Ca^{2+}$-binding proteins are involved in the regulation and processing of intracellular $Ca^{2+}$. They include such nonmembranous proteins, as calmodulin, troponin C, calcium binding protein and parvalbumin. They are often considered as cytosolic buffering structures, but their main role is probably to act as calcium-modulated proteins (multiple conformational changes secondary to calcium binding), involved in modulating the activities of numerous cytosolic enzymes and cellular processes.

### *2.2.3. Hard tissues*

As constituents of endoskeleton in vertebrates, hard tissues (with the exception of teeth) provide the internal support of the body and the attachment of the muscles and tendons essential for locomotion. As do other connective tissues, hard tissues consist of fibres and ground substance produced by specialized cells. But unlike the other tissues, the extracellular components of hard tissues are impregnated with solid Ca-P salts providing them with mechanical and structural properties enabling the performance of the major biological function of the skeleton. If the external shape and the internal architecture of a bone is genetically influenced, an internal adaptable structure is achieved by modelling (during growth) and internal remodelling in response to stresses and forces applied to the skeleton during locomotion and functional posture under gravitational force. As stated by Wolff (1892), a relationship exists between the form and function of bone: 'Every change in the form and function of bones or in their functions alone is followed by certain definite changes in their internal architecture and equally definite changes in their external conformation in accordance with mathematical laws'. Thus, bone cellular activities, which are primarily devoted to the morphogenesis of bones (external and internal structural organization and development), are linked to the sensitivity of bone cells to biophysical events such as mechanical stress (Frost, 1982, 1987), pressure, and piezoelectricity (Bassett, 1968). Bone cell activities are also regulated by hormonal systems and local factors. Hard tissue turnover involves the activities of two distinct cell populations: (i) osteoblasts and chondrocytes which lay down the organic matrix; (ii) chondroclast and osteoclasts which degrade the calcified tissues. These cells are involved in skeletal growth and modelling, i.e. establishment of a bone's shape and architecture within the growing skeleton, and skeletal remodelling, i.e. internal reconstruction of pre-existing bone. These skeletal metabolic processes are associated with important calcium movements coming from and going to the ECF, and are directly involved in the overall dynamics of calcium metabolism.

Another major function of bone is its role in mineral, especially calcium, homeostasis; here, bone serves as an endogenous ion reservoir for the transport of calcium to and from the ECF. A simplistic, but current view of the role of bone in extracellular calcium regulation consists in the hormonal modulation of the calcium fluxes linked to bone modelling and remodelling for the benefit of plasma calcium homeostasis. The ambiguity of such a schema of regulation must, however, be stressed. Indeed, any change in these calcium fluxes has obvious repercussions on the internal organization of bone with its primary function for mechanical support, unlike the intestine or kidney which are only concerned with the relationships of calcium with the *milieu extérieur*. This is precisely the reason why the evidence for calcium dynamics specific to bone, but partly distinct from the calcium movements associated with bone formation and resorption, have been carefully investigated as events especially adapted to ensure plasma calcium homeostasis (Neuman and Ramp, 1971; Talmage et al., 1978). Initially proposed by Neuman, this kind of calcium dynamics implies mechanisms of self-regulation (Neuman, 1975a) and takes into account the physico-chemical properties of the interface between the solution phase and the solid phase at the bone surface. This bone surface beneath the so-called bone membrane covers an area much larger than that formed by active accretion or resorption zones (Matthews and Martin, 1971).

Glimcher (1987) stated that the two major biological functions of the bone 'depend on the precise chemical composition, physical chemical properties, and crystal structure of the mineral phase'. This fairly static viewpoint does not place sufficient emphasis on the contribution of some purely dynamic principles which are used by hard tissues to develop their spatio-temporal organization. These principles account for the peculiar relationship linking the mineral material in hard tissues with the ECF. Before dealing with the complexities and peculiarities of calcified cartilage or bone as organs, we have examined the physico-chemical processes implicated in solute ion-solid phase transition phenomena.

*2.2.3.1. Physico-chemical properties of the solute ion-solid phase system*

Our aim is not to reduce calcification in hard tissues to its physical dimension alone. On the contrary, we shall consider how, at different levels of organization (from local to systemic), hard tissues are able to optimally exploit the complexity of dynamic events involved in (i) the formation of a solid phase from an ionic solution or vice versa and (ii) the maintenance of a solution phase/solid phase ($s\phi/S\phi$) system scattered on a large area. The role of the cellular system is to produce an organic structural framework, so that an overall dynamic behaviour appropriate to the diversity of bone functions emerge from the various mineral reactions taking place inside hard tissues.

*2.2.3.1.1. Phase transition from solute ions.* The Ca-P solid phase in hard tissues is a calcium-deficient apatite [biological hydroxyapatite (bHA) with a Ca/P molar ratio less than the stochiometric ratio (1.66) of hydroxyapatite (HA)]. Structurally, bHA is microcrystalline and never forms crystals of dimension larger than a few hundred angstroms. The mineral in hard tissues is remarkable for its heterogeneity of crystal size and shape as well as the diversity of the chemical composition. The constituent ions come more or less directly from the ECF and, conversely, they are sooner or later, restored to the ECF. For a solid phase to form spontaneously from an aqueous solution, ions or groups of ions must break away from their binding with water and come together with sufficient collision energy to consolidate within a crystalline structure. Such a process requires a solution supersaturated in respect to the constituents of the precipitate and an overcoming of the activation energy barrier. The activation energy for precipitation of a solid from solution is related directly to the surface energy and inversely to the solution supersaturation. The same parameters, i.e. surface effects and solution concentration, are involved in the reverse process of crystal dissolution.

*(a) Nucleation and solid phase growth:* In purely chemical systems, there are two major stages ongoing from a homogeneous supersaturated solution to the state of thermodynamic equilibrium (defined by the solubility product) of an s$\phi$/S$\phi$ system: primary nucleation, and solid mass increment due to crystal growth or secondary nucleation. (i) The higher the concentration of solutes, the greater the probability that the chemical materials form unstable clusters or aggregates, so that further growth occurs, accompanied by formation of a nucleus of critical size, i.e. a stable solid phase of the smallest possible size. This schema of primary nucleation is also applied to heterogeneous cases, i.e. in the presence of compounds other than solute ions, as it is in the biological milieu. These external agents may be considered as catalysts or inhibitors depending on whether they facilitate or slow down certain steps of the reaction. Catalysts are agents which fit into the nucleating crystal lattice so well that nuclei are obtained at a lower degree of supersaturation. Inversely, inhibitors react or compete with pre-existing aggregates preventing growth to the critical size and thus prevent solid phase precipitation. Many of the biochemical molecules present in hard tissues possess nucleating ability. The most prominent of these are type I collagen (Glimcher, 1959), phospholipid-calcium-$P_i$ complexes (Boskey and Posner, 1977), phosphoproteins (Glimcher, 1984), osteonectin (Termine et al., 1981). $F^-$, citrate, $Mg^{2+}$, ATP, $HCO_3^-$, $PP_i$ (Fleisch, 1981) are inhibitors. (ii) As soon as the first nuclei appear and as long as the solubility product is not reached, the other two steps, crystal growth and secondary nucleation, take place. The kinetics of these steps are more complex since not only must the concentration product of solutes be considered, but also the specific effect of the solid phase acting as a catalyst for its own production. A nonlinear autocatalytic process is involved, whatever the mode of solid mass increment, i.e. either by growth in size or by multiplication of crystal numbers (Garside and Davey, 1980; Nancollas, 1984). According to the classical theory (Walton, 1965), growth occurs by addition of ions at growth sites (kink, step) on the crystal surface and by *in situ* formation of a two-dimensional critical nucleus. The energy barrier to be overcome is smaller than that required for primary nucleation (formation of a free three-dimensional critical nucleus), and crystal growth operates at a lower supersaturation level. Factors such as crystal surface roughness and fluid shear forces determine whether secondary nucleation or crystal growth predominates. In most cases, the rate of solid phase growth is a function of the amount of solid already formed as a first or lower order. Therefore, at a high solid concentration, i.e. under conditions in which secondary nucleation may be induced by crystal-crystal contact, an autocatalytic process of order closer to 2 than 1 occurs (Garside and Davey, 1980). Interestingly, the process of crystal-crystal contact may explain the aggregates of 'fused' crystals recently found in bone (Wiener and Price, 1986). The two mechanisms for crystal multiplication and growth in size interplay during mineral increment in mature bone. There are two distinct steps: (i) an initial primary mineralization by multiplication of microcrystals which accounts for 70% of mass increment (mostly secondary nucleation) and (ii) a later secondary mineralization with increase in size of the pre-existing

crystals (Glimcher, 1981). Several products interact with the crystal growth process; there are mainly inhibitors, acting as stabilizers for already formed crystals (e.g. bone gla-protein: Price and Williamson, 1981).

*(b) Clustering:* Numerous experimental results and theoretical considerations have led to revise the classical concept describing the s$\phi$/S$\phi$ system as formed by only one solution and one solid phase. Explicit consideration of a size-dependent decrease in Gibbs' free energy implies stabilization of clusters of subcritical size (Larson and Garside, 1986; Söhnel and Garside, 1988), i.e. the existence of ordered chemical species belonging to solution phase (clustering). There is increasing experimental evidence for a certain continuum between the fully ordered solid state and the fully disordered solute ion phase. A self-sustained mechanism for futher clustering in solution has been proposed, based on the increased probability of clusters coming into contact and then coalescing (Larson and Garside, 1986). These clusters are the species diffusing to the surface of a growing crystal and they could form a dynamic layer able either to reorder itself so as to fit into the crystal lattice or to provide the major source of secondary nuclei. This recent theory provides an interesting continuity from the steps preceding primary nucleation to solid phase growth; it could be relevant to bone calcification, solute clusters displaying properties of the bulk solid. For instance, a nonlinear autocatalytic rate of cluster formation could be possibly influenced by various nucleators and inhibitors. Also, due to their larger size than ions, the rate at which the solute clusters diffuse within the extracellular matrix may become a determining factor in the overall dynamics of bone calcification. Eventually, such clusters could be locally produced during crystal dissolution and re-used for new solid phase formation or as growth units for pre-existing crystals, at some distance away.

*2.2.3.1.2. Solid phase(s)/solution phase(s) system.* In addition to the dynamics of phase transition, some physico-chemical properties inherent to a s$\phi$/S$\phi$ system and governing the dynamic behaviour of the overall system may be of major importance for calcium metabolism *in vivo*. The controversy focuses on the problem of equilibrium (or nonequilibrium) condition of an s$\phi$/S$\phi$ and on its pertinence to the relationships that bone solid phase(s) maintain(s) with its aqueous environment.

*(a) Equilibrium conditions:* Most of the dynamic studies on s$\phi$/S$\phi$ have been carried out in a closed system. In such a situation, s$\phi$/S$\phi$ tends spontaneously towards its thermodynamic equilibrium where, at any given time, mass transfer from solid to solution equals mass transfer from solution to solid. The significant parameters, at this point, are the activity of the ion constituents in solution (ion activity product defines the solubility product) and the particle size and shape of the solid phase, as an homogeneous population. The activity product of constituent solute ions (mainly $Ca^{2+}$, $HPO_4^{2-}$ and $H_2PO_4^-$ in plasma has been discussed by several authors. They have used the notion of solubility product as the basis for fascinating investigations into the mineral organization of bone (Neuman and Neuman, 1958). For instance, it

has been suggested that bone may contain one specific extracellular fluid (bone fluid compartment) whose ionic composition differs from plasma (Neuman and Ramp, 1971), or salts other than HA (Neuman, 1975b, 1982) (such as brushite, DCDP, or octocalcium phosphate, OCP). Nevertheless, the use of this solubility product concept has been severely criticized. Indeed, as with nucleation or crystal growth, the solubility of the bone solid phase may be very different from that of a given calcium-phosphate crystal in a purely chemical system. Hence, the concept of a biological solubility which takes into account the influence of biologial constraints was introduced (McLean and Urist, 1955). In theory, the solubility product also presupposes that the overall system is in equilibrium (Best, 1959). But if, a long time after the initial steps of primary nucleation and crystal growth, the solution phase behaves as if it is in quasi-equilibrium (no significant variation of solute ions concentration), ion movements still exist. These ions movements, seen in isotopic studies, are, to some extent, related to phenomena of recrystallization and ripening inside the bulk solid phase (Misra, 1979).

These dynamic processes are clearly important for bone. Since bone is under continuous renewal by successive waves of formation and resorption, crystals of different ages always coexist so that no equilibrium can be reasonably expected within the bone solid phase (Bonard et al., 1983). This is even more true if the initially deposited solid phase is a metastable precursor, e.g. DCPD (Roufosse et al., 1979), OCP (Brown et al., 1981), or even a noncrystalline form such as ACP (amorphous Ca-P) (Termine and Posner, 1966; Betts et al., 1981), and if these intermediary species are stabilized as DCPD-HA mixture (Neuman et al., 1982) or directly associated with crystalline HA particles, as an OCP layer at the HA crystal surface (Brown and Chow, 1983).

The concept of interface is intimately connected to the dynamic expressions of an s$\phi$/S$\phi$ system. The interface, which involves both solvent and solid, defines the structural arrangement specific to the boundary zone between the bulk solution (fully disordered) and the bulk solid (fully ordered) phases. Isotopic studies of HA in aqueous solution *in vitro,* conducted under equilibrium conditions, revealed complex calcium transport kinetics. Classical interpretation consists of attributing these calcium movements to ionic exchanges between the bulk solution and not only the surface layer, but also a special water structure(s) at the crystal surface, the hydration layer (Weikel et al., 1954). A similar mechanism has been proposed for calcium exchange at bone surfaces *in vivo* (Groer and Marshall, 1973). However, a different explanation has been provided from a s$\phi$/S$\phi$ system other than HA (Binsma and Kolar, 1984). According to this view, the kinetic complexity stems from the diversity of bonding strengths in the building units, which depends on their position in the surface layer (kink, step, etc), i.e. it rests on the mechanisms directly involved in the formation and dissolution processes themselves. Other complexities in the interfacial properties of HA have been invoked as the basis for interpreting many experimental results (incongruent dissolution of HA and its electro-chemical properties). Brown and Chow (1983) suggest the existence of an intermediary layer, made of half unit cell of OCP, between hydration shell and HA surface. This model could present dynamic similarities with the recent theory of clustering and its application to crystal growth and secondary nucleation.

*(b) Nonequilibrium conditions:* Spatio-temporal dynamic behaviours other than steady-state may be expected in an open system (see Section 1.1.2), taking into account the nonlinearities inherent in the autocatalytic processes of clustering, growth or secondary nucleation. In fact, oscillatory behaviours in space or time have been reported for numerous chemical systems directly related to the reaction of phase transition. This kind of dynamic self-organized expression is explained using the concepts of far from equilibrium system (dissipative structures) and nonlinear processes linked to the formation of intermediate reactional products, such as clusters or colloidal particles (Kai et al., 1982). The literature is extensive, but those publications on the periodic precipitation process known as Liesegang rings (Hatschek, 1920), the oscillatory growth rate of a single crystal growing under diffusional control (Garcia-Ruiz et al., 1987), and the intermittent formation of secondary nuclei in supersaturated solutions (Mullin and Leci, 1972) can provide a framework for our propositions (see Section 5.1.1) on calcium metabolism *in vivo*. Various organic materials of hard tissues acting as catalysts, inhibitors, etc., may maintain intermediary mineral species, directly involved in nonlinear autocatalytic processes, and able, at least in theory, to generate self-sustained oscillations under suitable conditions.

### *2.2.3.2. Calcified cartilage*

The calcification of cartilage is one of the two forms of ossification during growth (the other being intramembranous ossification). Classically, it is thought that calcified cartilage serves as a support for endochondral ossification during bone elongation; thus this tissue is used as template which is shaped into the model of specific bones and its dynamic organization is reported as highly dependent upon self-regulated processes.

*2.2.3.2.1. Tissue.* It is generally agreed that cartilage and bone forming cells originate from a common progenitor pool (stromal mesenchymal cells), but mechanisms underlying the expression of bone or cartilage phenotypes are not clear. Growth plate cartilage is organized into a series of zones. The first zone contains proliferating chondrocytes, and is in charge of matrix synthesis (mainly type II collagen and proteoglycans, rich in chondroitin sulphate). A region of hypertrophic chondrocyte follows which contains numerous matrix vesicles (extracellular membrane-bound structures rich in alkaline phosphatase and phospholipid-calcium-$P_i$ complexes). The third zone is made of columns of hypertrophic cells where rapid calcification of cartilage takes place. Calcified cartilage appears as spicules oriented parallel to the direction of growth. Vascular invasion occurs in this area whereas a part of the cartilage is resorbed by chondroclasts. The remainder serves as a calcified support for the preosteoblast-osteoblast population. New bone (primary spongiosa) is deposited along the spicules by active osteoblasts while preosteoblasts migrate with the velocity of organ growth to maintain the osteogenic population in newly-added tissue (Kimmel and Jee, 1980). Endochondral ossification is similar for any type of bone originating from a cartilaginous anlage (Balmain et al., 1983). Caplan and Pechak (1987), on the basis of embryonic osteogenesis, suggest that, in contrast to classical concepts, chondrogenesis and osteogenesis are independent events, osteogenesis being the main morphogenetic and developmental component. Cartilage should guide the replacement by marrow/vasculature and all structural bone formation should be associated with the direct conversion of mesenchymal cells into osteoblast in a cartilage-independent process.

*2.2.3.2.2. Organic-mineral relationships.* Calcification involves cellular calcium efflux (Wuthier, 1982), metabolic regulation of phosphorus pools (Kakuta et al., 1985), matrix vesicles (Anderson, 1985), special calcium-binding-proteins (chondrocalcin: Poole et al., 1984) and sulphated-proteoglycans, these later molecules concentrate Ca and superpose Ca with P in a ratio Ca/P = 1, suggesting an intermediate formation of DCPD (Arsenault and Ottensmeyer, 1983). Changes in proteoglycan aggregates also occur during cartilage mineralization. Their large hydrodynamic molecular size interferes with the diffusion rate of ions and Ca-P clusters, thereby controlling mineral deposition in cartilage (Buckwalter et al., 1987). The mobilization of $Ca^{2+}$ to form Ca-P salts occurs at the expense of $Ca^{2+}$ bound to the proteoglycan; this process is probably related to the swelling in the region of chondrocyte hypertrophy and the associated increase in proteoglycan degradation (Campo, 1988). The Ca-P phase does not seem to be associated with collagen (Boyde, 1981a). The mineral phase is poorly crystallized, with a relatively high phosphate content and a low Ca/P molar ratio (Legros et al., 1977).

*2.2.3.2.3. Regulatory processes.* The first level of regulation results from the strong 'dynamic reciprocity' that exists between the extracellular matrix and chondrogenesis (Bissell et al., 1982). Thus, chondrogenesis can be induced by signal(s) associated with bone extracellular matrix (Nogami and Urist, 1974; Sampath et al., 1984). In this respect, diffusible (bone morphogenic protein: Urist et al., 1983) and extractable (Sampath et al., 1984) substances have been identified. It also seems that osteogenic and chondrogenic cells may be interconvertible (Kahn and Simmons, 1977). The second level of regulation is based on the important influence of physical characteristics, such as diffusion, swelling, on the properties of cartilage. For instance, chondrocytes respond directly *in vitro* to intermittent compressive force by increasing their rates of differentiation and maturation, which result in an increased deposition of Ca-P salts in the matrix (Veldhuijzen et al., 1986). The third level of regulation is provided by systemic factors. A direct effect of GH on differentiation of chondroprogenitor cells has been firmly established and, *in vitro,* cartilage growth is stimulated by numerous factors, including CT (Burch, 1984), PTH (Burch and Lebovitz, 1983), and 1,25-

$(OH)_2D$ (Burch et al., 1988). Pines and Hurwitz (1988) reported that avian chondroprogenitor cells are targets for PTH action.

*2.2.3.3. Bone*

Although modelling and remodelling of the bone may stem from only two events, formation and resorption, the diversity of their spatial and temporal organization leads to the development of a highly heterogeneous tissue. (i) Macroscopically, two kinds of bone are recognized: cortical and trabecular bone. Cortical bone has a dense arrangement. It is made up of osteons: concentric layers of bone surrounding a canal which contains at least one blood vessel, the Harvesian system. Trabecular bone is mainly found in flat bones and within the epiphyses and metaphyses of long bone. It has an internal architecture of fine calcified trabeculae traversing the marrow cavities, and provides large spaces for blood vessels. (ii) Microscopically, the degree of internal organization in bone seems to be inversely correlated with its rate for formation. Thus, when bone growth is rapid, as in fetal life, only woven (immature) bone is formed. This woven bone is composed of calcified collagen fibrils which form a felt-like web with no preferential orientation. Conversely in the adult, bone is almost exclusively lamellar (mature bone) as a result of the regular arrangement of its calcified collagen fibrils.

*2.2.3.3.1. Tissue.* Bone formation and bone resorption may or may not be geographically separated (bone modelling or remodelling).

*(a) Formation:* The creation of a suitable micro-environment seems to be required for osteodifferentiation from osteoprogenitor cells giving rise to preosteoblasts which may still show mitotic activity. Final active osteoblasts secrete the organic matrix, 90% of which is type I collagen. The remaining 10% is made up of ground substance or non-collagenous bone protein (NCBP: Linde et al., 1983), comprising phosphoproteins (Glimcher, 1984), gla-containing proteins (such as osteocalcin: Hauschka et al., 1975), bone gla-protein (Price et al., 1976) and osteonectin (Termine et al., 1981) plus small quantities of proteoglycans and lipids. Some distance away (osteoid width in $\mu$m range), the bone tissue calcifies. As bone formation progresses, some of the active osteoblasts become osteocytes. They make cytoplasmic contact, recognized as gap junctions (Jeansonne et al., 1979; Doty, 1981), with each other through minute channels (canaliculi) in the bone and, except in resorptive zones, with the other cells at the bone surface (Matthews et al., 1976). A cellular continuum composed of the preosteoblasts-osteoblast-osteocyte-lining cells (surface inactive osteoblasts: Miller and Jee, 1987) is formed. Around the lacunae and canaliculi, there is a thin layer of non mineralized matrix which separates the cellular processes from the mineralized wall. Most of the free bone surfaces in rapidly growing young animals are either forming or resorbing. In adult man, 80% of the free bone surface is quiescent and covered by bone-lining cells (Parfitt, 1984).

Immature bone is produced by the rapid and uncoordinated action of very active osteoblasts (Jones et al., 1985). Osteocytes are very frequent and their distribution bears no relationship to vascular canals. The lacunar volume is high and blood flow is greater than that of mature bone (Schnitzer et al., 1982). Immature bone is normally replaced by lamellar bone through internal 'remodelling'. Mature bone is formed in apposition to existing bone. Each osteoblast is coordinated with its neighbours for the relatively slow secretion of nascent collagen fibrils which further away from the cellular layer mature and closely pack. Thus, through a specific relationship between ground substance coating and the collagen periodicity, a very well-organized (crystalline collagen structure) pattern of bone matrix emerges, which parallels the subjacent lamellar bone (Fornasier, 1981).

*(b) Resorption:* Osteoclast formation is a complex multistep process, including proliferation, differentiation and fusion of cells (for review see: Mundy and Roodman, 1987). In contrast to osteoblasts, osteoclasts are not bone-derived and are derived from a bone marrow stem cell. There are two schools of thought about the osteoclast progenitors. One school claims that they form from a cell lineage that is separate from the lineage of conventional blood cells (Horton et al., 1985). The other holds that the granulocyte-macrophage colony-forming cell could be ancestral to osteoclast. According to Mundy and Roodman (1987), the promonocytes (under the influence of interleukin-I and transforming growth factors) should differentiate to the early preosteoclasts which further differentiate and fuse to form the multinucleated osteoclasts. Active osteoclasts are found immediately adjacent to bone with intimate contact with the calcified matrix through ruffled cell borders. They show continuous cytoplasmic mobility which seems to be required for exocytosis or endocytosis (Chambers et al., 1984). As bHA is a stable form with regard to ECF, bone resorption requires the production of a local milieu. Classically, it is assumed that bone mineral is released first and this is followed by matrix degradation. Mineral release may be correlated with a local production by osteoclasts of hydrogen ions (local low pH: Fallon, 1984) via a proton pump ATPase (Baron et al., 1985) or via the activity of carbonic anhydrase (Kenny, 1985). At the acid pH reported for osteoclast resorption fluid, Neuman et al. (1987) suggest that the resorbing mineral may revert to precursor form or cluster, thus contributing to the maintenance of metastable Ca-P forms at the bone surface. Local release of the calcium chelator, hyaluronic acid, could also help in mineral removal while producing an environment in which osteoclasts can move freely across the bone surface (Lubens et al., 1974). The relationship between osteoclastic activity and collagenase production is unclear. Heersche (1978) suggests that bone collagen resorption requires the contribution of other cell types, 'helper cells' such as osteoblasts which are the only cells in bone in which collagenase has been identified (Puzas and Brand, 1979). The recent observation that bone matrix can be digested by osteoblastic collagenase to produce a layer of fragile and easily dislodged bone mineral supports this suggestion (Sakamoto and Sakamoto, 1985). Nevertheless,

osteoclasts are capable of resorbing bone without assistance from any other cell type (Chambers et al., 1984). Lysosomal enzymes could start resorption by breaking proteoglycans or other protective noncollagen products, then mineral (as ions, cluster or small crystals) could be released and lysosomal enzymes could cause further degradation of the underlying collagenous matrix (Eilon and Raisz, 1978). The resorptive cells penetrate into bone via a path which may be partly governed by the orientation of collagen bundles and by the state of bone mineral (Ride, 1986).

*(c) Remodelling:* All growing bony skeletons are subjected to internal remodelling which involves the maturation of immature bone. The primary spongiosa is replaced by secondary mature bone spongiosa in the metaphysis. It has been suggested that this remodelling is due to piecemeal resorption of immature bone by successive waves of osteoclasts followed by gradual replacement by mature bone (Parfitt, 1976), but this mechanism is not clear.

Another type of internal remodelling, which occurs in large, long-lived animals and begins in humans during the first year of postnatal life is mature bone turnover. This type of remodelling is important in human pathology, and its organization and operation was first described 25 years ago by Frost (1964); recent reviews of this process can be found (Baron et al., 1983; Parfitt, 1984). Mature bone turnover concerns bone mostly covered by lining cells and consequently in a quiescent state. It occurs in focal and discrete packets (quantum concept of the bone structural unit) and takes a finite period of time. Such a local process results in adult bone being continually broken down and reformed on trabecular surfaces and in Haversian systems. The quiescent old bone becomes activated and there is local recruitment of osteoclasts. This is followed by a short stage (about 10 days) of bone resorption, and a long latent stage of reversal (about 3 months) during which mononuclear cells deposit a thin layer of highly mineralized bone matrix. Finally, there is an active stage of new bone formation and a return to quiescence. Note that remodelling, as a carefully coordinated sequence of cellular events, depends on self-regulatory mechanisms underlying the coupling between osteoclastic bone resorption and bone formation.

*2.2.3.3.2. Organic-mineral relationships.* Bone calcification is mainly an extracellular process which involves a series of interactions between organic and mineral components. It is the site of the highly nonlinear mineral reactions summarized in Section 2.2.3.1. The mechanism of calcification may vary considerably, depending on the nature of the bone itself. (i) Calcification is diffuse in immature bone with no precise relation to the collagen fibrils, and the process is similar to that of cartilage calcification (e.g. via matrix vesicles and involving of sulphated-glycosaminoglycans: Arsenault and Ottenmeyer, 1984). Both collagen and the ground substance seems fully mineralized in a single wave of calcification (Boyde, 1981a). (ii) Mature bone calcification occurs in osteoid after a certain maturation time. The increase in mineral mass during primary mineralization is principally due to secondary nucleation (see Section

2.2.3.1). No matrix vesicles have been detected. Mineral deposits are initially centred on fibrils; the ground substance apparently remains unmineralized until a later stage of maturation (Boyde, 1981a). The contribution of the physico-chemical properties of collagen (role of holes, pores, diffusion process) has also received considerable attention (Glimcher, 1987) and a diagrammatic representation of a multistep pathway in the nucleation of bHA by collagen from ions in solution has been proposed (Wadkins et al., 1974). The coupling of osteonectin to collagen enhances the ability of the latter to bind mineral (Termine et al., 1981). Furthermore, according to Katz (1969), the presence of collagen reduced by a factor of approximately 2 the number of ions required to obtain a first cluster of HA. During further maturation of the tissue, secondary mineralization occurs with, in addition, modification in mineral chemical composition.

*2.2.3.3.3. Regulatory processes.* Bone regulatory processes may be associated with three general features of the tissue. (i) The multiplicity of its cell population, each with its distinctive properties and capabilities. Activity of certain cells may be coupled (osteoblast-osteoclast coupling), as during bone remodelling, or they may act in concert, either via cell-cell communications (preosteoblast-osteoblast-osteocyte-lining cell complex) or via their distribution as morphologically interacting layers at the bone surface (Rodan and Martin, 1981: model for osteoblast-osteoclast). (ii) The complexity of both extracellular-intracellular and purely extracellular interactions taking place inside bone. (iii) The functional significance of the skeleton as a tissue that adjusts its architecture according to its functional load bearing and the strains induced by these loads. The mechanostat recently proposed by Frost (1988), provides a good indication of how mechanical factor influence bone and contribute to its regulation.

*(a) Local regulation:* This large diversity implies that the dynamic processes of bone regulation cannot be explained simply in terms of systemic effectors and suggests such factors as self-organization originating from extracellular mineral-organic interactions and local agents are involved. Osteoblasts, or osteoclasts or both osteoblasts and osteoclasts produce coupling factors. A series of bone-derived growth factors (i.e. non-collagenous protein components of bone matrix that act, *in vitro,* to increase the proliferation rate of preosteoblasts), could be released in active form during bone resorption, and cause local increase in the proliferation of preosteoblasts (Canalis et al., 1980; Drivdahl et al., 1982; Sampath et al., 1982). Local factors are also derived from macrophage-monocyte and lymphocyte (Rifas et al., 1984). Thus, interleukin-I (which is also produced by an osteoblast-rich population (Amano et al., 1988)) stimulates bone resorption (Gowen et al., 1983) and acts as a regulator of bone formation (Ikeda et al., 1988). Shape change and gap junction formation induced by prostaglandins (Shen et al., 1986) may be important events in the initiation of the remodelling cycle. Because it is chemotactic for monocyte and bone cells (Malone et al., 1982), osteocalcin, a circulating NCBP synthesized by osteoblast but mostly ad-

sorbed onto bHA crystals, participates in the attraction and attachment of precursor cells to bone surface. However, as outlined by Mundy and Roodman (1987) the humoral hypothesis has been questioned by Boyde: the continuous layer of osteoblast separated from inactive osteoclast could be sufficient to explain the cellular events of remodelling (principle of bone cellular self-organization).

*(b) Systemic regulation:* **PTH:** The skeletal effects of PTH have been recently reviewed by Wong (1986). Stimulation of osteoclastic bone resorption was first shown *in vivo* by Barnicot (1948), then demonstrated in organ culture (Gaillard, 1961) and the effect of PTH on osteoclastic bone resorption was associated with the hypocalcaemia produced by PTX. The intensity of PTH-induced bone resorption may be dependent on the presence of other hormones, e.g. vitamin D metabolites (Garabedian et al., 1974) or CT (Milhaud and Moukhtar, 1966). There is so far no evidence that mature multinucleated osteoclasts possess PTH receptors, and PTX newborn rats retain normal numbers of functional osteoclasts (Kruckowski and Kahn, 1980). Nevertheless, PTH increases the number of osteoclasts both *in vivo* and *in vitro* (as early as 30 min after PTH administration in the rat: Burger et al., 1986) and these osteoclasts have an increased volume of ruffled border (Holtrop et al., 1974). Such rapid changes point to PTH acting on osteoclast precursors by stimulating their fusion. There is also indirect evidence that PTH can regulate preosteoclast proliferation; thus PTH would act as a growth factor for the osteoclast lineage (Nijweide et al., 1986). Interestingly, receptors for PTH have been found on mononuclear phagocytes and leukocytes (Kahn et al., 1978; Perry et al., 1948a), but there is still no evidence that osteoclast precursors possess receptors for PTH. PTH receptors have been demonstrated on osteoblasts and their immediate precursors (Silve et al., 1982; Rouleau et al., 1988). The reported effects of PTH on bone formation *in vivo* and *in vitro* are contradictory; these paradoxical effects appear to be dose- and time-dependent. High doses of PTH inhibit *in vivo* bone formation in short-term experiments (Bingham et al., 1969; Milhaud et al., 1971), while low, intermittent doses of PTH given for longer periods stimulate bone formation (Tam et al., 1982; Gunness and Hock, 1984). PTH inhibits the synthesis of collagen (Kream et al., 1980) and bone gla-protein (Lian et al., 1984) *in vitro.* But alkaline phosphatase, a classical marker for the osteoblast phenotype, may be either inhibited (Majeska and Rodan, 1982) or stimulated (Puzas and Brand, 1985) by PTH. The acute effects of PTH may represent its action on the pre-existing population of osteoblasts, whereas the intermittent and long-term effects result from changes in the population of cells belonging to osteoblastic cell line (osteoprogenitor-preosteoblast-lining cell-osteocyte) and the de-differentiating effect of PTH on the osteoblasts. Rodan and Martin (1981) explained the stimulatory action of PTH on bone resorption, by postulating that PTH interacts with a receptor on a cell of osteoblast lineage. PTH should thus induce either a morphological change in the osteoblasts lining the bone surface (Jones and Boyde, 1976) or activation of pre-existing osteoclasts (Perry et al., 1984b; Wong, 1984), which should permit osteoclasts to resorb bone. Finally,

Talmage and his colleages (Norimatsu et al., 1982) suggested that the rapid mobilization of skeletal calcium by PTH is independent of osteoclastic resorption and is correlated with a calcium efflux controlled by the osteocyte-lining cell complex covering bone. The preosteoblast is a target cell for PTH (Rouleau et al., 1988) and has multiple cytoplasmic extensions which may abut on both bone matrix and vascular surfaces. It could be in a unique position to mediate the PTH action suggested by Talmage. PTH treatment of bone cultures increases cAMP (Chase and Aurbach, 1970), which suggests stimulation of adenylate cyclase (type I receptor). cAMP and calcium are involved in stimulation of alkaline phosphatase by PTH in cultured bone cells (Yee et al., 1986) and PTH-dependent modulation of type II [IP3, diacylglycerol (DAG)-calcium messenger system] has been described in osteoblast-like cell (Reid et al., 1987). A two-receptor model for the interaction of PTH with osteoblasts has been proposed (Lowik et al., 1985) which correlates well with the results of recent studies showing that PTH effects both cAMP and DAG in osteoblast-like cells, with a resulting drop in cytosolic pH (Reid et al., 1988). The authors speculate on the physiological role(s) of the PTH-induced lowering of intracellular pH, and make two suggestions: (i) a reduction in junctional communication between cells of osteoblast lineage with, as predicted by Rodan and Martin model, liberation of osteoclasts, or (ii) inhibition of the $Na^+/H^+$ exchanger (Redhead and Baker, 1988), with a resulting increase in the pH immediately outside the cell, activation of alkaline phosphatase and modification of the Ca-P forms located at the bone surface under the osteoblast-osteocyte cellular complex.

**Vitamin D:** In synergy with PTH, 1,25-$(OH)_2$D stimulates bone resorption and increases plasma calcium concentration in thyroparathyroidectomized (TPTX) rats (Garabedian et al., 1974). The 1,25-$(OH)_2$D-induced increase in the number of osteoclasts is independent of PTH (Holtrop et al., 1981), but receptors for 1,25-$(OH)_2$D have not yet been identified in mature osteoclasts (Merk et al., 1986). It is suggested that 1,25-$(OH)_2$D regulates the differentiation and fusion of osteoclast progenitors, and thus mediates bone resorption. This suggestion arises from recent studies with leukaemia cells (Abe et al., 1981) and bone marrow cultures (Ibbotson et al., 1984), but depends on the assumption that macrophages and osteoclast precursors are similar. Low concentration of 1,25-$(OH)_2$D enhances the fusion of marrow mononuclear cells to form cells with some osteoclastic characteristics. 1,25-$(OH)_2$D could also indirectly stimulate the final stages of osteoclast differentiation by acting on T lymphocytes: T cells contain 1,25-$(OH)_2$D receptors (Provedini et al., 1983), can convert 25-OHD to 1,25-$(OH)_2$D, and at least one of the regulated lymphokines can elicit macrophage fusion to form giant multinucleate osteoclast-like cells (Abe et al., 1983). 1,25-$(OH)_2$D-responsive cells in the immune system thus appear to play a central role in the function of 1,25-$(OH)_2$D in bone resorption, and raises the question of the interaction between the immune system and osteoclastic bone resorption (Labat and Milhaud, 1986; Suda et al., 1986). Osteoblasts and preosteoblasts contain 1,25-$(OH)_2$D receptors (Chen et al., 1983) and 1,25-$(OH)_2$D seems to be required for normal bone matrix synthesis *in vivo.* The amount of serum bone gla-protein increases 12 h after administration of 1,25-$(OH)_2D$ in both young and old rats (Price, 1985). 1,25-$(OH)_2D$ modifies both alkaline phosphatase activity and collagen formation *in vitro.* Its effects may be inhibitory (Rowe and Kream, 1982) or stimulatory (Manologas et al., 1981), depending upon the differentiation status of the cells (Rodan and Rodan, 1984).

**CT:** The hormone was discovered by the rapid hypocalcaemia elicited by its administration to the rat. The mechanisms of this effect were assessed by Milhaud et al. (1965b) on the basis of calcium kinetics using $^{45}Ca$ performed *in vivo.* The hypocalcaemia and hypophosphatemia result from the inhibition of bone destruction by the hormone. For the first time, bone resorption could be suppressed by a physiological agent. A relationship was established linking the rate of pre-existing bone resorption to the magnitude of the hypocalcaemic effect elicited by CT (Milhaud et al., 1967). The suppression of hydroxyproline release by CT administration supports this mechanism of action (Klein and Talmage, 1968). The hypocalcaemic effect of CT is antagonized by PTH, although the two hormones lower plasma phosphate level synergistically (Milhaud and Moukhtar, 1966). The evidence from these experiments performed *in vivo* was confirmed by studies *in vitro* in the presence or absence of other bone resorbing agents (Friedman and Raisz, 1965). Specific CT-binding sites have been found on rat bone osteoclasts *in situ* (Warshawsky et al., 1980) and in isolated osteoclasts (Nicholson et al., 1986). *In vivo,* CT administration first decreases the number of nuclei per osteoclast and then the number of osteoclasts, suggesting a disaggregation into mononuclear cells (Baron and Vignery, 1982). CT causes striking morphological changes in isolated osteoclasts (Chambers and Magnus, 1982), decreasing mobility and altering specific components of the osteoclast cytoskeleton (actomyosin interaction may be involved in the early stages of cytoplasmic retraction: Warshafsky et al., 1985). CT action requires the activation of adenylate cyclase (Heersche et al., 1974). It inhibits the effects of PTH on the proliferation of newly formed osteoclasts from precursors in organ culture and may block the fusion of osteoclast precursors (Feldman et al., 1980). CT receptors have been detected on mononuclear cells, probably osteoclast precursors (Nicholson et al., 1986). CT effect on bone formation is controversial. Milhaud et al. (1966) and Baylink et al. (1969) concluded that repeated administration of large doses of CT to rats inhibits bone formation. But, low dose of CT is reported to increase bone formation in rats (Wase et al., 1967), and in man (Krane et al., 1973; Milhaud et al., 1975; Weiss et al., 1981; Gruber et al., 1984). In a study by Farley et al. (1988), it is suggested that CT increases osteoblastic cell proliferation. Bone cells of osteoblastic lineage have CT receptors (Rao et al., 1981; Morel et al., 1985; Forrest et al., 1985). This finding reinforces the proposition of Talmage et al. (1983) that the reduction of calcium efflux from bone surfaces by the lining cell-osteocyte complex contributes to the hypocalcaemic effect of this hormone.

**$Ca^{2+}$:** Nevertheless, extracellular calcium concentration plays a major role in the rate of bone formation. Thus, normalization of plasma calcium concentration in vitamin D-deficient rat (Howard and Baylink, 1980; Underwood and DeLuca, 1984), as in children suffering from hereditary resistance to 1,25-$(OH)_2D$ (Balsan et al., 1986), promotes normal bone growth and mineralization. Similarly, most of the bone abnormalities seen in TPTX rat (thyroxine supplemented) disappear when the animals are fed a high calcium diet, which corrects the hypocalcaemia (Burnell et al., 1977).

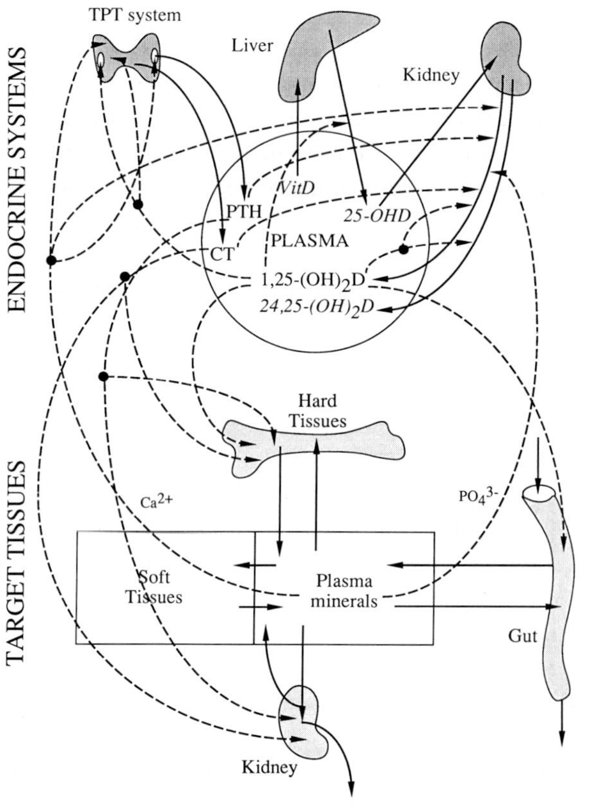


Fig. 1. Schema of the events involved in regulation of plasma calcium homeostasis, consisting of both calcium metabolism and the regulating hormonal system, and the interactions taking place within and between these two systems. Lower part of the figure: hard tissues, kidney and gut generate the calcium fluxes (——) into and out of plasma exchanging with soft tissues calcium. These organs are targets for PTH, 1,25-$(OH)_2D$, and CT (– – –). Upper part of the figure: the thyroparathyroid system, liver and kidney are involved in calcium-regulating hormone biosynthesis and secretion rate in plasma (——) and are eventually target organs for the calcium-regulating hormones (– – –). $Ca^{2+}$, $PO_4^{3-}$, PTH, CT and vitamin D metabolites plasma concentrations are related to one another through a set of relationships (– – –). See Section II for detailed descriptions.

## 3. Understanding the dynamic organization and regulation of calcium metabolism

The outline presented in Fig. 1 incorporates the main metabolic events of both the regulating hormonal system and calcium metabolism itself, and the interactions taking place within and between these two systems. This outline is intended to provide a simple description of our current knowledge of calcium homeostasis without any causal implications. Each arrow represents a number of highly regulated elementary processes whose integration at a higher level of organization (required to understand calcium homeostasis) is not obvious. Moreover, since the concept involves a division between regulated and regulating systems, any biological view of calcium homeostasis clearly depends upon the internal dynamic properties of each of these systems. Intuitive reasoning is excluded with such a complicated schema unless it is over-simplified. Mathematical and engineering models have therefore become important in this type of scientific problem. The numerous models used for calcium metabolism and their continuing development provide clear evidence for the place of modelling in this biological field. Although there is often no clear-cut boundary between the biological and theoretical aspects, the understanding of calcium metabolism proceeds from the mathematical analyses of kinetic data on the dynamic organization of calcium metabolism itself, and from the formalization, within theoretical (mainly cybernetic) models, of the biological view of calcium homeostasis.

### 3.1. Models of the dynamic organization of calcium metabolism

As emphasized by McIntosh and McIntosh (1980), 'The mathematical concept of linearity is very important in modeling biological systems because the linearity of a system determines both the kinds of behaviours available to it, and the mathematical approaches which can be used in investigating these. Only certain kinds of interaction are linear, producing responses which can be readily characterized and predicted. Nonlinear interactions have the potential to give rise to complex, non-intuitive behaviours which are of great interest in biology because of their rich variety of form'. The earliest models of the dynamic organization of calcium metabolism (Aubert and Milhaud, 1960; Bauer et al., 1961; Marshall, 1964) are all linear and analytically solvable. The best known model is the compartmental model, based on the approximation to a sum of exponential terms of the tracer dilution curve in plasma. The development of numerical and theoretical modelling methods has spawned more recent models of calcium metabolism (Neer et al., 1967; Burkinshaw et al., 1969; Charkes and Makler, 1983; Reeve et al., 1983). None of these models, except those developed by the present authors (Perault-Staub et al., 1975a, 1984; Staub et al., 1977, 1981) (See Section 5) has taken into account either the nonlinear properties or the rhythmic behaviour of calcium metabolism.

### 3.1.1. *Compartmental analysis*

#### 3.1.1.1. *Formalism*

It is generally agreed that calcium metabolism *in vivo* falls within the widely accepted conceptual framework of compartmental systems (Jacquez, 1972; Godfrey, 1983), as the principal dynamic components are transport or transformation processes, i.e. transfer processes. Although compartmental formalism is applicable to the temporal behaviour of dynamic systems of relatively general nature (see Section 5.1 for use of this formalism under its nonlinear form), classical compartmental analysis has restricted its application to very special conditions (steady-state approximation) as follows.

*3.1.1.1.1. General ordinary differential system.* Let $X_i(t)$, $i = 1, 2, \ldots, n$, the amount of material in the $i$th compartment, and consider compartment as an instantaneously homogeneous kinetic entity. Then, the general form of a set of ordinary differential equations defining the temporal behaviour of a nonlinear system (to which any biological system may be compared), is:

$$dX_i/dt = -X_i \sum_{\substack{j=0 \\ j \neq i}}^{n} K_{ji}(\underline{X}, t) + \sum_{\substack{j=1 \\ j \neq i}}^{n} K_{ij}(\underline{X}, t)\, X_j + T_{i0}(\underline{X}, t) \qquad (1)$$

$$X_i(0) = X_{iI}$$

where $K_{ji}(\underline{X}, t)$ is the fractional transfer function (FTF) from compartment $i$ to $j$; $\underline{X}$ is the $n$-dimensional vector whose components are $X_i$; $T_{i0}(\underline{X}, t)$ is the flow of material into compartment i from the external environment, denoted 0. The values of $K$, $\underline{X}$, $T$ are assumed to be positive at any time.

If a tracer-based modelling is used and if we denote $Q_i$ and $q_i$ as the respective amounts of tracee and tracer (ideal in the sense that it cannot be distinguished by the system from the substance being traced, tracee) in the $i$th compartment, the mass balance equations derived from Eqn. (1) for tracer and tracee are of the form:

$$dQ_i/dt = -Q_i \sum_{\substack{j=0 \\ j \neq i}}^{n} K_{ji}(\underline{X}, t) + \sum_{\substack{j=1 \\ j \neq i}}^{n} K_{ij}(\underline{X}, t)\, Q_j + F_{i0}(\underline{X}, t) \qquad (2)$$

$$Q_i(0) = Q_{iI},\ \underline{X} = \underline{Q} + \underline{q}$$

$$dq_i/dt = -q_i \sum_{\substack{j=0 \\ j \neq i}}^{n} K_{ji}(\underline{X}, t) + \sum_{\substack{j=1 \\ j \neq i}}^{n} K_{ij}(\underline{X}, t)\, q_j + f_{i0}(\underline{X}, t) \qquad (3)$$

$$q_i(0) = q_{iI},\ \underline{X} = \underline{Q} + \underline{q}$$

where $T_{i0}$ $(\underline{X}, t)$ of Eqn. (1) becomes $F_{i0}$ $(\underline{X}, t)$ for the tracee and $f_{i0}$ $(\underline{X}, t)$ for the tracer. Assuming that $q_{iI}$ is a negligibly small quantity compared to $Q_{iI}$, $\underline{X}$ can be set approximately equal to $\underline{Q}$, then:

$$dQ_i/dt = -Q_i \sum_{\substack{j=0 \\ j \neq i}}^{n} K_{ji} (\underline{Q}, t) + \sum_{\substack{j=1 \\ j \neq i}}^{n} K_{ij} (\underline{Q}, t)\, Q_j + F_{i0} (\underline{Q}, t) \tag{4}$$

$$Q_i (0) = Q_{iI}$$

$$dq_i/dt = -q_i \sum_{\substack{j=0 \\ j \neq i}}^{n} K_{ji} (\underline{Q}, t) + \sum_{\substack{j=1 \\ j \neq i}}^{n} K_{ij} (\underline{Q}, t)\, q_j + f_{i0} (\underline{Q}, t) \tag{5}$$

$$q_i (0) = q_{iI}$$

From a formal point of view, solution of Eqns. (4) and (5) requires specifying all *a priori* nonlinear transfer functions $K_{ij}$ $(\underline{Q}, t)$, $F_{i0}$ $(\underline{Q}, t)$ and $f_{i0}$ $(\underline{Q}, t)$. Since no general analytical solution exists for this system, a solution has to be obtained, numerically, by simultaneous integration of Eqns. (4) and (5): kinetic behaviour of tracer directly depends upon the time variation of tracee $(\underline{Q})$. There is no functional dependence of $K_{ij}$ on $\underline{Q}$, in linear compartmental models because $K_{ij}$ is either a constant parameter ($K_{ij} = k_{ij}$, a fractional transfer coefficient, FTC) or, in the time-varying model, an explicit function of time. Then, the two systems of differential equations may generally be treated analytically, but independently. Only the input functions $F_{i0}$ $(t)$ and $f_{i0}$ $(t)$ and the initial conditions $Q_{iI}$ and $q_{iI}$ make the kinetic behaviours of tracee and tracer different.

*3.1.1.1.2. Steady-state approximation.* According to the formalism expressed here, Eqn. (5) is linear with respect to tracer quantities $(q_i)$ whatever the nature (linear or nonlinear) of the differential system [Eqn. (4)] corresponding to tracee dynamics may be. This property makes the use of tracer particularly advantageous in the dynamic studies of a biological system, since as soon as tracee quantities $(Q_i)$ are constant over time (steady-state approximation), then the kinetics of tracer distribution can be described by a strictly linear differential system:

$$dQ_i/dt = 0 \tag{6}$$

$$Q_i (t) = Q_{iI}$$

$$dq_i/dt = -q_i \sum_{\substack{j=0 \\ j \neq i}}^{n} k_{ji} + \sum_{\substack{j=1 \\ j \neq i}}^{n} k_{ij} q_j + f_{i0}(t) \tag{7}$$

$$q_i(0) = q_{i\mathrm{I}}$$

In this form, linear compartmental model building has been carried out by statistically fitting the kinetic tracer data with numerically integrated responses of models and varying, within well-defined structures, both the number of compartments and the arrangement of relationships between them. The theoretical and practical parameter identifiability must also be studied by appropriate methods developed for linear models (DiStefano, 1976; Walter, 1982). Nevertheless, classical compartmental analysis goes further with the mathematical properties of such linear differential systems dealing with its analytical solution, i.e. the sum of exponential terms. Indeed, if for simplicity we consider $f_{i0}(t) = 0$, a condition fulfilled by introducing, for instance, the tracer as a bolus injection, then Eqn. (7) in matrix form becomes,

$$d\underline{q}/dt = -\underline{M}\,\underline{q}$$

where

$\underline{M}$ has $\sum_{\substack{j=0 \\ j \neq i}}^{n} k_{ji}$ for diagonal components and $-k_{ij}$ elsewhere,

and admits as analytical solution a sum of exponential terms having the general form:

$$\underline{q}(t) = \sum_{i=1}^{n} c_i \underline{A}_i e^{-\lambda_i t} \tag{8}$$

where, $\underline{A}_i$, the eigen vectors and, $\lambda_i$, the eigen values of matrix $\underline{M}$ are combination of FTC, and $c_i$ are constant values such as:

$$q_{i\mathrm{I}} = \sum_{i=1}^{n} c_i \underline{A}_i$$

The analysis of tracer kinetic data made by fitting the general analytical form of Eqn. (8) presents serious advantages (e.g. computational time) since it allows the determination of quantitative characteristics of tracer distribution. Thus, the compartmental model can be chosen *a posteriori* and the value of its parameter recalculated by establishing the relationships between $k_{ij}$ of a given compartmental structure and the value of $\underline{A}_i$ and $\lambda_i$ of the exponential form.

*3.1.1.2. Application to calcium metabolism*

Calcium dynamics *in vivo* have been classically analyzed against such a theoretical background. The method of choice in compartmental analysis consists of fitting experimental specific activity data, $q_i/Q_i$ ($Q_i$ constant over the experimental time) present in the plasma after a bolus intravenous injection of radioactive calcium at $t = 0$, to a minimal, but necessary number of exponential terms. The models obtained typically revealed 2 to 5 compartments either mammillary (such as the one presented in Fig. 2 according to Aubert and Milhaud, 1960) or catenary in structure (Neer et al., 1967). Such an analysis, together with other chemical measurements, such as ingested calcium, urinary and fecal calcium excretion, provides quantitative estimation of parameters, such as bone accretion and resorption, which are inaccessible to direct measurement.

One important result was the effective calcium mass dynamically involved in the body: these models indicated that only few percent of the total calcium mass (about 1% in the adult man, and less than 10% in the young growing rat) is exchangeable. This calcium is probably directly associated with soft tissues, although experiments show that bone surface constitutes a non-negligible part of the exchange with ECF. Thus, most of the skeletal calcium is not included in the rapidly turning over compartments. The models assume that the rapidly exchanging calcium pool is in a steady-

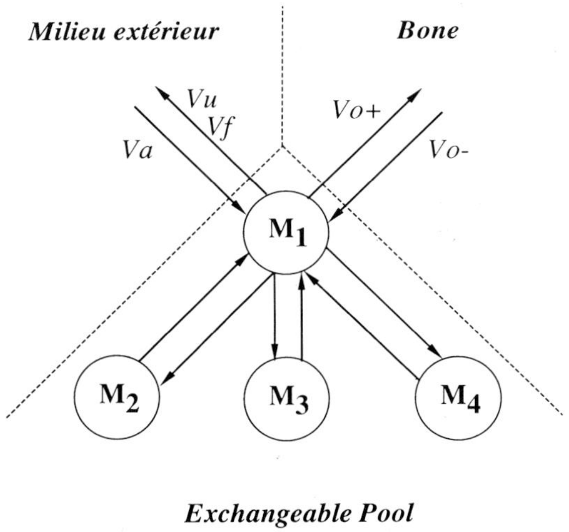


Fig. 2. Classical schema of calcium metabolism from a compartmental analysis, exemplified by a mammillary 4-compartment representation. Each arrow represents a linear flux. Calcium mass in each compartment is constant, $M_1$ including plasma calcium mass and the three other compartments, calcium exchangeable pool (soft tissues + few percent of bone calcium). The steady-state of the system results from an instantaneous equilibrium between the net constant calcium flux through the intestinal and renal cellul interface separating the *milieu extérieur* from the plasma ($V_{a-}(V_u + V_f) = \Delta$) and the net constant calciu flux resulting from bone turnover, i.e. bone formation and resorption ($V_{o+} - V_{o-} = \Delta$).

state, while a non-steady-state (e.g. increase of bone calcium mass linked to growth) may characterize the 'nonexchangeable' part of the body calcium.

### *3.1.2. Other models of in vivo calcium dynamics*

The sum of exponential terms is not the only function which adequately fits tracer data in the plasma pool. Some investigators have criticized the compartmental approach on the grounds that simpler (involving fewer parameters) and computationally more tractable models can be formulated using other mathematical functions, such as power functions or integral equations (Reeve et al.,1976). Thus, other mathematical models have been successfully applied to kinetic tracer data and a critical analysis of the methods used for analyzing human calcium kinetics (Jung et al., 1978) suggests that the choice of an analytical model for calcium metabolism remains heuristic, rather than conceptual. In fact, all the models studied yield relatively similar estimations of accretion rate and exchangeable pool values, the only differences affecting the precision of parameter estimation or the effective distinction between rates of bone formation and long-term exchange.

## 3.2. Biological view of plasma calcium homeostasis

Plasma calcium homeostasis is generally considered to result from a sequence of events which is initiated in response to a change of plasma calcium concentration in either direction from its normal value. Bone, kidney and the intestine are, as target organs of calcium-regulating hormones, involved in the control of plasma calcium concentration. However, there is disagreement about the relative contribution of these organs to the overall process of maintaining plasma calcium concentration within the normal limits. Relatively simple views of plasma calcium regulation take into consideration only one organ, supposed to be the main regulator of plasma calcium homeostasis.

### *3.2.1. Kidney*

Nordin and his colleages (Nordin and Peacock, 1969; Nordin et al., 1972) proposed that, under normal circumstances, serum calcium level is determined by calcium absorption and excretion, the main regulator being the kidney, via PTH mediated-tubular reabsorption of calcium (with bone acting as a calcium reservoir when serum calcium cannot be maintained by the gut and kidneys alone). They described a relationship between the serum calcium concentration and changes in urinary calcium excretion (per 100 ml glomerular filtration rate, GFR) derived from oral load and intravenous calcium infusion in normal subjects. The difference between the serum calcium concentrations in hypoparathyroid, normal and many hyperparathyroid subjects can largely be accounted for by promoting tubular reabsorption of calcium by PTH. Minute-to-minute control of the serum ionized calcium concentration could invoke a change in plasma calcium concentration leading to a reverse change in tubular calcium reabsorption via modification in the circulating PTH concentration. Thus, the tubular maximum for distal calcium reabsorption should be a function of circulating PTH. However, data from many pathological (renal or endocrine) and experimental studies, plus the fact that the determining factor is the absolute calcium excretion, have persuaded others (Massry, 1982; Parfitt, 1987) that this view overemphasizes the importance of the kidneys. Moreover, ever since the initial propositions of Nordin, other hormones have been shown to influence tubular calcium reabsorption, which complicates this regulatory schema. For instance, CT, like PTH, increases tubular calcium reabsorption, but its secretion is inversely linked to fluctuations in plasma calcium concentration. In sum, while the loss of calcium by urine and its control by PTH may be important, it alone is not sufficient to explain plasma calcium homeostasis. Broadus (1981) proposed a simple schema in which the effect of PTH on the kidney is largely responsible for minute-to-minute calcium homeostasis, but in conjunction with bone: the PTH-induced mobilization of skeletal $Ca^{2+}$ into ECF coupled with renal $Ca^{2+}$ retention may be sufficient to correct transient hypocalcaemia. Furthermore, the phosphaturic effects of PTH, which act over the same time frame, handle the phosphate mobilized from bone along with $Ca^{2+}$.

### *3.2.2. Bone*

#### *3.2.2.1. Resorption*

The rate of osteoclastic bone resorption has, since the initial proposal by McLean and Urist (1955), been considered to be the major determining factor for both the physiological plasma calcium concentration and its maintenance at a nearly constant value. PTH played a major role because, according to this initial schema, PTH alone raised the plasma calcium above the level found in absence of parathyroid glands by osteoclastic resorption and regulated this bone parameter in the face of fluctuations in the calcium supply. The inclusion of 1,25-$(OH)_2$D has made the schema of plasma calcium regulation now slightly more complex. Short-term hypocalcaemia is prevented by an increased in PTH secretion which stimulates osteoclastic bone resorption, whereas the reverse occurs to prevent hypercalcaemia. PTH has little effect on 1,25-$(OH)_2$D synthesis over a period of hours. In prolonged abnormalities of plasma calcium concentration, the bone scenario is the same, but both PTH and 1,25-$(OH)_2$D participate in bone resorption. A complete schema requires the inclusion of CT as an agent sensitive to plasma calcium change and inhibitor of osteoclastic bone resorption. In fact, while the physiological maintenance of a normal plasma calcium concentration clearly requires PTH, the role of PTH-stimulated osteoclastic resorption in plasma calcium regulation has become less obvious than initially proposed: (i) PTH target cells include the osteoblasts and bone formation and resorption are coupled. Consequently, there can be no simple relationship between osteoclastic bone resorption and plasma calcium regulation in such a complex system. As emphasized by Parfitt (1979) and Mundy and Roodman (1987) from clinical observations, there is indeed no evidence for a direct correlation between plasma calcium concentration, the rate of bone resorption and the level of circulating PTH. (ii) The major role assigned to osteoclastic bone resorption rests on the simple schema in which bone is simply a calcium reservoir with only two one-way fluxes of calcium (see compartmental analysis Section 3.1.1.2), linked to bone formation and resorption. This classical schema ignores the fact that there are $Ca^{2+}$ fluxes between bone and the ECF, which are independent of bone osteoclastic resorption, and that the reported rates of bone modelling and remodelling (bone formation and bone resorption) provide insufficient $Ca^{2+}$ for moment-to-moment plasma calcium regulation (Doty et al., 1965; Canas et al., 1969; Neuman et al., 1977).

*3.2.2.2. Blood/bone disequilibrium, equilibrium*

Explicit consideration of mineral physico-chemical properties (see Section 2.2.3.1) has led to a new approach of the homeostasis function of bone. According to Neuman and Neuman (1958), the bone mineral phase must be normally in moment-to-moment equilibration with its own fluid environment, except in zones of osteoclastic bone resorption. At that time, bone was known to be in a single mineral solid phase, HA; it followed that, in contrast to ECF, the bone fluid could not be supersaturated with respect to HA. Thus, a rational explanation for the apparent incompatibility between the ionic composition of the ECF and the physico-chemical properties of bone mineral was that there are two different fluids, bone fluid compartment (BFC) and ECF (Neuman and Ramp, 1971). The maintenance of such a blood/bone compartmentation was suggested to be under the control of a cellular activity, producing a disequilibrium between the ECF and BFC by local modifications of pH, secretion of calcium complexer and active pumping of free $Ca^{2+}$ out of bone. The concept of a bone membrane pump became popular some years ago, based on such data as: the existence of a $Ca^{2+}$ efflux from living bone *in vitro,* which cannot be explained in terms of bone resorption (Neuman et al., 1977), the demonstration of a high concentration of $K^+$ in bone which was shown to be under cellular control (Canas et al., 1969) and the anatomical evidence for an osteoblast-osteocyte-lining cell complex (Matthews et al., 1976). Some authors (Talmage et al., 1978; Matthews et al., 1980) proposed that the bone surface cell-complex was responsible for bone calcium efflux, operating at a rate 15 times greater than bone resorption and, under the control of PTH and CT, producing moment-to-moment equilibration of the reverse, passive, bone calcium influx. Thus, according to this theory, the nonequilibrium blood/bone would be largely under cellular and hormonal control.

At the same time, Scarpace and Neuman (1976) focussed on the regulatory potential of the physico-chemical properties of the bone surface. They revised their initial concept of a blood/bone disequilibrium, which was inconsistent with the minor concentration differences of $Ca^{2+}$ and $P_i$ in BFC and ECF and the largely passive bone calcium efflux. Contemporary thinking now favours a blood/bone equilibrium (Neuman, 1982; Neuman et al., 1982) with the equilibrium state involving that one percent or less of the bone calcium which forms an unstable soluble Ca-P phase at the bone surface. This phase, acting as calcium-buffering phase for calcium homeostasis, would be DCPD or one of the less soluble intermediates between it and HA. On one side, it would be maintained by proteins synthesized by osteoblasts and present in bone matrix (slowing the rate of transformation or changing the crystal surface) and, on the other side, it would be converted autocatalytically and irreversibly to HA. The residual 99% of calcium in bone would be unavailable to the ECF (deep HA). Neuman et al. (1987) suggested that the mineral phase located at the bone surface (under the osteocyte-lining cell complex), receives a continual supply of soluble phases during the perpetual process of bone formation and resorption. The existence of an active influx of protons in the cells of the periosteal layer might be at least partly responsible for controlling mineral solubility at bone surface (McGrath et al., 1986) and its regulation by PTH (Peterson et al., 1985). However, even if the influence of living cells is important for this bone homeostatic function, it is noteworthy that the extracellular stabilizing and solubilizing agents play, themselves, a major role because a part of the buffering capacity of bone is preserved after cell death (Neuman et al., 1987).

An examination of the characteristics of different clinical cases of hypercalcaemia, led Parfitt (1979) to propose that the equilibrium hypercalcaemia is linked to a disturbance of the large bidirectional fluxes of calcium at the quiescent bone surfaces. For the homeostatic function of bone in normal adult man, he suggested a compromise between Neuman and Talmage theories: a large part of this homeostatic system should be governed by the blood-bone equilibrium, at quiescent bone surfaces and some function of the osteocyte-bone lining cell complex should be stimulated by PTH.

### *3.2.3. Gut*

All environmental calcium enters the organism via intestinal absorption. In this respect, it may be considered as a disturbing signal of calcium homeostasis (Aubert and Bronner, 1965). However, the efficiency of calcium absorption varies inversely with calcium intake, suggesting a regulation according to the needs of the organism (Nicolaysen et al., 1953). 1,25-$(OH)_2$D is now known to be the main regulator of intestinal absorption. This absorption is said to affect plasma calcium homeostasis as follows: a change in plasma calcium causes PTH secretion to vary in the opposite direction; PTH induces a change in the rate of 1,25-$(OH)_2$D production, leading to a corresponding change in intestinal calcium absorption. However, because calcium absorption involves a nonsaturable process, some authors prefer to classify intestinal calcium input in the rat as a disturbing signal (Bronner, 1984). Hurwitz et al. (1984a) concluded from experimental data obtained in chickens fed varying dietary calcium that the 1,25-$(OH)_2$D-regulated component of calcium absorption acts as a regulatory agent for plasma calcium homeostasis via an adequate adaptation of calcium absorption to dietary calcium. This last property, in addition to the fact that the plasma calcium concentration of vitamin D-deficient animals can be normalized by feeding an appropriate Ca-P diet (Underwood and DeLuca, 1984), underlines the important physiological homeostatic function of intestinal calcium absorption over a wide range of dietary calcium.

### 3.3. Models of calcium homeostasis

Models of calcium homeostasis bring together two types of models, cybernetic and simulation models. Both explicitly formalize the relationships between calcium-regulating hormones and calcium metabolic pathways. However, simulation models appeared only recently, with the development of efficient numerical and computational methods for handling very complex systems while the cybernetic models, initially proposed 25 years ago, are constrained by the requirement of analytical solutions, leading to emphasizing the place of linear control systems.

#### *3.3.1. Cybernetic models*

Aubert and Bronner (1965) built a symbolic model for the regulation of plasma calcium concentration in the rat. This model was based on the control principles developed by Goldman (1960) and previously commented on in Section 1. The simplest version considers the blood plasma concentration as a controlled system, the intestinal calcium absorption rate as a disturbing signal, and the bone as a controlling system acting via the signal $\Delta$, which is the net difference between bone accretion and resorption. As with any model of this type, the activity of the control system rests on the action of the error in the plasma calcium concentration (the difference between a reference value and the real concentration), a null error being, by definition, characteristic of the steady-state of calcium metabolism in the 'homeostatic' condition. Aubert and Bronner used compartmental analysis for quantification of the calcium metabolism parameters in normal and TPTX rats ingesting various amounts of dietary calcium. They established linear relationships between these parameters and between them and circulating PTH. From the first study and more detailed later ones (Bronner, 1973, 1982) they state that: bone (mainly bone resorption), and kidney respond in a proportional way to positive or negative errors in plasma calcium concentration – PTH is released in proportion to a negative error and contributes by adding an integral error correction, which accounts for the greater stability of plasma calcium concentration in normal than in TPTX rats. If explicitly introduced, CT is thought to be released in proportion to the derivative of the positive error of the plasma calcium concentration and to act on bone to inhibit bone resorption. According to the authors, this cybernetic schema does not demonstrate that the organism derives any benefit from the CT-induced faster correction of the plasma calcium error. Other models considered the responses of both CT and PTH as being linearly related to the error signal (proportional control: Powell, 1972; Phang and Weiss, 1976). PTH appears to be more important than CT in regulating plasma calcium in normal human beings. A regulatory schema tentatively including vitamin D as a controlling system has been suggested (Bronner, 1982). But there are some difficulties due to the regulatory effect of 1,25-$(OH)_2D$ on the 'disturbing signal', i.e. intestinal calcium absorption. Riggs (1966) and Hausmann and Riggs (1966) used a mathematical approach to estimate the regulatory efficacy of PTH (measurement of the homeostatic index) through its action on bone in dog: the most important function of PTH is not plasma calcium regulation, but rather the maintenance of a higher concentration than that prevailing in the absence of PTH.

### *3.3.2. Simulation models*

Another kind of model of calcium homeostasis has been developed in a different conceptual framework. These models of simulation bring together the mechanisms involved in the dynamic organization of calcium metabolism, the effects of calcium-regulating hormones on metabolic pathways, and the interactions between both calcium and hormonal metabolism itself, and the different regulating hormones, in a single formalized schema. Such complex mathematical models require numerous variables and parameters whose values are either estimated outside the model or identified using appropriated experimental data. Complex relationships between variables, including nonlinearities, are also *a priori* taken into account.

The first simulation model was developed by Jaros et al. (1980) as a complex analog-digital simulation model to handle the short-term regulation of calcium-ion concentration. It includes four classes of systems, three dealing with calcium metabolism itself: (i) kidney and intestine, at the interface with the environment; (ii) the extracellular fluid, viewed as a distribution system and (iii) hard tissues composed of two bone compartments, i.e. fluid bone (and not bone fluid) containing recently formed unstable Ca-P salts, and solid bone containing stable HA. The fourth class concerns PTH, CT and vitamin D which control plasma calcium homeostasis via complex feedback mechanisms. This model was used to support the hypothesis, formulated by Neuman and Talmage (see Section 3.2.2.2), that bone, with the buffering properties of its fluid compartment, is the main organ involved in short-term plasma calcium homeostasis. The same model (Jaros et al., 1984) tested the assumption that the regulatory mechanisms of calcium homeostasis are arranged in a hierarchical fashion. The fast calcium regulatory process involves a direct CT-induced control of bone-lining cells, followed by the PTH effects at the bone surface; later, vitamin D acts on intestinal absorption and finally, PTH and CT, on bone resorption.

There is another model, distinguishing also between bone surface fluid and deep bone surface, but with a different structural arrangement: this model was developed by Dawes et al. (1984). It focuses on the mechanisms by which PTH controls plasma ionized calcium concentration. Only one of a series of candidate models was considered valid: it includes an exhaustive store of PTH which is drawn on during periods of depressed plasma calcium, and agrees with a study of PTH metabolism in calves (Jung et al., 1982).

The model established by Hurwitz et al. (1983) in chickens incorporates detailed relationships between PTH and kidney 1$\alpha$-hydroxylase activity and compartmentalization of 1,25-$(OH)_2D$ between blood and the intestinal mucosa. Kidney and bone respond within minutes to a change in plasma calcium whereas the intestinal response is delayed for several hours. This model stresses the importance of the vitamin D-intestinal axis in the regulation of plasma calcium (Hurwitz et al., 1984b). The animal adapts to wide fluctuations in calcium intake by forming bone at a close-to-normal rate and by maintaining plasma calcium at a suitable level. This model has been extended to include growth and its associated processes (Hurwitz et al., 1987). Computer simulation predicted spontaneous oscillations in plasma calcium and its major regulatory processes.

## 4. Oscillatory behaviours associated with calcium dynamics and regulation

The classical understanding of calcium metabolism and its dynamic organization and regulation is based on a conceptual framework largely influenced by steady-state behaviours, linear or linearized models and feedback mechanisms. However, such a 'steady-state' picture of calcium metabolism is an oversimplification. Most variables involved in calcium metabolism are not constant. Frequent measurements of these variables over a protracted period of time indicate that there are oscillatory, mainly periodic, changes in man and in many other species. It is difficult to point to a variable which has no oscillatory behaviour, mainly a circadian rhythm. Furthermore, while little is still known about the mechanisms responsible for these events and their mutual internal synchronization, there is good evidence that all these rhythms are generated endogenously. Therefore (see Section 1), a conceptual change is needed to integrate these results and to build a 'more realistic' schema of plasma calcium homeostasis which is unfettered by the 'steady-state' picture. We shall report (i) a selection of the experimental evidence for the oscillatory behaviour of parameters linked to both calcium metabolism (organ and plasma) and calcium-regulating hormones and (ii) an analysis of their consequences for the concept of calcium homeostasis.

## 4.1. Experimental evidence

### *4.1.1. Oscillatory behaviour of plasma calcium*

Jubiz et al. (1972) demonstrated, in man, the existence of a circadian rhythm of total serum calcium concentration which is not altered by prolonged fasting. This finding was explained by a dilution of serum proteins by circadian modification of blood volume. Five years later, Kanabrocki et al. (1977) studied the effects of meal timing on daily chronograms of total serum calcium concentrations in healthy young men. They observed dramatic circadian difference between individuals. Interested by the sleep stage cycles, Kripke et al. (1978) observed high frequency variations in total plasma calcium, possibly related to circulating PTH or to sleep stage. Finally, in 1981, a circadian rhythm of blood ionized calcium concentration was clearly demonstrated in young men (Markowitz et al., 1981) and confirmed in healthy teenagers (Markowitz et al., 1984) and adults (Ishida et al., 1983; Markowitz et al., 1985). The U-shaped curve (daily amplitude of about 6%) indicates that the concentration of $Ca^{2+}$ fell during the day and rose late in the evening. The circadian profile has been correlated with changes in the total calcium by some authors, while others have found no correlation. This behaviour reflects an integration of multiple intrinsic factors. The parenteral administration of single, physiological doses of 1,25-$(OH)_2D_3$ causes no major disturbances in the circadian $Ca^{2+}$ pattern (Markowitz et al., 1985). The circadian rhythm of the ionized plasma calcium concentration persists in postmenopausal women, but, in contrast to young men, the ionized calcium peaks in the late evening (Perry et al., 1986). The absence of effect of meals on ionized calcium, leads the authors to 'believe that this diurnal variation is related to intrinsic rather than extrinsic cause(s)'.

A small, but significant circadian variation in the total plasma calcium concentration of rats fed *ad libitum* was first shown by our group (Milhaud et al., 1972) and has been confirmed by many other authors (Hunt and Perris, 1974; Talmage et al., 1975a; McEachron et al., 1982; Shinoda and Seto, 1985). The daily amplitude reaches 7 – 10%, and the variation pattern parallels that of plasma ionized calcium concentration (Hunt and Perris, 1974; Staub et al., 1979). The $Ca^{2+}$ plasma concentration is maximal in the early afternoon, begins to fall before the dark period, and reaches its lowest value at the end of the first part of the dark phase (Perault-Staub et al., 1974; Talmage et al., 1975a). Since rats feed mainly during the dark period, the circadian profile in plasma ionized calcium concentration is the reverse to that expected from a passive dependence on intestinal calcium entry; the fall before food intake favours 'anticipatory regulation' (Perault-Staub et al., 1974). The circadian rhythm occurs in both young and adult rats, and persists regardless of whether the rats are (i) fed ad libitum or on a regulated schedule; (ii) in a light/dark cycle or in constant darkness; (iii) hypophysectomized, parathyroid auto-transplanted, 6-day thyroidectomized (Perault-Staub et al., 1975b; Hirsch and Hagaman, 1982) or adrenalectomized rats

(Russell et al., 1984a). In hypocalcaemic, calcium-deficient rat, the circadian fluctuation in plasma (total and ionized) calcium concentration not only persists with the same pattern, but is considerably amplified since, after three weeks of deficient diet, the daily amplitude reaches 30% (Staub et al., 1979). These results clearly establish that extrinsic factors (light/dark cycle and intermittent calcium intake) as well as intrinsic factors (pituitary gland or CT) are not essential for rhythmic expression of plasma calcium concentration. Nevertheless, they influence the circadian rhythm of plasma calcium concentration: for instance, (i) after 10 to 30 days of constant illumination, circadian variations in plasma calcium, as with locomotor activity, became less distinct, as these phenomena are probably related (Shinoda and Seto, 1985); (ii) the circadian rhythm of plasma calcium concentration is entirely reversed, within 10 – 15 days (i.e. at a time when more general circadian behaviours are recovered), if the 24 h-light/dark cycle is shifted from 12 h in rats.

There is a marked effect in TPTX (not thyroxine-deprived) rats maintained on a regular diet (Talmage, 1975; Perault-Staub et al., 1975b). In these hypocalcaemic animals, plasma calcium fluctuates 30% per day, increasing during the dark-fed period and decreasing during the light-unfed period. The plasma calcium concentration seems to behave passively, depending on the periodic calcium input from the intestine. Nevertheless, the circadian changes in serum calcium are not mediated *in toto* by PTH and CT: TPTX rats made normocalcaemic by feeding a high calcium diet present a smaller daily variation (10%) in spite of the increased periodic intestinal calcium intake (Staub et al., 1979).

Plasma is the fluid irrigating all the organs in the body and, therefore, its dynamic behaviour 'integrates', at a high level of organization, all the functions which are converging on or coming from it. Thus, explanations for the oscillatory behaviour of plasma calcium concentration must be based on periodic events associated with the main metabolic pathways of calcium metabolism.

### *4.1.2. Circadian behaviours at the interface with the milieu extérieur*

In physiological terms, plasma calcium homeostasis refers to the capacity of the organism to maintain a 'constant' plasma calcium concentration, despite daily variations in exogenous calcium input via dietary intake. Regardless of the zeitgeber role played by the alternation of light and dark or social habits, both feeding and sleep/wake behaviours share a large endogenous nature (self-regulated eating and activity patterns, role of suprachiasmatic or ventral hypothalamic nuclei, of global metabolic rate etc.: Boulos et al., 1980; Even et al., 1988; Sakaguchi et al., 1988) and influence the circadian relationships that the organism has with its *milieu extérieur*. However, the circadian rhythms of calcium intestinal absorption and renal excretion are controlled by mechanisms which do not passively depend on (i) external synchronizers, (ii) behavioural patterns of feeding and activity or (iii) hormonal systems. They are potentially independent oscillators, and thus of great importance for plasma calcium homeostasis.

#### 4.1.2.1. *Intestinal calcium absorption*

Wrobel and Nagel (1979) demonstrated that the active calcium transport along the small intestine of the rat displays daily rhythmic variations of considerable amplitude, the highest transport being achieved 4 h after the onset of darkness, regardless of dietary calcium intake. The amplitude of diurnal changes in the adult rat intestine is of the same order as its adaptative responses to growth, pregnancy or dietary intake. Although the light-dark cycle and the time of food presentation act as synchronizers of this rhythm, it persists in rats exposed to constant illumination and in fasted or adrenalectomized or vitamin D-treated rats, indicating the endogenous nature of the rhythm (Wrobel, 1983). No statistically significant daily changes in CaBP activity were detected and Wrobel concludes that the circadian rhythmicity originates from a mechanism different from intestinal adaptation to dietary calcium. These findings illustrate that intestinal calcium absorption with its precise temporal organization differs from the 'disturbing signals' considered in classical schema of plasma calcium homeostasis.

Brush border enzyme activities peak at night in the rat small intestine, in synchronization with the periodicity in calcium intestinal absorption (Saito et al., 1978). The epithelial cells and the pericryptal fibroblast sheath of the murine small intestine, caecum and colon proliferate (peak at about 03.00 a.m.) according to distinct circadian rhythms (Neal and Potten, 1981). The rates of mouse intestinal cell movement also changed over a 24-h period. There is a steady increase in villus cell migration during food intake (Kaur and Potten, 1986a) while crypt cell migration follows a biphasic daily profile and requires protein synthesis (Kaur and Potten, 1986b).

#### 4.1.2.2. *Renal excretion*

Renal calcium excretion has a diurnal rhythm with a day-time maximum and a nocturnal minimum in human subjects on a normal day-night routine (Carruthers et al., 1964; Halloran et al., 1985). Subjects either active throughout the day and night or fasting or eating standard 3-hourly meals display an intrinsic rhythm with maximal calciuria early in the morning. This peak coincides with the maxium of the diurnal rhythm of cortisol secretion (Moore-Ede et al., 1972).

In rat, there are diurnal renal excretions of phosphorus, calcium and sodium, with a peak during the first part of the dark phase for phosphorus and a similar peak during the last part of the dark phase for sodium and calcium. Continuous intragastric feeding does not change rhythmic patterns for phosphorus and sodium excretion and elicits a slight phase shift for calcium so that the maximum occurs during the first part of the light phase. These renal rhythms do not reflect the intermittent food and mineral intake (Roelfsema et al., 1982). After PTX, or thyroidectomy (thyroxine infused), the urinary rhythms of phosphorus and calcium are still present, so neither PTH nor CT are a prerequisite (Roelfsema, 1983).

It therefore appears that circadian behaviours of calcium metabolism predominate at the interface of the organism with the *milieu extérieur*. It does not seem that the periodic events of intestinal absorption and renal excretion are in phase (as would be expected in the classical regulation schema, i.e. kidney excretes calcium excess when calcium absorption is maximal), implying the involvement of other endogenous regulatory processes.

### *4.1.3. Periodic behaviours in hard tissues*

Numerous periodic behaviours related to hard tissues have been described since the first report by Simmons (1962), 25 years ago. There are only few results on the biological rhythms in human hard tissues: e.g. (i) a periodicity of 3 days for human bone growth estimated from *in vivo* time-spaced tetracycline markers (Swinson et al., 1975); (ii) a circadian change in hydroxyproline urinary excretion probably reflecting hard tissue turnover (Radom et al., 1972); (iii) a significant diurnal variation in human alveolar bone turnover rate (Petrovic et al., 1981; Stutzmann et al., 1981); (iv) seasonal variation in the calcium balance of adult humans (Malm, 1958). A circadian rhythmicity in circulating osteocalcin (an indicator of the rate of bone turnover, synthesized by osteoblast, the excess being released during bone resorption) was found in man. There is a nocturnal peak which is not correlated with ionized calcium or inorganic phosphate in the plasma (Gundberg et al., 1985). A single physiological dose of $1,25(OH)_2D_3$ phase-shifts the osteocalcin circadian rhythm (Markowitz et al., 1987). The longitudinal bone growth of rabbits was described as a regular cyclic event as early as 1940, with a period of 24 h (Okada and Mimura, 1940; Hansson et al., 1974) or 48 h (Tam et al., 1974).

Most studies of rhythmic variations in hard tissues have been done on rodents. Several parameters have been assessed.

#### *4.1.3.1. Cellular proliferation*

A maximum number of cells in growing tissue express their proliferative potential, at particular times during the 24-h day: (i) cells of rat periodontal ligament, the source of osteoblasts for adjacent alveolar bone, proliferate during the 12 h light period. The circadian rhythm of jaw mechanical function during feeding may be an important regulator of this phenomenon (Roberts et al., 1979, 1984). (ii) Rat epiphyseal cartilage, diaphyseal and metaphyseal cells proliferate at the onset of the dark period. This peak is closely correlated with the serum corticosterone rhythm and abolished by adrenalectomy. The burst of cell proliferation induced by dexamethasone in tissue culture (McCulloch and Tenenbaum, 1986) is consistent with this correlation between skeletogenesis and corticosterone. PTX does not alter the proliferation activity of epiphyseal cartilage cells (Russell et al., 1984a). (iii) A circadian rhythm of chondroblast proliferation rate persists in organ cultures of rat cartilage (Stulzmann and Petrovic, 1979), underlining the endogenous component of the growth rate of an individual cartilage. Here, hormonal and environmental variations act as synchronizers of a potentially autonomous oscillator.

Circadian variation in mitotic activity in rat bone marrow closely parallels that of ionized calcium in plasma: it is maximum at the middle of the light period and abolished by PTX (Hunt and Perris, 1974).

*4.1.3.2. Enzyme activities*

Simmons et al. (1979) found that the enzyme activity of the cells in cartilage and bone show a circadian pattern: (i) the highest concentrations of enzymes active in matrix synthesis occurred in the middle of the light-unfed period in the epiphyseal cartilage and metaphysis while the concentration of matrix alkaline phosphatase was highest during the night, suggesting that mineralization occurs most actively at night in the growth apparatus. (ii) Metabolic cellular activity in diaphyseal bone was highest during the first 4 h of darkness. Immobilization (2 days) abolished the rhythmic growth patterns.

*4.1.3.3. Collagen and noncollagen protein synthesis*

Collagen and noncollagen protein (NCP) have different circadian profiles (Russell et al., 1984a). NCP synthesis occurs at the onset of the dark period in epiphyseal cartilage and in metaphyseal and diaphyseal bone, while peak collagen synthesis occurs during the middle of the light period. PTX greatly modifies the rhythms of collagen and NCP synthesis. Dietary Ca-lactate supplements, which raise serum Ca levels towards normal in PTX rats, do not normalize bone collagen and NCP synthesis values. The authors conclude that PTH *per se* is essential for the maintenance of normal rhythms of collagen and NCP synthesis.

*4.1.3.4. Mineralization*

The maximal mineralization of metaphyseal bone during night was confirmed by density gradient fractionation and measuring the percentage of newly deposited Ca-P salts (Russell et al., 1984b). Tetracycline studies also demonstrated that diaphyseal bone formation peaks at night (Rosenberg et al., 1979). In summary, mineralization of the epiphyseal cartilage and bone of growing rats seem to occur actively at night, at a time when the animals exhibit the greatest motor activity (Simmons et al.,1983). As newly formed collagen must undergo extracellular maturation before nucleation, the peak of collagen synthesis during the light period and mineralization during the night suggest that the delay time(s) between matrix synthesis and mineralization must be an integer of 12 h.

*4.1.3.5. Calcium relationships between bone and plasma*

The plasma $^{45}$Ca concentration of rats (Perault-Staub and Milhaud, 1970; Perault-Staub et al., 1973; Talmage et al., 1975a) or dogs (Wong and Klein, 1984) prelabelled with single pulses or repeated injections of $^{45}$Ca show clear circadian variations. The skeleton rapidly becomes the main source of radionuclide whatever the mode of labelling. Consequently, these daily changes in plasma radionuclide concentration reflect a circadian relationship between the bone and the plasma. The circadian variations of plasma $^{32}P$ and $^{45}Ca$ are parallel in rats given a single injection of the two radionuclides (Talmage et al., 1975a).

The amplitude of daily changes in $^{45}Ca$ was much greater than that in stable calcium plasma concentrations (50 and 7%, respectively) in young rats. $^{45}Ca$ concentration increases during the 12-h light-unfed period peaking during the latter part of this period, then falling toward a minimum at the middle of the next 12-h dark-fed period. A circadian variation in the plasma $^{45}Ca$ curve appears significant as early as 2 days after labelling (Staub et al., 1979) suggesting that it originates from the circadian relationship between plasma and rapidly labelled mineral pool(s) in bone. The daily pattern of changes in plasma $^{45}Ca$ is preserved in young hypophysectomized or parathyroid auto-transplanted rats kept in constant darkness. It is also maintained, but with a smallest amplitude, in young 6-day thyroidectomized and in adult rats (Perault-Staub et al., 1975b; Talmage et al., 1975a).

$^{45}Ca$ plasma rhythmicity is greatly reduced in PTX as in TPTX (not thyroxine deprived) rats (Perault-Staub et al., 1975b; Talmage, 1975a). Only a small peak occurs at the middle of the light-unfed period. From this result, Talmage concluded that the $^{45}Ca$ rhythmicity was directly dependent on PTH and CT. However, we demonstrated that normal daily fluctuations in plasma $^{45}Ca$ were restored in normocalcaemic TPTX rats fed a high-calcium diet (Staub et al., 1979). Hence, these fluctuations can operate in the absence of PTH and CT.

Diurnal fluctuations in plasma $^{45}Ca$ also occur in young normal rats fed a calcium-deficient diet for 3 weeks. The amplitude and pattern of the daily fluctuations remain essentially unchanged and there is a significant correlation between plasma ionized calcium and $^{45}Ca$ concentration in this situation. These results strongly favour the idea that, at least in rats, the rhythmic relationship between bone and plasma has a strong endogenous potential (Staub et al., 1979).

Hormonal or dietary changes seem to have different effects on the rhythmic behaviour of $^{45}Ca$ in the dog (Wong and Klein, 1984). The circadian variation in plasma $^{45}Ca$ concentration that occurs in normal dogs was abolished in TPTX animals fed a regular diet but was not recovered in calcium-supplemented TPTX or one-week calcium-deficient dogs. Moreover, there were no circadian changes in either total or ionized plasma calcium in any of these conditions. As emphasized by the authors, these experiments do not indicate whether the $^{45}Ca$ circadian variation in dogs is inherently endogenous or is related only to diurnal feeding patterns. The apparent discrepancies between the circadian behaviours in dogs and rats should be interpreted with care because, as stressed by Moore-Ede et al. (1982), cats and dogs 'do not possess the same circadian organization as humans and most other mammalian species'.

### *4.1.4. Oscillatory behaviour of calcium regulating hormones*

The calcium-regulating hormones deserve attention as (i) potentially self-oscillatory systems; (ii) possibly related to other oscillatory factors such as ionized plasma calcium or other hormones; (iii) oscillatory agents acting on target organ which may itself be oscillatory.

#### *4.1.4.1. Parathyroid hormone*

Pulsatile, ultradian, circadian and seasonal variations have been reported for PTH either in circulating plasma level or in secretion rate at the gland level. A circadian variation in circulating iPTH concentration (native hormone plus smaller peptides) in human subjects was demonstrated for the first time by Jubiz et al. (1972): PTH levels rise after 8.00 p.m., reaching the highest levels between 2.00 and 4.00 a.m. and falling to baseline by 8.00 a.m. This nocturnal rise in PTH was independent of serum total calcium concentrations within the normal range and was not altered by prolonged fasting. This nocturnal iPTH peak was also found in cases of primary hyperparathyroidism (Dube et al., 1972; Sinha et al., 1975), but no clear relationship between plasma PTH and plasma calcium concentrations was detected. Kripke et al. (1978), using a C-terminal radioimmunoassay, disclosed several high-frequency nocturnal peaks in iPTH concentration. Depending on the frequencies, iPTH was either in phase with plasma calcium concentration or related to sleep stages and calcium-independent. These patterns also suggested interactions between PTH and the neural system. No similar high frequency fluctuations in serum iPTH during daylight hours has been demonstrated by Robinson et al. (1982), using an antiserum specific for the intact PTH molecule.

Pulsatile glandular iPTH secretion in man (Harms et al., 1987) has been described. Episodic secretion of iPTH was found earlier in dog, with significant cycles of about 12-min period (Fox et al., 1981). As emphasized by the authors and illustrated by Hesch et al. (1988), the pulse amplitude of PTH could govern hormone receptor interaction in the osteoblast (highly nonlinear and self-oscillating model), and be of great physiological importance. It could also explain such phenomena as the receptor down-regulation observed under continuous PTH administration.

A seasonal rhythm in the human plasma iPTH level displays an increase in winter and a decrease in summer which might reflect an homeostatic adaptation to the decreased synthesis of vitamin D metabolites in winter (Agnusdei et al., 1988).

The existence of diurnal periodicity in circulating iPTH in normal rats is controversial, due to the very low level of circulating PTH and the limit of detectability of radioimmunoassays. Three studies, all using assays based on bovine PTH, showed no circadian iPTH rhythm (Russell et al., 1983), a maximum during the night (Stromberg and Simmons, 1981; Kalu et al., 1982), or at the middle of the light period of the day (McEachron et al., 1982). Radioimmunoassay recognizing the mid-region of human PTH did not detect circadian or seasonal fluctuations in serum iPTH

(Wong et al., 1983). Lausson et al. (1984), using a radioimmunoassay for 1 – 34 hPTH, found two daily peaks in plasma iPTH occurring at transition times between feeding and resting period: furthermore, the mean iPTH level increased in severely hypocalcaemic calcium-deficient rats with no notable change in the daily iPTH fluctuations.

*4.1.4.2. Calcitonin*

Hillyard et al. (1977) reported a significant circadian variation in the plasma iCT levels of normal subjects, with a peak at or after noon. This peak was not detected in fasting subjects. *A priori,* this result might be predictable from the pharmacological effect of several gastrointestinal hormones on CT secretion (Owyang et al., 1978). Much more sensitive assay methods did not confirm such a noon-time peak: there was no evidence for rhythmic event during the daylight hours and serum iCT was unaffected by food ingestion in both normal males and male insulin-dependent diabetics (Robinson et al., 1982; Funch-Jensen et al., 1980; Emmertsen et al., 1983).

There is a general consensus concerning the existence of a circadian rhythm in plasma iCT concentration in rats. Early results (Milhaud et al., 1972) demonstrated a diurnal rhythm in the acute effect of thyroidectomy on plasma calcium and phosphate levels and in the magnitude of responses to exogenous CT. We therefore suggested that there was a diurnal rhythm in CT function which was maximal during the night, minimal during the light hours. We also suggested that CT function slightly increased at the usual light/dark transition independent of food access, which should preclude any stimulus from absorbed calcium or from the excitation of feeding (Perault-Staub et al., 1973). The first relatively insensitive radioimmunoassay studies done in 1975 only detected iCT shortly after animals had begun to eat (Talmage et al., 1975b), leading the authors to assume that CT was secreted in response to an intestinal-stimulus and not by a rise in plasma calcium concentration. Improved radioimmunoassays (Roos et al., 1980; Lausson et al., 1985) led to the unequivocal circadian variation in circulating iCT, with an acute increase just before and during feeding. The daily iCT fluctuation retains the same circadian profile after acute or prolonged fasting. These results, together with these of Hirsch and Hagaman (1982) show that marked differences in feeding patterns do not modify the diurnal patterns of iCT and raise doubts about the direct feeding or food-stimulated gastrointestinal involvement in daily CT secretion.

The iCT circadian variation persists in severely hypocalcaemic calcium-deficient rats and has a similar amplitude around a similar mean daily value (Lausson et al., 1985). But it undergoes an important phase shift: the major iCT peak occurs at the end of the light period and iCT remains low during the dark feeding period. This profile persists during 24-h fasting in spite of major changes in plasma calcium concentration (suppression of the 30% fall in plasma calcium concentration which occurs during the dark-fed period in control calcium-deficient animals). Thus, as in normal rats, there is no simple cause-effect relationship between plasma iCT and calcium concentration in calcium-deficient rats. These observations indicate self-sustained rhythms linked to CT metabolism and possibly entrained by zeitgebers to a 24-h period.

Finally, seasonal variation of circulating iCT were detected in male and female rat, levels being higher in spring than in autumn (Petko and Kovacs, 1981). Seasonal differences in the structure of C cells and in their distribution and number in spring and in autumn were observed (Petko, 1978).

#### *4.1.4.3. Vitamin D metabolites*

Serum concentrations of 25-(OH)D and 24,25-$(OH)_2$D in man show a highly significant seasonal variation with maximum in August-September and June-July respectively. 1,25-$(OH)_2$D reveals no seasonal variation (Overgaard et al., 1988). In preliminary studies, the serum concentration of 1,25-$(OH)_2$D was shown to undergo high frequency (2.2 and 3.6 h) fluctuations of large amplitude in healthy men (Markowitz et al., 1982). Later observations are conflicting: 1,25-$(OH)_2$D does not largely fluctuate during the day, but is maintained within approximately 20% of its overall 24-h mean (Adams et al., 1979; Prince et al., 1983). According to Halloran et al. (1985), variance analysis established on five men suggests significant daily variations in the hormone concentration, but significant circadian rhythm with a peak at early afternoon was only detected in two subjects. The reason for a detectable circadian rhythm in some men but not others is not clear. Circadian variation in serum 1,25-$(OH)_2$D was in no case correlated with diurnal changes in serum Ca and Pi concentrations.

No detectable daily change in plasma 25-(OH)D has been observed in the adult rat whereas plasma 24,25-$(OH)_2$D fluctuates with a decrease before the light-dark transition coinciding with the rhythmic fall in plasma calcium and the increased intestinal calcium transport activity (Wrobel and Ghazarian, 1982). Miller and Norman (1979) demonstrated circadian fluctuation in the activity of 25-(OH)D-1$\alpha$-hydroxylase in the chick. Since then, these authors (Norman et al., 1980; Miller and Norman, 1982) have found evidence for circadian rhythms in the serum levels of CaBP with a minimum at mid-morning and a maximum at the end of the night. Chicks, raised under inverse lighting, have a reverse CaBP circadian profile, demonstrating that light/dark schedule and the associated meal feeding schedule act as efficient zeitgebers.

### 4.2. Consequences for calcium homeostasis

Diurnal variations in the functions of some components of calcium metabolism, such as the intestine and kidney are well-established, although they are currently excluded from formal schemas of calcium homeostasis. The periodic behaviours of calcium-regulating hormones are considered as being either at the origin of, or secondary to, these metabolic variations. But, it is the experimental evidence for a well-defined temporal pattern for plasma calcium concentration that raised questions about the conceptual framework of calcium homeostasis. The fact that the plasma calcium concentration in the rat varies and drops in anticipation of feeding, calls to mind the idea of time-keeping associated with calcium regulation. This leads to a more integrative view of calcium homeostasis than the minute-to-minute schema, avoiding explicit consideration of perturbing signals and resulting error. In support of the concept of intrinsic periodicity, Parfitt (1987) proposed a schema for plasma calcium homeostasis in adult man that locates the homeostatic system at the quiescent bone surface: 'the complex system of lining cells, bone fluid and variety of ions, macromolecules and crystals . . . provides a means of anticipating circadian fluctuations in calcium supply'. In fact, as early as 1974 – 1975, the same concepts of anticipation, diurnal variations and calcium dynamics at the bone surface had led to a renewal in plasma calcium homeostasis in rat: (i) the present authors (Milhaud et al., 1972; Perault-Staub et al., 1974, 1975b), proposed to relate calcium homeostasis to 'on the one hand the existence of internal dynamic changes which are rhythmic in nature, and on the other hand the introduction of behavioural responses as part of the process of homeostasis'. (ii) In comparison of our findings to their own, Talmage et al. (1975a) preferred to think of the existence of 'a conditioned, Pavlovian-type response aiding processes which would be produced by food itself reaching the digestive tract'. The initial conceptual differences led the two groups to formulate quite different schemas for plasma calcium homeostasis while starting with similar data (daily variations in rat plasma calcium and $^{45}Ca$ concentration).

### *4.2.1. Talmage's theory*

Talmage et al. (1980) chose to disregard the intrinsic nature of the rhythmic behaviours associated with calcium and hormonal dynamics. Six steps should occur from the time a calcium-containing meal is consumed until that portion of calcium stored in bone fluid is utilized during unfed period to help maintain plasma calcium concentration. (i) CT secretion is stimulated by feeding and subsequent digestive processes. (ii) Postprandial secretion of CT restricts the efflux of calcium from bone fluid to blood, thereby maintaining PTH secretion. (iii) Both PTH and CT are secreted postprandially and act in concert on calcium homeostasis. (iv) CT actively moves phosphate into bone and prevents its loss from bone fluid to blood. (v) Postprandial storage of calcium with phosphate (colloid form) occurs in bone fluid. (vi) This labile storage form of calcium is the first to be utilized during the following daily unfed period. Such a schema includes a set of new experimental results and conceptual insights into the actions of PTH and CT on cells lining the surfaces of bone (Talmage et al., 1978). It attributes an important physiological role for CT (Talmage et al., 1983). Nevertheless, the calcium-regulating hormones were assigned a major role, generating, under the influence of various secretagogues, any dynamic changes reflected in calcium metabolism. This role was focussed on the conceptual novelty of anticipatory regulation, the secretion of CT by C-cells being conditioned by gastrointestinal or/and neurogenic stimuli during the prandial period. Unfortunately, such considerations do not fit with the endogenous nature of oscillatory behaviours of hormonal and calcium metabolism systems.

### 4.2.2. Our proposal

Oscillatory behaviours confer functional advantages such as anticipatory or predictive regulation to the biological system and its regulation (see Section 1.1.2). We chose to focus on the intrinsic nature of oscillatory variations and to build a new schema of plasma calcium homeostasis around this concept. Three reasons led to this choice: (i) the idea that the oscillatory behaviour of calcium metabolism can be thought of as property of dissipative structures in the sense of Prigogine (see Section 1), i.e. of a dynamic nonlinear system maintained out of its thermodynamic equilibrium condition; (ii) the plasma $^{45}Ca$ circadian variations occur irrespective of the thyroparathyroid system, i.e. in normocalcemic TPTX rats (Staub et al., 1979); (iii) the highly nonlinear nature of mineral reactions (see Section 2.2.3.1) occurring during nucleation and crystal growth, with their 'theoretical' ability (Sel'kov, 1968; Nicolis and Prigogine, 1977) to generate self-oscillatory behaviours. Autocatalytic processes are known to adequately describe the oscillatory behaviour of some biological systems (Tyson and Kauffman, 1975; Goldbeter and Nicolis, 1976; Meinhardt, 1982; Meyer and Stryer, 1988). We then suggested the circadian calcium movements between bone and ECF arising from relevant nonlinear processes located at the bone surface. A preliminary schema is as follows (Staub et al., 1979): (i) calcium metabolism is an open system maintained in a non-steady-state and the quasi-constancy of plasma calcium level results from the interplay of a set of circadian calcium fluxes linked to the main metabolic functions. Figure 3 illustrates the new 'complementarity concept' of plasma calcium homeostasis. At the plasma, a strict or quasi-complementarity results from combination of circadian net calcium fluxes coming through the two interfaces separating ECF from the *milieu extérieur* (intestine and kidney) and from the deep bone. (ii) Little calcium is excreted daily in the urine of normal rats. Plasma calcium homeostasis results from a nearly perfect harmony of intestinal and bone rhythmic events operating in phase opposition in rats. The large variations in plasma calcium concentration in both hypocalcaemic TPTX and calcium-deficient rats, with their daily opposite profiles, reinforce this assumption. In the first case, the rhythmic event coming from bone is so damped that plasma calcium depends on calcium input via the intestine; the situation is reversed in calcium-deficient rats where the periodic calcium input via the intestine is very depressed. (iii) Hormonal systems, especially calcium-regulating hormones, act as internal mediators optimizing the intrinsic dynamics of calcium metabolism. As pacemaker and/or transducer, it could coordinate and synchronize metabolic oscillators by acting either directly on intestinal, renal and bone cells, or indirectly, through behavioural control (feeding and activity habits). (iv) This schema includes modulation by extracellular calcium concentration of hormone secretions or biosynthesis via feedback loops of control. Extrinsic periodic events such as light/dark, food and activity cycles behave as primary zeitgebers.

We therefore, like Talmage, assigned to mineral metabolism in bone a major role in plasma calcium homeostasis, but according to Neuman's blood/bone equilibrium

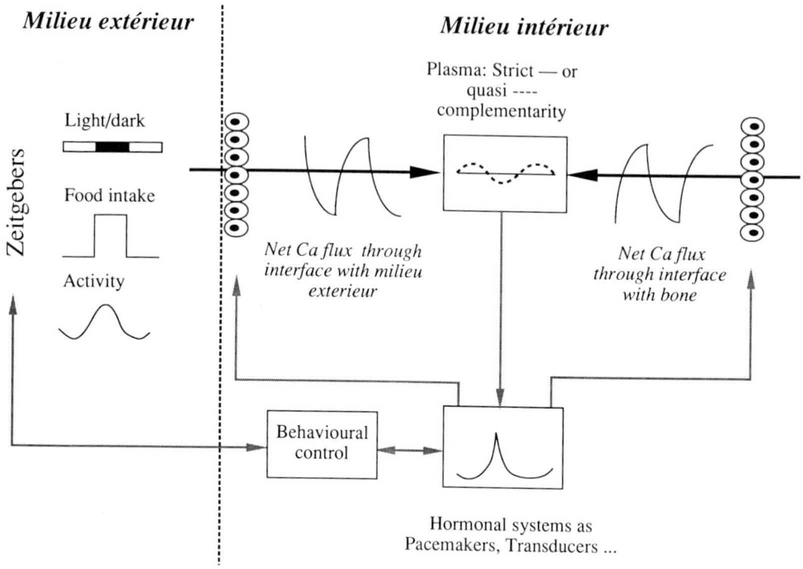


Fig. 3. Illustration of the 'complementarity concept' for plasma calcium homeostasis. The nearly constant behaviour observed at plasma level results from quasi-complementarity between two periodic events: net calcium flux through the intestinal and renal cellular interface separating the *milieu extérieur* from the plasma, and net calcium flux through the cellular interface separating bone from plasma. The hormonal system, with its possible periodic profile, could act either directly on target organs or indirectly, via behavioural modifications, as pacemaker and/or transducer to coordinate and synchronize the metabolic oscillators. The effects of zeitgebers and the interactions between plasma calcium concentration and the hormonal system are included.

latest concept (Neuman, 1982; intermediary calcium phosphate forms located at bone surface) rather than to his first blood/bone disequilibrium theory (Neuman, 1975a: bone fluid compartment). At variance with Talmage's theory, both calcium metabolic pathways and calcium-regulating hormones are potentially autonomous oscillators, able to be mutually synchronized and/or entrained by external or internal events.

## 5. A temporal self-organized model for calcium metabolism in the rat

In theory, simple dynamic systems (having few variables and nonlinearities) generate temporal organizations of varying complexity – from the simple steady-state to complex oscillatory behaviours. In this respect, the overall schema elaborated from the current knowledge of calcium metabolism and its regulation (Fig. 1) includes so many variables and interactions that, *a priori,* it is capable of explaining, at least qualitatively, any temporal expressions describing calcium metabolism or its control (hormonal) system. Hence, our assumptions must be formally tested by: (i) using experimental data pertinent to the dynamic properties of calcium metabolism and collected at a level of organization *(in vivo)* appropriate to calcium homeostasis; (ii) selecting a strategy which allows both the elaboration of a 'simplifying theory' of the dynamic organization of calcium metabolism (self-regulation included), and the integration of additional complexities introduced by the regulatory system. The physico-chemical properties underlying the mineral reactions have been chosen as the origin of the dynamic expressions of calcium metabolism. The biological environment constrains the system's temporal expression by specifying the conditions in which the mineral reactions occur.

We developed (Staub et al., 1988) a nonlinear self-oscillatory model for rat calcium metabolism which correctly fitted the experimental kinetic data from which the propositions were developed, i.e. both plasma calcium and $^{45}Ca$ concentration. Typical kinetic data obtained in young normal rats maintained under physiological conditions are shown in Fig. 4. These data account for the overall internal dynamics of tracer distribution in the body (dilution curve) as well as for the associated circadian behaviour. Periodic variations in $^{45}Ca$ are significant from the second day, reaching about 50% amplitude at the end of the experimental period (7 days).

### 5.1. Formalism and specification

We used the compartmental formalism presented in Section 3.1.1, but we disregarded the steady-state approximation ($dQ_i/dt \neq 0$) currently used in calcium metabolism. The set of nonlinear differential systems, Eqn. (4) and (5), relates to tracee ($^{40}Ca$)

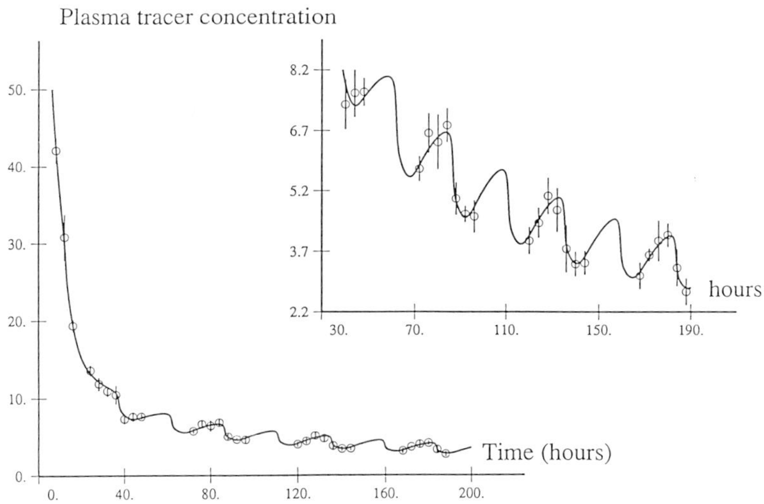


Fig. 4. Time-course of plasma $^{45}Ca$ concentration in 2-month-old rats fed a normal diet, on a 12:12 h light-dark schedule and labelled intravenously at time 0. The experimental data (O, with SD given as vertical bars) are compared to the simulated behaviour (——) of compartment 1, including plasma in the self-oscillatory model shown in Fig. 5. The oscillatory pattern obtained from 30-h postlabelling is enlarged in the upper part of the figure.

and tracer ($^{45}Ca$), respectively. The theoretical and technological aspects used for the model building (including the integration method, optimization procedures, statistical tests of the goodness of fit and identifiability study) have been described (Staub et al., 1988). In its general form, the Eqn. (4) and (5) differential system is useless. The nonlinearities must be explicitly formulated, and the model structure, i.e. number of compartments and their relationships with each other and with the environment, must be specified before integrating the differential system. Additional statements are required to define the nonlinear process at the origin of the circadian variations and the way in which any internal dynamics may be damped, if not suppressed, at plasma level (homeostasis).

### *5.1.1. The nonlinear process at the origin of the periodic behaviour*

The circadian periodicity associated with tracer data kinetics is directly related to temporal variations in bone mineral metabolism. As described in Section 2.2.3.1, one of the remarkable properties of the phase transition involved in hard tissues calcification is its nonlinearity due to the autocatalytic processes of clustering, crystal growth or secondary nucleation. This kind of nonlinearity elicits spontaneous oscillatory behaviours in numerous chemical (Nicolis and Prigogine, 1977) and precipitating systems (Kai et al., 1982). Very simple bidimensional models having a single nonlinearity can, for given relationships between parameters, induce instabilities of the associated steady-state(s) leading to asymptotically stable periodic behaviours, provided that the nonlinearity is an autocatalytic process of order two (Sel'kov, 1968). Since autocatalysis seems pertinent to the process of calcification, the minimal hypothesis implies that the nonlinear part of the compartmental structure consists of two compartments (2 and 3 in Fig. 5). This nonlinear structure exchanges calcium with another compartment (compartment 1) which includes at least the plasma calcium pool. All internal fluxes are defined by FTC ($k_{ij}$), i.e. are linear, except for the compartment 3 formation flux, FTF $K_{32}$, which is defined as:

$$K_{32} = {}^{1}k_{32} + {}^{2}k_{32}\, Q_3^{2}, \tag{9}$$

compartment 3 is formed from compartment 2 by a strictly linear process (defined by ${}^{1}k_{32}$) plus an autocatalytic mechanism of order 2 with the parameter ${}^{2}k_{32}$ having the dimensions time$^{-1}$ · mass$^{-2}$, i.e. a process dependent on the square of the calcium mass present in compartment 3.

### *5.1.2. Complementarity in the plasma*

The plasma calcium concentration in the normal rat has a significant circadian variation. For simplicity, let us neglect this small amplitude variation, i.e. retain the classical hypothesis of constant plasma calcium concentration. This allows direct com-

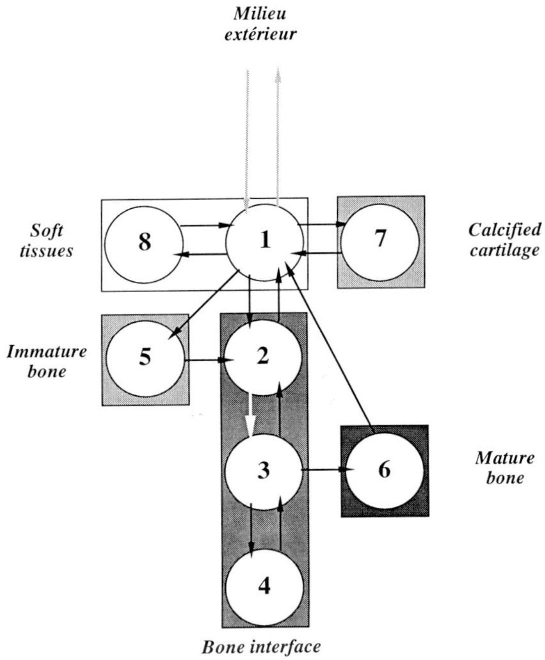


Fig. 5. Schema of calcium metabolism according to self-oscillatory 8-compartment model. Each solid line arrow represents a linear flux. The white line arrow represents the autocatalytic process occurring at bone surface [see Eqn. (9) in text] and the two dashed line arrows, the nonlinear relationships of the system with its *milieu extérieur* [see Eqn. (10) in the text]. Physiological significance of the compartments, as analyzed in the text, are reported.

putation of the quantity of calcium coming from the environment, i.e. entry of $^{40}$Ca into compartment 1, from:

$$dQ_1/d_t = F_{10} - \sigma = 0 \tag{10}$$

where

$$\sigma = K_{01}\, Q_{1I} + Q_{1I} \sum_{j=2}^{n} k_{j1} - \sum_{j=2}^{n} k_{1j}\, Q_j$$

Since $F_{10}$ cannot be negative, such as when the actual value of the sum of influxes into compartment 1 exceeds the sum of effluxes from this compartment ($\sigma < 0$), then:

if $\sigma \geq 0$, $F_{10} = \sigma$ and $K_{01} = k_{01}$

$$\text{but if } \sigma < 0,\ F_{10} = 0 \text{ and } K_{01} = \left( \sum_{j=2}^{n} k_{1j} Q_j - Q_{1I} \sum_{j=2}^{n} k_{j1} \right) / Q_{1I}$$

Thus, in a correct model having 24-h periodic variation of calcium fluxes originating from substructure 2-3, $F_{10}$ should have a circadian profile coherent with intestinal calcium absorption. Our model should then have at most 3 nonlinear fluxes, one describing internal transformation [$K_{32}$ in Eqn. (9)], and the other two concerning the relationships of the system with its environment [$F_{10}$ and $K_{01}$, Eqn. (10)].

### 5.2. Dynamic and physiological properties

The self-oscillatory compartmental model for rat calcium metabolism includes 8 compartments and 16 parameters (Fig. 5). With this structure and the identified parameter values, at none of the experimental times the predicted values of $^{45}$Ca plasma concentration (in compartment 1) differ significantly from the experimental mean values (see Fig. 4), so that the compartmental nonlinear formalism and the explicitly introduced nonlinearities quantitatively describe the kinetic data. Moreover, the asymptotic self-oscillatory behaviour is globally stable, i.e. the circadian behaviour is the only stable one for the identified parameter values (Staub et al. 1988). This first step overcome, let us now analyse the properties of the model in looking for (i) some of its global behaviours; (ii) the predicted internal distribution of calcium mass; (iii) the predicted model of temporal organization over a 24-h period.

#### 5.2.1. Asymptotic and transitory behaviours: age-related growth

This model may first be analysed for its stable asymptotic regime, as for linear compartmental models (the only behaviour studied in this case). But, in contrast to linear models, only numerical simulation can assess the overall properties of the periodic asymptotic behaviour. Table 1 summarizes the main characteristics of the model after a very long simulation time: the constant or mean asymptotic, if periodic, value is reported for each compartment. The result predicts a total calcium mass (4 g) which is much greater than the calcium mass of the experimental rat. In fact, this value is a good approximation of the total calcium mass of the adult rat. This finding, plus the predicted mean periodic values of $F_{10}$ and the total exit, which are equal (about 11 mg/day) at this time, suggests that the asymptotic behaviour of the model does not fit with calcium metabolism of the young growing rat, but has similarities with the behaviour of the adult rat (Milhaud et al., 1963).

Analysis of the trajectory predicted by the model, starting from initial zero mass values, leads to the determination of a point (working point) which fits well with the behaviour of the young rat from which the data were collected. At this point, only compartment 6 and 4 masses are significantly lower than their asymptotic values

TABLE 1. Mass values (mg) of the 8-compartment self-oscillatory model

| | Mass values (mg) | | |
|---|---|---|---|
| | Asymptotic (extrema) | Identified (± SD) | Working point |
| 1 | 3.0 | 3.0 | 3.0 |
| 2 | 21.4 (32.2/5.4) | 26.3 (± 5.4) | 24.1 |
| 3 | 7.8 (26.0/2.4) | 4.0 (± 0.6) | 2.5 |
| 4 | 136.0 (137.2/134.2) | 76.9 (± 18.8) | 77.9 |
| 5 | 342.2 | 340.6 (± 73.6) | 342.2 |
| 6 | 3354.6 (3362.5/3344.2) | | 706.0 |
| 7 | 53.8 | | 53.8 |
| 8 | 25.8 | | 25.8 |
| Total mass | 3944.6 | | 1235.3 |
| Period (h) | 22.5 | 24.2 | 24.4 |
| $F_{10}$ (mg/d) | 10.7 | | 42.0 |
| $\Delta$ (mg/d) | 0.0 | | 38.5 |

Mean asymptotic values are reported in the first column with, for self-oscillatory compartments, variation domain defined by 2 extrema. Identified initial mass values (± SD) are reported in middle column. Initial mass values at the working point, as described in the text, are shown in the last column. Estimates of period, $F_{10}$ and $\Delta$ at both asymptotic regime and working point are given.

(Table 1). The sum of the calcium masses within the model (1.2 g) approximates the real calcium mass of the young rats. The daily growth (increase in the mass of compartment 6, see Fig. 6) averages 38.5 mg/day, which agrees with the chemically assessed calcium balance ($\Delta$) (Milhaud et al., 1963). Simulation towards the asymptotic regime produces a correct approximation of this regime after 420 simulated days (14-month-old rat) and a progressive decrease in $\Delta$ is observed from around the working point (corresponding to a 2-month-old rat). This finding agrees with the physiological age-related rate of calcium mass increase.

### *5.2.2. Physiological significance of the internal distribution*

Besides these general dynamic features, there are six distinct compartments whose size range from a few milligrams to grams (Table 1). They are equivalent to calcium in bone (compartment 6: deep mature bone; compartments 2, 3 + 4: interface ECF/mature bone, and compartment 5: immature bone) or in calcified cartilage (compartment 7), while calcium in soft tissues involves only two rapidly exchangeable pools, (compartment 1: extracellular and compartment 8: intracellular; (Fig. 5). These compartments can be described in more detail using current knowledge of calcium metabolism (see Section 2).

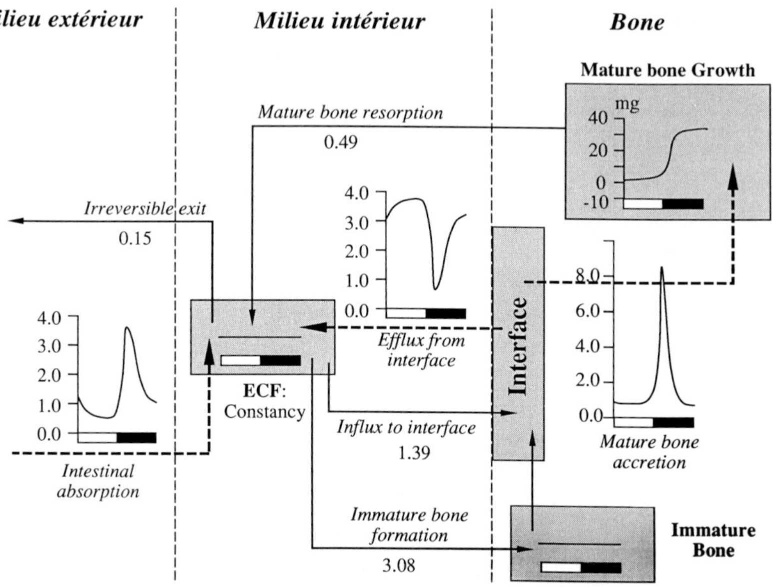


Fig. 6. 24-h temporal order within the self-oscillatory model of calcium metabolism. Three kinds of temporal behaviours coexist: constancy in the ECF (compartment 1) and immature bone, rhythmicity at bone interface (compartment 2 – 4) and growth in deep mature bone (compartment 6). The values of the constant calcium fluxes (straight solid line) are expressed in mg/h. The daily profile of the periodic calcium fluxes (straight dashed line) is shown over 24 h.

(i) **Compartment 1** (3.0 mg), can be directly compared to the mass of calcium in the ECF, including the plasma. $F_{10}$, with its average value of 42 mg/day and its circadian pattern (see Fig. 6) peaking during the first part of the dark-fed period is consistent with intestinal calcium absorption while the exit flux agrees with the sum of urinary and endogenous fecal calcium excretion (3.5 mg/day)

(ii) **Compartment 8** (25.8 mg) has an exchange rate of more than 200 mg/day and might well represent the soft tissue calcium pool. Indeed, the soft tissues are thought to contain about 1 – 2% of the total body calcium mass and calcium fluxes between ECF and soft tissues are considered to be very rapid.

(iii) **Compartment 6,** the largest in size, is far from its asymptotic regime. It has a low mean transit time (55 days) and probably represents calcium in mature bone. The irreversible flux feeding this compartment from compartment 3, with its average value of 53 mg/day, may be identified to the irreversible process of mature bone formation (cortical or trabecular lamellar bone). Its circadian periodicity (see Fig. 6), with a maximum at the time of food intake, corresponds to the experimentally observed circadian pattern of bone mineralization (Russell et al., 1984b). Conversely, the slightly rhythmic flux of calcium from compartment 6 to the ECF (15.5 mg/day) may be readily compared to mature bone resorption (action of osteoclasts involved in endosteal resorption and formation of the medullary cavity in long bones). Irreversible fluxes linked to compartment 6 may be considered as representative of calcium movements linked to mature bone modelling and remodelling.

(iv) **Compartment 5,** relatively large, with a mean transit time of 4.5 days, a rapid rate of formation (74 mg/day) from the ECF, is homologous with the calcium deposited in the newly formed areas of bone replaced by lamellar bone some days later (immature bone remodelling). The model predicts that the conversion from immature to mature requires an internal reutilization of bone calcium via irreversible flux from compartment 5 to compartment 2. This raises the question of the mechanism responsible for this conversion of immature to mature bone. Perhaps the steps leading from 'unstable to a stable form' of bone are quasi continuous and involve differential rate of maturation for the cellular, mineral and organic components. The rate of matrix production might exceed its maturation rate in zones of rapid bone formation. The conservation of osteoid several microns thick is then linked to the provisional accumulation of mineral within the immature osteoid, producing a poorly organized bone structure. The utilization of this mineral reserve would be postponed until the tissue reaches a degree of maturation. This would induce a destabilization of the initial association (poorly crystallized bHA randomly distributed throughout collagen, vesicle-derived mineral clusters) in favour of the production of a mature bone structure. While such a schema does not exclude the contributions of osteoblasts and osteoclasts, immature bone matrix may contain 'a built-in, self-destruct mechanism' which would aid in the self-organization of bone, as proposed for fetal bone (Boyde et al., 1978).

(v) **Compartment 7** (54 mg, mean transit time of 1.5 days) may represent the metabolism of calcified cartilage. According to the model of matrix-induced bone formation (Reddi, 1981), calcifying cartilage has a time-lag of about 2 days. This structure lacks matrix-mineral organization like immature bone, but does not mature and is irreversibly destroyed by chondroclasts. Compartment 7 accounts for all these criteria.

(vi) **Compartments 2, 3** and **4,** are the self-oscillatory substructure fundamental for the dynamic peculiarities of the overall model: it has a reversible exchange with ECF, a central nonlinear process (second-order autocatalytic production of 3 from 2), reversible internal transformations, and thus acts as the interface between the ECF and mature bone. This role of interface seems to be justified because, if the substructure was distributed (with HA density) over the osteoid-lacunar-canalicular bone surface (Boyde, 1981b), it would be at most 2 $\mu$m thick, a value close to that estimated by calcium exchange (Groer and Marshall, 1973). As previously suggested, the self-oscillatory substructure could involve the transformations, at the bone surface, of Ca-P associations that are the precursors of the ultimate solid phase, bHA. The prediction from our model of the presence of small amounts of Ca-P forms that differ from bHA is reminiscent of the second theory of blood/bone equilibrium proposed by Neuman (1982). Yet, disregarding the chemical nature of these Ca-P associations, we suggested applying a general schema of nucleation and crystal growth such as that developed by Larson and Garside (1986) (see Section 2.2.3.1). The self-oscillatory substructure should be coherent with the maintenance of Ca-P associations, ranging from primitive aggregates (compartment 2) to semi-ordered clusters or prenuclei (compartment 3), between osteoblast-osteocyte-lining cells complex and deep mature bone.

These pre-nuclei arise from primitive aggregates, and contribute to their own production. They should redissolve or be used for either formation of mirocrystals, whose growth is prevented by adsorption of biological material and which retain a reversible relationship with other Ca-P associations at the bone surface (compartment 4), or as 'growth units' for the irreversible growth of compartment 6. The complex system of cells at the bone surface and macromolecular components of bone extracellular matrix should play an important role in controlling these processes.

### *5.2.3. 24-Hour temporal order: self-regulatory process*

The model has the remarkable property of simultaneously accounting for the three features of temporal behaviour inherent in young rat calcium metabolism: rhythmicity, constancy and growth, as illustrated in Fig. 6.

The ECF/mature bone interface is the locus of special dynamic behaviour. It provides temporal coordination of calcium metabolism on both sides of the bone surface by generating: (i) a rhythmic calcium efflux from the bone surface to the ECF, which is in phase opposition with the circadian flux of calcium coming from the *'milieu extérieur'* by intestinal calcium absorption; (ii) an irreversible circadian efflux from surface towards deep mature bone which is approximately in phase with calcium absorption: as if the net calcium movement produced by calcium absorption was simultaneously integrated for the benefit of mature bone growth. As for plasma calcium concentration, there are only small (less than 10%) daily variations in the total calcium mass of bone interface, while, if considered separately, compartment 2 or 3 has more than 100% daily fluctuation. The interface includes the active zones of mature bone formation, in opposition to the view of Talmage (Talmage et al., 1980) or Parfitt (1987), and the dynamic daily organization predicted by the model does not require significant daily variations in mature bone resorption.

This brief presentation of the dynamic properties of calcium metabolism supports the initial idea that the temporal behaviours are largely dictated by the properties of an autocatalytic process involved in bone mineral transformation at the ECF/bone interface. This process acts as a master event within a network of metabolic pathways, leading to a self-sustained periodic behaviour for the overall system, with its consequences for understanding calcium homeostasis (see Section 4.2). Nevertheless, the conceptual leap rests not only on the passage from constant to circadian behaviour, but mainly on likening calcium metabolism to a nonlinear system with its potential to give rise to a set of complex non-intuitive behaviours.

## 6. Heuristic potential of the nonlinear model for calcium metabolism

The dynamic organization of biological system can best be understood in terms of spatio-temporal expressions that nonlinear systems can produce. Progress in this field is depending upon the development of mathematical theories and methods enabling a rational analysis of these systems (Gukenheimer and Holmes, 1983). In this respect, correct use of the heuristic potential of the nonlinear calcium metabolism model lies in the diversity of the temporal expressions this model can show beyond the identified circadian behaviour. These temporal expressions can be divided into two categories: (i) constant and simple periodic behaviours which are applied to calcium metabolism and its regulation and (ii) complex periodic or aperiodic oscillatory behaviours, till now rarely observed for calcium metabolism or its associated hormonal systems. Theoretical experience on complex behaviours can be most useful in broadening our view of calcium metabolism and the interpretation of new and, if necessary, old data. Experimental protocols are generally developed for situations where only constant or synchronous simple periodic behaviours are expected.

The nonlinear sub-structure (compartments 2, 3 and 4) describing the interface ECF/mature bone was analysed by Tracqui et al. (1985). This study involved continuously varying some parameter values of the nonlinear sub-structure to determine, by a combination of analytical and numerical methods, the critical points at which the theoretical behaviour of the system is qualitatively modified (bifurcation point). Qualitative modifications concern the stability and/or the type of the asymptotic temporal behaviour (steady-state, periodic or aperiodic oscillations). The theoretical results could be of interest in several areas: (i) in comparative studies between species for which the dynamic processes involved in bone calcium metabolism are suspected to be of similar nature but quantitatively different; (ii) to explain, for given species, the behavioural modifications due to a continuous drift of some parameter values during, e.g. growth or age; (iii) to account for the temporal response to an acute 'perturbation', i.e. the transient variation of a variable or parameter value induced, e.g. by calcium load or transient hormonal action.

Temporal expressions describing the relationships between bone surface and ECF deal directly with plasma calcium homeostasis. So, without entering into the details of the bifurcation diagram (Tracqui et al., 1987), let us examine some of the general properties predicted from this study (Staub et al., 1989).

### 6.1. Simple temporal behaviours

#### *6.1.1. Constant behaviour*

Calcium metabolism is generally assumed in this situation, i.e. the asymptotic behaviours of all variables are constant (steady-state). The first complexity involves the number of real steady-states: the ordinary differential system equivalent to the nonlinear substructure may have up to two stable steady-states for a given set of parameter values.

When the parameter values produce a system with only one stable steady-state, the situation might be identical to that in which classical compartmental analysis of calcium metabolism was done. In such a situation, the system can be linearized on the basis of tracer kinetic data (see Section 3.1.1), and the bone interface is a part of the exchangeable calcium pool.

If there are two stable steady-states, special dynamic properties evolve from switching back and forth between these steady-states. Assume that the nonlinear substructure is in one steady-state during feeding or fasting part of the day, and is subject to circadian perturbations (for instance hormonal) of small amplitude and duration. The substructure could drift from this state towards the other and leave this later state as a result of a reverse perturbation. Explicit consideration of such behaviours could enhance the efficiency of previous schema for generating circadian variations in rat calcium metabolism. The cyclic action of CT on bone surface, as suggested in the Talmage theory, would be a good example (see Section 4.2.1).

### *6.1.2. Simple periodic behaviour*

Let us now consider the conditions in which our study of calcium metabolism in the normal rat was done, i.e. those for the self-generation of periodic solutions. At this relatively low level of complexity, the role of calcium-regulating hormones in calcium homeostasis can be discussed. As previously suggested (Fig. 3), it is attractive to consider the hormonal system as controlling the amplitude, period and/or phase of both the main oscillators in rat, intestinal absorption and bone efflux. Circadian variations modulate the capacity of calcium transport by the rat small intestine (Wrobel and Nagel, 1979), feeding habits being a major zeitgeber. Thus, the main argument for control of this periodic phenomenon lies in its amplitude. 1,25-$(OH)_2$D, with its direct effect on intestinal absorption, could adjust the amplitude of this parameter. The osteoblast-type cells covering the bone surface are targets for all three hormones, 1,25-$(OH)_2$D, PTH and CT which are probably involved in the control of the self-oscillatory nonlinear substructure. The hormonal effects could concern three levels of control: (i) the very existence of the periodic variation at the bone interface might depend upon the mean circulating level of some regulating hormones. (ii) PTH and/or CT, via the circadian profiles of their plasma concentrations, might act as pacemakers to ensure phase control and period entrainment of spontaneous periodic bone calcium efflux. (iii) 'Defaults' in complementarity could elicit variations in plasma calcium concentration, inducing, in reaction, changes in hormonal secretion. The hormones should act here as transducers, able to detect errors in internal synchronization and to reset the implicated oscillators. (iv) Interrelationships, at central nervous system level, between hormonal system and behavioural control (Fig. 3) could interfere with calcium homeostasis in two ways: behavioural effect on the periodic expression of the hormones (phase shifts induced by modification of zeitgebers) and the reverse action of the hormonal system on the behavioural control. The latter could account for the suggested effect of CT on feeding behaviour (Freed et al., 1979; Clementi et al., 1983).

Although this view of calcium homeostasis is supported by considerable experimental evidence, it raises questions about the mechanisms underlying the hormonal periodicity. In fact, the mechanisms controlling biosynthesis, cellular metabolism and secretion of the hormone possess *a priori* a sufficient level of complexity (see Section 2.1.2) to produce self-oscillatory behaviours. Furthermore, coupling between metabolic and hormonal oscillators might be more subtle than the classical feedback mechanisms which may be disclosed by new experimental approaches, such as constant versus pulsatile infusion of exogenous hormones.

The situation identified in the young growing rat is the simplest case (see Section 5.2): a single unstable steady-state associated with a globally stable periodic (circadian) solution. However, there are somewhat more complex situations involving multistability. For instance, a periodic behaviour can be associated with either a stable steady-state or another periodic behaviour (birhythmicity: Tracqui and Staub, 1987). Thus, the disappearance or the major changes in $^{45}$Ca circadian behaviour induced by fasting (Talmage, 1975) may be newly interpreted: a transient perturbation may shift the system from its circadian behaviour to another one with quite different properties.

### 6.2. Complex temporal behaviours

The theoretical study of the complex behaviours for the nonlinear sub-structure is still under investigation. Preliminary results (Staub et al., 1989) demonstrate its ability for generating behaviours either periodic with more than one maximum or minimum (composite features including large variations associated with varying numbers of 'small' amplitude variations), or aperiodic, the so-called chaotic oscillations.

Most of the examples of a complex temporal behaviour come from outside calcium metabolism (Goldbeter and Decroly, 1983; Rapp, 1984), but some data on calcium metabolism and its regulation may concern this type of phenomena: e.g. the observation of high-frequency variations in the total plasma calcium concentration in man (Kripke et al., 1978), or a model for osteoporosis based on the modification of the pulsatile pattern of PTH secretion (Harms et al., 1987).

## 7. Conclusion and suggestions for future directions

The goal of this chapter was to summarize the highlights of plasma calcium homeostasis and to develop several new proposals. Major progress have been made concerning the cellular and mineral events underlying the temporal organization of calcium metabolism and calcium-regulating hormones. However, the gap remains striking between the increasing complexity of the new data and the relative *status quo* of the concepts currently presented for understanding calcium regulation. As a consequence, it is not surprising that the orchestration of the events involved in plasma calcium homeostasis remains poorly understood. A conceptual renewal is required to evaluate the capacity of self-organization of calcium metabolism both in time and in space. This conceptual framework is in line with the proposals made by Best and Hearon (1960) and fits with the physical biology of bone developed by Richelle and Onkelinx (1969). But it gains by the developments of theoretical and numerical methods for nonlinear systems analysis and advances in bone cellular organization and physico-chemical properties of its mineralization.

Our aim is to examine calcium metabolism as a nonlinear system that is far from equilibrium and to disclose the connection between the calcium dynamics intrinsic to each organ and their ultimate composition at plasma level. The explicit consideration of some nonlinear reactions which act as master pieces for the internal organization of calcium and its hormonal regulation, represents a break with the classical viewpoint. Consequently, the reader should discard from now current notions of plasma calcium homeostasis based on the exclusive use of cybernetic diagrams and on the representation of calcium metabolism by a linear system that is maintained in a steady-state. He is invited to adopt the contemporary view on the phenomena highly relevant for biological systems such as those of self-replication, -organization and -regulation, peculiarities of nonlinear systems which are exemplified by the behaviours of simple theoretical or physico-chemical systems. The basic concepts of the dynamic organization of biological system and their evolution since Claude Bernard were surveyed, paying special attention to oscillatory behaviours. As example, we developed a self-oscillatory model for rat calcium metabolism and its homeostatic regulation, characterized by four major features: First, the nonlinear reactions qualifying calcium-phosphate transformations under the osteoblast-osteocyte-lining cell complex at bone surface (self-replication of precrystalline structures) are the key processes for the spontaneous generation of oscillatory behaviours. They affect directly the rates of mature bone formation and calcium efflux from the bone surface to ECF. Second, plasma calcium homeostasis involves small circadian variation in the rat, resulting from the quasi-complementarity of two major circadian functions: bone calcium efflux and intestinal calcium entrance. Third, period, amplitude and phase of these oscillatory events are adjusted to ensure the delicate timing necessary for plasma calcium homeostasis and the 24-h temporal organization of calcium functions in the body. The osteoblast phenotype of cells covering bone may be the target cells for the hormonal control of the self-oscillatory mineral dynamics at bone surface, and consequently, essential for plasma calcium homeostasis. Fourth, an attractive hypothesis is that regulation of plasma calcium homeostasis is achieved by coupling between oscillators (exogenous, metabolic, hormonal, or neural), with their inherent flexibility in response to challenge. The biosynthesis, secretion, and mutual interactions of the calcium-regulating hormones are such complex processes that they might behave as potentially independent oscillators.

Future research might extend this study in at least three directions: First, our theoretical studies show that, if the circadian periodicity is predominant in normal rat, numerous other oscillatory behaviours are expected at the bone surface, from a single constant behaviour to much more complex behaviours (e.g. complex aperiodic features) with the possibility of transition from a state into another one. Potentiality for such a diversity of self-oscillatory behaviours illustrates how the calcium homeostasis must be formulated differently and how experimental and formal approaches must be interconnected since these behaviours cannot be intuitively predicted. Fortunately, the physico-mathematical modelling of complex systems are now entering the biological field. Second, we focussed the attention on the processes of phase transition associated with calcium-phosphate reactions, but further improvement of our model will include other types of nonlinear reactions, acting in cooperation with these mineral reactions. Thus, our proposals can be extended to other topics, e.g. cellular and biochemical findings. Third, our current theoretical approach of calcium metabolism, with its impact on the understanding of extracellular calcium homeostasis, emphasizes the role of Ca-P associations at bone surface in generating specific endogenous temporal structures. However, physical properties other than reactional such as diffusion of chemical species (ions, cluster or precrystalline forms of Ca-P associations) inside the extracellular matrix covering the bone surface may be suggested as determining factors of the overall (i.e. spatio-temporal) dynamic organization. One of the most extensively developed models for pattern formation is the reaction-diffusion theory, which has been successfully applied to a number of questions related to the generation of complex shapes and patterns. In view of the great similarities between (i) the physico-chemical mechanisms postulated for the generation of spatial structures in precipitating systems and those proposed here for the temporal organization of bone mineral metabolism, (ii) the mathematical formulation of the nonlinear substructure of our model and that of the autocatalytic models describing morphogenesis during biological development and pattern formation (Meinhardt and Klinger, 1987), a theoretical study of the conditions in which the nonlinear substructure of calcium metabolism might generate spatio-temporal organization is required. It could be linked to generation of primitive bone shape and provide basic information on the local regulation of bone cellular activities through, for instance, chemotactic substances associated with mineral materials. These results, in turn, will contribute (i) to support the recent suggestion for a direct morphogenetic role of osteogenic cells during bone formation (Caplan and Pechak, 1987); (ii) to a better understanding of extracellular calcium homeostasis which, at its high level of organization, integrates all the spatio-temporal dynamics of calcium metabolism, including spatio-temporal homogeneity at plasma level.

## Acknowledgements

The authors wish to acknowledge Dr. P. Tracqui and S. Lausson who participated in some of the studies described herein.

## References

Abe E, Miyaura C, Sakagami H, et al. Differentiation of mouse myeloid leukemia cells induced by 1,25-dihydroxyvitamin D3. Proc Natl Acad Sci USA 1981;78:4990 – 4994.

Abe E, Miyaura C, Tanaka H, et al. 1,25-dihydroxyvitamin D3 promotes fusion of mouse alveolar macrophages both by a direct mechanism and by a spleen cell-mediated indirect mechanism. Proc Natl Acad Sci USA 1983;80:5585 – 5587.

Adams ND, Gray RW, Lemann J. The effects of oral CaCO3 loading and dietary calcium deprivation on plasma 1,25-dihydroxyvitamin D concentrations in healthy adults. J Clin Endocrinol Metab 1979;48:1008 – 1016.

Agnusdei D, Montagnani M, Gennari C. Seasonal variations of serum parathyroid hormone in patients with postmenopausal osteoporosis. J Endocrinol Invest 1988;11(Suppl 2):31.

Ali-Rachedi A, Varndell IM, Facer P, et al. Immunocytochemical localization of katacalcin, a calcium lowering hormones cleaved from the human calcitonin precursor. J Clin Endocrinol Metab 1983; 57:680 – 682.

Aloia RC. Membrane fluidity in biology. General Principles, New York: Vol. 2. Academic Press, 1983.

Amano S, Hanazawa S, Hirose K, Ohmori Y, Kitano S. Stimulatory effect on bone resorption of interleukin-I-like cytokine produced by an osteoblast-rich population of mouse calvaria cells. Calcif Tissue Int 1988;43:88 – 91.

Amara SG, Jonas V, Rosenfeld MG, Ong ES, Evans RM. Alternative RNA processing in calcitonin gene expression generates mRNA encoding products. Nature 1982;298:240 – 244.

Amara SG, Evans RM, Rosenfeld MG. Calcitonin/calcitonin gene related peptides transcription unit: tissue-specific expression involves selective use of alternative polyadenylation sites. Mol Cell Biol 1984;4:2151 – 2160.

Ammann P, Rizzoli R, Fleisch H. Calcium absorption in rat large intestine in vivo: availability of dietary calcium. Am J Physiol 1986;251:G14 – G18.

Anderson HC. Matrix vesicle calcification: Review and update. In: Peck WA, ed. Bone and Mineral Research, Vol. 3. Amsterdam: Elsevier, 1985;109 – 149.

Ardaillou R, Sizenenko P, Meyrier A, Vallée G, Geaugas C. Metabolic clearance rate of radioiodinated human calcitonin in man. J Clin Invest 1970;49:2345 – 2352.

Arsenault AL, Ottenmeyer FP. Quantitative spatial distributions of calcium, phosphorus, and sulfur in calcifying epiphysis with high resolution electron spectroscopic imaging. Proc Natl Acad Sci USA 1983;80:1322 – 1326.

Arsenault AL, Ottenmeyer FP. Visualization of early intramembranous ossification by microscopic and spectroscopic imaging. J Cell Biol 1984; 98:911 – 921.

Aschoff J. Circadian rhythms: general features and endocrinological aspects. In: Krieger D, ed. Endocrine Rhythms, Vol. 19. New York: Raven Press, 1979:1 – 61.

Aubert JP, Bronner F. A symbolic model for the regulation by bone metabolism of the blood calcium level in rats. Biophys J 1965;5:349 – 358.

Aubert JP, Milhaud G. Méthode de mesure de principales voies du métabolisme calcique chez l'homme. Biochim Biophys Acta 1960;39:122 – 132.

Aurbach GD, Marx SJ, Spiegel AM. Calcium homeostasis. Parathyroid hormone, calcitonin, and the calciferols. In: Wilson JD, Foster DW, eds. Textbook of Endocrinology. Philadelphia: Saunders Co,

1985;1137 - 1217.

Balmain N, Moscofian A, Cuisinier-Gleizes P. Metaphyseal pattern: Uniqueness of this structure in growing gones originating from cartilaginous anlage. A microradiographic study. Calcif Tissue Int 1983;35:225 - 231.

Balsan S, Garabedian M, Larchet M, et al. Long-term nocturnal calcium infusion can cure ricket and promote normal mineralization in hereditary resistance to 1,25-dihydroxyvitamin D. J Clin Invest 1986;77:1661 - 1667.

Baran DT, Milne ML. 1,25-dihydroxyvitamin D increases hepatocyte cytosolic calcium levels: A potential regulator of vitamin D-25-hydroxylase. J Clin Invest 1986;77:1622 - 1626.

Barnicot NA. The local action of the parathyroid and other tissues on the bone in intracerebral grafts. J Anat 1948;82:233 - 248.

Baron R, Vignery A. Behavior of osteoclasts during a rapid change in their number induced by high doses of parathyroid hormone or calcitonin in intact rats. Metab Bone Dis Rel Res 1982;2:339 - 346.

Baron R, Vignery A, Horowitz M. Lymphocytes, macrophages and the regulation of bone remodeling. In: Peck WA, ed. Bone and Mineral Research, Vol. 2. Amsterdam: Elsevier, 1983;175 - 244.

Baron R, Neff L, Louvard D, Courtoy P. Acidification and bone resorption: immunocytochemical localization of a lysosomal membrane protein at the ruffled border of osteoclasts. J Cell Biol 1985;101:2210 - 2222.

Bassett C. Biologic significances of piezoelectricity. Calcif Tissue Res 1968;1:252 - 272.

Bauer GCH, Carlsson A, Lindquist B. Metabolism and homeostatic function of bone. In: Comar CL, Bronner F, eds. Mineral Metabolism, Vol. I. New York: Academic Press, 1961;609 - 676.

Baylink D, Morey E, Rich C. Effect of calcitonin on the rates of bone formation and resorption in the rat. Endocrinology 1969;84:261 - 269.

Bell NH. Vitamin D-endocrine system. J Clin Invest 1985;76:1 - 6.

Bell NH, Shaw S, Turner RT. Evidence that 1,25-dihydroxyvitamin D3 inhibits the hepatic production of 25-hydroxyvitamin D in man. J Clin Invest 1984; 74:1540 - 1544.

Bell PA, Kodicek E. Investigations on metabolites of vitamin D in rat bile. Separation and partial identification of a major metabolite. Biochem J 1969;115:663 - 669.

Belousov BP. A periodic reaction and its mechanism. Published in 1951 and translated into English by Maloney PG, Field RJ. In: Field RJ, Burger M, eds. Oscillations and Travelling Waves in Chemical Systems, 1985;605 - 613.

Bernard C. Leçons sur les phénomènes de la Vie Communs Aux Animaux et Aux Végétaux, Vol. 1. Paris: Ballière, 1878;113 - 121.

Berridge MJ, Irvine RF. Inositol triphosphate, a novel second messenger in cellular signal transduction. Nature 1984;312:315 - 321.

Best JB. Some theoretical considerations concerning crystal with relevance to the physical properties of bone. Biochim Biophys Acta 1959;32:194 - 202.

Best JB, Hearon JZ. Thermodynamic principles and concepts. In: Comar CL, Bronner F, eds. Mineral Metabolism, Vol. I. New York: Academic Press, 1960;11 - 60.

Betts F, Blumenthal NC, Posner AS. Bone mineralization. J Cryst Growth 1981;53:63 - 73.

Bikle DD, Zolock DT, Morrissey RL, Herman RH. Independence of 1,25-dihydroxyvitamin D3-mediated calcium transport from de novo RNA and protein synthesis. J Biol Chem 1978;253:484 - 488.

Bingham PJ, Brazell IA, Owen M. The effect of parathyroid extract on cellular activity and plasma calcium levels in vivo. J Endocrinol 1969;45:387 - 400.

Binsma JJM, Kolar Z. Study of the dynamic equilibrium in the CaF2/aqueous solution system using $45Ca^{2+}$ as radiotracer. Farady Disc Chem Soc 1984;77:257 - 263.

Birnbaum RS, Mahoney WC, Burns DM, O'Neil JA, Miller RE, Roos BA. Identification of procalcitonin in a rat medullary thyroid carcinoma cell line. J Biol Chem 1984;259:2870 - 2876.

Bissell MJ, Hall HG, Parry G. How does the extracellular matrix direct gene expression? J Theor Biol 1982;99:31 - 68.

Bonard LC, Roufosse AH, Sabine WK, Grynpas MD, Glimcher MJ. X-ray diffraction studies of the crystallinity of bone mineral in newly synthesized and density fractionated bone. Calcif Tissue Int 1983;35:202 – 209.

Booth BE, Tsai HC, Morris RC. Vitamin D status regulates 25-hydroxyvitamin D3-1$\alpha$-hydroxylase and its responsiveness to parathyroid hormone in the chick. J Clin Invest 1985;75:155 – 161.

Boskey AL, Posner AS. In vitro nucleation of hydroxyapatite by a bone calcium-phospholipid complex. Calcif Tissue Res 1977;22(Suppl):197 – 200.

Bouizar Z, Rostene WM, Moukhtar MS, Milhaud G. Characterization and quantitative topographical distribution of salmon calcitonin-binding sites in rat kidney section. FEBS Lett 1986;196:19 – 22.

Boulos Z, Rosenwasser AM, Terman M. Feeding schedules and the circadian organization of behavior in the rat. Behav Brain Res 1980;1:39 – 65.

Bourdeau JE, Burg MG. Effect of parathyroid hormone on calcium transport in the cortical thick ascending limb of Henle's loop. Clin Res 1979;27:410 – 416.

Boyde A. Electron microscopy of the mineralizing front. In: Jee WSS, Parfitt AM, eds. Bone Histomorphometry. Paris: Montagu, Armour. 1981a;69 – 79.

Boyde A. Evidence against 'osteocytic osteolysis'. In: Lee WSS, Parfitt AM, eds. Bone Histomorphometry. Paris: Armour Montagu, 1981b;239 – 257.

Boyde A, Banes AJ, Dillaman RM, Mechanic GL. A morphological study of an avian bone disorder caused by myeloblastosis-associated virus. Metab Bone Dis Rel Res 1978;1:235 – 242.

Boyle IT, Gray RW, DeLuca HF. Regulation by calcium of in vivo synthesis of 1,25-dihydroxycholecalciferol and 24,25-dihydroxycholecalciferol: Proc Natl Acad Sci USA 1971;68: 2131 – 2134.

Brasitus TA, Dudeja PK, Eby B, Lau K. Correction by 1,25-dihydroxycholecalciferol of the abnormal fluidity and lipid composition of enterocyte brush border membranes in vitamin D-deprived rats. J Biol Chem 1986;261:16404 – 16409.

Broadus AE. Mineral metabolism. In: Felig P, Baxter JD, Broadus AE, Frohman LA, eds. Endocrinology and Metabolism. New York: MacGraw-Hill, 1981;963 – 1079.

Bronner F. Kinetic and cybernetic analysis of calcium metabolism. In: Irving JT, ed. Calcium and Phosphorus Metabolism. New York: Academic Press, 1973;149 – 186.

Bronner F. Quantitative aspects of calcium metabolism and homeostasis. In: Kuhlencordt F, Kruse HP, eds. Calcium Metabolism, Bone and Metabolic Bone Diseases. Berlin: Springer-Verlag, 1975;1 – 24.

Bronner F. Calcium homeostasis. In: Bronner F, Coburn JW, eds. Disorders of Mineral Metabolism: Calcium Physiology, Vol. 2. New York: Academic Press, 1982;43 – 102.

Bronner F. Role of intestinal calcium absorption in plasma calcium regulation of the rat. Am J Physiol 1984;246:R680 – R683.

Bronner F, Pansu D, Bosshard A, Lipton JH. Calcium uptake by isolated rat intestinal cells. J Cell Physiol 1983;116:322 – 328.

Brown EM, Gardner DG, Windeck RA, Aurbach GD. Relationship of intracellular 3′-5′-adenosine monophosphate accumulation to parathyroid hormone release from dispersed bovine parathyroid cells. Endocrinology 1978;103:2323 – 2333.

Brown EM, LeBoff MS, Oetting M, Posillico JT, Chen C. Secretory control in normal and abnormal parathyroid tissue. Recent Prog Horm Res 1987;43:337 – 381.

Brown WE, Chow LC. Surface equilibria of sparingly soluble crystals. Colloids Surf 1983;7:67 – 80.

Brown WE, Mathew M, Tung MS. Crystal chemistry of octacalcium phosphate. Prog Cryst Growth Charact 1981;4:59 – 87.

Brumbaugh PF, Haussler MR. Specific binding of 1,25-dihydroxycholecalciferol to nuclear components of chick intestine. J Biol Chem 1975;250:1588 – 1594.

Buckwalter JA, Rosenberg LC, Ungar R. Changes in proteoglycan aggregates during cartilage mineralization. Calcif Tissue Int 1987;41:228 – 236.

Burch WM. Calcitonin stimulates growth and maturation of embryonic chick pelvic cartilage in vitro. Endocrinology 1984;114:1196 – 1202.

Burch WM, Lebovitz HE. Parathyroid hormone stimulates growth of embryonic chick pelvic cartilage in vitro. Calcif Tissue Int 1983;35:526 – 532.

Burch WM, Lopez-Claros M, Uskokovic MR, Drezner MK. 1,25-dihydroxyvitamin D3 stimulates avian and mammalian cartilage growth in vitro. J Bone Mineral Res 1988;3:87 – 91.

Burger EH, Boonekamp PM, Nijweide PJ. Osteoblast and osteoclast precursors in primary cultures of calvaria bone cells. Anat Rec 1986;214:32 – 40.

Burkinshaw L, Marshall DH, Oxby CB, Spiers FW, Nordin BEC, Young MM. Bone turnover model based on a continuously expanding exchangeable calcium pool. Nature 1969;222:146 – 148.

Burnell JM, Teubner E, Korn D, Miller A. Role of calcium in bone maturation arrest after thyroparathyroidectomy in the rat. Am J Physiol 1977;232:F33 – F41.

Burton AC. The properties of the steady states compared to those of the equilibrium as show in characteristic biological behavior. J Cell Comp Physiol 1939;14:327 – 349.

Bushinsky DA, Riera GS, Favus MJ, Coe FL. Evidence that blood ionized calcium regulates serum 1,25-(OH)2D3 independently of parathyroid hormone and phosphorus in the rat. J Clin Invest 1985;76:1599 – 1604.

Campo RD. Effects of cations on cartilage structure: swelling of growth plate and degradation of proteoglycans induced by chelators of divalent cations. Calcif Tissue Int 1988;43:108 – 121.

Canalis E, Peck WA, Raisz LG. Stimulation of DNA and collagen synthesis by autologous growth factor in cultures fetal rat calvaria. Science 1980;210:1021 – 1023.

Canas F, Terepka AR, Neuman WF. Potassium and the milieu interieur of bone. Am J Physiol 1969;217:117 – 120.

Cannon WB. Organization for physiological homeostasis. Physiol Rev 1929;9:399 – 431.

Cantley LK, Russell J, Lettieri D, Sherwood LM. 1,25-dihydroxyvitamin D3 suppresses parathyroid secretion from bovine parathyroid cells in tissue culture. Endocrinology 1985;117:2114 – 2119.

Caplan AI, Pechak DG. The cellular and molecular embryology of bone formation. In: Peck WA, ed. Bone and Mineral Research, Vol. 5. Amsterdam: Elsevier, 1987;117 – 184.

Carafoli E. Intracellular calcium homeostasis. Ann Rev Biochem 1987;56:395 – 433.

Care AD, Sherwood LM, Potts JT, Aurbach GD. Evaluation by radioimmunoassay of factors controlling the secretion of parathyroid hormone. Perfusion of the isolated parathyroid gland of the goat and sheep. Nature 1966;209:55 – 57.

Care AD, Cooper CW, Duncan T, Orimo H. A study of thyrocalcitonin secretion by direct measurement of in vivo secretion rates in pig. Endocrinology 1968;83:161 – 169.

Care AD, Bates RFL, Gitelman HJ. A possible role for the adenyl cyclase system in calcitonin release. J Endocrinol 1970;48:1 – 15.

Carruthers BM, Copp DH, McIntosh HW. Diurnal variation in urinary excretion of calcium and phosphate and its relation to blood levels. J Lab Clin Med 1964;63:959 – 968.

Cecchetin B, Tarquini B, Miolo M, Conte N. The endogenous secretion rate of human calcitonin in normal conditions. Biomed Pharmacotherapy 1985;40:19 – 24.

Chambers TJ, Magnus CJ. Calcitonin alters behavior of isolated osteoclasts. J Pathol 1982;136;27 – 39.

Chambers TJ, Revell PA, Fuller K, Athanasou NA. Resorption of bone by isolated rabbit osteoclast. J Cell Sci 1984;66:383 – 399.

Chance B, Pye K, Higgins J. Wave form generation by enzymatic oscillators. IEEE spectrum 1967;4:79 – 86.

Chandler JS, Pike JW, Haussler MR. 1,25-dihydroxyvitamin D3 receptors in rat kidney cytosol. Biochem Biophys Res Commun 1979;90:1057 – 1063.

Charkes ND, Makler PT. Computer-simulated radionuclide bone scans in health and disease using compartmental analysis techniques. Proc Summer Computer Conference, Vancouver, 1983:738 – 743.

Chase LR, Aurbach GD. Parathyroid function and the renal excretion of 3′,5′-adenylic acid. Proc Natl Acad Sci USA 1967;58:518 – 526.

Chase LR, Aurbach GD. The effect of parathyroid hormone on the concentration of adenosine 3'5'-monophosphate in skeletal tissues in vitro. J Biol Chem 1970;245:1520 – 1526.

Chen C, Anast CS, Posillico JT, Brown EM. Effects of extracellular calcium and magnesium on cytosolic calcium concentration in fura-2-loaded bovine parathyroid cells. J Bone Mineral Res 1987;2:319 – 327.

Chen TL, Cone CM, Morey-Holton E, Feldman D. 1,25-dihydroxyvitamin D3 receptors in cultured rat osteoblast-like cells. J Biol Chem 1983;258:4350 – 4355.

Clementi G, Prato A, Bernardini R, et al. Behavioral and neuroendocrine effects of calcitonin. In: Endroczi E, et al. eds. Integrative Neurohumoral Mechanisms. Amsterdam: Elsevier, 1983;115 – 122.

Clements MR, Johnson L, Fraser DR. A new mechanism for induced vitamin D deficiency in calcium deprivation. Nature 1987;325:62 – 65.

Cohn DV, Etling JJ. Synthesis and secretion of parathormone and secretory protein-I by the parathyroid gland. In: Peck WA, ed. Bone and Mineral Research, Vol. 2. Amsterdam: Elsevier, 1983;1 – 64.

Colston KW, Evans IMA, Spelsberg TC, MacIntyre I. Feedback regulation of vitamin D metabolism by 1,25-dihydroxycholecalciferol. Biochem J 1977;164:83 – 89.

Cooper CW, McGuigan JE, Schwesinger WH, Brubaker RL, Munson PL. Correlation between levels of gastrin and thyrocalcitonin in pig thyroid venous blood. Endocrinology 1974;95:302 – 307.

Copp DH, Cameron EC, Cheney BA, Davidson AGF, Henze KG. Evidence for calcitonin-a new hormone from the parathyroid that lowers blood calcium. Endocrinology 162;70:638 – 649.

Corlett SC, Chaudhary MS, Tomlinson S, Care AD. The involvement of intracellular calcium ion concentration and calmodulin in the 25-hydroxylation of cholecalciferol in ovine and rat liver. Cell Calcium 1987;8:247 – 258.

Dawes MW, Carson ER, Reeve J. Modelling the endocrine control structure of calcium metabolism. Endocrine-Metabolic systems. II. In: IFAC 9th Triennial Word Congress, 1984;3109 – 3114.

De Rouffignac C, Elalouf JM, Roinel N, Bailly C, Amiel C. Similarity of the effects of antidiuretic hormone, parathyroid hormone, calcitonin, and glucagon on rat kidney. In: Robinson RR, ed. Proceedings of the 9th International Congress of Nephrology. Berlin: Springer-Verlag, 1984;340 – 357.

DeLuca HF. Metabolism and Mechanism of Action of VitaminD-1982. In: Peck WA, ed. Bone and Mineral Research, Vol. 1. Amsterdam: Elsevier, 1983;7 – 73.

Desplan C, Benicourt C, Jullienne A, et al. Cell free translation of mRNA coding for human and murine calcitonin. FEBS Lett 1980;117:89 – 92.

De Bella FP, Gilkinson JB, Flueck J, Arnaud CD. Carboxyl-terminal fragments of human parathyroid tumors: unique new source of immunogens for the production of antisera potentially useful in the radioimmunoassay of parathyroid hormone in human serum. J Clin Endocrinol Metab 1978;46:604 – 612.

DiStefano JJ III. Tracer experiment design for unique identification of nonlinear physiological systems. Am J Physiol 1976;230:476 – 485.

Doty SB. Morphological evidence of gap junctions between bone cells. Calcif Tissue Int 1981;33:509 – 512.

Doty SB, Yates CW, Lotz WE, Kisecleski W, Talmage RV. Effects of short term alpha irradiation on parathyroid activity and osteoclast numbers. Proc Soc Exp Biol Med 1965;114:77 – 81.

Drivdahl RH, Howard GA, Baylink DJ. Extracts of bone contain a potent regulator of bone formation. Biochim Biophys Acta 1982;714:26 – 33.

Dube WM, Goldsmith RS, Arnaud CD. Circadian rhythmicity of serum parathyroid hormone concentration in man: role of phosphate and ionized calcium. Clin Res 1972;20:425 – 429.

Düzgünes N, Papahadjopoulos D. Ionotropic effects on phospholipid membranes: calcium/magnesium specificity in binding, fluidity, and fusion. In: Aloia RC, ed. Membrane Fluidity in Biology, Vol. 2. New York: Academic Press, 1983;187 – 216.

Edmunds LN. Cellular and Molecular Bases of Biological Clocks. New York: Springer-Verlag, 1988.

Eilon G, Raisz LG. Comparison of the effects of stimulators and inhibitors of resorption on the release of lysosomal enzymes and radioactive calcium from fetal bone in organ culture. Endocrinology 1978;103:1969 – 1975.

Elalouf JM, Roinel N, de Rouffignac C. Stimulation by human calcitonin of electrolyte transport in distal tubules of rat kidney. Pflugers Arch 1983;399:111 – 118.

Emmertsen K, Christensen SE, Schmitz O, Marqversen J. Diurnal pattens of serum immunoreactive calcitonin in healthy males and in insulin dependent diabetics. Clin Endocrinol 1983;19:533 – 537.

Epstein PA, Prentki M, Attie MF. Modulation of intracellular $Ca^{2+}$ in the parathyroid cell. FEBS Lett 1985;188:141 – 144.

Esvelt RP, Schnoes KK, DeLuca HF. Isolation and characterization of 1α-hydroxy-tetranorvitamin D-23-carboxylic acid: a major metabolite of 1,25-dihydroxyvitamin D3. Biochemistry 1979;18:3977 – 3983.

Even P, Couland H, Nicolaidis, S. Integrated metabolic control of food intake after 2-deoxyglucose and nicotinic acid injection. Am J Physiol 1988;255:R82 – R89.

Fallon MD. Bone resorbing fluid from osteoclasts in acidic- an in vitro micropuncture study. In: Cohn DV, Fujita T, Potts JT, Talmage RV, eds. Endocrine Control of Bone and Calcium Metabolism. Amsterdam: Excerpta Medica, 1984;144 – 150.

Farley JR, Tarbaux LM, Hall SL, Linkhart TA, Baylink DJ. The anti-bone-resorptive agent calcitonin also acts in vitro to directly increase bone formation and bone cell proliferation. Endocrinology 1988;123:159 – 167.

Favus MJ, Langman CB. Evidence for calcium-dependent control of 1,25-dihydroxyvitamin D3 production by kidney proximal tubules. J Biol Chem 1986;261:11224 – 11229.

Favus MJ, Mangelsdorf DJ, Tembe V, Coe BJ, Haussler MR. Evidence for in vivo upregulation of the intestinal Vitamin D receptor during dietary calcium restriction in the rat. J Clin Invest 1988;82:218 – 224.

Feldman D, McCain TA, Hirst MA, Chen TL, Colston KW. Characterization of a cytoplasmic receptor-like binder for 1,25-dihydroxycholecalciferol in rat intestinal mucosa. J Biol Chem 1979;254:10378 – 10384.

Feldman RS, Krieger NS, Tashjian AH. Effects of parathyroid hormone and calcitonin on osteoclast formation in vitro. Endocrinology 1980;107:1137 – 1143.

Field RJ. Chemical organization in time and space. Am Sci 1985;73:142 – 150.

Field RJ, Noyes RM. Oscillations in chemical systems. IV. Limit cycle oscillations in a model of a real chemical reaction. J Chem Phys 1974;60:1877 – 1884.

Fischer JA, Oldham, SB, Sizemore GW, Arnaud CD. Calcitonin stimulation of parathyroid hormone secretion in vitro. Horm Metab Res 1971;3:223 – 224.

Fleisch H. Inhibitors of calcium phosphate precipitation and their role in biological mineralization. J Cryst Growth 1981;53:120 – 134.

Fornasier VL. Transmission electron microscopy studies of osteoid maturation. In: Jee WSS, Parfitt AM, eds. Bone Histomorphometry. Paris: Armour Montagu, 1981;103 – 108.

Forrest SM, Ng KW, Findlay DM, et al. Characterization of an osteoblast-like clonal cell which responds to both parathyroid and calcitonin. Calcif Tissue Int 1985;37:51 – 56.

Fox J, Offord K, Heath H. Episodic secretion of parathyroid hormone in the dog. Am J Physiol 1981;241:E171 – E177.

Fraser DR, Kodicek P. Unique biosynthesis by kidney of a biologically active vitamin D metabolite. Nature 1970;228:764 – 766.

Freake HC, McIntyre I. Specific binding of 1,25-dihydroxycholecalciferol in human medullary thyroid carcinoma. Biochem J 1982;206:181 – 184.

Freed WJ, Perlow MJ, Wyatt RJ. Calcitonin: inhibitory effect on eating in rats. Science 1979:206:850 – 853.

Fried RM, Tashjian AH. Unusual sensitivity of cytosolic free $Ca^{2+}$ to changes in extracellular $Ca^{2+}$ in rat C-cells. J Biol Chem 1986;261:7669 – 7674.

Friedman J, Raisz LG. Thyrocalcitonin: inhibitor of bone resorption in tissue culture. Science 1965;150: 1465 – 1467.

Frost HM. Mathematical Elements of Lamellar Bone Remodelling. Springfield. Illinois: Thomas CC, 1964.

Frost HM. Review article: Mechanical determinants of bone modeling. Met Bone Dis Rel Res 1982;4:217 – 229.

Frost HM. The mechanostat: a proposed pathogenic mechanism of osteoporoses and the bone mass effects of mechanical and nonmechanical agents. Bone Mineral 1987;2:73 – 85.

Frost HM. Vital biomechanics: proposed general concepts for skeletal adaptations to mechanical usage. Calcif Tissue Int 1988;42:145 – 156.

Funch-Jensen P, Nielsen HE, Christensen CK, et al. Food-stimulation serum calcitonin concentrations in patients with ulcer negative dyspepsia, duodenal ulcer and in controls. Digestion 1980;20:137 – 140.

Gaillard PJ. Parathyroid and bone tissue in culture. In: Greep RO, Talmage RV, eds. The Parathyroids. Springfield, Illinois: Thomas CC, 1961;20 – 45.

Garabedian M, Holick MF, DeLuca HF, Boyle IT. Control of 25-hydroxycholecalciferol metabolism by parathyroid glands. Proc Natl Acad Sci USA 1972;69:1673 – 1676.

Garabedian M, Tanaka Y, Holick MF, DeLuca HF. Response of intestinal transport and bone calcium mobilization to 1,25-dihydroxyvitamin D3 in thyroparathyroidectomized rats. Endocrinology 1974;94: 1022 – 1027.

Garcia-Ruiz JM, Santos A, Alfaro EJ. Oscillatory growth rates in single crystal growing under diffusional control. J Cryst Growth 1987;84:555 – 558.

Garside J, Davey RJ. Secondary contact nucleation: kinetics, growth and scale-up. Chem Eng Commun 1980;4:393 – 424.

Ghijsen WEJM, DeJong MD, van Os CH. ATP-dependent calcium transport and its correlation with $Ca^{2+}$-ATPase activity in basolateral plasma membranes of rat duodenum. Biochim Biophys Acta 1982;689:327 – 336.

Ghijsen WEJM, DeJong MD, van Os CH. Kinetic properties of $Na^{+}/Ca^{2+}$ exchange in basolateral plasma membranes of rat small intestines. Biochim Biophys Acta 1983;730:85 – 94.

Gittes RF, Toverud SU, Cooper CW. Effects of hypercalcemia and hypocalcemia on the thyrocalcitonin content of rat thyroid glands. Endocrinology 1968;82:83 – 90.

Glimcher MJ. Molecular biology of mineralized tissues with particular reference to bone. Rev Mod Phys 1959;31:359 – 393.

Glimcher MJ. On the form and function of bone: from molecules to organs. Wolff's law revisited, 1981. In: Veis A, ed. The Chemistry and Biology of Mineralized Connective Tissues. Amsterdam: Elsevier, 1981;617 – 673.

Glimcher MJ. Recent studies of the mineral phase in bone and its possible linkage to the organic matrix by protein-bound phosphate bonds. Phil Trans R Soc London Ser B 1984;304:479 – 508.

Glimcher MJ. The nature of the mineral component of bone and the mechanism of calcification. In: Griffin PP, ed. American Academy of Orthopaedic Surgeons Instructional Course Lectures XXXVI, Park Ridge, 1987;49 – 69.

Godfrey K. Compartmental Models and Their Application. New York: Academic Press, 1983.

Goldberg , Agus ZS, Goldfard A. Renal Handling of phosphate, calcium and magnesium. In: Brenner BM, Rector FC, eds. Kidney, Vol. I. Philadelphia: Saunders, 1976;334 – 390.

Goldberger AG, West BJ. Chaos in physiology: Health or disease? In: Degn H, Holden AV, Olsen LF, eds. Chaos in Biological Systems, Vol. 138. New York: Plenum Press, 1987;1 – 5.

Goldbeter A, Decroly O. Temporal self-organization in biochemical systems: periodic behavior vs. chaos. Am J Physiol 1983;245:R478 – R483.

Goldbeter A, Nicolis G. An allosteric enzyme model with positive feedback applied to glycolytic oscillations. In: Rosen R, Snell FM, eds. Progress in Theoretical Biology, Vol. 4. New York: Academic Press, 1976:65 – 161.

Goldman S. Cybernetic aspects of homeostasis. In: Comar CL, Bronner F, eds. Mineral Metabolism Vol 1, Part A. New York: Academic Press, 1960;61 – 100.

Goldstein DA, Romoff M, Bogin E, Massry SG. Relationship between the concentrations of calcium and phosphorus in blood and cerebrospinal fluid. J Clin Endocrinol Metab 1979;49:58 – 62.

Goodwin BC. Biological stability. In: Waddington CH, ed. Towards a Theoretical Biology, Vol. 3. Drafts. Edinburgh: University Press, 1970;1 – 17.

Gowen M, Wood DD, Ihrie EJ, Mcgurie MKB, Russell GG. An interleukin 1-like factor stimulates bone resorption in vitro. Nature 1983;306:378 – 380.

Groer PG, Marshall JH. Mechanism of calcium exchange at bone surface. Calcif Tissue Res 1973;12: 175 – 192.

Gruber HE, Ivey J, Baylink DJ, et al. Long term calcitonin therapy in postmenopausal osteoporosis. Metabolism 1984;33:295 – 301.

Gukenheimer J, Holmes P. Nonlinear Oscillations, Dynamical Systems, and Bifurcations of Vector Fields. New York: Springer-Verlag, 1983.

Gundberg CM, Markowitz ME, Mizruchi M, Rosen JF. Osteocalcin in human serum: a circadian rhythm. J Clin Endocrinol Metab 1985;60:736 – 739.

Gunness M, Hock JM. Increased trabecular bone mass in rats treated with human synthetic parathyroid hormone. Metab Bone Dis Rel Res 1984;5:177 – 181.

Habener JF, Potts JT. Relative effectiveness of magnesium and calcium on the secretion and biosynthesis of parathyroid hormone in vitro. Endocrinology 1976;98:197 – 202.

Habener JF, Kemper B, Potts JT. Calcium-dependent intracellular degradation of parathyroid hormone: a possible mechanism for regulation of hormones stores. Endocrinology 1974;97:431 – 441.

Habener JF, Rosenblatt M, Potts JT. Parathyroid hormone: Biochemical aspects of biosynthesis, secretion, action, and metabolism. Physiol Rev 1984;64:985 – 1053.

Hadded JG. Traffic, binding, and cellular access of vitamin D sterols. In:Peck WA, ed. Bone and Mineral Research, Vol. 5. Amsterdam: Elsevier, 1987;281 – 308.

Halberg F. Chronobiology. Ann Rev Physiol 1969;31:675 – 725.

Haller-Brem S, Muff R, Petermann JB, Born W, Roos BA, Fischer JA. Role of cytosolic free calcium concentration in the secretion of calcitonin gene-related peptide and calcitonin from medullary thyroid carcinoma cells. Endocrinology 1987;121:1272 – 1277.

Halloran BP, Portale AA, Castro M, Morris RC, Goldsmith RS. Serum concentration of 1,25-dihydroxyvitamin D in the human: diurnal variation. J Clin Endocrinol Metab 1985;60:1104 – 1110.

Halloran BP, Bikle DD, Levens MJ, Castro ME, Globus RK, Holton E. Chronic 1,25-dihydroxyvitamin D3 administration in the rat reduces the serum concentration of 25-hydroxyvitamin D by increasing metabolic clearance rate. J Clin Invest 1986;78:622 – 628.

Hanley DA, Takatsuki K, Sultan, JM, Schneider AB, Sherwood LM. Direct release of parathyroid hormone fragments from functioning bovine parathyroid glands in vitro. J Clin Invest 1978;62:1247 – 1254.

Hansson LI, Stenstrom A, Thorngen KG. Diurnal variation of longitudinal bone growth in the rabbit. Acta Orthop Scand 1974;45:499 – 507.

Harary HH, Brown JE. Spatially nonuniform changes in intracellular calcium ion concentrations. Science 1984;224:292 – 294.

Harms H, Kapteina U, Kulpmann T, Hesch RD. The pulse amplitude and frequency modulation of PTH secretion in man. International Symposium on Osteoporosis (Abstract), Aalborg, Sweden, 1987;232.

Harrison HE, Harrison HC. Vitamin D and permeability of intestinal mucosa to calcium. Am J Physiol 1965;208:370 – 374.

Harrison LG. What is the status of reaction-diffusion theory thirty-four years after Turing? J Theor Biol 1987;125:369 – 384.

Hatschek E. A series of abnormal liesegang stratifications. Biochem J 1920;14:418 – 421.

Hauschka PV, Lian JB, Gallop PM. Direct identification of the calcium-binding aminoacid and $\gamma$-carboxyglutamate in mineralized tissue. Proc Natl Acad Sci USA 1975;72:3926 – 3929.

Hausmann E, Riggs DS. The effectiveness of negative feedback in regulating plasma calcium in the dog. J Theor Biol 1966;12:350 – 363.

Heersche JNM. Mechanism of osteoclastic bone resorption: a new hypothesis. Calcif Tissue Res 1978;26:81 – 84.

Heersche JNM, Marcus R, Aurbach GD. Calcitonin and the formation of 3′5′-AMP in bone and kidney. Endocrinology 1974;94:241 – 247.

Hennesy JF, Gray TK, Cooper CW, Ontjes DA. Stimulation of thyrocalcitonin secretion by pentagastrin and calcium in two medullary carcinoma. J Clin Endocrinol Metab 1973;36:200 – 203.

Henry HL, Midgett RJ, Norman AW. Regulation of 25-hydroxyvitamin D3-1-hydroxylase in vivo. J Biol Chem 1974;249:7584 – 7592.

Hermann RH. The principles of metabolic control. In: Hermann RH, Cohn RM, McNamara PD, eds. Principles of Metabolic Control in Mammalian Systems. New York and London: Plenum Press, 1980;1 – 61.

Hesch RD, Brabant G, Rittinghaus EF, Atkinson MJ, Harms H. Pulsatile secretion of parathyroid hormone and its action on a type I and type II PTH receptor: a hypothesis for understanding osteoporosis. Calcif Tissue Int 1988;42:341 – 344.

Hess B, Boiteux A. Oscillatory phenomena in biochemistry. Ann Rev Biochem 1971;40:237 – 258.

Hillyard CJ, Cooke TJC, Coombes RC, Evans IMA, MacIntyre I. Normal plasma calcitonin circadian variation and response to stimuli. Clin Endocrinol 1977;6:291 – 298.

Hillyard CJ, Abeyasekera G, Craig RK, Myers C, Stevenson JC, McIntyre I. Katacalcin: a new plasma calcium lowering hormone. Lancet 1983;i:646 – 648.

Hirsch P, Hagaman JR. Feeding regimen, dietary calcium, and the diurnal rhythms of serum calcium and calcitonin in the rat. Endocrinology 1982;110:961 – 968.

Hirsch P, Gauthier GF, Munson P. Thyroid hypocalcemic principle and recurrent laryngeal nerve injury as factors affecting the response to parathyroidectomy in rats. Endocrinology 1963;73:244 – 252.

Holick MF, MacLaughlin JA, Doppelt SA. Factors that influence the cutaneous photosynthesis of previtamin D3. Science 1981;211:590 – 592.

Hollings CS. Resilience and stability of ecosystems. In: Jantsch E, Waddington CH, eds. Evolution and Consciousness. London: Addison-Wesley Publ Co, 1976;73 – 92.

Holtrop ME, Raisz LG, Simmons HA. The effect of parathyroid hormone, colchicine and calcitonin on the ultrastructure and the activity of osteoclasts in organ culture. J Cell Biol 1974;60:346 – 355.

Holtrop ME, Cox KA, Clark MR, Hollick MF, Anast CS. 1,25-dihydroxycholecalciferol stimulates osteoclasts in rat bones in the absence of parathyroid hormone. Endocrinology 1981;108:2293 – 2301.

Horiuchi N, Suda T, Takahashi H, Shimazawa E, Ogata E. In vivo evidence for the intermediary role of 3′,5′-cyclic AMP in parathyroid hormone-induced stimulation of 1α-25-dihydroxyvitamin D3 synthesis in rats. Endocrinology 1977;101:969 – 974.

Horton MA, Rimmer EF, Moore A, Chambers TJ. On the origin of the osteoclasts: The cell surface phenotype of rodent osteoclasts. Calcif Tissue Int 1985;37:46 – 50.

Howard BA, Baylink DJ. Matrix formation and osteoid maturation in vitamin D-deficient rats made normocalcaemic by dietary means. Mineral Electr Metab 1980;3:44 – 50.

Hruska KA, Kopelman AR, Rutherford WE, Klahr S, Slatopolsky E. Metabolism of immunoreactive parathyroid hormone in the dog: the role of the kidney and the effects of chronic renal disease. J Clin Invest 1975;56:39 – 48.

Hughes MR, Maussler MR. 1,25-dihydroxycholecalciferol receptors in parathyroid glands. J Biol Chem 1978;253:1065 – 1069.

Hughes MR, Brumbaugh PF, Haussler MR, Wergedal JE, Baylink DJ. Regulation of serum 1α-25-dihydroxyvitamin D by calcium and phosphate in the rat. Science 1975;190:578 – 580.

Hunt NH, Perris AD. Calcium and the control of circadian mitotic activity in rat bone marrow and thymus. J Endocrinol 1974;62:451 – 462.

Hurwitz S, Fishman S, Bar A, Pines M, Riesenfeld G, Talpaz H. Simulation of calcium homeostasis: modeling and parameter estimation. Am J Physiol 1983;245:R664 – R672.

Hurwitz S, Fishman S, Bar A, Talpaz H. Role of the 1,25-dihydroxycholecalciferol-regulated component of calcium absorption in calcium homeostasis. In: Bronner F, Peterlik M, eds. Epithelial Calcium and Phosphate Transport: Molecular and Cellular Aspects. New York: Liss AH, Inc, 1984a;357 – 362.

Hurwitz S, Fishman S, Bar A, Talpaz H. Calcium metabolism in birds: computer simulation of response to 1,25-dihydroxycholecalciferol. Am J Physiol 1984b;246:R684 – R687.

Hurwitz S, Fishman S, Talpaz H. Model of plasma calcium regulation: system oscillations induced by growth. Am J Physiol 1987;252:R1173 – R1181.

Huwyler R, Born W, Ohnhaus EE, Fischer JA. Plasma kinetics and urinary excretion of exogenous human and salmon calcitonin. Am J Physiol 1979;236:E15 – E19.

Ibbotson KJ, Roodman GD, McManus LM, Mundy GR. Identification and characterization of osteoclast-like cells and their progenitors in cultures of feline marrow mononuclear cells. J Cell Biol 1984;99:471 – 480.

Ikeda E, Kasaka M, Hakeda Y, Yokota K, Kumegawa M, Yamamoto S. Effect of interleukin I beta on osteoblastic clone MC3T3-EI cells. Calcif Tissue Int 1988;43:162 – 166.

Ishida M, Seino Y, Yamaoka K, et al. The circadian rhythms of blood-ionized calcium in humans. Scand J Clin Lab Invest 1983;43(Suppl 165):83 – 88.

Jacobs JW. Calcitonin gene expression. In: Peck WA, ed. Bone and Mineral Research, Vol. 3. Amsterdam: Elsevier, 1985;151 – 180.

Jacobs JW, Potts JT, Bells H, Habener JF. Calcitonin precursor identified by cell-free translation of mRNA. J Biol Chem 1979;254:10600 – 10603.

Jacobs JW, Simpson E, Penschow J,Hudson P, Coghlan J, Niall H. Characterization and localization of calcitonin messenger ribonuclei acid in rat thyroid. Endocrinology 1983;113:1616 – 1622.

Jacquez JA. Compartmental Analysis in Biology and Medicine. Amsterdam: Elsevier, 1972.

Jaeger P, Jones W, Clemens TL, Hayslett J. Evidence that calcitonin stimulates 1,25-dihydroxyvitamin D production production and intestinal of calcium in vivo. J Clin Invest 1986;78:456 – 461.

Jaros GG, Guyton AC, Coleman TG. The role of bone in short-term calcium homeostasis: an analog-digital computer simulation. Ann Biomed Eng 1980;8:103 – 141.

Jaros GG, Belonge PC, van Hoorn-Hickman R, Newman E. Transient response of the calcium homeostatic system: effect of calcitonin. Am J Physiol 1984;246:R693 – R697.

Jeansonne BG, Feagin FA, McMinn RW, Shoemaker RL, Rehm WS. Cell-to-cell communication of osteoblasts. J Dent Res 1979;58:1415 – 1423.

Jonas V, Lin CR, Kawashima E et al. Alternative RNA processing events in human calcitonin/calcitonin gene-related peptide. Proc Natl Acad Sci USA 1985;82:1994 – 1998.

Jones RW. Principles of Biological Regulation: An Introduction to Feedback Systems. New York: Academic Press, 1973.

Jones SJ, Boyde A. Morphological changes of osteoblasts in vitro. Cell Tissue Res 1976;166:101 – 107.

Jones SJ, Boyde A, Ali NN, Maconnachie E. A review of bone cell and substratum interactions. Scanning 1985;7:5 – 24.

Jubiz W, Canterbury JM, Reiss E, Tyler FH. Circadian rhythm in serum parathyroid hormone concentration in human subjects: Correlation with serum calcium, phosphate, albumin, and growth hormone levels. J Clin Invest 1972;51:2040 – 2046.

Jullienne A, Calmettes C, Raulais D, Milhaud G, Moukthar, MS. Immunochemical characterization of calcitonin in human disorders. In: Copp DH, Talmage RV, eds. Endocrinology of Calcium Metabolism. Amsterdam: Excerpta Medica, 1978;55 – 63.

Jung A. Endocrine control of calcium metabolism. In: Cramp DG, ed. Quantitative Approaches to Metabolism. New York: John Wiley and Sons Ltd, 1982;219 – 246.

Jung A, Bartholdi P,Mermillod B, Reeve J, Neer R. Critical analysis of methods for analysing human calcium kinetics. J Theor Biol 1978;73:131 – 157.

Jung A, Mayer GP, Hurst JG, Neer R, Potts JT. Model for parathyroid hormone secretion and metabolism in calves. Am J Physiol 1982;242:R141 – R150.

Kahn AJ, Simmons DJ. Chondrocyte-to-osteocyte transformation in grafts of perichondrium-free epiphyseal cartilage. Clin Orthop Rel Res 1977;129:299 – 304.

Kahn AJ, Stewart CC, Teitelbaum SL. Contact-mediated bone resorption by human monocytes in vitro.

Science 1978;199:988 – 990.

Kai S, Müller SC, Ross J. Measurements of temporal and spatial sequences of events in periodic precipitation processes. J Chem Phys 1982;76:1392 – 1406.

Kakuta S, Golub EE, Shapiro IM. Morphochemical analysis of phosphorus pools in calcifying cartilage. Calcif Tissue Int 1985;37:293 – 299.

Kalu DN, Hardin RR, Murata I, Huber MB, Roos BA. Age-dependent modulation of parathyroid hormone action. Age 1982;5:25 – 29.

Kanabrocki EL, Brewer RL, Scheving LE, Pauly JE. Circadian fluctuations in urinary excretion of calcium and magnesium and in serum calcium in presumably healthy young soldiers: Effect of meal timing on the serum calcium rhythm. In: XII International Conference of International Society for Chronobiology. Milan: Il Ponte, 1977;29 – 38.

Katz EP. The kinetics of mineralization in vitro. I. The nucleation properties of 640 Ä collagen at 25°. Biochim Biophys Acta 1969;194:121 – 129.

Kaur P, Potten CS. Circadian variation in migration velocity in small intestinal epithelium. Cell Tissue Kinetics 1986a;19:591 – 599.

Kaur P, Potten CS. Effects of puromycin, cycloheximide and noradrenaline on cell migration within the crypts and on the villi of the small intestine. Cell Tissue Kinetics 1986b;19:611 – 625.

Kawashima H, Torikai S, Korukawa K. Calcitonin selectively stimulates 25-hydroxyvitamin D2-1$\alpha$-hydroxylase in proximal straight tubule of rat kidney. Nature 1981;291:327 – 329.

Kemper B, Habener JF, Mulligan RC, Potts JT, Rich A. Pre-proparathyroid hormone: a direct translation product of parathyroid messenger RNA. Proc Natl Acad Sci USA 1974;71:3731 – 3735.

Kenny AD. Role of carbonic anhydrase in bone: partial inhibition of disuse atrophy of bone by parenteral acetazolamide. Calcif Tissue Int 1985;37:126 – 133.

Kimmel DB, Jee WSS. Bone cell kinetics during longitudinal bone growth in the rat. Calcif Tissue Int 1980;32:123 – 133.

Klein DC, Talmage RV. Thyrocalcitonin suppression of hydroxyproline release from bone. Proc Soc Exp Biol Med 1968;127:95 – 99.

Knutson JC, DeLuca HF. 25-hydroxy-vitamin D3-24-hydroxylase: subcellular localisation and properties. Biochemistry 1974;13:1543 – 1548.

Krane SM, Harris ED, Singer FR, Potts JT. Acute effects of calcitonin on bone formation in man. Metabolism 1973;22:51 – 58.

Kream BE, Reynolds RD, Knutson JC, Eisman JA, DeLuca HF. Specific cytosol-binding protein for 1,25-dihydroxyvitamin D3 in rat intestine. J Biol Chem 1977;252:4501 – 4505.

Kream BE, Rowe DV, Gworek SC, Raisz LG. Parathyroid hormone alters collagen synthesis and procollagen mRNA levels in fetal rat calvaria. Proc Natl Acad Sci USA 1980;77:5654 – 5658.

Kripke DF, Lavie P, Parker D, Huey L, Deftos LJ. Plasma parathyroid hormone and calcium are related to sleep stage cycles. J Clin Endocrinol Metab 1978;47:1021 – 1027.

Kruckowski M, Kahn AJ. Normal osteoclast number and function in rat pups lacking parathyroid hormone. Experientia 1980;26:871 – 872.

Kumar R, Nagubandi S, Mattox VR, Londowski JM. Enterohepatic physiology of 1,25-dihydroxyvitamin D3. J Clin Invest 1980;65:277 – 284.

Labat ML, Milhaud G. Ostepetrosis and the immune deficiency syndrome. In: Peck WA, ed. Bone and Mineral Research, Vol. 4. Amsterdam: Elsevier, 1986;131 – 212.

Larson MA, Garside J. Solute clustering and interfacial tension. J Cryst Growth 1986;76:88 – 92.

Lasmoles F, Desplan C, Segond N et al. Cell-free translation of chicken calcitonin messenger RNA. FEBS Lett 1983;1:100 – 104.

Lausson S, Staub JF, Milhaud G. Relations between circadian variations of calcium, phosphate CT and PTH in rat. 7th International Congress of Endocrinology. Amsterdam: Excerpta Medica, 1984;832.

Lausson S, Staub JF, Milhaud G, Perault-Staub AM. Circadian variations in plasma calcium and calcitonin: effect of calcium deficiency and fasting. J Endocrinol 1985;107:389 – 395.

Le Grimellec C, Poujeol P, De Rouffignac C. H3 insulin and electrolyte concentrations in Bowman's capsule in rat kidney. Pflugers Arch 1975;354:117 – 131.

Lee DBN, Brautbar N, Kleeman CR. Disorders of phosphorus metabolism. In: Bronner F, Coburn JW, eds. Disorders of Mineral Metabolism, Vol 3. New York: Academic Press, 1981;284 – 388.

Legros R, Bonel G, Balmain N,Juster M. Etude systématique des variations de composition du constituant minéral de différents os de divers animaux suivant sa localisation. CR Acad Sci (Paris) Série D 1977;285:1519 – 1522.

Lemoullec JM, Jullienne A, Chenais J et al. The complete sequence of human preprocalcitonin. FEBS Lett 1984;167:93 – 97.

Levine BA, Williams RJP. Calcium binding to proteins and other large biological anion centers. In: Cheung WY, ed. Calcium and Cell Function, Vol. II. New York: Academic Press, 1982;1 – 38.

Lian JB, Coults M, Canalis E. Regulation of osteocalcin synthesis in cultured fetal rat calvariae. Calcif Tissue Int 1984;36:518 – 521.

Linde A, Jontell M, Lundgren T, Nilson B, Suanberg V. Non collagenous protein of rat compact bone. J Biol Chem 1983;258:1698 – 1705.

Lowik CWGM, Van Leuwen JPTM, Van der Meer JM, Van Zeeland JK, Scheven BAA, Herrmann-Erke MPM. A two receptor model for the interaction of parathyroid hormone on osteoblasts: a role for intracellular-free calcium and cAMP. Cell Calcium 1985;6:311 – 326.

Lubens RA, Goggins JF, Raisz LG. Stimulation of parathyroid hormone on bone hyaluronate synthesis in organ culture. Endocrinology 1974;94:737 – 745.

MacGregor RR, Jilka RL, Hamilton JW. Formation and secretion of fragments of parathormone. J Biol Chem 1986;261:1929 – 1934.

Majeska R, Rodan GA. Alkaline phosphatase inhibition by parathyroid hormone and isoproterenol in a clonal rat osteosarcoma cell line: possible mediation by cyclic AMP. Calcif Tissue Int 1982;34:59 – 66.

Malm OJ. Calcium requirement and adaptation in adult man. Scand J Clin Lab Invest 1958;10:1 – 290.

Malone JD, Teitelbaum SL, Griffin GL, Senior RM, Kahn AJ. Recruitment of osteoclast precursors by purified bone matrix constituents. J Cell Biol 1982;29:227 – 230.

Manning RM, Adami S, Papapoulos SE, et al. A carboxy-terminal assay for human parathyroid hormone. Clin Endocrinol 1981;15:439 – 449.

Manologas SC, Burton DW, Deftos LJ. 1,25-dihydroxyvitamin D3 stimulates the alkaline phosphatase activity of osteoblast-like cells. J Biol Chem 1981;256:7115 – 7117.

Markowitz M, Rotkin L, Rosen JF. Circadian rhythms of blood minerals in humans. Science 1981;213:672 – 674.

Markowitz M, Rosen JF, Laxminarayan S, Smith C, DeLuca HF. Periodic oscillations in serum 1,25-dihydroxyvitamin D in humans In: Norman AW, Schaefer K, Herrath DV, Gringoleit HG, eds. Vitamin D: Chemical Biochemical and Clinical Endocrinology of Calcium Metabolism. New York: de Gruyter, 1982;707.

Markowitz ME, Rosen JF, Laximinarayan S, Mizruchi M. Circadian rhythm of blood minerals during adolescence. Pediatr Res 1984;18:456 – 462.

Markowitz ME, Rosen JF, Mizruchi M. Effects of 1,25-dihydroxyvitamin D3 administration on circadian mineral rhythms in humans. Calcif Tissue Int 1985;37:351 – 356.

Markowitz ME, Gundberg CM, Rosen JF. The circadian rhythm of serum osteocalcin concentrations: effects of the 1,25-dihydroxyvitamin D administration. Calcif Tissue Int 1987;40:179 – 183.

Marshall JH. Theory of alkaline earth metabolism: The power function makes possible a simple but comprehensive model of skeletal systems. J Theor Biol 1964;6:386 – 392.

Marx SJ, Woodard C, Aurbach GD. Renal receptors for calcitonin. J Biol Chem 1973;16:4797 – 4802.

Massry SG. Renal Handling of calcium. In: Bronner F, Coburn JW, eds. Disorder of Mineral Metabolism, Vol. II. New York: Academic Press, 1982;189 – 235.

Matsumoto T, Fontaine O, Max E, Rasmussen H. Effect of 1,25-dihydroxyvitamin D3 on phospholipid metabolism in chick duodenal mucosal cell. J Biol Chem 1981;256:3354 – 3360.

Matthews JL, Martin JH. Intracellular transport of calcium andits relationship to homeostasis and mineralization. Am J Med 1971;50:589 – 597.

Matthews JL, Talmage RV, Martin JH, Davis WL. Osteoblasts, bone lining cell and the bone fluid compartment. In: Meunier PJ, ed. 2nd International Workshop on Bone Morphology. Paris: Armour Montagu, 1976;239 – 247.

Matthews JL, Talmage RV, Doppelt R. Responses of the osteocyte-lining cell complex, the bone cell unit, to calcitonin. Metab Bone Rel Res 1980;2:113 – 122.

Mayer GP, Hurst JG. Sigmoidal relationship between parathyroid hormone secretion rate and plasma calcium concentration in calves. Endocrinology 1978;102:1036 – 1042.

McCulloch CAG, Tenenbaum HC. Dexamethasone induces proliferation and terminal differentiation of osteogenic cells in tissue culture. Anat Rec 1986;215:397 – 402.

McEachron DL, Kripke DF, Hawkins R, Haus E, Pavlinac D, Deftos L. Lithium delays biochemical circadian rhythms in rats. Neuropsychobiol 1982;8:12 – 29.

McGrath KJ, Heideger WJ, Beach KW. Calcium homeostasis. III. The bone membrane potential and mineral dissolution. Calcif Tissue Int 1986;39:279 – 283.

McIntosh JEA, McIntosh RP. Mathematical Modelling and Computers in Endocrinology. New York: Springer-Verlag, 1980.

McLean FC, Hasting AB. Clinical estimation and significance of calcium ion in the blood. Am J Med Sci 1935;189:601 – 613.

McLean FC, Urist MR. Bone. An Introduction to the Physiology of Skeletal Tissue. Chicago: University of Chicago Press, 1955.

Meinhardt H. Models of Biological Pattern Formation. London: Academic Press Inc, 1982.

Meinhardt H, Klinger M. A model for pattern formation on the shells of molluscs. J Theor Biol 1987;126:63 – 89.

Merk J, Klaus G, Hugel U, Waldherr R, Ritz E. No 1,25-dihydroxyvitamin D3 receptors on osteoclasts of calcium-deficient chicken despite demonstrable receptors on circulating monocytes. J Clin Invest 1986;77:312 – 314.

Meyer T, Stryer L. Molecular model for receptor-stimulated calcium spiking. Proc Natl Acad Sci USA 1988;85:5051 – 5055.

Milhaud G, Moukhtar MS. Antagonistic and synergistic actions of thyrocalcitonin and parathyroid hormone on the levels of calcium and phosphate in the rat. Nature 1966;211:1186 – 1187.

Milhaud G, Hankiss J. Inactivation de la thyrocalcitonine par divers organes. CR Acad Sci (Paris) Série D 1969;268:124 – 127.

Milhaud G, Szlamska I. Specific calcitonin-binding proteins in man. Experientia 1971;27:1335 – 1336.

Milhaud G, Cherian AG, Moukhtar MS. Calcium metabolism in the rat studied with calcium-45: Effect of age. Proc Soc Exp Biol Med 1963;114:382 – 384.

Milhaud G, Moukhtar MS, Bourichon J, Perault AM. Existence et activité de la thyrocalcitonine chez l'homme. CR Acad Sci (Paris) 1965a;261:4513 – 4516.

Milhaud G, Perault AM, Moukhtar M. Etude du mécanisme de l'action hypocalcemiante de la thyrocalcitonine. CR Acad Sci (Paris) 1965b;261:813 – 816.

Milhaud G, Moukhtar MS, Cherian G, Perault AM. Effet de l'administration de thyrocalcitonine sur les principaux paramètres du métabolisme calcique du calcium du rat normal et du rat thyroparathyroidectomisé. CR Acad Sci (Paris) 1966;262:511 – 514.

Milhaud G, Perault-Staub AM, Moukhtar MS. Thyrocalcitonine: effet de l'âge sur l'hypocalcémie et l'hypophosphorémie CR Acad Sci (Paris) 1967;264:110 – 113.

Milhaud G, Le D, Perault-Staub AM. Mechanism of the rapid hypercalcemic effect of parathormone: inhibition of bone accretion. Eur J Clin Biol Res 1971;5:451 – 454.

Milhaud G, Perault-Staub AM, Staub JF. Diurnal variation of plasma calcium and calcitonin function in the rat. J Physiol (Lond) 1972;222:559 – 567.

Milhaud G, Talbot JN, Coutris G. Calcitonin treatment of postmenopausal osteoporosis. Evaluation of efficacy by principal component analysis. Biomedecine 1975;23:223 – 232.

Miller B, Norman AW. Studies on the metabolism of calciferol XIV: evidence of a circadian rhythm in the activity of the 25-hydroxyvitamin D3-1-hydroxylase. Biochem Biophys Res Commun 1979;88:730 – 734.

Miller B, Norman AW. Evidence for circadian rhythms in the serum levels of the vitamin D dependent calcium binding protein and in the activity of the 25-hydroxyvitamin D3-1-$\alpha$-hydroxylase in the chick. FEBS Lett 1982;141:242 – 244.

Miller JC, Jee WSS. The bone lining cell: A distinct phenotype? Calcif Tissue Int 1987;41:1 – 5.

Misra DN. Isoionic isotope exchange with hydroxylapatite and the dilution effect. J Res Natl Bur Stand 1979;84:395 – 406.

Moore-Ede MC. Physiology of the circadian timing system: predictive versus reactive homeostasis. Am J Physiol 1986;250:R735 – R752.

Moore-Ede MC, Faulkner MH, Trede BE. An intrinsic rhythm of urinary calcium excretion and the specific effect of bedrest on the excretion pattern. Clin Sci 1972;42:433 – 445.

Moore-Ede MC, Sulzman FM, Fuller Ca. The Clocks That Time Us. Harvard: University Press, 1982.

Morel F. Regulation of kidney functions by hormones: A new approach. Rec Prog Horm Res 1983;39:271 – 304.

Morel G, Boivin G, David L, Dubois PM, Meunier PJ. Immunochemical ecidence for endogenous calcitonin and parathyroid hormone in osteoblasts from calvaria of neonatal mice. Cell Tissue Res 1985;240:89 – 93.

Morrissey JJ, Cohn DV. Secretion and degradation of parathormone as a function of intracellular maturation of hormone pools: modulation by calcium and dibutyryl cyclic AMP. J Cell Biol 1979;83:521 – 528.

Mullin JW, Leci CL. Desupersaturation of seeded citric acid solutions in a stirred vessel. AIChE Symp Series 1972;121:8 – 20.

Mundy GR, Roodman GD. Osteoclast ontogeny and function. In: Peck WA, ed. Bone and Mineral Research, Vol. 5. Amsterdam: Elsevier, 1987;209 – 281.

Munson PL. Physiology and pharmacology of thyrocalcitonin: In: Greep RO, Astwood EB, eds. Endocrinology, Vol VII. Washington: American Physiological Society, 1976;443 – 464.

Nancollas GH. The nucleation and growth of phosphate minerals. In: Nriagu JO, Moore PB, eds. Phosphate Minerals. Berlin: Springer-Verlag, 1984;137 – 154.

Naveh-Many T, Silver J. Regulation of calcitonin gene transcription by Vitamin D metabolites in vivo in the rat. J Clin Invest 1988;81:270 – 273.

Neal JV, Potten CS. Circadian rhythms in the epithelial cells and the pericryptal fibroblast sheath in three different sites in the murine intestinal tract. Cell Tissue Kinetics 1981;14:581 – 587.

Neer R, Berman M, Fisher L, Rosenberg LE. Multicompartmental analysis of calcium kinetics in normal adult males. J Clin Invest 1967;46:1364 – 1379.

Nellans HN, Kimberg DV. Anamalous secretion of calcium in rat ileum: role of the paracellular pathway. Am J Physiol 1979;236:E473 – E481.

Neuman NW. Blood: bone equilibrium. Calcif Tissue Int 1982;34:117 – 120.

Neuman MW, Imai K, Kawase T, Saito S. The calcium-buffering phase of bone mineral: some clues to its form and formation. J Bone Mineral Res 1987;2:171 – 181.

Neuman WF. The milieu interieur of bone: Claude Bernard revisited. Fed Proc 1969;28:1846 – 1850.

Neuman WF. The extracellular control of cellular metabolism in bone. In: Slavkin HC, Greulich RC, eds. Extracellular Matrix Influences on Gene Expressioin. New York: Academic Press, 1975a;693 – 699.

Neuman WF. The presence of a soluble 'regulator' phase (secondary calcium phosphate) in bone. In: Talmage RV, Owen M, Parsons JA, eds. Calcium-Regulating Hormones. Amsterdam: Excerpta Medica, 1975b;297 – 302.

Neuman WF, Neuman MW. The Chemical Dynamics of Bone and Mineral. Chicago: University of Chicago Press, 1958.

Neuman WF, Ramp WK. The concept of bone membrane: some implications. In: Nichols G, Wasserman RH, eds. Cellular Mechanisms for Calcium Transfer and Homeostasis. New York:Academic Press,

1971;197 – 209.
Neuman WF, Neuman MW, Lane K, Miller LL, Sammon PJ. The metabolism of labeled parathyroid hormone. V. Collected biological studies. Calcif Tissue Res 1975;18:271 – 286.
Neuman WF, Brommage R, Meyers CR. The measurement of $Ca^{2+}$ effluxes from bone. Calcif Tissue Res 1977;24:113 – 117.
Neuman WF, Neuman MW, Diamond AG, Menanteau J, Gibbons WS. Blood: bone disequilibrium. VI. Studies of the solubility characteristics of brushite-apatite mixtures and their stabilization by noncollagenous proteins of bone. Calcif Tissue Int 1982;34:149 – 157.
Nicholson GC, Moseley JM, Sexton PM, Mendelsohn FAO, Martin TJ. Abundant calcitonin receptors in isolated rat osteoclasts. J Clin Invest 1986;78:355 – 360.
Nicolaysen R, Eeg-Larsen N, Malm OJ. Physiology of calcium metabolism. Physiol Rev 1953;33:424 – 444.
Nicolis G, Prigogine I. Self-Organization in Non-Equilibrium Systems. New York: Wiley, 1977.
Nijweide PJ, Burger EH, Feyen JHM. Cells of bone: proliferation, differentiation and hormonal regulation. Physiol Rev 1986;66:855 – 886.
Nogami H, Urist RM. Stubstrate prepared from bone matrix for chondrogenesis in tissue culture. J Cell Biol 1974;62:510 – 519.
Nordin BEC, Peacock M. Role of the kidney in regulation of plasma calcium. Lancet 1969;ii:1280 – 1283.
Nordin BEC, Peacock M, Wilkinson R. The relative importance of gut, bone, and kidney in the regulation of serum calcium. In: Talmage RV, Munson PL, eds. Calcium, Parathyroid Hormone and the Calcitonins. Amsterdam: Excerpta Medica, 1972;263 – 272.
Norimatsu H, Yamamoto T, Ozawa H, Talmage RV. Changes in calcium phosphate on bone surfaces and in lining cells after the administration of parathyroid hormone and calcitonin. Clin Orthop 1982;164:271 – 278.
Norman AW, Miller BE, Putkey JA. Evaluation of the diurnal production of 1,25-dihydroxyvitamin D and vitamin D's effects on intestinal membrane organization. Progr Biochem Pharmacol 1980;17:160 – 168.
Norman AW, Roth J, Orci L. The vitamin D endocrine system: steroid metabolism, hormone receptors, and biological response (calcium binding proteins). Endocrinol Rev 1982;3:331 – 366.
Okada M, Mimura T. Zur physiologie und pharmakologie der hartegewebe. Proc Jpn Pharmacol Soc IV, Pharmakology 1940;13:96 – 99.
Onishi T, Deftos LJ. Plasma calcitonin in rats with renal failure. Calcif Tissue Int 1988;42:181 – 184.
Overgaard K, Nilas L, Sidenius Johansen J, Christiansen C. Lack of seasonal variation in bone mass and biochemical estimates of bone turnover. Bone 1988;9:285 – 288.
Owyang C, Heath H, Sizemore GV, Go VLW. Comparison of the effects of pentagastrin and meal-stimulated gastrin on plasma calcitonin in man. Digest Dis 1978;23:1084 – 1088.
Palmer JD. An Introduction to Biological Rhythms. New York: Academic Press, 1976.
Pansu D, Bellaton C, Bronner F. The effect of calcium intake on the saurable and the nonsaturable components of duodenal calcium transport. Am J Physiol 1981;240:G32 – G37.
Papapoulos SE, Manning RM, Hendy GN, Lewin IG, O'Riordan JLH. Studies of circulating parathyroid hormone in man using an homologous aminoterminal specific immunoradiometric assay. Clin Endocrinol 1980;13:57 – 67.
Parfitt AM. A theoretical model of relationship between parathyroid cell mass and plasma calcium concentration in normal and uremic subjects: An analysis of the concept of autonomy and speculations on the mechanism of parathyroid hyperplasia. Arch Intern Med 1969;124:269 – 273.
Parfitt AM. The actions of parathyroid hormone on bone: relation to bone remodeling and turnover, calcium homeostasis, and metabolic diseases. I. Mechanisms of calcium transfer between blood and bone and their cellular basis; morphological and kinetic approaches to bone turnover. Metabolism 1976;25:809 – 844.
Parfitt AM. Equilibrium and disequilibrium hypercalcemia: New light on an old concept. Metab Bone Dis Rel Res 1979;1:279 – 293.

Parfitt AM. The cellular basis of bone remodeling: The quantum concept reexamined in light of recent advances in the cell biology of bone. Calcif Tissue Int 1984;36:S37 – S45.

Parfitt AM. Bone and plasma calcium homeostasis. Bone 1987;8(Suppl 1):S1 – S8.

Parthemore JG, Deftos J. Calcitonin secretion in normal human subjects. J Clin Endocrinol Metab 1978;47:184 – 188.

Pattee HH. The problem of biological hierarchy. In: Waddington CH, ed. Towards a Theoretical Biology, Vol. 3. Drafts. Edinburgh: University Press, 1970;117 – 136.

Pavlidis T. Populations of interacting oscillators and circadian rhythms. J Theor Biol 1969;22:418 – 436.

Pavlidis T. Biological oscillators: Their Mathematical Analysis. New York and London: Academic Press, 1973.

Perault-Staub AM, Milhaud G. Homéostasie et variation du métabolisme calcique du rat au cours de la digestion. CR Acad Sci (Paris) 1970;270:2682 – 2685.

Perault-Staub AM, Staub JF, Milhaud G. Thyrocalcitonin and the physiological unstability of plasma calcium and phosphate in the rat. In: Czitober H, Eschberger J, eds. Calcified Tissue 1972. Vienna: Facta-Publication, 1973;393 – 397.

Perault-Staub AM, Staub JF, Milhaud G. A new concept of plasma calcium homeostasis. Endocrinology 1974;95:480 – 484.

Perault-Staub AM, Lefevre C, Staub JF, Brezillon P, Milhaud G. A time-varying model for calcium metabolism including diurnal variations. In: Kuhlencordt F, Kruse HP, eds. Calcium Metabolism, Bone and Metabolic Diseases. Berlin: Springer-Verlag, 1975a;25 – 30.

Perault-Staub AM, Staub JF, Milhaud G. Constancy and rhythmicity, a dual concept for homeostasis exemplified by 24 hour plasma calcium regulation in the rat. In: Talmage RV, Owen M, Parsons JA, eds. Calcium-Regulating Hormones. Amsterdam: Excerpta Medica, 1975b;229 – 238.

Perault-Staub AM, Brezillon P, Tracqui P, Staub JF. A self-organized temporal model for rat calcium metabolism: mineral nonlinear reaction, circadian dynamics and its control. In: The Institute of Measurement and Control. ed. Oscillations in Physiological Systems: Dynamics and Control. London, 1984;55 – 60.

Perry HM, Chappel JC, Bellorin-Font E, Tamao J, Martin KJ, Teitelbaum SL. Parathyroid hormone receptors in circulating human mononuclear leukocytes. J Biol Chem 1984a;259:5531 – 5535.

Perry HM, Dunn J, Chappel JC, Kahn AJ, Teitelbaum SL. Partial characterization of a parathyroid hormone stimulated osteoblast produced resorptive factor. Calcif Tissue Int 1984b;36:468.

Perry HM, Province MA, Droke DM, Kim GS, Shahed S, Avioli LV. Diurnal variation of serum calcium and phosphorus in postmenopausal women. Calcif Tissue Int 1986;38:115 – 118.

Peterson DR, Heideger WJ, Beach KW. Calcium Homeostasis: The effect of parathyroid hormone on bone membrane electrical potential difference. Calcif Tissue Int 1985;37:307 – 311.

Petko M. Seasonal variations of rat thyroid C cell population. Acta Biol Acad Sci Hung 1978;29:367 – 373.

Petko M, Kovacs L. Seasonal and sex differences in the serum calcitonin levels of the rat. Acta Biol Acad Sci Hung 1981;32:123 – 127.

Petrovic A, Stutzmann J, Oudet C. Turnover of human alveolar bone removed either in the day or in the night. J Interdiscipl Cycle Res 1981;12:161 – 166.

Phang JM, Weiss IW. Maintenance of calcium homeostasis in human beings. In: Greep RO, Astwood EB, eds. Handbook of Physiology, Endocrinology, Vol. 7. London: American Physiological Society, 1976:157 – 168.

Pines M, Hurwitz S. The effect of parathyroid hormone and atrial natriuretic peptide on cyclic-nucleotides production and proliferation of avian epiphyseal growth plate chondrogenitor cells. Endocrinology 1988;123:360 – 366.

Pittendrigh CS. On temporal organization in living systems. Harvey Lect 1961;56:93 – 125.

Poincaré H. Sur le problème de trois corps et les équations de la dynamique. Acta Mathematica Vol. 7, 1890.

Ponchon G, Kennan AL, DeLuca HF. Activation of vitamin D by the liver. J Clin Invest

1969;48:2032 – 2037.

Poole AR, Pidoux I, Reiner A, Choi H, Rosenberg LC. Association of an extracellular protein (chondrocalcin) with the calcification of cartilage in endochondral bone formation. J Cell Biol 1984;98:54 – 65.

Posner AS, Betts F. Molecular control of tissue mineralization. In: Veis A, ed. The Chemistry and Biology of Mineralized Connective Tissues, Vol. 22, Amsterdam: Elsevier, 1981:257 – 266.

Powell T. A mathematical model for calcium homeostasis. Bull Math Biophys 1972;34:483 – 502.

Price PA. Vitamin K-dependent formation of bone Gla-protein (osteocalcin) and its function. Vitam Horm 1985;42:65 – 108.

Price PA, Williamson MK. Effects of warfarin on bone. Studies on the vitamin K-dependent protein of rat bone. J Biol Chem 1981;256:12760 – 12766.

Price PA, Otsuka AS, Poser JW, Kristaponis J, Raman N. Characterization of a $\gamma$-carboxyglutamic acid containing protein from bone. Proc Natl Acad Sci USA 1976;73:1447 – 1451.

Prigogine I, Balescu R Phénomènes cycliques dans la thermodynamique des processus irréversibles. Acad R Belg Bull Class Sci 1956;42:256 – 265.

Prince RL, Wark JD, Omond S, Opie JM, Eagle MR, Eisman JA. A test of 1,25-dihydroxyvitamin D secretory capacity in normal subjects for application in metabolic bone diseases. Clin Endocrinol 1983;18:127 – 131.

Provedini DM, Tsoukas CD, Deftos LJ, Manolagas SC. 1,25-dihydroxyvitamin D3 receptors in human leukocytes. Science 1983;22:1181 – 1183.

Puzas JE, Brand JS. Parathyroid hormone stimulation of collagenase secretion by isolated bone cells. Endocrinology 1979;104:559 – 568.

Puzas JE, Brand JS. Bone cell phosphotyrosine phosphatase: characterization and regulation by calcitropic hormones. Endocrinology 1985;116:2463 – 2468.

Radom S, Zulawski M, Dahlig E. Circadian rhythm of total urinary hydroxyproline excretion and 3H-hydroxyproline test. Clin Chem Acta 1972;39:277 – 278.

Rao LG, Heersche JNM, Marchuk LL, Sturtridge W. Immunohistochemical demonstration of calcitonin binding to specific cell types in fixed rat bone tissue. Endocrinology 1981;108:1972 – 1978.

Rapp PE. The biological applications of control theory. In: Segel LA, ed. Mathematical Models in Molecular and Cellular Biology. Cambridge: University Press, 1980;146 – 247.

Rapp PE. Chaotic behaviour in physiological systems. In: The Institute of Measurement and Control, ed. Oscillations in Physiological Systems: Dynamics and Control. London, 1984:97 – 102.

Rapp PE. Why are so many biological systems periodic? Progr Neurobiol 1987;29:261 – 273.

Rapp PE, Berridge MJ. Oscillations in calcium-Cyclic AMP control loops form the basis of pacemaker activity and other high frequency rhythms. J Theor Biol 1977;66:497 – 525.

Rasmussen H, Barrett PQ. Calcium messenger system: An integrated view. Physiol Rev 1984;64:938 – 984.

Rasmussen H, Fontaine O, Max EE, Goodman DBP. The effect of 1$\alpha$-hydroxyvitamin D3 administration on calcium transport in chick intestine brush border membrane vesicles. J Biol Chem 1979;254:2993 – 2999.

Reddi AH. Cell biology and biochemistry of endochondral development. Cell Res 1981;1:209 – 226.

Redhead CR, Baker PF. Control of intracellular pH in rat calvaria osteoblast: coexistence of both chloride-bicarbonate and sodium-hydrogen exchange. Calcif Tissue Int 1988;42:237 – 242.

Reeve J, Wooton R, Hesp R. A new method for calculating the accretion rate of bone calcium and some observations on the suitability of strontium-85 as a tracer for bone calcium. Calcif Tissue Res 1976;20:121 – 135.

Reeve J, Green JR, Maletskos CJ, Neer RM. Skeletal retention of 45Ca and 85Sr compared: further studies on intravenously injected 85Sr as a tracer for skeletal calcium. Calcif Tissue Int 1983;35:9 – 15.

Reid IR, Civitelli R, Halstead LR, Avioli LV, Hruska KA. Parathyroid hormone acutely elevates intracellular calcium in osteoblast-like cells. Am J Physiol 1987;253:E45 – E51.

Reid IR, Civitelli R, Avioli LV, Hruska KA. Parathyroid hormone depresses cytosolic pH and DNA synthesis in osteoblast-like cells. Am J Physiol 1988;255:E9 – E15.

Reinberg A, Halberg F. Chronopharmacology. Advances in the Biosciences, Vol. 19. London: Pergamon Press, 1979.

Richelle LJ, Onkelinx C. Recent advances in the physical biology of bone and other hard tissues. In: Comar CL, Bronner F, eds. Mineral Metabolism, Vol. 3. New York: Academic Press, 1969;123 – 190.

Ride S. Effect of mineral content of human bone in vitro resorption. Anat Embryol 1986;174:225 – 234.

Rifas L, Shen V, Mitchell K, Peck WA. Macrophage-derived growth factor for osteoblast-like cells and chondrocytes. Proc Natl Acad Sci USA 1984;81:4558 – 4562.

Riggs DS. A quantitative hypothesis concerning the action of the parathyroid hormone. J Theor Biol 1966;12:364 – 372.

Riggs DS. Control Theory and Physiological Feedback Mechanisms. Baltimore: Williams and Wilkins, 1970.

Ringer S. A further contribution regarding the influence of the different constituents of the blood on the contraction of the heart. J Physiol (Lond) 1883;4:29 – 42.

Rizzoli R, Fleisch H, Bonjour JP. Effect of thyroparathyroidectomy on calcium metabolism in the rat. Role of 1,25-dihydroxyvitamin D3. Am J Physiol 1977;223:E160 – E164.

Roberts WE, Aubert MM, Sparaga JM, Smith RK. Circadian periodicity of the cells kinetics of rat molar periodontal ligament. Am J Orthod 1979;76:316 – 323.

Roberts WE, Klinger E, Mozsary PG. Circadian rhythm of mechanically mediated differentiation of osteoblasts. Calcif Rissue Int 1984;36:S62 – S66.

Robertson WG, Marshall RW. Ionized calcium in body fluids. Crit Rev Clin Lab Sci 1981;85 – 125.

Robinson MF, Body JJ, Offord KP, Heath H. Variation of plasma immunoreactive parathyroid hormone and calcitonin in normal and hyperparathyroid man during daylight hours. J Clinical Endocrinol Metab 1982;55:538 – 544.

Roche C, Bellaton C, Pansu D, Miller A, Bronner F. Localization of vitamin D-dependent active $Ca^{2+}$ transport in rat duodenum and relation to CaBP. Am J Physiol 1986;251:G314 – G320.

Rodan GA, Martin TJ. Role of osteoblasts in hormonal control of bone resorption – a hypothesis. Calcif Tissue Int 1981;33:349 – 351.

Rodan GA, Rodan SB. Expression of the osteoblastic phenotype. In: Peck WA, ed Bone and Mineral Research, Vol. 2. Amsterdam: Elsevier, 1984;244 – 285.

Roelfsema F, van der Heide D, Smeenk D. The influence of continuous intragastric feeding of liquid food (vivonex) on the diurnal excretion of electrolytes and urea in rats. J Interdiscip Cycle Res 1982;13:89 – 96.

Roelfsema F, van der Heide D, Poulis J, Smeenk D. Diurnal urinary calcium and phosphate excretion patterns in parathyroidectomized rats. J Interdiscip Cycle Res 1983;14:305 – 314.

Roos BA, Bundy LL, Miller EA, Deftos LJ. Calcitonin secretion by monolayer culture of human C-cells derived from medullary thyroid carcinoma. Endocrinology 1975;97:39 – 43.

Roos BA, Cooper CW, Frelinger AL, Deftos LJ. Acute and chronic fluctuations of immunoreactive and biologically active plasma calcitonin in the rat. Endocrinology 1978;103:2180 – 2186.

Roos BA, Yoon M, Cutshaw SV, Kalu DN. Calcium regulatory action of endogenous rat calcitonin demonstrated by passive immunization with calcitonin antibodies. Endocrinology 1980;107:1320 – 1326.

Roos BA, O'Neil JA, Muszynski M, Birnbaum RS. Noncalcitonin secretory products of calcitonin gene expression. In: Cohn DV, Fujita T, Potts JT, Talmage RV, eds. Endocrine Control of Bone and Calcium Metabolism. Asterdam: Elsevier, 1984;169 – 176.

Rosenberg GD, Simmons DJ, Halberg F, Burstein A. Skeletal effects of alternate day and daily corticosteroid regimens in the rat. Orthop Trans 1979;2:108 – 109.

Rosenfeld MG, Mermod JJ, Amara SG, et al. Production of a novel neuropeptide encoded by the calcitonin gene via tissue-specific RNA processing: Nature 1983;304:129 – 135.

Roufosse AH, Landis WJ, Sabine WK, Glimcher MJ. Identification of brushite in newly deposited bone mineral from embryonic chicks. J Ultrastruct Res 1979;68:235 – 255.

Rouleau MF, Mitchell J, Goltzman D. In vivo distribution of parathyroid hormone receptors in bone: evidence that a predominant osseous target cell is not the mature osteoblast. Endocrinology 1988;123:187 – 191.

Rowe DW, Kream BE. Regulation of collagen synthesis in fetal rat calvaria by 1,25-dihydroxyvitamin D3. J Biol Chem 1982;257:8007 – 8015.

Russell JE, Simmons DJ, Huber B, Roos BA. Meal timing as a Zeitgeber for skeletal deoxyribonucleic acid and collagen synthesis rhythms. Endocrinology 1983;113:2035 – 2042.

Russell JE, Walker WV, Simmons DJ. Adrenal/parathyroid regulation of DNA, collagen and protein synthesis in rat epiphysial cartilage and bone. J Endocrinol 1984a;103:49 – 57.

Russell JE, Grazman B, Simmons DJ. Mineralization in rat metaphyseal bone exhibits a circadian stage dependency. Proc Soc Exp Biol Med 1984b;176:342 – 345.

Saito M, Sato Y, Suda M. Circadian rhythm and dietary response of disaccharidase activities in isolated rat jejunum. Gastroenterology 1978;75:828 – 834.

Sakaguchi T, Takahashi M, Bray GA. Diurnal changes in sympathetic activity. Relation to food intake and to insulin injected into the ventromedial or suprachiasmatic nucleus. J Clin Invest 1988;82:282 – 286.

Sakamoto S, Sakamoto M. On the possibility that bone matrix collagen is removed prior to bone mineral during active cell-mediated resorption In: Ornoy A, Harell A, Sela S, eds. Current Advances in Skeletogenesis. Amsterdam: Elsevier, 1985;65 – 70.

Sampath TK, DeSimone DP, Reddi AH. Extracellular bone matrix-derived growth factors. Exp Cell Res 1982;142:460 – 464.

Sampath TK, Nathanson MA, Reddi AH. In vitro transformation of mesenchymal cells derived from embryonic muscle into cartilage from embryonic muscle into cartilage in response to extracellular matrix components of bone. Proc Natl Acad Sci USA 1984;81:3419 – 3423.

Scarpace PJ, Neuman WF. The blood: bone disequilibrium. II. Evidence against the active accumulation of calcium or phosphate into the bone extracellular fluid. Calcif Tissue Res 1976;20:151 – 158.

Schnitzer JE, McKinstry P, Light TR, Ogden JA. Quantification of regional chrondroosseous circulation in canine tibia and femur. Am J Physiol 1982;242:H365 – H375.

Schrödinger E. What is life? Cambridge: University Press, 1945.

Seamon KB, Kretsinger RH. Calcium-modulated proteins. In: Spiro TG, ed. Calcium in Biology. Vol. 6. New York: John Wiley & Sons, 1983;1 – 52.

Segel LA. Modeling Dynamic Phenomena in Molecular and Cellular Biology. Cambridge: University Press, 1984.

Segond N, Jullienne A, Lasmoles F, Desplan C, Milhaud G, Moukhtar MS. Rapid increase of calcitonin-specific mRNA after acute hypercalcemia. Eur J Biochem 1984;139:209 – 215.

Segond N, Legendre B, Tahri EH, et al. Increased level of calcitonin mRNA after 1,25-dihydroxyvitamin D3 injection in the rat. FEBS Lett 1985;184:268 – 272.

Sel'kov EE. Self-Oscillations in glycolysis. 1. A simple kinetic model. Eur J Biochem 1968;4:79 – 86.

Selye H, Rosch PJ. Integration of endocrinology. In: Glandular Physiology and Therapy. Lippincott: Philadelphia, 1954;1 – 10.

Shareghi GR, Stoner LC. Calcium transport across segment of the rabbit distal nephron in vitro. Am J Physiol 1978;235:F367 – F372.

Shen V, Rifas L, Kohler G, Peck WA. Prostaglandins change cell shape and increase intercellular gap junctions in osteoblasts cultured from rat fetal calvaria. J Bone Mineral Res 1986;1:243 – 249.

Shinoda H, Seto H. Diurnal rhythms in calcium and phosphate metabolism in rodents and their relations to lighting and feeding schedules. Mineral Electrolyte Metab 1985;11:158 – 166.

Shoback DM, Membreno LA, McGhee JG. High calcium and other divalent cations increase inositol trisphosphate in bovine parathyroid cells. Endocrinology 1988;123:382 – 389.

Silve CM, Hradek GT, Jones AL, Arnaud CD. Parathyroid hormone receptor in intact embryonic chicken bone: characterization and cellular localization. J Cell Biol 1982;94:379 – 386.

Silver J, Russell J, Lettieri D, Sherwood LM. Regulation by vitamin D metabolites of messenger ribonucleic acid for preproparathyroid hormone in isolated bovine parathyroid cells. Proc Natl Acad Sci USA 1985;82:4270 – 4273.

Silver J, Naveh-Many T, Mayer H, Schmelzer HJ, Popovtzer MM. Regulation by vitamin D metabolites of parathyroid hormone gene transcription in vivo in the rat. J Clin Invest 1986;78:1296 – 1301.

Simmons DJ. Diurnal periodicity in epiphyseal cartilage. Nature 1962;195:82 – 83.

Simmons DJ, Whiteside LA, Whitson SW. Biorhythmic profiles in the rat skeleton. Metab Bone Dis Rel Res 1979;2:49 – 64.

Simmons DJ, Arsenis C, Whitson SW, Kahn SE, Boskey AL, Gollub N. Mineralization of rat epiphyseal cartilage: a circadian rhythm. Mineral Electrolyte Metab 1983;9:28 – 37.

Sinha TK, Miller S, Fleming J, et al. Demonstration of a diurnal variation in serum parathyroid hormone in primary and secondary hyperparathroidism. J Clin Endocrinol Metab 1975;41:1009 – 1013.

Soodak H, Iberall AS. Homeokinetics: a physical science for complex systems. Science 1978;201:579 – 582.

Söhnel O, Garside J. Solute clustering and nucleation. J Cryst Growth 1988;89:202 – 208.

Spencer R, Charman M, Wilson P, Lawson DEM. Vitamin D-stimulated intestinal calcium absorption may not involve calcium-binding protein directly. Nature 1976;263:161 – 163.

Staub JF, Brezillon P, Lefevre C, Milhaud G, Perault-Staub AM. Variations circadiennes, conception de l'homeostasie et modélisation du métabolisme calcique chez le rat. In: Lassmann G, Seitelberger F, eds. Rhythmische Funktionen in Biologischen Systemenen. Vienna: Facultas-Verlag, 1977;169 – 180.

Staub JF, Perault-Staub AM, Milhaud G. Endogenous nature of circadian rhythms in calcium metabolism. Am J Physiol 1979;237:R311 – R317.

Staub JF, Brezillon P, Perault-Staub AM, Milhaud G. Nonlinear modelling of calcium metabolism. First attempt in the calcium deficient rat. Trans Inst MC 1981;3:89 – 97.

Staub JF, Tracqui P, Brezillon P, Milhaud G, Perault-Staub AM. Calcium metabolism in the rat: A temporal self-organized model. Am J Physiol 1988;254:R134 – R149.

Staub JF, Tracqui P, Lausson S, Milhaud G, Perault-Staub AM. A physiological view of in vivo calcium dynamics: The regulation of a nonlinear self-organized system. Bone 1989;10:77 – 86.

Stewart AF, Broadus AE. Mineral metabolism. In: Felig P, Baxter JD, Broadus AE, Frohman LA, eds. Endocrinology and Metabolism. New York: McGraw-Hill: Book Co 1987;1317 – 1454.

Stromberg B, Simmons DJ. Circadian changes in the calcemic response of intact and parathyroidectomized rats to EDTA infusion. In: Walker CA, Winget CW, Soliman KFA, eds. Chronopharmacology and Chronotherapeutics. Florida University Foundation, 1981;303 – 313.

Stutzmann J, Petrovic A. Persistence in organ culture of a growth rate circadian rhythm. In: Reinberg A, Halberg I, eds. Chronopharmacology. New York: Pergamon Press, 1979;89 – 100.

Stutzmann J, Petrovic A, Malan A. Seasonal variations of the human alveolar bone turnover. A quantitative evaluation in organ culture. J Interdiscip Cycle Res 1981;12:177 – 180.

Suda T, Miyaura C, Abe E, Kuroki T. Modulation of cell differentiation, immune responses and tumor promotion by vitamin D compounds. In: Peck WA, ed. Bone and Mineral Research, Vol. 4. Amsterdam: Elsevier, 1986;1 – 48.

Sutton RAL, Dirks JH. Renal handling of calcium. Fed Proc 1978;37:2112 – 2119.

Swinson DR, Tam CS, Reed R, Hoffman D, Little AH, Cruickshank B. Bone growth kinetics IV: a preliminary investigation on a biorhythm in human osteogenesis. J Pathol 1975;116:13 – 17.

Talmage RV. Effect of fasting and parathyroid hormone injection on plasma $^{45}$Ca concentrations in rats. Calcif Tissue Res 1975;17:103 – 112.

Talmage RV, Roycroft JH, Anderson JJB. Daily fluctuations in plasma calcium phosphate, and their radionuclide concentrations in the rat. Calcif Tissue Res 1975a;17:91 – 102.

Talmage RV, Doppelt SH, Cooper CW. Relationship of blood concentrations of calcium, phosphate, gastrin and calcitonin to the onset of feeding in the rat. Proc Soc Exp Biol Med 1975b;149:855 – 859.

Talmage RV, Grubb SA, Vanderwiel CJ, Doppelt SH, Norimatsu H. The demand for bone calcium in maintenance of plasma calcium concentration. In: Horton J, Tarpley T, Davis W, eds. Mechanisms of Localized Bone Loss. Washington: Information retrieval, Inc 1978;73 – 92.

Talmage RV, Grubb SA, Norimatsu H, Van der Wiel CJ. Evidence for an important physiological role for calcitonin. Proc Natl Acad Sci USA 1980;77:609 – 613.

Talmage RV, Cooper CW, Toverud SU. The physiological significance of calcitonin. In: Peck WA, ed. Bone and Mineral Research, Vol I. Amsterdam: Excerpta Medica, 1983;74 – 143.

Tam CS, Reed R, Swinson DR, Little AH, Cruickshank B. Bone growth kinetics III: A biorhythm in bone growth in the rabbit. J Pathol 1974;114:127 – 133.

Tam CS, Heersche JNM, Murray TM, Parsons JA. Parathyroid hormone stimulates the bone apposition rate independently of its resorptive action: differential effects of intermittent and continual administration. Endocrinology 1982;110:506 – 512.

Tanaka Y, DeLuca HF. The control of 25-hydroxyvitamin D metabolism by inorganic phosphorus. Arch Biochem Biophys 1973;154:566 – 574.

Tanaka Y, DeLuca HF. Stimulation of 1,25-dihydroxyvitamin D3 production by 1,25-dihydroxyvitamin D3 in the hypocalcaemic rat. Biochem J 1983;214:893 – 897.

Taylor AN, Wasserman RH. Vitamin D3-induced calcium-binding protein: Partial purification, electrophoretic visualization, and tissue distribution. Arch Biochem Biophys 1967;119:536 – 540.

Termine JD, Posner AS. Infrared analyses of rat bone: age dependency of amorphous and crystalline mineral fractions. Science 1966;153:1523 – 1525.

Termine JD, Kleinman HK, Withson SW, Conn KL, McGarvey ML, Martin GR. Osteonectin, a bone-specific protein linking mineral to collagen. Cell 1981;26:99 – 105.

Theofan G, Nguyen AP, Norman WA. Regulation of calbindin-D28K gene expression by 1,25-dihydroxyvitamin D3 is correlated to receptor occupancy. J Biol Chem 1986;261:16943 – 16947.

Thom R. The basic ideas of biology (Comments by René Thom). In: Waddington CH, ed. Towards a Theoretical Biology, Vol. 1: Prolegomena. Edinburgh: University Press, 1968;32 – 41.

Thom R. Structural Stability and Morphogenesis. Benjamin WA, ed. Massassuchetts: Reading, 1975.

Tracqui P, Staub JF. Multiple stable periodic solutions of a vector field on R2 characterized by a monomial of degree 3. CR Acad Sci (Paris) 1987;305:331 – 336.

Tracqui P, Brezillon P, Staub JF, Perault-Staub AM, Milhaud G. Diversity and complexity of temporal dynamic behavior for a simple autocatalytic model. CR Acad Sci (Paris) 1985;300:253 – 258.

Tracqui P, Perault-Staub AM, Milhaud G, Staub JF. Theoretical study of a two-dimensional autocatalytic model for calcium dynamics at the extracellular fluid-bone interface. Bull Math Biol 1987;49:597 – 613.

Turing AM. The chemical basis of morphogenesis. Phil Trans R Soc (Lond) B 1952;237:37 – 72.

Tyson JJ, Kauffman S. Control of mitosis by a continuous biochemical oscillation: Synchronization, spatially inhomogeneous oscillations. J Math Biol 1975;1:289 – 310.

Tyson JJ, Othmer HG. The dynamics of feedback control circuits in biochemical pathways. In: Rosen R, Snell FM, eds. Progress in Theoretical Biology, Vol 5. New York: Academic Press, 1978;1 – 62.

Ullrich KJ, Rumrick G, Kloss C. Acute $Ca^{2+}$ reabsorption in the proximal tubule of the rat kidney. Pflugers Arch 1976;364:223 – 228.

Underwood JL, DeLuca HF. Vitamin D is not directly necessary for bone growth and mineralization. Am J Physiol 1984;246:E493 – E498.

Urist MR, DeLange RJ, Finerman GAM. Bone cell differentiation and growth factors. Science 1983;220:680 – 686.

Veldhuijzen JP, Klein-Nulend J, Burger EH. In vitro differentiation of growth plate chondrocytes of long-bone rudiments is enhanced by compressive force. In: Hurwitz S, Sela J, eds. Current Advances in Skeletogenesis, Vol. 3. Jerusalem: Heiliger Publishing, 1986;54 – 59.

Waddington CH. The basis ideas of biology. In: Waddington CH, ed. Towards a Theoretical Biology Vol. 1: Prolegomena. Edingburgh: University Press, 1968;1 – 32.

Wadkins CL, Luben R, Thomas M, Humphreys R. Physical biochemistry of calcification. Clin Orthop Rel Res 1974;99:246 – 266.

Walling MW, Kimberg DV. Active secretion of calcium by adult rat ileum and jejunum in vitro. Am J Physiol 1973;225:415 – 422.

Walling MW, Kimberg DV. Calcium absorption or secretion by rat ileum in vitro: effect of dietary calcium intake. Am J Physiol 1974;226:1124 - 1130.

Walter E. Identifiability of State Space Models. Berlin: Springer-Verlag, 1982.

Walton AG. Nucleation of crystal from solution. Science 1965;148:601 - 607.

Warshafsky B, Aubin JE, Heersche JNM. Cytoskeleton rearrangements during calcitonin-induced changes in osteoclast mobility in vitro. Bone 1985;6:179 - 185.

Warshawsky H, Goltzman D, Rouleau MF, Bergeron JJM. Direct in vivo demonstration by autoradiography of specific binding sites for calcitonin in skeletal and renal tissues of the rat. J Cell Biol 1980;85:682 - 694.

Wase AW, Solewski J, Riches E, Seidenberg J. Action of thyrocalcitonin on bone. Nature 1967;214: 383 - 384.

Wasserman RH, Chandler JS. Molecular mechanisms of intestinal calcium absorption. In: Peck, WA, ed. Bone and Mineral Research, Vol.3. Amsterdam: Elsevier, 1985;181 - 212.

Wasserman RH, Taylor AN. Some aspects of the intestinal absorption of calcium with special reference to Vitamin D. In: Comar CL, Bronner F, eds. Mineral Metabolism, Vol. 3. New York: Academic Press, 1969;321 - 403.

Wasserman RH, Taylor AN, Kallfez FA. Vitamin D and transfer of plasma calcium to intestinal lumen in chicks and rat. Am J Physiol 1966;211:419 - 423.

Wecksler WR, Mason RS, Norman AW. Specific cytosol receptors for 1,25-dihydroxyvitamin D3 in human intestine. J Clin Encodrinol Metab 1979;48:715 - 717.

Weikel JH, Neuman WF, Feldman I. The surface chemistry of bone. VIII. On the mechanism of ionic exchange. J Am Chem Soc 1954;76:5202 - 5207.

Weiss RE, Singer FS, Gorn AH, Hofer DP, Nimmi ME. Calcitonin stimulates bone formation when administrated prior to osteogenesis. J Clin Invest 1981;68:815 - 818.

Wiener N. Cybernetics or Control and Communication in the Animal and the Machine. New York; MIT Press and John Wiley & Sons, 1948.

Wiener S, Price PA. Disaggregation of bone into crystals. Calcif Tissue Int 1986;39:365 - 375.

Williams RJP. The biochemistry of sodium, potassium, magnesium and calcium. Q Rev Chem Soc 1970;24:331 - 365.

Winfree AT. Biological rhythms and the behaviour of populations of coupled oscillators. J Theor Biol 1967;16:15 - 42.

Winfree AT. The Timing of Biological Clocks. San Francisco and London: Freeman WH, 1987.

Wolf F, Scarpa A. Calcium binding by parathyroid cell plasma membranes. Cell Calcium 1987;8:171 - 183.

Wolff J. Das Gesetz der Transformation der Knochen. Quarto, Berlin, 1892.

Wong CC, Dohler KD, Atkinson MJ, Geerlings H, Hesch RD, von zur Muhlen A. Influence of age, strain and season on diurnal periodicity of thyroid stimulating hormone, thyroxine, triiodothyronine and parathyroid hormone in the serum of male laboratory rats. Acta Endocrinol 1983;102:377 - 385.

Wong G. Paracrine interactions in bone-secreted products of osteoblasts permit osteoclasts to respond to parathyroid hormone. J Biol Chem 1984;259:4019 - 4021.

Wong GL. Skeletal effects of parathyroid hormone In: Peck WA, ed. Bone and Mineral Research, Vol 4. Amsterdam: Elsevier, 1986;103 - 130.

Wong KM, Klein L. Circadian variations in contributions of bone and intestine to plasma calcium in dogs. Am J Physiol 1984;246:R688 - R692.

Wrobel J. Diurnal variations of calcium transport in the small intestine of adrenalectomized, nephrectomized, and vitamin D-treated rats. Calcif Tissue Int 1983;35:352 - 356.

Wrobel J, Ghazarian JG. Diurnal rhythmicity in plasma 24, 25-dihydroxyvitamin D3: correlation with intestinal calcium transport and plasma minerals. Biochem Biophys Res Commun 1982;106:1233 - 1239.

Wrobel J, Nagel G. Diurnal rhythm of active transport in rat intestine. Experientia 1979;35:1581 - 1582.

Wuthier RV. A review of the primary mechanism of endochondral calcification with special emphasis on the role of cells, mitochondria and matrix vesicles. Clin Orthop Rel Res 1982;169:219 - 242.

Yates FE. Outline of a physical theory of physiological systems. Can J Physiol Pharmacol 1982a;60:217 – 248.

Yates FE. System analysis of hormone action. Principles and strategies. In: Goldberger RF, Yamamoto KR, eds. Biological Regulation and Development. New York: Plenum Press, 1982b;25 – 97.

Yee JA, Sutton JK, Shew RL, Olansky L. Parathyroid hormone stimulation of alkaline phosphatase activity in cultured neonatal mouse calvaria bone cells: involvement of cyclic AMP and calcium. J Cell Physiol 1986;128:246 – 250.

Yoon PS, DeLuca HF. Purification and properties of chick renal mitochondrial ferredoxin. Biochemistry 1980;19:2165 – 2171.

*Bone and Mineral Research/7*
*Johan N.M. Heersche and John A. Kanis, editors*



# Calcium and hypertension

David A. McCarron

*Division of Nephrology and Hypertension, Institute for Nutrition and Cardiovascular Research, Department of Medicine, Oregon Health Sciences University, 3181 S.W. Sam Jackson Park Road, Portland, OR 97201, U.S.A.*

## I. Introduction

The hypothesis that an impairment in calcium homeostasis is a contributing factor in the development of hypertension was initially presented nearly a decade ago [1]. While it remains to be proven unequivocally and therefore continues to be a subject of controversy [2, 3], there is a broad and expanding body of evidence that supports this relationship between calcium metabolism and blood pressure control. The evidence comes from a variety of scientific endeavors, including epidemiologic analyses, animal investigations, and clinical trials in humans. This chapter provides a summary of the data that have accumulated during the past decade relating both calcium nutrition and metabolism to blood pressure regulation [4, 5].

## II. Epidemiologic analyses

### A. Biochemical parameters

In our initial study we observed slightly higher circulating parathyroid hormone levels in untreated patients with essential hypertension compared to normotensive subjects despite similar serum total calcium concentrations [1]. The increase could not be attributed to renal dysfunction, but was associated with an inappropriate increase in urinary calcium excretion when indexed against simultaneous urinary sodium excretion. This latter finding was characterized as a 'renal calcium leak' in hypertension. Other investigators have also noted an increase in urinary calcium excretion in hypertension [6 – 8], and of these, one group speculated and later confirmed [7, 8] lower dietary calcium intakes in hypertensive subjects in the study population.

Several studies have reported increased parathyroid hormone (PTH) levels in hypertension [9 – 12]. Grobbee et al. [12] documented that PTH values were positively correlated with blood pressure after adjustment for weight in a study of young males. In another group of individuals with early mild hypertension, these investigators found a continuous, positive relationship between PTH and blood pressure, independent of weight. The ratio of calcium and ionized calcium to PTH was related to blood pressure in a smaller study by Zachariah [13], suggesting abnormal regulation of PTH activity. A simultaneous increase in PTH, urinary cyclic AMP, and urinary calcium excretion in hypertension was confirmed by Strazzullo and co-workers [6] in a metabolic balance study, as well as by Ellison et al. [14].

Serum total calcium concentration has been positively correlated with blood pressure in many studies, although higher serum albumin concentrations may account for this relationship in some of them [7, 15]. Serum ionized calcium values, however, have been reported to be identical, modestly decreased, or increased in hypertensive as compared to normotensive subjects. We initially reported significantly lower ionized calcium levels in hypertension versus normotension [16], and this was confirmed by Folsom and coworkers [17] who found that ultrafilterable calcium ($p = 0.01$) and serum ionized calcium ($p = 0.7$) tended to be lower in individuals with higher blood pressure. This relationship may be continuous as an inverse correlation between ionized calcium and blood pressure was demonstrated in a general population [10, 18], as well as in adolescent [19] and elderly populations [20].

Resnick and colleagues [21] reported that any relationship between ionized calcium and blood pressure is dependent upon renin status; patients with low renin hypertension have lower ionized calcium as compared to patients with high renin hypertension who have higher ionized calcium values. This dependence was even more pronounced in an older age group [20]. Strazzullo et al. [22] noted that although baseline serum ionized calcium was nearly identical between normotensive and hypertensive subjects, this measurement increased less in hypertensive subjects following a calcium infusion.

In contrast, other epidemiologic studies, most with larger sample sizes, have demonstrated no relationship between blood pressure and ionized calcium levels [23 – 27]. An increase in serum ionized calcium concentration in hypertensive as compared to normotensive subjects has been reported [28, 29]. Although not described in many reports, methodologic variation may explain this discrepancy. Ionized calcium is difficult to measure accurately and is easily affected by a number of factors. Though the technology is improving, ionized calcium electrodes vary between manufacturers in their adjustment for pH alterations, and in the interference of protein and sodium. Measurements can also be affected by aerobic versus anaerobic technique, storage time and temperature, venepuncture with a tourniquet, and collection from fasting subjects. Many reports did not indicate whether antihypertensive medications were used by any study participants; in particular, thiazide diuretics may increase serum ionized calcium values when used chronically.

Serum phosphorus, on the other hand, has a more consistent relationship with high blood pressure. A number of studies have identified lower serum phosphorus values in subjects with hypertension or a continuous inverse correlation between serum phosphorus and arterial pressure [1, 30].

Measurements of vitamin D metabolism have been made only recently in hypertension. Sowers et al. [31] reported a significant inverse relationship between dietary vitamin D and blood pressure, independent of other factors; it was suggested that perhaps the regulation of calcium absorption from the gut or an interaction with PTH could explain the mechanism of effect. These same investigators reported that in 373 women, serum levels of $1,25(OH)_2D_3$ were directly related to blood pressure, and explained 7% of blood pressure variation. Calcium metabolism does differ between genders and such variations could account for the discrepancies in surveys of hypertensive populations.

Resnick et al. [21] have reported that not only does ionized calcium vary by renin status, but PTH levels and $1,25(OH)_2D_3$ are higher in low renin hypertension, with the opposite in high renin hypertension as compared to normal blood pressure. Renin status has not been reported in most other studies, and few simultaneously measured urinary calcium, ionized calcium, PTH, and $1,25(OH)_2D_3$ in hypertension and normotension. Overall, the subtle pattern of biochemical abnormalities is consistent with an abnormal regulation of the PTH-vitamin D axis in the clinical setting of high blood pressure.

### B. Dietary calcium

In a study we conducted at Oregon in 1982, hypertensive subjects had significantly lower dietary calcium intake as compared to normotensive subjects [32]. Of the nutrients measured, only calcium intake differed between the two groups. Our analysis of the database from the National Health and Nutrition Examination Survey I (NHANES I), a U.S. population survey conducted in the early 1970s, confirmed this observation [33]. In that survey, of the nutritional factors assessed, dietary calcium was the best predictor of the presence of hypertension. At higher levels of dietary calcium consumption, there was a lower probability of having blood pressure in the hypertensive range.

More than 20 reports have now identified an inverse relationship between dietary calcium intake and blood pressure status (Table 1), including six others that utilized the NHANES I database. Although the statistical analysis varied, most reported a significant relationship between dietary calcium and blood pressure either overall or in certain subgroups. Gruchow et al. [34], who initially reported the absence of this relationship, later published an alternative analysis which did indicate that the relationship between lower dietary calcium intake and higher blood pressure was dependent upon consumption of a high sodium diet. Several lines of evidence now suggest a potentially important overlap between the effects of sodium chloride on blood pressure and those of dietary calcium.

The association between dietary calcium intake and blood pressure appears to be

TABLE 1 Epidemiologic studies of calcium and hypertension

| Author | Population | Dietary data* | Subjects | |
|---|---|---|---|---|
| | | | No. | Age (yrs) |
| McCarron [32] | Portland, OR | 24-h recall | 96 | 25 – 65 |
| McCarron [33] | NHANES I | 24-h recall | 10 419 | 18 – 74 |
| Ackley [202] | San Diego, CA | Questionnaire | 5050 | 30 – 79 |
| Garcia-Palmieri [203] | Puerto Rico | 24-h recall | 7932 | 45 – 64 |
| Harlan [204] | NHANES I | 24-h recall | 2055 | 25 – 74 |
| Nichaman [205] | Chicago, IL | diet history | 1652 | 40 – 56 |
| Gruchow [196] | NHANES I | 24-h recall | – | 18 – 74 |
| Harlan [206] | NHANES I | 24-h recall | 3854 | 25 – 74 |
| Harlan [207] | NHANES I | 24-h recall, food frequency | 5305 | 12 – 74 |
| Johnson [208] | Wisconsin | Food record | 113 | 35 – 65 |
| Kromhout [197] | Netherlands | Diet history | 605 | 45 – 70 |
| McCarron [160] | Portland, OR | 24-h recall | 80 | 25 – 70 |
| Reed [209] | Honolulu, HI | 24-h recall | 6496 | 46 – 65 |
| Sempos [210] | NHANES I | 24-h recall | 5858 | 18 – 74 |
| Yamamoto [211] | Pittsburgh, PA | Food frequency | 1937 | 34 – 56 |
| Caggiula [212] | MRFIT | 24-h recall | – | – |
| Folsom [17] | Minnesota | Food frequency | 56 | 25 – 74 |
| Kok [144] | The Netherlands | Diet history | 2291 | 40 – 65 |
| Trevisan [213] | Italy | Food frequency | 6699 | 20 – 59 |
| Liebman [199] | SE U.S.A. | 24-h recall | 532 | 14 – 16 |
| Sempos [200] | NHANES I, II | 24-h recall | 11 330 | 40 – 74 |
| Joffres [35] | Honolulu, HI | 24-h recall | 615 | 46 – 65 |
| Witteman [36] | Boston nurses | 24-h recall | 58 218 | 34 – 59 |
| McGarvey [214] | Providence, RI | Questionnaire | 212 | 0 – 01 |
| Kesteloot [8] | Belgium | 24-h recall | 4055 | 25 – 74 |

* ETOH = alcohol; PUFA = polyunsaturated fatty acid; MRFIT = Multiple Risk Factor Intervention Trial.

independent of age, gender, race, socioeconomic status, geography, and weight. This correlation of dietary calcium with blood pressure has tended to be stronger with systolic than diastolic pressures. Most importantly, there is a suggestion that this relationship with blood pressure may be more pronounced below a threshold of 400 – 500 mg of calcium per day [33, 35, 36].

While these biochemical, nutritional, and clinical observations suggest that in settings where there is evidence of failure to adequately regulate calcium homeostasis, hypertension is more likely to be present, they do not support a cause-and-effect relationship. This can only be established on the basis of investigations in experimental models of hypertension, cellular and subcellular experiments that identify the mechanisms, and clinical trials in hypertensive subjects.

## III. Experimental models of hypertension

### A. Systemic calcium metabolism

Hypertensive animals and humans demonstrate several alterations in calcium ($Ca^{2+}$) metabolism at the systemic level which may affect $Ca^{2+}$ balance. These include: low serum ionized $Ca^{2+}$ concentrations, elevated serum PTH levels, inappropriate renal calcium losses, and alterations of intestinal calcium absorption and $1{,}25(OH)_2$ vitamin $D_3$ metabolism. Ultimately these disturbances affect total body and bone $Ca^{2+}$ balance.

Calcium metabolism has been best characterized in the laboratory in the spontaneously hypertensive rat (SHR), although substantial data also exist for several other experimental models of hypertension and for human essential hypertension. Blood pressure and calcium handling, like other physiologic processes, change as the hypertensive animal matures, and also vary by gender. Therefore, the age and sex of the animals in the SHR studies are emphasized here for a more clear understanding of the evolution of the abnormalities of calcium metabolism associated with arterial hypertension.

*1. Serum calcium.* A low serum ionized calcium concentration ($[Ca^{2+}]_s$) in the SHR, relative to its normotensive control the Wistar-Kyoto rat (WKY), was found at 5 and 13 weeks of age in female rats [37] and at 8, 10, 16, 24, 33, 40, and 45 weeks in males [38 – 40]. On average, $[Ca^{2+}]_s$ in WKY exceeded that in SHR by approximately 0.15 mEq/l. It was generally not specified whether the specimens were taken from fasting or non-fasting animals, and this could account for variability in findings. Wright et al. [41] also found decreased $[Ca^{2+}]_s$ in SHR as compared with normotensive Sprague-Dawley rats.

In contrast, Lau et al. [42] reported higher post-absorptive $[Ca^{2+}]_s$ in 25-week-old female SHR and no difference in fasting $[Ca^{2+}]_s$ between 26-week-old female SHR and WKY. However, these experiments were performed on parathyroidectomized rats. The same authors found that fasting plasma ultrafilterable $Ca^{2+}$ was lower in parathyroid-intact, 23-week-old female SHR. After parathyroidectomy, there was no difference in plasma ultrafilterable $Ca^{2+}$ between SHR and WKY. Plasma ultrafilterable $Ca^{2+}$ includes ionized calcium (~ 80%) as well as complexed, non-protein bound $Ca^{2+}$ (~ 20%). Thus, $[Ca^{2+}]_s$ may be decreased in the parathyroid-intact SHR compared to the WKY, but the difference is eliminated following parathyroidectomy. More recently, these investigators reported no difference in $[Ca^{2+}]_s$ between 25-day-old parathyroid-intact SHR and WKY of both genders [43]. Similarly, Bukoski et al. [44] reported no differences in serum ionized $Ca^{2+}$ in 12-week-old SHR and WKY, although serum $Ca^{2+}$ did reflect $Ca^{2+}$ content of the diet in younger rats. The uninephrectomized DOCA-salt hypertensive rat also exhibits low $[Ca^{2+}]_s$, as does the Dahl salt-sensitive rat; the one-kidney, one-clip and two-kidney, one-clip rat models of renovascular hypertension do not [37].

Total serum calcium is not altered in SHR in any consistent direction. The combination of low $[Ca^{2+}]_s$ and normal total serum calcium implies an increase in serum protein-bound $Ca^{2+}$ in SHR. Direct measurements in humans with essential hypertension confirm decreased serum ionized, complexed, and ultrafilterable $Ca^{2+}$ and increased protein-bound $Ca^{2+}$ [17]. Other investigators have also reported low $[Ca^{2+}]_s$ in human essential hypertension [16, 45] and in patients with primary aldosteronism [46].

*2. Parathyroid hormone and urinary cyclic AMP.* Generally, serum PTH levels are elevated in the SHR, presumably as a secondary response to the low $[Ca^{2+}]_s$. Stern et al. [39] found that carboxy-terminal PTH was detectable in 43% of 6-week-old and 55% of 10-week-old male SHR, whereas all of the WKY of the same ages had undetectable C-terminal PTH levels. In this study, $[Ca^{2+}]_s$ was significantly lower in 10-week-old SHR than in the WKY. Bindels et al. [38] also found elevated immunoreactive PTH and decreased $[Ca^{2+}]_s$ in 8-week-old SHR although another assay for intact PTH showed no difference between SHR and WKY. McCarron et al. [40] found that amino-terminal PTH was significantly elevated in male SHR at 18, 24, and 29 weeks of age. A C-terminal assay also revealed higher serum PTH in the SHR at 29 weeks. Again, $[Ca^{2+}]_s$ was significantly lower in the SHR at these ages. A mid-molecule PTH assay failed to detect a difference between the SHR and WKY [47]. SHR were shown to have hyperplasia of the parathyroid glands providing anatomical evidence for chronic stimulation of their parathyroid tissue [48].

While serum PTH levels may be appropriately elevated in the SHR in response to decreased $[Ca^{2+}]_s$, end-organ responsiveness may be abnormal. Basal nephrogenous cyclic AMP is lower in 11- to 17-week-old male SHR than in WKY [49]. Total urinary cyclic AMP has been reported to be decreased [42, 49] or normal [50] in 13- to 16-week-male SHR. Normal or decreased urinary cyclic AMP in the face of elevated serum PTH is consistent with renal unresponsiveness to the peptide hormone. Further evidence for reduced renal response to PTH in the SHR includes elevated $U_{Ca}V$ in the setting of higher PTH levels [40] and a subnormal increment in $1,25(OH)_2$ vitamin D production in response to PTH infusion [51]. Further, PTH infusion caused a smaller increment in $[Ca^{2+}]_s$ in 13-week-old male SHR than in WKY [52]. *In vitro* studies also suggest abnormal cyclic AMP generation as adenylate cyclase activity of isolated renal membranes from 5- and 16-week-old SHR was reduced in response to $PGE_2$ although the response to other stimuli and basal activity were normal [53]. Thus, the SHR's ability to compensate for a low $[Ca^{2+}]_s$ by renal mechanisms is compromised.

*3. Calcium excretion.* Urinary calcium excretion is increased in the mature SHR although there is disagreement as to whether this reflects primary intestinal hyperabsorption or a primary renal calcium leak. Preadolescence, 24-h urinary calcium has been variously reported as decreased [38, 43], not different [40, 42, 52, 54] and increased [42, 54, 55]. As the SHR reaches maturity, its urinary calcium excretion exceeds that of the WKY. Longitudinal studies indicate that hypercalciuria develops in male SHR by 17 weeks of age and in females by 25 – 26 weeks. McCarron et al. [40] reported significantly increased calcium excretion in 17-, 22-, 28- and 43-week-old male SHR with concurrently low $[Ca^{2+}]_s$ and elevated serum PTH concentrations. The hypercalciuria was interpreted to reflect a renal calcium leak similar to that noted in humans. That is, the kidneys of maturing and mature SHR fail to normally reabsorb calcium despite a lower filtered calcium load and a higher level of serum PTH. The latter should stimulate renal $Ca^{2+}$ reabsorption. These early studies were recently confirmed in a longitudinal study in our laboratory [56]. On a low $Ca^{2+}$ diet, hypercalciuria was enhanced in 18- to 20-week-old male SHR [55], providing further evidence for a renal leak.

Lau et al. [42] found higher 24-h calcium excretion beginning at 25 weeks of age in the female SHR. Parathyroidectomy enhanced hypercalciuria in the 25-week-old female SHR. Urinary calcium excretion after fasting has been reported to be decreased in 23-week-old females, and in 8- to 14-week-old males [50]. The relevance of these findings, however, is questionable as 24-h urinary calcium excretion is only increased in older SHR. Nonetheless, based on low fasting calcium excretion and normal urinary cyclic AMP (PTH was not measured), the 24-h hypercalciuria was felt to result from increased intestinal calcium absorption [42] and not from diminished renal tubular calcium reabsorption.

Because of differences in sex and age of animals used in various studies and in actual measurements of calcium balance, the distinction between absorptive and renal hypercalciuria remains unsettled. A further complication arises because the SHR may have defective calcium metabolism involving several organs which prevents anticipated compensatory responses. Expected findings with a primary renal calcium leak include: fasting hypercalciuria and ionized hypocalcemia; elevated serum PTH, urinary cyclic AMP, and serum $1,25(OH)_2D_3$; parathyroid hyperplasia; and negative (or neutral) calcium balance relative to WKY [57]. Thus, renal hypercalciuria is consistent with whole animal calcium deficiency in SHR. Absorptive hypercalciuria predicts normal fasting urinary and serum ionized calcium, suppressed parathyroid function and gland size, and positive (or neutral) Ca balance relative to WKY [57]. Pure absorptive hypercalciuria therefore indicates calcium surfeit rather than deficit.

Hypercalciuria is also found in the uninephrectomized, DOC-treated rat model fed sodium chloride but not sodium bicarbonate [58]. In this model, hypercalciuria precedes the onset of hypertension. Similarly, urinary calcium excretion is increased in the Dahl salt-sensitive hypertensive rat [59] and in the Milan rat strain of spontaneous hypertension [60] compared to their respective controls. Hypercalciuria appeared to be on a renal basis in both the DOC and Milan hypertensive strains. Thus, hypercalciuria is common to several forms of experimental hypertension. A possible explanation for the hypercalciuria may be decreased renal adenylate cyclase response to PTH as described for Dahl salt-sensitive and DOC-NaCl hypertensive rats [61].

The Milan hypertensive strain also exhibits decreased renal $Ca^{2+}$-ATPase activity [62]. Either end-organ response failure to PTH's actions or reduced $Ca^{2+}$ pump activity could account for the renal leak of calcium.

*4. Calcium absorption.* Intestinal calcium transport and net absorption have been studied by several techniques with seemingly conflicting results. The *in vitro* everted duodenal sac preparation estimates net active and passive transfer of radiolabeled $Ca^{2+}$ from the mucosal to the serosal surface. Several investigators have found no difference in duodenal $Ca^{2+}$ absorption in 5- and 10-week-old male SHR [39, 63], increased absorption in 12-week-old male SHR [63], and decreased absorption in 5- and 12-week-old male SHR [64]. Schedl et al. [65] reported lower intestinal calcium transport in SHR obtained from three different breeders as compared with their normotensive controls. Similarly, *in vivo* techniques for measuring duodenal radioactive $Ca^{2+}$ transfer have indicated both increased absorption in 12-week-old male [63] and 50-week-old female SHR [42], as well as decreased absorption in 12-week-old male SHR [64]. These discordant findings may reflect variations in techniques, gender or age of the animal, and/or diet preparation.

The modified Ussing chamber technique, another *in vitro* approach, provides a direct measurement of active $Ca^{2+}$ flux across isolated intestinal segments. Using this technique, the unidirectional mucosal-to-serosal $Ca^{2+}$ flux was shown to be significantly reduced in 12- to 14-week-old male SHR compared to WKY [66, 67]. $Ca^{2+}$ secretion (serosal-to-mucosal flux) was not different between SHR and WKY. Thus, net duodenal $Ca^{2+}$ flux across the isolated duodenal segment was reduced in the adolescent SHR. An impairment of mucosal-to-serosal $Ca^{2+}$ flux has been identified in the 6-week-old male SHR, even in the face of increased $1,25(OH)_2$ vitamin $D_3$ levels (unpublished observations). By contrast, Ussing studies on 24- [67] and 35-week [68] -old male animals revealed no difference between SHR and WKY in unidirectional and net $Ca^{2+}$ flux across duodenum and colon on a normal $Ca^{2+}$ diet, although duodenal flux was reduced in 24-week-old SHR on a low $Ca^{2+}$ diet [67].

Isolated duodenal enterocytes provide another technique for assessment of $Ca^{2+}$ metabolism in intestinal epithelium. With this method, influx of radiolabelled $^{45}Ca$ was decreased in enterocytes isolated from the proximal duodenum of 12- to 14-week and 28- to 32-week-old male SHR as compared with age-matched WKY [69]. Also, $^{45}Ca$ efflux was decreased in enterocytes from 12- to 14-week-old SHR [70]. While isolated cellular flux data do not measure actual transmucosal $Ca^{2+}$ flux, they do indicate that one step of intestinal $Ca^{2+}$ transport is reduced in both the growing and the mature male SHR.

Because *in vitro* and segmental *in vivo* techniques may not fully account for differences in paracellular and segmental intestinal calcium absorption, measurements of whole animal $Ca^{2+}$ absorption have been attempted. Stern et al. [39] performed balance studies on male SHR and WKY from 6 to 10 weeks of age and reported no significant difference in cumulative $Ca^{2+}$ intake and mean daily urinary and fecal calcium excretion. Over the 4-week study, SHR retained 180 ± 15 mg $Ca^{2+}$ as compared with 218 ± 24 mg $Ca^{2+}$ in WKY, suggesting a trend for reduced $Ca^{2+}$ absorption and less cumulative balance in the growing SHR. Similarly, Lau et al. [42] found reduced fractional $Ca^{2+}$ absorption and a trend for reduced absolute $Ca^{2+}$ absorption and $Ca^{2+}$ retention in 10-week-old male SHR in a 6-day balance study. By contrast, Bindels et al. [38] found no difference in $Ca^{2+}$ absorption in 6- and 8-week-old male SHR, and Hsu et al. [50] reported increased $Ca^{2+}$ absorption in 13- to 16-week-old male SHR based upon increased urinary $Ca^{2+}$ excretion following an oral load of either cold or radiolabelled $Ca^{2+}$. Increased $Ca^{2+}$ absorption was also found in balance experiments performed on 3.5-week-old pre-hypertensive male and female SHR [43] and in mature hypertensive 25-week and 50-week-old female SHR [42]. Drüeke et al. [71] followed male SHR from 6 to 12 weeks of age, and reported a deterioration in net calcium balance compared to WKY.

These data from several laboratories using different diets indicate that male SHR malabsorb $Ca^{2+}$ during maturation and the developmental phase of their hypertension. Calcium malabsorption becomes less apparent as the SHR ages. In very early life, male SHR may exhibit increased calcium absorption. Female SHR hyperabsorb calcium at all ages studied (3.5, 25, and 50 weeks). There is currently no explanation for these differences between sexes.

*5. Bone mineralization.* Because bone is the largest store of $Ca^{2+}$ in the body, bone mineralization should provide a more accurate index of whole animal $Ca^{2+}$ balance. Bone mineralization reflects net $Ca^{2+}$ retention as determined by intestinal absorption and urinary excretion of calcium and the net action of PTH and $1,25(OH)_2D_3$, as well as other $Ca^{2+}$ regulating hormones. In male SHR and WKY, bone $Ca^{2+}$ content (mg Ca/g fat-free dry weight) was the same at 6 and 18 weeks of age [38, 50], but was significantly decreased at 23 [67] and 54 [72] weeks of age. Similarly, ash weight/volume, and ash weight/dry weight of the femoral bone were unchanged in 6-week-old male SHR [38], but were reduced in 26-week-old male SHR [73]. Bone cortical thickness was also reduced in the 26-week-old animal. Yamori et al. [74] have also reported reduced bone mineral content in the stroke-prone SHR.

By contrast, a study of hydralazine-treated female SHR reported increased fractional bone mass and $Ca^{2+}$ density at one year of age [42]. Thus, bone $Ca^{2+}$ content is normal early in the life of the male SHR, but is less than that observed in the WKY as the animals reach late adolescence. Reduced bone $Ca^{2+}$ content in SHR is consistent with reduced $Ca^{2+}$ retention over time. These differences are not apparent in the female SHR.

*6. Vitamin D.* Vitamin D metabolism is abnormal in the SHR, which may partially account for the decreased intestinal $Ca^{2+}$ absorption. Altered vitamin D regulation may also be involved in the increased renal excretion of $Ca^{2+}$ and altered cellular $Ca^{2+}$ metabolism associated with hypertension. Serum levels of $1,25(OH)_2D$ are reported to be elevated [38, 43] or unchanged [39, 64, 75, 76] in young male SHR from 3 to 13 weeks of age. However, a number of laboratories have detected low basal serum $1,25(OH)_2D$ concentration in SHR as early as 11 weeks of age [51, 67, 76 – 78]. That is, low serum $1,25(OH)_2D$ levels are found just as the SHR is developing hypertension and $Ca^{2+}$ malabsorption. Low or even normal serum $1,25(OH)_2D$ levels are clearly inappropriate since the SHR have low $[Ca^{2+}]_s$, low serum phosphorus [39, 55], and elevated PTH. Serum 25(OH)D tends to be elevated in the SHR, indicating that vitamin D intake or substrate availability is not compromised and therefore cannot account for the inappropriately low $1,25(OH)_2D$ [64, 76, 79].

Altered vitamin D metabolism in the SHR is also indicated by subnormal increments in serum $1,25(OH)_2D_3$ in response to PTH administration [51, 75], cyclic AMP stimulation [51], and phosphate depletion [51, 78]. The response of serum $1,25(OH)_2D$ to a low $Ca^{2+}$ diet has been reported to be both decreased [67] and normal [76] in the SHR. The low basal and PTH-stimulated serum $1,25(OH)_2D$ in SHR can be accounted for by a reduced production rate since metabolic clearance of $1,25(OH)_2D$ is not different in SHR and WKY [47]. Further evidence for abnormal vitamin D metabolism is the observation that SHR, but not WKY, develop hypocalcemia and low serum $1,25(OH)_2D$ when placed on a vitamin D deficient diet between the ages of 4 and 13 weeks [79]. Serum 25(OH)D falls to undetectable levels in both groups, although only WKY are able to maintain $1,25(OH)_2D$ and $Ca^{2+}$ homeostasis.

The mechanism of abnormal $1,25(OH)_2D$ production in the SHR is unknown. Intrinsic 1-$\alpha$-hydroxylase enzyme activity of isolated renal mitochondria appears to be normal or even enhanced [75]. Cyclic AMP generation is involved in PTH-stimulation of $1,25(OH)_2D$ production [80]. Although urinary cyclic AMP generation is decreased in SHR, cyclic AMP infusion results in a smaller increment in serum $1,25(OH)_2D_3$ in SHR than in WKY, suggesting that an additional defect is involved [51]. Increased intracellular or mitochondrial concentration of $Ca^{2+}$, inorganic phosphate, or hydrogen ion could suppress activity of the 1-$\alpha$-hydroxylase enzyme in renal proximal tubules as these are postulated regulators of the enzyme. There is some evidence for systemic acidosis [81] and phosphate retention [38, 82] in SHR. Cytosolic free $Ca^{2+}$ is elevated in some cells of the SHR, but preliminary reports indicate unchanged or low levels in renal proximal tubules [83, 84].

While some studies have suggested that SHR display intestinal resistance to the effects of $1,25(OH)_2D_3$ [63, 64], more recent work demonstrates normal [67] or increased [85] intestinal response to the hormone. Lucas et al. [67] found that $Ca^{2+}$ flux across isolated duodenal segments measured by Ussing apparatus is normalized in SHR when they are given short-term supplemental $1,25(OH)_2D_3$. In contrast, the low $^{45}Ca$ influx reported in SHR isolated enterocytes is not fully corrected by $1,25(OH)_2D_3$ administration [69]. The calcemic response to systemic PTH infusion is blunted in SHR and is normalized when the animals are given $1,25(OH)_2D_3$ [52]. Thus, it appears that the defective vitamin D metabolism observed in the SHR is of possible functional importance.

### B. Cellular calcium metabolism

Whether organ level disturbances in $Ca^{2+}$ metabolism in humans with essential hypertension and in the SHR reflect a primary alteration in cellular calcium metabolism and whether these cellular defects play a causal role in chronically elevated blood pressure are pertinent questions. One would predict that $Ca^{2+}$ metabolism of vascular smooth muscle is abnormal in the hypertensive state if indeed this cell type is involved in a primary fashion in the pathogenesis of the disease as opposed to playing a passive role. Because direct investigation in the human situation is complicated by difficulties in obtaining appropriate tissue samples and cell types, most information has come from studies on formed elements of the blood from humans with essential hypertension or vascular tissue isolated from animal models of hypertension.

*1. Vascular smooth muscle.* One hypothesis put forth to account for hypertension of vascular origin is that there is a defect in the ability of the vascular smooth muscle cell to maintain normal levels of intracellular free $Ca^{2+}$. Cellular $Ca^{2+}$ metabolism has been studied using a variety of techniques including measurement of flux of $^{45}Ca$ into intact tissues and isolated membrane preparations, enzymatic analysis of pumps or carriers believed to play a role in regulating intracellular levels of $Ca^{2+}$, and more recently, using intracellular indicators to assess free levels of intracellular $Ca^{2+}$.

Studies of vascular smooth muscle isolated from the SHR that have examined $^{45}Ca$ influx into whole tissue have shown either an increase [86], no change [87], or a decrease in influx [88]. These results are dependent upon the age of the animal, the time course over which influx was determined, and the method of defining intracellular vs. extracellular $^{45}Ca$. Only limited conclusions about specific pools of $Ca^{2+}$ or binding sites can be drawn from these investigations. While early studies focused on conduit arteries, Cauvin et al. [89] have examined unidirectional influx of $^{45}Ca$ into mesenteric resistance vessels of the SHR and observed enhanced influx of $Ca^{2+}$ under both basal and norepinephrine-stimulated conditions. These studies derive support from the finding of Mulvany et al. [90] that resistance arteries of the mesenteric bed have an increased sensitivity to extracellular $Ca^{2+}$.

Combined with the observations that $Ca^{2+}$ channel blockers have a greater blood pressure-lowering effect and vasodilator action in essential hypertension than in control subjects, these results have been interpreted to indicate that the cell membrane of vascular smooth muscle is more permeable to $Ca^{2+}$ in the hypertensive state [91 – 93]. A report by Rusch and Hermsmeyer [94] demonstrated an increased distribution of the *L*-type channel in the vascular smooth muscle cell of the SHR when compared to the WKY. This abnormal distribution of L/T $Ca^{2+}$ channel ratio in patch-clamp studies of azygous vein derived from vascular smooth muscle cells of the SHR provides a possible electrophysiologic basis for the putative membrane leak of $^{45}Ca$ reported to be present in the vascular tissue of the SHR. Given the role of membrane-bound $Ca^{2+}$ in regulating its own channel, this observation provides a pathophysiologic basis for why dietary $Ca^{2+}$ or $Ca^{2+}$ antagonist might both prove to be effective antihypertensive interventions.

Studies of $Ca^{2+}$ transport by isolated membrane fractions of vascular smooth muscle show a consistent trend that suggests a depressed ability of the smooth muscle cell membrane to actively transport $Ca^{2+}$. When ATP-supported $Ca^{2+}$ uptake was measured in microsomal fractions of aorta isolated from SHR [86, 95, 96] or from cell membrane enriched fractions of mesenteric arteries of SHR [97, 98], uptake was attenuated compared with fractions isolated from normotensive controls. This decrease in uptake may be a reflection of an abnormal cell membrane $Mg^{2+}/Ca^{2+}$-ATPase pump.

A more rigorous approach would combine $Ca^{2+}$ uptake studies using isolated membrane vesicles with kinetic analyses of the purified $Mg^{2+}/Ca^{2+}$-ATPase. While this enzyme has been purified from both aortic muscle of the cow [99] and smooth muscle of the pig antrum [100, 101], it has not been possible to purify it from vascular smooth muscle of the rat. Therefore, the enzyme has not been well characterized in experimental hypertension. On the other hand, $Mg^{2+}/Ca^{2+}$-ATPase isolated from other smooth muscle systems has been shown to be activated by calmodulin; has a requirement for $Mg^{2+}$, $Ca^{2+}$ and ATP; and is similar to membrane associated $Ca^{2+}$-ATPase from other organ systems, i.e. skeletal and cardiac muscle [102]. Therefore, it may be inferred that the enzyme is similar in the various smooth muscle types, but knowledge of potential differences in either its activity or activation characteristics in the setting of elevated arterial pressure does not exist. Another defect in the vascular tissue calmodulin-Ca ATPase system in the SHR is an increase in tissue activator of calmodulin. Huang et al. [103] reported an apparent increased recovery of calmodulin content from cardiac tissue as well as the kidney of the SHR. The biochemical characteristics of the activator remain uncertain, although it does appear to be a lipid and is favorably influenced by dietary $Ca^{2+}$ and increased by NaCl (personal communication). This observation offers a molecular basis for explaining part of dietary calcium's antihypertensive action in the laboratory setting.

The $Na^{+}$-$Ca^{2+}$ exchange carrier may also play a role in the regulation of intracellular $Ca^{2+}$. At least two groups have detected the presence of this carrier in cell membrane enriched fractions of vascular smooth muscle [104, 105]. In the former study, a comparison of $Na^{+}$-$Ca^{2+}$ exchange activity of cell membrane enriched fractions of mesenteric arteries of the SHR and WKY was carried out and no differences were detected.

Besides these transport systems which are directly involved in $Ca^{2+}$ transport, the $Na^{+}$,$K^{+}$-ATPase/sodium pump system may play a role in the regulation of intracellular $Ca^{2+}$ levels by its electrogenic contribution to the membrane potential and thus an indirect effect on potential-operated $Ca^{2+}$ channels [106]. The sodium pump also regulates levels of intracellular sodium and may help set the level of, and interface with, intracellular $Ca^{2+}$ via the $Na^{+}$-$Ca^{2+}$ exchange mechanism discussed above. Several models of experimental hypertension show depressed sodium pump function when assessed indirectly via either $^{86}Rb$ uptake [107] or potassium-induced relaxation of isolated vessels [108]. However, when the number of pump sites in aorta of SHR and WKY was determined using [$^{3}H$]ouabain binding, no differences were detected [109], indicating that the pumps may be different physiologically but perhaps not enzymatically or biochemically.

The $Na^{+}$-$H^{+}$ exchanger is a second transport system that may be linked to $Ca^{2+}$ regulation via alterations in intracellular $Na^{+}$. This carrier has been identified in membrane preparations of vascular smooth muscle [110] and is activated by the diacyl glycerol arm of the phosphatidylinositol pathway [111]. While is it suggested to provide a major $Na^{+}$ influx pathway [112], it has not been studied to date in vascular smooth muscle of the SHR or its normotensive control.

Considering the various systems involved in the regulation of intracellular $Ca^{2+}$ levels, the question remains as to whether intracellular $Ca^{2+}$ concentration is altered under basal or stimulated conditions. Studies using $^{45}Ca$ allow some estimation of influx rates and total exchangeable $Ca^{2+}$ binding sites, but do not allow delineation between bound and free $Ca^{2+}$. An advancement in this area has been the application of the intracellular $Ca^{2+}$ dyes Quin-2, Fura-2, and Indo-1 to both smooth muscle and formed elements. Several studies have examined intracellular $Ca^{2+}$ levels in vascular smooth muscle during hypertension using a $Ca^{2+}$-sensitive dye. Nabika et al. [113] examined monolayers of aortic smooth muscle cells grown on coverslips and found no differences in basal levels of intracellular $Ca^{2+}$ between the SHR and WKY, whereas agonist-induced increases were greater in SHR. In contrast, Sugiyama et al. [114] examined both primary and passaged smooth muscle cells and found that intracellular $Ca^{2+}$ was higher in vascular smooth muscle cells of 12-week-old SHR.

Bukoski et al. [115] reported that resting intracellular-free $Ca^{2+}$ levels are not different in intact mesenteric arteries of SHR compared to WKY. Erne and Hermsmeyer [116] have also reported no differerence in total free [$Ca^{2+}$] values, but have detected a significant difference in the subcellular distribution of free $Ca^{2+}$. The vascular smooth muscle cells of the SHR exhibit greater peripheral subsarcolemmal concentrations of the cation. Isolated renal tubular cells have also been used to determine intracellular free $Ca^{2+}$ values in the SHR [48]. Similar to the results in vascular tissue, no differences were observed between hypertensive and normotensive animals.

*2. Platelets.* Studies of $Ca^{2+}$ metabolism in formed elements of the blood of humans with essential hypertension and SHR have been conducted with the expectation that differences observed in these cell types reflect differences present in vascular smooth muscle cells or that the same (humoral or pharmacologic) factors that induce changes in formed elements are also operative in vascular smooth muscle cells and resistance vessels. Platelets have been most extensively studied, because of the relative ease and quantity in which they are obtained, and their similarity to vascular smooth muscle in terms of second messenger responses [117].

An increase in the intracellular levels of $Ca^{2+}$ in platelets derived from people with essential hypertension using Quin-2 has been reported by several groups [118 – 122] and Fura-2 [123] as an intracellular indicator. A positive relationship between blood pressure and intracellular $Ca^{2+}$ concentration has been demonstrated [118, 121]. Erne et al. [118] reported a fall in intracellular $Ca^{2+}$ when blood pressure was lowered with antihypertensive therapy. This may be interpreted to indicate that either the humoral profile of the plasma compartment was altered to provide for a lowering of intracellular $Ca^{2+}$ in the platelet or that the platelets themselves were affected in a manner parallel to that of the vascular smooth muscle.

In addition to intracellular $Ca^{2+}$ concentration, platelet $Ca^{2+}$-ATPase has been examined in essential hypertension. Overall $Ca^{2+}$-ATPase activity was greater in platelets of hypertensive subjects, while calmodulin stimulated the ATPase to a lesser extent than in controls [124]. While these results do not readily explain the elevated levels of intracellular $Ca^{2+}$ reported in platelets, these investigators suggest that the elevated $Ca^{2+}$-ATPase capacity reflects a negative feedback control mechanism by which the cell protects itself from a $Ca^{2+}$ overload.

*3. Erythrocytes.* Postnov et al. [125] examined $Na^+$ permeability and $Ca^{2+}$ binding capacity or erythrocytes (defined as the pool removable by incubation with EDTA), and found that $Na^+$ flux was elevated while extracellular $Ca^{2+}$ binding capacity was depressed during hypertension. Furthermore, intracellular $Ca^{2+}$ was observed to have an inhibitory action on $Na^+$-$K^+$-ATPase function in red cells in essential hypertension. This has been interpreted to reflect a depressed inner cell membrane binding capacity. In another study, this group [126] re-affirmed the findings of depressed binding of $Ca^{2+}$ to outer membranes of red cell ghosts as well as studying the $Ca^{2+}$-ATPase activity of erythrocytes obtained from humans with essential hypertension. They found that upon depletion of thc preparation of calmodulin, no differences in $Ca^{2+}$-ATPase activity were observed between hypertensive subjects and normotensive controls. Upon re-addition of calmodulin, however, the erythrocyte $Ca^{2+}$-ATPase from hypertensive subjects was stimulated to a lesser degree, while there was no difference in the distribution of calmodulin in red cells of the two groups. Combined with the report of a biochemical characterization of calmodulin isolated from the brains of SHR and WKY which showed no differences in the affinity of the activation protein for $Ca^{2+}$ or in its ability to stimulate phosphodiesterase activity [127], these results indicate that a defect in the enzyme that is specific to the enzyme's capacity to be stimulated by calmodulin may be present in hypertension. Thus, again the basic science literature suggests that some as yet unidentified defect exists in the regulation of the $Ca^{2+}$ pump in animals and humans with essential hypertension. Since the $Ca^{2+}$ pump is regulated by both $Ca^{2+}$ and calmodulin, such a defect would afford a cellular mechanism whereby increasing dietary $Ca^{2+}$ might reverse a cell abnormality associated with high blood pressure.

In a study of $Ca^{2+}$-ATPase activity of red cells of hypertensive and normotensive humans, basal $Ca^{2+}$-ATPase activity, defined as ATPase activity resistant to inhibition by the calmodulin inhibitor trifluoroperazine, was found to be depressed in those with high blood pressure, while maximal stimulated activity was not different [128]. While these data do not appear to agree with those of Postnov et al. [129], a study by Olorunsogo et al. [130] reported that maximum red cell $Ca^{2+}$-ATPase activity was depressed with hypertension, but activation by calmodulin was normal.

*4. Other formed elements.* Intracellular $Ca^{2+}$ levels have been examined in neutrophils by Lew et al. [131] and no differences were observed between normotensive and hypertensive individuals. These authors concluded that not all cell types demonstrate elevated levels of intracellular $Ca^{2+}$ during hypertension. Using SHR lymphocytes, Bruschi et al. [132] observed a higher concentration of free intracellular $Ca^{2+}$ compared with cells derived from controls, but the level of intracellular $Ca^{2+}$ was not influenced by alterations in extracellular $Ca^{2+}$ or by the addition of ouabain or catecholamines. These latter, negative findings suggest that a problem existed with the *in vitro* cell preparation.

*5. Summary of cellular $Ca^{2+}$ metabolism.* Vascular smooth muscle in experimental hypertension may exhibit changes in basic mechanisms of $Ca^{2+}$ regulation. The picture in human vascular tissue is unclear at this time. It may be that changes in the cellular $Ca^{2+}$ metabolism of the formed elements reflect altered physiology of the organism in terms of responses to humoral factors; but the degree to which they reflect similar changes in vascular muscle, particularly in humans, remains to be determined and may be unrelated to the pathogenesis of elevated peripheral vascular resistance and arterial pressure.

Figure 1 depicts the relationships among a defect in cell calcium transport, renal reabsorption of calcium, intestinal calcium absorption, vascular smooth muscle calcium handling, and the development of hypertension. This figure is based on data from studies in both experimental and human studies, and provides a theoretical description of how findings in these two areas may be linked. With reduced dietary calcium intake, hypertensive individuals may experience a simultaneous impairment in their ability to retain calcium. Because of either a genetic defect or an effect of inadequate calcium intake, an abnormality in cell calcium transport may develop which impairs intestinal absorption and renal reabsorption of calcium. This is followed by alterations in biochemical parameters, reducing retained calcium and bone density. Shifts in cell calcium permeability, transport, storage, and release in the vascular smooth muscle could develop which would potentially alter optimal vascular smooth muscle function, resulting in increased peripheral resistance and arterial pressure.

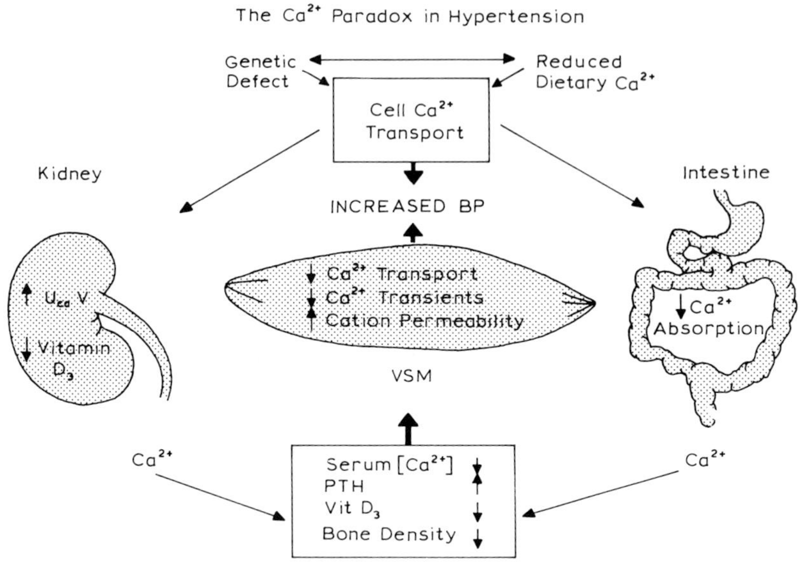


Fig. 1. The theoretical physiologic relationships involved in the development of hypertension. (From Kidney Int 1989;35:717 – 736.)

## IV. Effect of dietary calcium on blood pressure in experimental hypertension

Increased dietary calcium has been demonstrated to have an antihypertensive effect in a number of hypertensive and normotensive rat strains. The hypertensive models include the SHR [39, 40, 54], the salt-sensitive SHR (Taconic Farms) [133], the DOCA-saline rat [134, 135], the Dahl sodium chloride-dependent genetic model [136], the two-kidney, one-clip renovascular model [137], and the stroke-prone SHR [138]. In the normotensive strains, the blood pressure-lowering effect of dietary calcium has been reported in WKY [139], Wistar [140], Fisher 344 [141], and Sprague-Dawley rats [142].

In addition to studies to characterize the blood pressure response to increased calcium, several studies have examined the effects of calcium restriction on blood pressure [40, 139]. Normal calcium composition of a rat diet is 0.5 – 1% by weight. Our early studies showed a reduction in blood pressure on a high (4%) calcium diet [40]. When the diet was reduced to 2% calcium we observed a similar antihypertensive effect [66, 143]. Karanja et al. [143] reported that there is a dose-response curve for dietary calcium in the SHR; a maximum antihypertensive effect was identified at 1.5% calcium with only minimal further reduction in blood pressure at higher levels of calcium. Conversely, an acceleration of hypertension was noted at levels below 0.5%. Similar to observations in humans [32, 144], the relationship between dietary calcium content and blood pressure response is nonlinear in the SHR; in the male

SHR the steepest portion of the curve lies below the 0.5% dietary calcium range [143].

Although Lau et al. [42] have reported a consistent blood pressure-lowering effect in the female SHR, we have not been able to confirm this. Hatton et al. [145] have demonstrated an effect of modifying calcium intake *in utero* and during the first 3 weeks post-partum. These manipulations have produced significant effects on the development of hypertension in the young SHR. Besides the dose of calcium utilized, a time dependency of the calcium antihypertensive effect has been identified. When introduced into the diet of the very young animal, the antihypertensive effects emerge more rapidly. When introduced during adolescence, a longer period (up to 10 weeks) may be necessary before blood pressure reduction is observed.

There appear to be critical nutrient interactions with the calcium effect on blood pressure in the SHR. Sodium restriction impairs the antihypertensive effect of increasing dietary calcium, whereas modest sodium supplementation enhances calcium's antihypertensive action [66, 146]. Of the various calcium salts that have been studied, carbonate salt has been used most commonly; calcium phosphate [140], lactate, gluconate, citrate, and chloride [147] have also been shown to lower blood pressure in experimental models.

In the Dahl sodium chloride-dependent genetic model of hypertension, providing a 2% calcium diet has prevented the rise in blood pressure typically observed in this animal [103]. In the DOCA-saline model of experimental hypertension, supplemental calcium also prevents the expected rise in its blood pressure when exposed to the higher NaCl intake and mineralocorticoid hormone [134, 135]. In the renovascular model, the two-kidney, one-clip hypertensive rat, calcium supplementation of relatively short duration (4 – 6 weeks) has been shown to prevent the rise in blood pressure [137]. Further, the diet reverses a number of the hormonal responses previously characterized in this model. The salt-sensitive SHR (Taconic Farms) does not experience a rise in blood pressure if calcium is added to its diet at the same time the sodium chloride content is increased [133]. Not only is blood pressure regulation maintained normally in this model by supplemental calcium, but central nervous system defects in blood pressure regulation that have previously been reported are altered by this intervention. Recently, Furspan et al. [138] and McCarron and coworkers (unpublished observations) have demonstrated dramatic blood pressure reductions in the stroke-prone SHR fed a calcium-rich diet.

These observations in both hypertensive and normotensive animals whose genetic backgrounds differ and whose primary pathological mechanisms vary greatly suggest a generic action of calcium in lowering blood pressure. All of these models demonstrate an increase in their peripheral vascular resistance. The fact that increased calcium intake lowers blood pressure in each of these models suggests that dietary calcium either modifies circulating factors which control peripheral vascular tone or the vascular smooth muscle cells' response to circulating factors. Long-term effect on cell growth and hypertrophy must also be considered, as well as the possibility that the calcium is correcting a primary defect in intracellular calcium metabolism.

## V. Effect of dietary calcium on blood pressure in human hypertension

The critical test of the hypothesis that calcium metabolism is a factor in hypertension is whether or not changes in dietary calcium intake will influence blood pressure in humans. The clinical relevance of epidemiologic analysis and animal investigations ultimately depends upon demonstration of an antihypertensive effect of calcium in controlled clinical studies. Table 2 summarizes the published trials of calcium supplementation to date. Although a number of these lacked a placebo phase or a control group, 13 included both random allocation and a placebo control. The most common intervention has been 1.0 – 1.5 g/day of calcium supplementation, although from 0.4 to 2.0 g/day has been used. The studies have utilized the calcium salt most frequently, but calcium citrate, gluconate and lactogluconate, yeast, and dietary calcium have also been employed. The trials have ranged from 5 days to one year.

A significant blood pressure reduction was observed in at least a segment of the population in three-quarters of these trials, with no significant blood pressure changes reported in the remainder. Blood pressure reduction with calcium supplementation has ranged from 2 to 10 mmHg. The studies reporting the most convincing blood pressure reduction have included more than 50 subjects overall, and were randomized, placebo-controlled studies. In many of the reports the sample size was insufficient to detect the small blood pressure reductions generally observed with nonpharmacologic interventions.

Duration of the intervention may be critical to determining an effect of calcium on blood pressure. A significant blood pressure reduction was observed in our initial clinical study after 8 weeks of supplementation, but not after 6 weeks; whereas two of the trials reporting no effect [148, 149] were only 4 weeks in length. Although two brief trials (1 – 2 weeks) did report positive results, these reductions were likely detected either because of a higher level of supplementation [150] or more intensive observation within a metabolic ward [151].

Both hypertensive and normotensive populations have demonstrated blood pressure reductions with increased calcium. With one exception [152], studies of hypertensive subjects have chiefly included individuals with borderline-mild hypertension. Not surprisingly, somewhat greater blood pressure reductions have been achieved in hypertensive populations. These studies are noteworthy for the absence of adverse reactions; in particular, there has been no report to date of a subject developing renal calculi during calcium supplementation. Many reports have emphasized the potential benefits of adequate calcium intake for important subpopulations including blacks [153, 154], pregnancy-induced hypertensive subjects [155], and salt-sensitive subjects [156].

It is important to note that while the blood pressure reductions observed in these clinical trials have been modest (3 – 6 mmHg), when projected upon the general population, these changes could represent significant benefits in overall cardiovascular morbidity and mortality [157]. The response to calcium supplementation is Gaussian,

TABLE 2 Clinical trials of calcium supplementation and blood pressure

| Author | Subjects | | | Design | Dose | Significant blood pressure response |
|---|---|---|---|---|---|---|
| | No. | Age (yrs) | Sex | | | |
| Belizan [150] | 57 | 18 – 35 | – | Randomized, placebo | 1 g Ca ($CaCO_3$) × 22 wks | Yes |
| Resnick [161] | 10 | – | – | Uncontrolled | 2 g Ca ($CaCO_3$) × 5 days | Yes |
| Johnson [208] | 95 | 35 – 65 | F | Placebo | 1.5 g Ca ($CaCO_3$, citrate) × 8 wks | Yes |
| McCarron [160] | 80 | 22 – 70 | – | Randomized, crossover, placebo | 1 g Ca ($CaCO_3$, citrate) × 8 wks | Yes |
| Meese [215] | 27 | – | – | Randomized, crossover, placebo | 800 mg Ca ($Ca^{2+}$, citrate) × 8 wks | No |
| Grobbee [162] | 90 | 18 – 27 | – | Randomized, placebo | 1 g Ca ($CaCO_3$) × 12 wks | Yes |
| Luft [151] | 16 | 22 – 56 | – | Randomized, crossover, placebo | 1 g Ca ($CaCO_3$) × 8 days | Yes |
| Tabuchi [152] | 8 | $\bar{x}$ = 73 | – | Placebo | 2 g Ca (gluconate) × 2 wks | Yes |
| Bloomfield [148] | 32 | 18 – 75 | – | Randomized, placebo | 1.5 g Ca ($CaCO_3$) × 4 wks | No |
| Siani [216] | 8 | – | – | Randomized, crossover, placebo | 1 g $CaCO_3$ × 3 wks | No |
| Siani [217] | 15 | – | – | Randomized, crossover | 400 mg vs. 1400 mg dietary Ca × 4 wks | No |
| Lyle [159] | 75 | 19 – 52 | M | Randomized, placebo | 1.5 g Ca ($CaCO_3$) × 12 wks | Yes |
| Strazzullo [164] | 17 | $\bar{x}$ = 43 | M | Randomized, crossover, placebo | 1 g Ca (lactogluconate + carbonate) × 15 wks | Yes |
| Bierenbaum [218] | 200 | 21 – 56 | – | Uncontrolled | 1.4 g Ca as milk × 6 mth | Yes |
| Gilliland [219] | 24 | 57 ± 10 | F | Uncontrolled | 400 mg Ca as $CaCO_3$ × 24 wks | Yes |
| Thomsen [220] | 28 | – | F | Randomized, placebo | 2000 mg Ca × 1 yr | No |
| Vinson [221] | 15 | 19 – 24 | M | Randomized, placebo | 500 mg Ca as Ca gluconate or 500 mg Ca as Ca yeast × 7 wks | Yes |
| Cappuccio [149] | 18 | 28 – 65 | – | Randomized, placebo | 1600 mg/day Ca as Ca lactate glucose × 4 wks | No |
| Van Beresteyn [222] | 58 | 20 – 23 | F | Randomized, placebo | 1500 mg Ca as $CaCO_3$ powder × 6 wks on Ca-restricted diet (500 mg/day) | No |
| Bierenbaum [223] | 50 | 21 – 65 | – | Crossover | 1.15 g dietary calcium | Yes |
| Nowson [224] | 95 | 22 – 77 | MF | Randomized, placebo | 400 or 800 mg Ca as $CaCO_3$ × 8 wks | No |

representing larger changes in blood pressure for some individuals. Similarly, as with most antihypertensive interventions, some individuals are either resistant to the treatment or actually experience a blood pressure rise. The heterogeneous response to calcium supplementation is similar to that observed with sodium restriction and potassium supplementation [158].

## VI. Predictors of a blood pressure response in humans

Various demographic, biochemical, and nutritional parameters have been examined in an effort to identify predictors of blood pressure response to calcium supplementation. While male subjects appear to be slightly more sensitive than females, this difference is not firmly established. In a trial with both black and white subjects, no difference was seen in blood pressure response based upon race [159].

Of the biochemical parameters, serum ionized calcium has not been a predictor of a blood pressure response although in our initial trial those subjects who had the smallest change in ionized calcium had the largest drop in blood pressure [160]. Resnick and Laragh [161] have reported that blood pressure reduction is dependent on renin status, and high renin hypertensive subjects may experience a pressor effect, although this has not been confirmed in other studies.

Grobbee and Hofman [162] reported that subjects below the median for serum total calcium had a greater blood pressure response compared to those above the median. Similarly, subjects in their study who were above the median parathyroid hormone level had greater reductions in blood pressure. Lyle and co-workers [163] also observed this relationship for PTH as well as for serum total calcium values. Strazzullo et al. [164] found that higher urinary calcium excretion at baseline was inversely associated with blood pressure reduction with calcium supplementation. Baseline dietary calcium intake has not been a predictor of blood pressure response in any trials [160, 165, 166].

## VII. Mechanisms of dietary calcium's antihypertensive action

A number of mechanisms have been investigated to determine how dietary calcium affects blood pressure in experimental animals and humans (Fig. 2). The following discussion focuses primarily on the intrinsic properties of the resistance arterioles or circulating factors that are known to modify vascular smooth muscle contractility, and several non-vascular mechanisms that must be considered.

### A. Vascular smooth muscle

On the basis of earlier work of Bohr [167], we initially postulated a membrane-

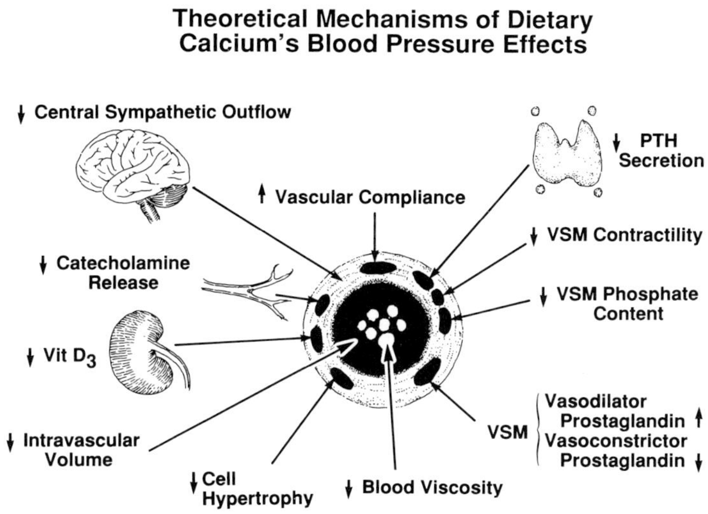


Fig. 2. Potential mechanisms by which altered dietary calcium intake might impair vascular smooth muscle function and arterial pressure. (From Kidney Int 1989;35:717 – 736.)

stabilizing effect of dietary calcium that would reduce vascular sensitivity to circulating vasoconstrictors [168] which has since been tested by Bukoski et al. [44, 169]. No consistent shift has been identified in the sensitivity of either aortic or mesenteric vascular rings to exogenous norepinephrine in animals fed a calcium supplemented diet. We have also tested the hypothesis that dietary calcium impairs pressor responses of intact animals to infusions of norepinephrine and thereby lowers blood pressure. The results indicate that quite the reverse is true. In the SHR, supplementing the diet with calcium produces an increase in the maximal contractility thereby normalizing the previously reported impairment of maximal contractility in this model. Scrogin et al. [170] have reported that while maximal vasoconstrictor response to norepinephrine is not decreased by calcium supplementation, the time to recovery is significantly improved. A membrane effect has been identified by Furspan and Bohr [138] who noted that the inappropriate membrane permeability to $Na^+$ and $K^+$ was reversed by the higher $Ca^{2+}$ diet in the stroke-prone SHR.

Using isolated cultured aortic vascular smooth muscle cells from the WKY and SHR, we have assessed the effect of 7-day exposure to increasing extracellular calcium within the physiologic range on cell $^{45}Ca$ uptake [171]. We have observed that prolonged exposure to higher extracellular calcium produces a greater $^{45}Ca$ uptake of the isolated vascular smooth muscle cells from the SHR, while no effect is observed in the WKY.

Passive properties of the vascular smooth muscle must also be considered. Vascular smooth muscle hypertrophy has long been known to develop in the hypertensive animal in concert with the rise in blood pressure [172]. The SHR's vascular smooth muscle cells proliferate faster than those of WKY. However, there are no data regarding direct effects of modifying calcium intake on cell growth and hypertrophy, although in one study we observed a favorable reduction in cardiac hypertrophy [66].

Passive elastic properties of the vasculature also contribute to blood pressure regulation. As we have reported, vascular aortic rings isolated from the supplemented SHR do not exhibit the typical age-related increase in wall stiffness, and is perhaps an effect of lowered blood pressure [169].

### B. Calcium-regulating hormone

Receptors for both PTH and 1,25$(OH)_2$ vitamin D have now been demonstrated in vascular tissue [173, 174]. Both circulating parathyroid hormone and vitamin D levels may be modified by the changes in dietary calcium. As postulated by Resnick [175] and by Bukoski and McCarron [168], the calcium-regulating hormones must be considered as potentially important mediators of dietary calcium's antihypertensive effect. From current studies we have been able to demonstrate a direct effect on vascular smooth muscle free intracellular $Ca^{2+}$ by both of these calcium-regulating hormones in intact mesenteric resistance arteries. For example, Bukoski et al. [176] have shown that short-term incubation of intact mesenteric resistance vessels with 1,25$(OH)_2$ vitamin $D_3$ increases the $Ca^{2+}$ transient induced by norepinephrine in the SHR, while PTH significantly depresses this parameter. No effects were seen in the WKY. These findings suggest direct effects of the calcium-regulating hormones on $Ca^{2+}$ metabolism of intact resistance vessels. They further suggest that the observed response to the calcium-regulating hormones differs based upon whether the vascular tissue is isolated from the normal or hypertensive animal.

The mechanisms by which 1,25$(OH)_2$ vitamin $D_3$ modifies cell calcium uptake, calcium transients, or vascular reactivity are unknown. In contrast, it is known that PTH can increase cyclic AMP levels of smooth muscle and presumably alters $Ca^{2+}$ metabolism through a cyclic AMP-protein kinase-linked mechanism.

### C. Central nervous system effects

Several lines of evidence suggest that dietary calcium supplementation favorably modifies central nervous system sympathetic outflow. It has been demonstrated by Hatton et al. [117, 178] that both acute and chronic stress-induced elevations in blood pressure were lessened by supplementation of the SHR diet with calcium. Yang et al. [133] have shown that the salt-sensitive SHR which exhibits an altered central nervous system response to sodium chloride loading is protected by calcium supplementation of the diet. Finally, Peuler et al.[136] have demonstrated in the Dahl salt-sensitive animal that sympathetic outflow is favorably modified by calcium supplementation concurrent with the reduction in blood pressure. Baksi [142] has reported that feeding $Ca^{2+}$ reduces central catecholamine levels in the Sprague-Dawley rat.

Hatton and co-workers [179] measured peripheral catecholamine levels in the calcium-loaded SHR and observed that circulating catecholamine levels are, if anything, slightly elevated on the higher calcium diets. This finding must be reconciled with the observation that central nervous system outflow is reduced following dietary calcium supplementation in the SHR and Dahl rat. These investigators suggested that calcium loading affects catecholamine receptor-binding in vascular tissue.

### D. Phosphate depletion

Lau and co-workers [180] have proposed that phosphate depletion accounts for the blood pressure-reducing effects of dietary calcium. Several pieces of evidence argue against this theory. First, at lower levels of supplemental calcium in the range of 2%, changes in serum phosphorus are well within the normal range [66]. Second, the observation that maximal vascular contractility is improved in the vascular tissue of the supplemented hypertensive animal indicates that vascular smooth muscle contraction is not diminished on an increased calcium diet [169]. Third, Bindels et al. [181] have demonstrated that supplementing the SHR's diet with phosphate results in a blood pressure reduction during mid-adolescence. Phosphate metabolism, however, must remain an active area of investigation in efforts to better understand how calcium supplementation lowers blood pressure.

### E. Non-vascular mechanisms

Non-vascular mechanisms must also be considered. First, a reduction in intravascular volume as a consequence of a natriuretic action of calcium supplementation has been proposed based upon the observation of several investigative groups [39, 182]. This hypothesis has been addressed directly in humans by Luft and co-workers [162] who were unable to demonstrate any change in sodium balance in a metabolic study of normal subjects and hypertensive individuals supplemented with calcium for 1 to 2 weeks. Second, Lau et al. [180] have observed that vascular volume is increased in the supplemented SHR whose blood pressure has been reduced. In younger animals fed additional calcium, Hatton et al. [183] found no change in plasma volume. Finally, the most compelling evidence against a natriuretic action are the observations from our laboratory [66] and from that of Hamet et al. [146] which have demonstrated that calcium's antihypertensive action is enhanced by simultaneous sodium chloride supplementation. Collectively, these various observations argue strongly against a change in intravascular volume, and thereby overall sodium balance, being induced by chronic calcium supplementation. Short-term calcium supplementation may facilitate the acute response to a sodium load [39, 156], but this adjustment need not account for the long-term blood pressure changes observed.

Another non-vascular mechanism that might be affected by dietary calcium is change in blood viscosity. Hatton et al. [184] have measured changes in hematocrit that occur with calcium supplementation as an indirect assessment of viscosity. The changes in blood pressure observed with the higher calcium intake are independent of changes in the animal's hematocrit. Thus, it appears that central and direct peripheral mechanisms are involved in the blood pressure reduction noted with calcium supplementation.

## VIII. Potential clinical applications

Dietary calcium's blood pressure-lowering effect may be of particular importance to several subpopulations at risk of developing hypertensive cardiovascular disease. Kurtz and co-workers [185] have demonstrated that sodium chloride-sensitive hypertensive subjects develop increased urinary calcium excretion similar to that observed in the DOCA-saline and Dahl sodium chloride-dependent experimental models [59]. Oshima and colleagues [186] have reported a remarkable relationship between salt sensitivity and an increase in the intracellular concentration of calcium. Their findings provide a subcellular link between salt sensitivity in human hypertension and cellular calcium metabolism. The observation that calcium supplementation will lower blood pressure in various animal models of sodium chloride-related hypertension [134, 136] provides compelling evidence that in the laboratory provision of adequate calcium may afford protection against sodium chloride-induced hypertension. This proposition has recently been tested and confirmed by Saito et al. [156].

Pregnancy-induced hypertension is another clinical problem for which the concepts outlined in this review may have a future application. Several disturbances of calcium metabolism have been identified in human pregnancy [187 – 189], many of which are similar to those observed in essential hypertension. Furthermore, several intervention trials have already demonstrated that during the third trimester of pregnancy, calcium supplementation significantly reduces either blood pressure or the incidence of pregnancy-induced hypertension [189 – 192].

Alcohol-associated hypertension may be another productive area of investigation. Chronic alcohol ingestion induces several alterations in cell calcium homeostasis [193, 194] and ultimately results in significant bone mineral loss [195], the mechanisms of which are unclear. An interaction among alcohol consumption, dietary calcium intake, and blood pressure has been reported in two of the epidemiologic studies noted above [196, 197]. In addition, Criqui et al. [198] have reported that compared to other nutrient-blood pressure relations, the association of dietary calcium to blood pressure was evident only at low levels of alcohol intake, suggesting an effect of alcohol on blood pressure effects of dietary calcium.

Alterations in calcium metabolism may be particularly important for the pathogenesis of hypertension in black subjects [153, 154]. Dietary calcium intake among blacks in this country is significantly less than that observed in whites [199, 200]. One epidemiologic study has demonstrated that after correcting for differences in dietary calcium intake one can account for a large proportion of variation in blood pressure between adolescent white and black females [199]. The sentinel observations of Zemel and co-workers [153, 154] suggest a beneficial effect of calcium intake on blood pressure control and cardiovascular regulation in hypertensive black diabetic patients.

Perhaps the most important application of this hypothesis is the extent to which maintenance of the recommended daily allowance (RDA) for calcium will prevent the blood pressure increase occurring with age in industrialized societies, and the subsequent morbidity and mortality. Based upon one prospective study, it would seem possible to reduce the rise in blood pressure and the prevalence of hypertension that emerges with aging. This may be particularly true in groups with chronic underconsumption of dietary calcium such as women and blacks.

## IX. Summary

Pathologic alterations in calcium metabolism are a factor in blood pressure regulation in some humans and selected experimental models. A consistent nutrient/blood pressure association has been demonstrated in epidemiological studies. An additional lifestyle intervention has been identified that holds the potential to lower blood pressure in a subset of individuals at risk. We now know that calcium-regulating hormones may have important direct cardiovascular actions that, in part, may account for the mechanisms whereby dietary calcium lowers blood pressure in experimental animals and humans. We have also witnessed the development of a new theoretical explanation for sodium-chloride sensitivity from the research in this area. Finally, a potential mechanism(s) has emerged that may provide a pathophysiologic link between hypertension and certain high risk populations.

At present, the primary clinical application of the findings in the area of a relationship between calcium metabolism and the development of blood pressure is clearly related to adequate dietary calcium intake. In patients being treated for mild to moderate hypertension, it seems prudent that their level of dietary calcium intake be assessed. Where appropriate, these patients should be encouraged to maintain calcium intake at the level 800 to 1000 mg/day, the current recommended daily allowance of the National Academy of Science. As the evidence that has accumulated during the past decade suggests, efforts to prevent calcium deficiency rather than attempts to increase dietary calcium to some level above the current RDA, should be a major objective in the treatment of patients with essential hypertension [33, 201], or individuals who are at risk of developing this common medical disorder.

## Acknowledgments

The author's original research cited in this article has been supported by the National Dairy Promotion and Research Board, M.J. Murdock Charitable Trust, American Heart Association and Oregon Affiliate to the American Heart Association, National Dairy Council, National Kidney Foundation; a General Clinical Research Center (GCRC) grant from the U.S. Public Health Service; a Senior Fellowship of the Fogarty International Center of the National Institutes of Health; a GCRC Clinical Associate Physician Award, RR00334 2152; and grant 5R01 HL40005-02 from the National Heart, Lung, and Blood Institute. The author is indebted to his colleagues in the Division of Nephrology and Hypertension at the Oregon Health Sciences University, including, Richard D. Bukoski, Ph.D., R. Kent Hermsmeyer, Ph.D., Eric W. Young, M.D., Cynthia D. Morris, Ph.D., Daniel C, Hatton, Ph.D., Njeri Karanja, Ph.D., and William M. Bennett, M.D., for collaboration in and support of the original research cited; and to Molly Reusser for editorial expertise in the preparation of this chapter.


## References


1 McCarron DA, Pingree PA, Rubin RJ, Gaucher SM, Molitch M, Krutzik S. Enhanced parathyroid function in essential hypertension: a homeostatic response to a urinary calcium leak. Hypertension 1980;2:162 – 168.

2 Kolata G. Does lack of calcium cause hypertension? Several recent studies link calcium and high blood pressure but the medical community is divided on how to interpret them. Science 1984;225:705 – 706.

3 McCarron DA. Is calcium more important than sodium in the pathogenesis of essential hypertension? Hypertension 1985;7:607 – 627.

4 McCarron DA. Calcium metabolism and hypertension. Kidney Int 1989;35:717 – 736.

5 Morris CD, Hatton DC, Young EW, Karanja N, McCarron Da. Calcium nutrition and metabolism and blood pressure control. In: Rapaport E, ed. Cardiology Update. New York: Elsevier, 1990;175 – 211.

6 Strazzullo P, Nunziata V, Cirillo M, et al. Abnormalities of calcium metabolism in essential hypertension. Clin Sci 1983;65:137 – 141.

7 Kesteloot H, Geboers J. Calcium and blood pressure. Lancet 1982;i:813 – 815.

8 Kesteloot H, Joossens JV. Relationship of dietary sodium potassium, calcium, and magnesium, with blood pressure: Belgian Interuniversity Research on Nutrition and Health. Hypertension 1988;12:594 – 599.

9 Wessels F, Hoffmann D, Wagner H, Zumkley H. Influence of family history of hypertension on the relationships between blood pressure, body weight, electrolyte metabolism, renin, prolactin and parathormone. Clin Sci 1981;61:359s – 369s.

10 Hvarfner A, Bergstrom R, Morlin C, Wide L, Ljunghall S. Relationships between calcium metabolic indices and blood pressure in patients with essential hypertension as compared with a healthy population. J Hypertens 1987;5:451 – 456.

11 Grobbee DE, Hackeng WHL, Birkenhager JC, Hofman A. Intact parathyroid hormone (I-84) in primary hypertension. Clin Exp Hypertens 1986;A8:299 – 308.

12 Grobbee DE, Hackeng WHL, Birkenhager JC, Hofman A. Raised plasma intact parathyroid hormone concentrations in young people with mildly raised blood pressure. Br Med J 1988;296: 814 – 816.

13 Zachariah PK, Schwartz GL, Strong CG, Ritter SG. Parathyroid hormone and calcium: a relationship in hypertension. Am J Hypertens 1988;1:79S – 82S.

14 Ellison DH, Shneidman R, Morris C, McCarron DA. Effects of calcium infusion on blood pressure in hypertensive and normotensive humans. Hypertension 1986;8:497 – 505.

15 Kotchen TA, Kotchen JM, Guthrie GP, McKean HE. Serum calcium and hypertension. N Engl J Med 1982;307:1525 – 1525.

16 McCarron DA. Low serum concentrations of ionized calcium in patients with hypertension. N Engl J Med 1982;307:226 – 228.

17 Folsom AR, Smith CL, Prineas RJ, Grimm RH Jr. Serum calcium fractions in essential hypertensive and matched normotensive subjects. Hypertension 1986;8:11 – 15.

18 Hvarfner A, Ljunghall S, Morlin C, Wide L. Calcium metabolism and arterial blood pressure in a healthy population sample and in hypertensive men. Am J Nephrol 1986;6(Suppl. 1):14 – 15.

19 Alpert BS, Murphy JK, Stapleton FB, Biddle JB, Willey ES, Sexton JE. Calcium and blood pressure: a study of healthy adolescents. Circulation 1987;76(Suppl. IV):IV-360

20 Zozaya JLG, Viloria MP, Castro A. The relationship between low plasma renin activity, low serum ionic calcium, and elevated systolic arterial tension in the normotensive elderly. Am J Hypertens 1988;1:393 – 396.

21 Resnick LM, Muller FB, Laragh JH. Calcium regulating hormones in essential hypertension. Relation to plasma renin activity and sodium metabolism. Ann Intern Med 1986;105:649 – 654.

22 Strazzullo P, Galletti F, Cirillo M, et al. Altered extracellular calcium homeostasis in essential hypertension: a consequence of abnormal cell calcium handling. Clin Sci 1986;71:239 – 244.

23 Kesteloot H, Van Schaftingen E, Van Hoof R, Geboers J. Relationship between ionized serum calcium and blood pressure. Circulation 1983;68(Suppl. III):III-90.

24 Buckley BM, Smith SC, Beevers M, Beevers DG, McKiernan MJ. Lack of evidence of low ionized calcium levels in systemic hypertension. Am J Cardiol 1987;59:878 – 880.

25 Haller H, Ludersdorf M, Lenz T, Philipp T, Distler A. Is there a correlation between extracellular and intracellular calcium disturbances in essential hypertension? Clin Exp Hypertens 1987;A9:183.

26 Shore AC, Booker J, Sagnella GA, Markandu ND, MacGregor GA. Serum ionized calcium and pH: effects of blood storage, some physiological influences and a comparison between normotensive and hypertensive subjects. J Hypertens 1987;5:499 – 505.

27 Cooper RS, Shamsi N. Ionized serum calcium in black hypertensives: absence of a relationship with blood pressure. J Clin Hypertens 1987;3:514 – 519.

28 Fogh-Andersen N, Hedegaard L, Thode J, Siggaard-Andersen O. Sex-dependent relation between ionized calcium in serum and blood pressure. Clin Chem 1984;30:116 – 118.

29 Tillman DM, Semple PF. Calcium and magnesium in essential hypertension. Clin Sci 1988;75:395 – 402.

30 Rosenthal FD, Roy S. Hypertension and hyperparathyroidism. Br Med J 1972;4:396 – 397.

31 Sowers MR, Wallace RB, Lemke JH. The association of intakes of vitamin D calcium with blood pressure among women. Am J Clin Nutr 1985;42:135 – 142.

32 McCarron DA, Morris CD, Cole C. Dietary calcium in human hypertension. Science 1982;217:267 – 269.

33 McCarron DA, Morris CD, Henry HJ, Stanton JL. Blood pressure and nutrient intake in the United States. Science 1984;224:1392 – 1398.

34 Gruchow HW, Sobocinski KA, Barboriak JJ. Threshold effects of dietary calcium on blood pressure. J Hypertens 1986;4(Suppl. 5):s355 – s357.

35 Joffres MR, Reed DM, Yano K. Relationship of magnesium intake and other dietary factors to blood pressure: the Honolulu Heart Study. Am J Clin Nutr 1987;45:469 – 475.

36 Witteman JCM, Willett WC, Stampfer MJ, et al. Dietary calcium and magnesium and hypertension: a prospective study. Circulation 1987;76(Suppl. IV):IV-35.

37 Wright GL, Rankin GO. Concentrations of ionic and total calcium in plasma of four models of

hypertension. Am J Physiol 1982;243:H365 – H370.
38 Bindels RJM, Van Den Broeck LAM, Jongen MJM, Hackeng WHL, Lowik CWGM, Van Os CH. Increased plasma calcitonin levels in young spontaneously hypertensive rats: role in disturbed phosphate homeostasis. Pflügers Arch 1987;408:395 – 400.
39 Stern N, Lee DBN, Silis V, et al. Effects of high calcium intake on blood pressure and calcium metabolism in young SHR. Hypertension 1984;6: 639 – 646.
40 McCarron DA, Yung NN, Ugoretz BA, Krutzik S. Disturbances of calcium metabolism in the spontaneously hypertensive rat. Hypertension 1981;3(Suppl. I):I162 – I167.
41 Wright GL, Toraason MA, Barbe JS, Crouse W. The concentration of ionic and total calcium in plasma of the spontaneously hypertensive rat. Can J Physiol Pharmacol 1980;58:1494 – 1499.
42 Lau K, Zikos D, Spirnak J, Eby B. Evidence for an intestinal mechanism in hypercalciuria of spontaneously hypertensive rats. Am J Physiol 1984;247:E625 – E633.
43 Lau K, Langman CB, Gafter U, Dudeja PK, Brasitus TA. Increased calcium absorption in prehypertensive spontaneously hypertensive rats. Role of serum 1,25-dihydroxyvitamin $D_3$ levels and intestinal brush border membrane fluidity, J Clin Invest 1986;78:1083 – 1090.
44 Bukoski RD, Xue H, McCarron DA. Mesenteric artery contractile properties during dietary calcium manipulation in spontaneously hypertensive and Wistar Kyoto normotensive rats. Am J Hypertens 1989;2:440 – 448.
45 Resnick LM, Laragh JH, Sealy JE, Alderman MH. Divalent cations in essential hypertension. Relations between serum ionized calcium, magnesium, and plasma renin activity. N Engl J Med 1983;309:888 – 891.
46 Resnick LM, Laragh JH. Calcium metabolism and parathyroid function in primary aldosteronism. Am J Med 1985;78:385 – 390.
47 Young EW, Hsu CH, Patel S, Simpson RU, Komanicky P. Metabolic degradation and synthesis of calcitriol in spontaneously hypertensive rat. Am J Physiol 1987;252:E778 – E782.
48 Merke J, Lucas PA, Szabo A, et al. Hyperparathyroidism and abnormal calcitriol metabolism in the spontaneously hypertensive rat. Hypertension 1989;13:233 – 242.
49 Hsu CH, Yang C-S, Patel SR, Stevens MG. Calcium and vitamin D metabolism in spontaneously hypertensive rats. Am J Physiol 1987;253:F712 – F718.
50 Hsu CH, Chen P-S, Smith DE, Yang C-S. Pathogenesis of hypercalciuria in spontaneously hypertensive rats. Miner Electrol Metab 1986;12:130 – 141.
51 Young EW, Patel SR, Hsu CH. Plasma $1,25(OH)_2D_3$ response to parathyroid hormone, cyclic adenosine monophosphate, and phosphorus depletion in the spontaneously hypertensive rat. J Lab Clin Med 1986;108:562 – 566.
52 Hsu CH, Patel S, Young EW. Calcemic response to parathyroid hormone in spontaneously hypertensive rats: role of calcitriol. J Lab Clin Med 1987;110:682 – 689.
53 Umemura S, Smyth D, Pettinger W. Defective renal adenylate cyclase response to prostaglandin E2 in spontaneously hypertensive rats. Kidney Int 1984;25:338.
54 Ayachi S. Increased dietary calcium lowers blood pressure in the spontaneously hypertensive rat. Metabolism 1979;28:1234 – 1238.
55 Hsu CH, Chen PS, Caldwell RM. Renal phosphate excretion in spontaneously hypertensive and normotensive Wistar Kytoto rats. Kidney Int 1984;25:789 – 795.
56 Young E, Martin AS, Metz J, Walczyk M, McCarron D. Urinary calcium excretion in the adult spontaneously hypertensive rat (abstract). Sixth International Symposium on SHR and Related Studies, Iowa City IA, May 1989.
57 Coe FL, Favusm MJ. Disorders of stone formation. In: Brenner BM, Rector FC., eds. The Kidney. Philadelphia: Ardmore Medical Books, 1986;1403 – 1422.
58 Kurtz TW, Morris RC Jr. Dietary chloride as a determinant of disordered calcium metabolism in salt-dependent hypertension. Life Sci 1985;36:921 – 929.
59 Umemura S, Smyth DD, Nicar M, Rapp JP, Pettinger WA. Altered calcium homeostasis in Dahl

hypertensive rats: physiological and biochemical studies. J Hypertens 1986;4:19 – 26.

60 Cirillo M, Galletti F, Corrado MF, Strazzullo P. Disturbances of renal and erythrocyte calcium handling in rats in of the Milan hypertensive strain. J Hypertens 1986;4:443 – 449.

61 Umemura S, Smyth DD, Pettinger WA. Renal adenylate cyclase in Dahl and DOC-Na hypertensive rats: defective response to parathyroid hormone with calcium leak. J Hypertens 1986;4(Suppl. 3):s291 – s293.

62 Bianchi G, Ferrari P, Salvati P, et al. A renal abnormality in the Milan hypertensive strain of rats and in humans predisposed to essential hypertension. J Hypertens 1986;4(Suppl. 3):s33 – s36.

63 Toraason MA, Wright GL. Transport of calcium by duodenum of spontaneously hypertensive rat. Am J Physiol 1981;241:G344 – G347.

64 Schedl HP, Miller DL, Pape JM, Horst RL, Wilson HD. Calcium and sodium transport and vitamin D metabolism in the spontaneously hypertensive rat. J Clin Invest 1984;73:980 – 986.

65 Schedl HP, Wilson HD, Horst RL. Calcium transport and vitamin D in three breeds of spontaneously hypertensive rats. Hypertension 1988;12:310 – 316.

66 McCarron DA, Lucas PA, Shneidman RJ, Lacour B, Drüeke T. Blood pressure development of the spontaneously hypertensive rat after concurrent manipulations of dietary $Ca^{2+}$ and $Na^{+}$: relation to intestinal $Ca^{2+}$ fluxes. J Clin Invest 1985;76:1147 – 1154.

67 Lucas PA, Brown RC, Drüeke T, Lacour B, Metz JA, McCarron DA. Abnormal vitamin D metabolism, intestinal calcium transport, and bone calcium status in the spontaneously hypertensive rat compared with its genetic control. J Clin Invest 1986;78:221 – 227.

68 Gafter U, Kathpalia S, Zikos D, Lau K. Ca fluxes across duodenum and colon of spontaneously hypertensive rats: effect of $1,25(OH)_2D_3$. Am J Physiol 1986;251:F278 – F282.

69 Roullet CM, Young EW, Roullet J-B, Drüeke T, McCarron DA. Calcium uptake by duodenal enterocytes isolated from young and mature SHR and WKY rats. Am J Physiol 1989;257:F574 – F579.

70 Lucas PA, Roullet CM, Lacour B, Dang P, McCarron DA, Drüeke T. Decreased duodenal enterocyte calcium flux rates in the spontaneously hypertensive rat. Am J Hypertens 1989;2:86 – 92.

71 Drüeke T, Nabarra B, Ben Nasr L, Thomasset M, Lacour B, McCarron DA. Ultrastructural and functional abnormalities of intestinal and renal epithelium in the spontaneously hypertensive rat (SHR). Am J Hypertens 1989;2:27A.

72 Metz JA, Karanja N, McCarron DA. Bone density in two hypertensive strains: effects of dietary sodium. Clin Res 1988;36:139A.

73 Izawa Y, Sagara K, Kadota T, Makita T. Bone disorders in spontaneously hypertensive rat. Calcif Tissue Int 1985;37:605 – 607.

74 Yamori Y, Fukuda S, Tsuchikura S, Ikeda K, Nara Y, Horie R, Stroke-prone SHR (SHRSP) as a model for osteoporosis (abstract). Sixth International Symposium on SHR and Related Studies, Iowa City IA, May 1989.

75 Kawashima H. Altered vitamin D metabolism in the kidney of the spontaneously hypertensive rat. Biochem J 1986;237:893 – 897.

76 Schedl HP, Miller DL, Horst RL, Wilson, HD, Natarajan K, Conway T. Intestinal calcium transport in the spontaneously hypertensive rat: response to calcium depletion. Am J Physiol 1986;250:G412 – G419.

77 Merke J, Slotkowski A, Mann H, Lucas PH, Drüeke T, Ritz E. Abnormal $1,25(OH)_2D_3$ receptor status in genetically hypertensive rats. Kidney Int 1987;31:303.

78 Kurtz TW, Portale AA, Morris RC Jr. Evidence for a difference in vitamin D metabolism between spontaneously hypertensive and Wistar-Kyoto rats. Hypertension 1986;8:1015 – 1020.

79 Hsu CH, Yang C-S, Patel SR, Stevens MG. Calcium and vitamin D metabolism in spontaneously hypertensive rats. Am J Physiol 1987;253:F712 – F718.

80 Horiuchi N, Suda T, Takahashi H, Shimazawa E, Ogata E. In vivo evidence for the intermediary role of 3′,5′-cyclic AMP in parathyroid hormone-induced stimulation of 1a,25-dihydroxyvitamin $D_3$ synthesis in rats. Endocrinology 1977;101:969 – 974.

81 Lucas PA, Lacour B, McCarron DA, Drüeke T. Disturbances of acid-base balance in the young spontaneously hypertensive rat. Clin Sci 1987;73:211 – 215.

82 Eby B, Salvi D, Lau K. Pathophysiology and consequence of reduced $PO_4$ excretion in the spontaneously hypertensive rat. Proc First Ann Meet Am Soc Hypertens 1986;29A.

83 Jacobs WR, Brazy PC, Mandel LJ. Fura 2 measurements of intracellular free calcium in renal cortical tubules from SHR and WKY rats. Kidney Int 1987;31:350.

84 Llibre J, LaPointe MS, Batlle DC. Free cytosolic calcium in renal proximal tubules from the spontaneously hypertensive rat. Hypertension 1988;12:399 – 404.

85 Gafter U, Eby B, Martin C, Lau K. Response of spontaneously hypertensive rats to $1,25(OH)_2D_3$ in vivo. Kidney Int 1986;30:497 – 512.

86 Bhalla RC, Webb RC, Singh D, Ashley T, Brock T. Calcium fluxes, calcium binding, and adenosine cyclic 3′5′-monophosphate-dependent protein kinase activity in the aorta of spontaneously hypertensive and Kyoto Wistar normotensive rats. Molec Pharmacol 1978;14:468 – 477.

87 Zsoter TT, Wolchinsky C, Henein NF, Ho LC. Calcium kinetics in the aorta of spontaneously hypertensive rats. Cardiovasc Res 1977;11:353 – 357.

88 Shibata S, Kuchii M, Taniguchi T. Calcium flux and binding in the aortic smooth muscle from the spontaneously hypertensive rat. Blood Vess 1975;12:279 – 289.

89 Cauvin C, Hwang O, Yamamoto M, Van Breemen C. Effects of dihydropyridines on tension and calcium-45 influx in isolated mesenteric resistance vessels from spontaneously hypertensive and normotensive rats. Am J Cardiol 1987;59:116B – 122B.

90 Mulvany MJ, Nyborg N. An increased calcium sensitivity of mesenteric resistance vessels in young and adult spontaneously hypertensive rats. Br J Pharmacol 1980;71:585 – 596.

91 Braunwald E. Mechanism of action of calcium channel blocking agents. N Engl J Med 1982;307:1618 – 1627.

92 Buhler FR, Hulthen UL, Kiowski W, Muller FB, Bolli P. The place of the calcium antagonist verapamil in antihypertensive therapy. J Cardiovasc Pharmacol 1982;4:s350 – s357.

93 Robinson BF, Dobbs RJ, Bayley S. Response of forearm resistance vessels to verapamil and sodium nitroprusside in normotensive and hypertensive men: evidence for a functional abnormality of vascular smooth muscle in primary hypertension. Clin Sci 1982;63:33 – 42.

94 Rusch NJ, Hermsmeyer RK. Calcium currents are altered on the vascular cell membrane of spontaneously hypertensive rats. Circ Res 1988;63:997 – 1002.

95 Aoki K, Yamashita K, Tomita N, Tazumi K, Hotta K. ATPase activity and $Ca^{++}$ binding ability of subcellular membrane of arterial smooth muscle in spontaneously hypertensive rat. Jpn Heart J 1974;15:180 – 181.

96 Webb RC, Bhalla RC. Altered calcium sequestration by subcellular fractions of vascular smooth muscle from spontaneously hypertensive rats. J Mol Cell Cardiol 1976;8:651 – 661.

97 Kwan C-Y, Belbeck L, Daniel EE. Abnormal biochemistry of vascular smooth muscle plasma membrane isolated from hypertensive rats. Mol Pharmacol 1980;17:137 – 140.

98 Kwan C-Y, Daniel EE. Arterial muscle membrane abnormalities of hydralazine-treated spontaneously hypertension rats. Eur J Pharmacol 1987;82:187 – 190.

99 Chiesi M, Gasser J, Carafoli E. Properties of the Ca-pumping ATPase of sarcoplasmic reticulum from vascular smooth muscle. Biochem Biophys Res Commun 1984;124:797 – 806.

100 Wuytack F, Raeymaekers L, Verbist J, De Smedt H, Casteels R. Evidence for the presence in smooth muscle of two types of $Ca^{2+}$-transport ATPase. Biochem J 1984;224:445 – 451.

101 Wuytack F, Casteels R. Demonstration of a ($Ca^{2+}$ = $Mg^{2+}$) -ATPase activity probably related to $Ca^{2+}$ transport in the microsomal fraction of porcine coronary artery smooth muscle. Biochim Biophys Acta 1980;595:257 – 263.

102 Carafoli E. Calcium-transporting systems of plasma membranes, with special attention to their regulation. Adv Cyclic Nucl Protein Phosph Res 1984;17:534 – 549.

103 Huang S-L, Wen YI, Kupranycz DB, et al. Abnormality of calmodulin activity in hypertension.

Evidence of the presence of an activator. J Clin Invest 1988;82:276 – 281.
104 Matlib MA, Schwartz A, Yamori Y. A $Na^+$-$Ca^{2+}$ exchange process in isolated sarcolemmal membranes of mesenteric arteries from WKY and SHR rats. Am J Physiol 1985;249:C166 – C172.
105 Daniel EE, Kwan CY. Control of contraction of vascular muscle — relation to hypertension. Trends Pharmacol Sci 1981;2:207 – 223.
106 Fleming WW. The electrogenic $Na^+$, $K^+$-pump in smooth muscle: physiologic and pharmacologic significance. Ann Rev Pharmacol Toxicol 1980;20:129 – 149.
107 Overbeck HW, Pamnani MB, Akera T, Brody TM, Haddy FJ. Depressed function of a ouabain-sensitive sodium-potassium pump in blood vessels from renal hypertensive dogs. Circ Res 1976;38(Suppl II):II-48 – II-52.
108 Webb RC, Bohr DF. Potassium relaxation of vascular smooth muscle from spontaneously hypertensive rats. Blood Vess 1979;16:71 – 79.
109 Wong SK, Westfall DP, Menear D, Fleming WW. Sodium-potassium pump sites, as assessed by [$^3$H]-ouabain binding, in aorta and caudal artery of normotensive and spontaneously hypertensive rats. Blood Vess 1984;21:211 – 222.
110 Kahn AM, Shelat H, Allen JC. $Na^+$-$K^+$ exchange is present in sarcolemmal vesicles from dog superior mesenteric artery. Am J Physiol 1986;250:H313 – H319.
111 Williamson JR. Inositol lipid metabolism and intracellular signaling mechanisms. News Physiol Sci 1986;1:72 – 76.
112 Little PJ, Cragoe EJ Jr, Bobik A. Na-H exchange is a major pathway for Na influx in rat vascular smooth muscle. Am J Physiol 1986;251:C707 – C712.
113 Nabika T, Velletri PA, Beaven MA, Endo J, Lovenberg W. Vasopressin induced calcium increases in smooth muscle cells from spontaneously hypertensive rats. Life Sci 1985;37:579 – 584.
114 Sugiyama T, Yoshizumi M, Takaku F, et al. The elevation of the cytoplasm calcium ions in vascular smooth muscle cells in SHR — measurement of the free calcium ions in single living cells by laser microfluorospectrometry. Biochem Biophys Res Commun 1986;141:340 – 345.
115 Bukoski RD, Dewan P, McCarron DA. Intracellular $Ca^{2+}$ in cultured aortic myocytes and mesenteric resistance vessels of spontaneously hypertensive and Wistar Kyoto rats. FASEB J 1988;2:A503.
116 Erne P, Hermsmeyer K. Intracellular vascular muscle $Ca^{2+}$ modulation in SHR/WKY hypertension. Hypertension 1989;14:145 – 151.
117 Erne P, Resink TJ, Burgisser E, Buhler FR. Platelets and hypertension. J Cardiovasc Pharmacol 1985;7(Suppl. 6):S103 – S108.
118 Erne P, Bolli P, Burgisser E, Buhler FR. Correlation of platelet calcium with blood pressure: effect of antihypertensive therapy. N Engl J Med 1984;310:1084 – 1088.
119 Bruschi G, Bruschi ME, Caroppo M, Orlandini G, Spaggiari M, Cavatorta A. Cytoplasmic free [$Ca^{2+}$] is increased in the platelets of spontaneously hypertensive rats and essential hypertensive patients. Clin Sci 1985;68:179 – 184.
120 Le Quang Sang KH, Benlian P, Duval C, Montenay-Garestier T, Meyer P, Devynck M-A. Platelet cytosolic-free calcium concentration in primary hypertension. J Hypertens 1985;3:539.
121 Le Quan Sang KH, Devynck M-A. Increased platelet cytosolic free calcium concentratioin in essential hypertension. J Hypertens 1986;4:567 – 574.
122 Lechi A, Lechi C, Bonadonna G, et al. Increased basal and thrombin-induced free calcium in platelets of essential hypertensive patients. Hypertension 1987;9:230 – 235.
123 Cooper RS, Shamsi N, Katz S. Intracellular calcium and sodium in hypertensive patients. Hypertension 1987;9:224 – 229.
124 Resink TJ. Tkachuk VA, Erne P, Buhler FR. Platelet membrane calmodulin-stimulated calcium-adenosine triphosphatase. Altered activity in essential hypertension. Hypertension 1986; 8:159 – 166.
125 Postnov YV, Orlov SN, Shevchenko A, Adler AM. Altered sodium permeability, calcium binding and Na-K-ATPase activity in the red blood cell membrane in essential hypertension. Pflügers Arch 1977; 371:263 – 369.

126 Postnov YV, Orlov SN, Pokudin NI. Decrease of calcium binding by the red blood cell membrane in spontaneously hypertensive rats and in essential hypertension. Pflügers Arch 1979;379:191 – 195.
127 Pokudin NI, Orlov SN, Ryashsky GG, Menshikov NY, Tkachuk VA, Postnov YV. Isolation and characteristics of calmodulin from the brain of rats with spontaneous genetic hypertension. Kardiologiia 1985;25:72 – 77.
128 Vincenzi FF, Morris CD, Kinsel LB, Kenny M, McCarron DA. Decreased in vitro $Ca^{2+}$ ATPase activity in red blood cells of hypertensive subjects. Hypertension 1986;8:1058 – 1066.
129 Postnov YV, Orlov SN, Reznikova MB, Rjazhsky GG, Pokudin NI. Calmodulin distribution and $Ca^{2+}$ transport in the erythrocytes of patients with essential hypertension. Clin Sci 1984;66:459 – 463.
130 Olorunsogo OO, Okudolo BE, Lawal SOA, Falase AO. Erythrocyte membrane $Ca^{2+}$ pumping ATPase of hypertensive humans: reduced stimulation by calmodulin. Biosci Rep 1985;5:525 – 531.
131 Lew PD, Favre L, Waldvogel FA, Vallotton MB. Cytosolic free calcium and intracellular calcium stores in neutrophils from hypertensive subjects. Clin Sci 1985;69:227 – 330.
132 Bruschi G, Bruschi ME, Caroppo M, Orlandini G, Pavarani C, Cavatorta A. Intracellular free $Ca^{2+}$ in circulating lymphocytes of spontaneously hypertensive rats. Life Sci 1984;35:535 – 542.
133 Yang R-H, Jin H, Chen Y-F, Oparil S, Wyss JM. Dietary $Ca^{2+}$ supplementation prevents the exaggerated responsiveness of anterior hypothalamic $\alpha_2$-adrenoceptors in NaCl-loaded spontaneously hypertensive rats. J Cardiovasc Pharmacol 1989;13:162 – 167.
134 Berthelot A, Gairard A. Parathyroid hormone- and deoxycorticosterone acetate-induced hypertension in the rat. Clin Sci 1980;0:365 – 371.
135 Kurtz TW, Morris RC Jr. Attenuation of deoxycorticosterone-induced hypertension by supplemental dietary calcium. J Hypertens 1986;4(Suppl. 5):s129 – s131.
136 Peuler JD, Morgan DA, Mark AL. High calcium diet reduces blood pressure in Dahl salt-sensitive rats by neural mechanisms. Hypertension 1987;9(Suppl. III):159:165.
137 Kageyama Y, Suzuki H, Arima K, Saruta T. Oral calcium treatment lowers blood pressure in renovascular hypertensive rats by suppressing the renin-angiotensin system. Hypertension 1987;10:375 – 382.
138 Furspan PB, Rinaldi GJ, Hoffman K, Bohr DF. Dietary calcium and cell membrane abnormality in genetic hypertension. Hypertension 1989;13:727 – 730.
139 McCarron DA. Blood pressure and calcium balance in the Wistar-Kyoto rat. Life Sci 1982;30:683 – 689.
140 Brommage R, Thomas D, Brady R, Lau K. Effects of dietary Ca deprivation on Ca absorption and serum $1,25(OH)_2D_3$ levels in young spontaneously hypertensive rats (SHR): evidence for deranged regulation of vitamin D metabolism. Clin Res 1986;34:541A.
141 Huie PE, Hatton DC, Muntzel MS, Metz JA, McCarron DA. Genetic variability in response to dietary calcium. Life Sci 1987;41:2185 – 2193.
142 Baksi N. Blood pressure and hypothalamic norepinephrine and dopamine in calcium-deficient rats. Am J Hypertens 1989;2:462 – 464.
143 Karanja N, Metz JA, Mercer LP, McCarron DA. Analysis of BP response and $Ca^{2+}$ metabolism using the saturation kinetics model. Am J Physiol 1987;253:R501 – R508.
144 Kok FJ, Vandenbroucke JP, Van Der Heide-Wessel C, Van Der Heide RM. Dietary sodium, calcium, and potassium, and blood pressure. Am J Epidemiol 1986;123:1043 – 1048.
145 Hatton DC, Huie PS, Muntzel MS, Metz JA, Karanja N, McCarron DA. Blood pressure development and serum calcium in suckling spontaneously hypertensive rat pups: effects of maternal dietary calcium. J Hypertens 1986;4(Suppl. 3):s465 – s467.
146 Hamet P, Skuherska R, Cherkaouil, Pang SC, Amer V, Tremblay J. Calcium levels and platelet responsiveness in spontaneously hypertensive rats on high calcium diet. J Hypertens 1986;4(Suppl. 6):S176.
147 Kurtz TW, Morris RC Jr. Dietary chloride and bicarbonate as determinants of desoxycorticosterone

hypertension. J Hypertens 1984;2(Suppl. 3):371 – 373.

148 Bloomfield RL, Young LD, Zurek G, Felts JH, Straw MK. Effects of oral calcium carbonate on blood pressure in subjects with mildly elevated arterial pressure. J Hypertens 1986;4(Suppl. 5):s351 – s354.

149 Cappuccio FP, Markandu ND, Singer DRJ, Smith SJ, Shore AC, MacGregor GA. Does oral calcium supplementation lower high blood pressure? A double blind study. J Hypertens 1987;5:67 – 71.

150 Belizan JM, Villar J, Pineda O, et al. Reduction of blood pressure with calcium supplementation in young adults. J Am Med Assoc 1983;249:1161 – 1166.

151 Luft FC, Aronoff GR, Sloan RS, Fineberg NS, Weinberger MH. Short-term augmented calcium intake has no effect on sodium homeostasis. Clin Pharmacol Ther 1986;39:414 – 419.

152 Tabuchi Y, Ogihara T, Hashizume K, Saito H, Kumahara Y. Hypotensive effect of long-term oral calcium supplementation in elderly patients with essential hypertension. J Clin Hypertens 1986;3:254 – 262.

153 Zemel MB, Gualdoni SM, Sowers JR. Reductions in total and extracellular water associated with calcium-induced natriuresis and the antihypertensive effect of calcium in blacks. Am J Hypertens 1988;1:70 – 72.

154 Zemel MB, Kraniak J, Standley PR, Sowers JR. Erythrocyte cation metabolism in salt-sensitive hypertensive blacks as affected by dietary sodium and calcium. Am J Hypertens 1988;1:386 – 392.

155 Belizan JM, Villar J, Zalzar A, Rojas L, Chan D, Bryce GF. Preliminary evidence of the effect of calcium supplementation on blood pressure in normal pregnant women. Am J Obstet Gynecol 1983;146:175 – 180.

156 Saito K, Sano H, Furata Y, Fukuzaki H. Effect of oral calcium on blood pressure response in salt-loaded borderline hypertensive patients. Hypertension 1989;13:219 – 226.

157 Blackshear JL, Garnic D, Williams GH, Harrington DP, Hollenberg NK. Exaggerated renal vasodilator response to calcium entry blockade in first-degree relatives of essential hypertensive subjects. Hypertension 1987;9:384 – 389.

158 Luft FC, Miller JZ, Lyle RM, et al. The effect of dietary interventions to reduce blood pressure in normal man. J Am Coll Nutr 1989;8:495 – 503.

159 Lyle RM, Melby CL, Hyner GC, Edmondson JW, Miller JZ, Weinberger MH. Blood pressure and metabolic effects of calcium supplementation in normotensive white and black men. J Am Med Assoc 1987;257:1772 – 1776.

160 McCarron DA, Morris CD. Blood pressure response to oral calcium in persons with mild to moderate hypertension. Ann Intern Med 1985;103:825 – 831.

161 Resnick LM, Laragh JH. The hypotensive effect of short-term oral calcium loading in essential hypertension. Clin Res 1983;31:334A.

162 Grobbee DE, Hofman A. Calcium supplementation lowers blood pressure in young mildly hypertensive subjects: A randomized, controlled trial. Lancet 1986;ii:703 – 707.

163 Lyle RM, Melby CL, Hyner GC. Metabolic differences between subjects whose blood pressure did or did not respond to oral calcium supplementation. Am J Clin Nutr 1988;47:1030 – 1035.

164 Strazzullo P, Siani A, Guglielmi S, et al. Controlled trial of long-term oral calcium supplementation in essential hypertension. Hypertension 1986;8:1084 – 1088.

165 Morris CD, McCarron DA. Calcium supplementation in hypertension: effect after 8 and 16 weeks of treatment. Second European Meeting on Hypertension, Milan, Italy, 1985.

166 Morris CD, Karanja N, McCarron DA. Dietary vs. supplemental calcium to reduce blood pressure. Clin Res 1988;36:A139.

167 Bohr DF. Vascular smooth muscle: dual effect of calcium. Science 1963;139:597 – 599.

168 Bukoski RD, McCarron DA. Calcium and hypertension. In: Baker PF, ed. Handbook of Experimental Pharmacology — Calcium in Drug Actions. Berlin: Springer-Verlag, 1987;465 – 485.

169 Bukoski RD, McCarron DA. Altered aortic reactivity and lowered blood pressure associated with high calcium intake. Am J Physiol 1986;251:H976 – H983.

170 Scrogin KS, Hatton DC, McCarron DA. Calcium and blood pressure in normotensive and hyperten-

sive rat pups. FASEB J 1989;3:765A.

171 Bukoski RD, Xue H, McCarron DA. Effect of 1,25(OH)$_2$ vitamin D$_3$ and ionized $Ca^{2+}$ on $^{45}Ca$ uptake by primary cultures of aortic myocytes of spontaneously hypertensive and Wistar Kyoto normotensive rats. Biochem Biophys Res Commun 1987;146:1330 – 1335.

172 Webb RC, Bohr DF. Recent advances in the pathogenesis of hypertension: consideration of structural, functional, and metabolic vascular abnormalities resulting in elevated arterial resistance. Am Heart J 1981;102:251 – 264.

173 Hirata Y, Takata S, Takagi Y, Yoshimi H, Fujita T. Parathyroid hormone receptors in vascular smooth muscle and endothelial cells. First International Conference on PTH, Kobe, Japan, 1987.

174 Kawashima H. Receptor for 1,25-dihydroxyvitamin D in a vascular smooth muscle cell line derived form rat aorta. Biochem Biophys Res Commun 1987;146:1 – 6.

175 Resnick LM, Calcium and hypertension: the emerging connection. Ann Intern Med 1985;103:944 – 945.

176 Bukoski RD, Xue H, Dewan P, McCarron DA. Calciotropic hormones and vascular calcium metabolism in experimental hypertension. In: Halpern W, et al., eds. Resistance Arteries. Ithaca, NY: Perinatology Press, 1988;320 – 328.

177 Hatton DC, Huie PE, Muntzel MS, Metz JA, McCarron DA. Stress-induced blood pressure responses in SHR: effect of dietary calcium. Am J Physiol 1987;252:R48 – R54.

178 Huie PE, Hatton DC, Muntzel MS, Metz JA, McCarron DA. Psycho-social stress, dietary calcium and hypertension in the SHR. Physiol Behav 1987;40:425 – 429.

179 Scrogin KE, Hatton DC, Metz JA, Muntzel MS, McCarron DA. Effect of dietary calcium on stress-induced catecholamine release and sensitivity in the spontaneously hypertensive rat. Proc Soc Neurosci Ann Meet 1987;13:1549.

180 Lau K, Chen S, Eby B. Evidence for the role of PO4 deficiency in antihypertensive action of a high-Ca diet. Am J Physiol 1984;246:H324 – H331.

181 Bindels RJM, Van Den Broek LAM, Hillebrand SJW, Wokke JMP. A high phosphate diet lowers blood pressure in spontaneously hypertensive rats. Hypertension 1987;9:96 – 102.

182 Kaplan NM, Meese RB. The calcium deficiency hypothesis of hypertension: a critique. Ann Intern Med 1986;105:947 – 955.

183 Hatton D, Muntzel M, McCarron D, Scrogin K, Pressley M, Bukoski R. Early influence of dietary calcium on blood pressure and plasma volume. Fed Proc 1987;46:1071.

184 Hatton D, Muntzel M, Absalon J, McCarron D. Dietary Ca and Fe interaction on hematoctrit in the SHR. FASEB J 1988;2:A969.

185 Kurtz TW, Al-Bander HA, Morris RC Jr. 'Salt-sensitive' essential hypertension in men. N Engl J Med 1987;317:1043 – 1048.

186 Oshima T, Matsuura H, Kido K, et al. Intralymphocytic sodium and free calcium and plasma renin in essential hypertension. Hypertension 1988;12:26 – 31.

187 Pedersen EB, Johannesen P, Kristensen S, Rasmussen AB, Emmertsen K. Calcium, parathyroid hormone and calcitonin in normal pregnancy and preeclampsia. Gynecol Obstet Invest 1984;18:156 – 164.

188 Taufield PA, Ales KL, Resnick LM, Druzin ML, Gertner JM, Laragh JH. Hypocalciuria in preeclampsia. N Engl J Med 1987;316:715 – 718.

189 Varner MW, Cruikshank DP, Pitkin RM. Calcium metabolism in the hypertensive mother, fetus and newborn. Am J Obstet Gynecol 1983;147:762.

190 Villar J, Repke J, Belizan JM, Pareja G. Calcium supplementation reduces blood pressure during pregnancy: results from a randomized controlled clinical trial. Obstet Gynecol 1987;70:317 – 322.

191 Marya RK, Rathee S, Manrow M. Effect of calcium and vitamin D supplementation on toxaemia of pregnancy. Gynecol Obstet Invest 1987;24:38 – 42.

192 Kawasaki N, Matsui I, Ito M, et al. Effect of calcium supplementation on the vascular sensitivity to angiotensin II in pregnant women. Am J Obstet Gynecol 1985;153:576 – 582.

193 Fulton M, Thomson G, Hunter R, Raab G, Laxen D, Hepburn W. Influence of blood lead on the ability and attainment of children in Edinburgh. Lancet 1987;i:1221 – 1226.

194 Ross DH. Chronic ethanol administration inhibits calmodulin-dependent $Ca^{++}$ uptake in synaptosomal membrane. Pharm Biochem Behav 1986;24:1659 – 1664.

195 Harland BF, Johnson RD, Blendermann EM, et al. Calcium, phosphorus, iron, iodine, and zinc in the 'Total Diet'. J Am Diet Assoc 1980;77:16 – 20.

196 Gruchow HW, Sobocinski KA, Barboriak JJ. Alcohol, nutrient intake, and hypertension in US adults. J Am Med Assoc 1985;253:1567 – 1571.

197 Kromhout D, Bosschieter EB, Coulander CL. Potassium, calcium, alcohol intake and blood pressure: the Zutphen Study. Am J Clin Nutr 1985;41:1299 – 1304.

198 Criqui MH, Langer RD, Reed DM. Dietary alcohol, calcium, and potassium: effects on blood pressure. CVD Epidemiol News 1988;43:30.

199 Liebman M, Chopin LF, Carter E, Clark AJ, Disney GW, et al. Factors related to blood pressure in a biracial adolescent female population. Hypertension 1986;8:843 – 850.

200 Sempos C, Cooper R, Kovar MG, Johnson C, Drizd T, Yetley E. Dietary calcium and blood pressure in National Health and Nutrition Examination Surveys I and II. Hypertension 1986;8:1067 – 1074.

201 McCarron DA, Morris CD. The calcium deficiency hypothesis of hypertension. Ann Intern Med 1987;107:919 – 922.

202 Ackley S, Barrett-Connor E, Suarez L. Dairy products, calcium, and blood pressure. Am J Clin Nutr 1983;38:457 – 461.

203 Garcia-Palmieri MR, Costas R Jr, Cruz-Vidal M, Sorlie PD, Tillotson J, Havlik RJ. Milk consumption, calcium intake, and decreased hypertension in Puerto Rico. Puerto Rico Heart Health Program Study. Hypertension 1984;6:322 – 328.

204 Harlan WR, Hull AL, Schmouder RL, Landis JR, Thompson RE, Larkin FA. Blood pressure and nutrition in adults. The National Health and Nutrition Examination Survey. Am J Epidemiol 1984;120:17 – 28.

205 Nichaman M, Shekelle R, Paul O. Diet, alcohol, and blood pressure in the Western Electric Study. Am J Epidemiol 1984;120:469 – 470.

206 Harlan WR, Hull AL, Schmouder RL, Landis JR, Larkin FA, Thompson FE. High blood pressure in older Americans. The First National Health and Nutrition Examination Survey. Hypertension 1984;6:802 – 809.

207 Harlan WR, Landis JR, Schmouder RL, Goldstein NG, Harlan LC. Blood lead and blood pressure: relationship in the adolescent and adult US populatioin. J Am Med Assoc 1985;253:530 – 534.

208 Johnson NE, Smith EL, Freudenheim JL. Effects on blood pressure of calcium supplementation in women. Am J Clin Nutr 1985;42:12 – 17.

209 Reed D, McGee D, Yano K, Hankin J. Diet, blood pressure, and multicollinearity. Hypertension 1985;7:405 – 410.

210 Sempos CT, Cooper RS, Johnson C, Drizd TA, Yetley EA. Association of dietary and serum calcium to blood pressure in adults 40 – 74 years. Am J Epidemiol 1985;122:548.

211 Yamamoto M, Kuller L. Calcium and elevated blood pressure — further evidence from the Three-Area Stroke Mortality Study. Am J Epidemiol 1985;122:512.

212 Caggiula AW, Milas NC, McKenzie JM, Sugars C. Nutrition intake and blood pressure in the multiple risk factor intervention trial. CVD Epidemiol News 1986;41:27.

213 Trevisan M. Relationship between total and varied sources of dietary calcium intake and blood pressure. Am J Epidemiol 1986;124:507.

214 McGarvey ST, Zinner SH, Rosner B, Willett WC. Maternal prenatal dietary calcium and magnesium intake and infant blood pressure. 28th Annual Conference on Cardiovascular Disease and Epidemiology, 1988.

215 Meese RB, Gonzalez DG, Casparian JM, Ram CVS, Pak CYC, Kaplan NM. Failure of calcium supplements to relieve hypertension. Clin Res 1986;34:A218.

216 Siani A, Strazzullo P, Guglielmi S, Mancini M. Clinical studies of the effects of different oral calcium intakes in essential hypertension. J Hypertens 1987;5:s311 – s313.

217 Siani A, Strazzullo P, Guglielmi S, et al. Controlled trial of low calcium versus high calcium intake in mild hypertension. J Hypertens 1988;6:253 – 256.

218 Bierenbaum ML, Wolf E, Raff M, Maginnis WP. The effect of dietary calcium supplementation on blood pressure and serum lipid levels: preliminary report. Nutr Rep Int 1987;36:1147 – 1157.

219 Gilliland M, Zawada ET, McClung D, TerWee J. Preliminary report: natriuretic effect of calcium supplementation in prehypertensive women over forty. J Am Coll Nutr 1987;6:139 – 143.

220 Thomsen K, Nilas L, Christiansen C. Dietary calcium intake and blood pressure in normotensive subjects. Acta Med Scand 1987;222:51 – 56.

221 Vinson JA, Mazur T, Bose P. Comparison of different forms of calcium on blood pressure of normotensive young males. Nutr Rep Int 1987;36:497 – 505.

222 Van Beresteyn ECH, Schaafsma G, De Waard H. Oral calcium and blood pressure: a controlled intervention trial. Am J Clin Nutr 1986;44:883 – 888.

223 Bierenbaum ML, Wolf E, Bisgeier G, Maginnis WP. Dietary calcium: a method of lowering blood pressure. Am J Hypertens 1988;1:149s – 152s.

224 Nowson C, Morgan T. Effect of calcium carbonate on blood pressure in normotensive and hypertensive people. Hypertension 1989;13:630 – 639.

*Bone and Mineral Research/7*
*Johan N.M. Heersche and John A. Kanis, editors*



# The pathogenesis of humoral hypercalcaemia of malignancy

STUART H. RALSTON

*University Department of Orthopaedic Surgery, Western Infirmary Glasgow G11, 6NT, U.K.*

## I. Introduction and historical aspects

Hypercalcaemia was first recognised to be a complication of malignant disease between the 1920 and 1930s, mainly in patients with advanced breast cancer and myeloma who had evidence of extensive metastatic bone disease (Gutman et al. 1936). From these observations, it was naturally assumed that hypercalcaemia most commonly arose as the result of excessive skeletal calcium release by the invading tumour (Gutman et al. 1936) — a view which has prevailed until relatively recently (Mundy and Martin 1982). Although there were occasional reports of hypercalcaemia occurring in the absence of bone metastases (Gutman et al. 1936; Zondek 1924), the concept that hypercalcaemia in malignancy might arise as the result of a humoral mechanism was not put forward until 1941, when Albright suggested that hypercalcaemia and hypophosphataemia associated with a renal cell carcinoma may have been due to the 'ectopic' release of a PTH-like substance (Case records of MGH 1941).

Following this, several reports of hypercalcaemia occurring in the absence of bone metastases appeared in the literature forming the syndrome of 'pseudohyperparathyroidism' (Fry 1962), which more recently has been termed the humoral hypercalcaemia of malignancy (HHM) (Martin and Atkins 1977). In a review of 50 patients with pseudohyperparathyroidism, Lafferty defined three main criteria for its diagnosis: the absence of bone metastases, identified either on radiographs or at post mortem, the biochemical features of hypercalcaemia and hypophosphataemia and correction of these by tumour resection (Lafferty 1966).

On the basis of these criteria, humoral mechanisms of hypercalcaemia were considered to be relatively rare, and confined to patients with solid tumours such as lung carcinoma and renal carcinomas which were unassociated with bone metastases (Lafferty 1966; Mundy and Martin 1982). Whilst there had been isolated reports of pseudohyperparathyroidism as defined above, occurring in patients with breast carcinoma (Mavligit et al. 1971; Hirshorn et al. 1979; Sztern et al. 1981), local osteolytic mechanisms of hypercalcaemia have generally been considered to prevail in this situation and also in myeloma where osteolytic lesions are also generally present by the time hypercalcaemia has developed (Mundy and Martin 1982).

From clinical observations made initially in late 1960s (Gardner 1969) and again in the early 1980s (Ralston et al. 1982), it became apparent that the presence of metastatic bone disease was insufficient to account for hypercalcaemia in many cancer patients. Neither the presence nor the extent of metastatic bone disease as assessed radiographically (Gardner 1969), or by the more sensitive technique of radionuclide bone scanning (Ralston et al. 1982) could be shown to correlate with the occurrence or severity of hypercalcaemia or other biochemical indices of bone resorption in cancer patients (Ralston et al. 1984a). From these and other observations concerning the nephrogenous production of cyclic adenosine monophosphate (NcAMP) — a biochemical index of PTH-like activity (Broadus et al. 1977) — it has now become apparent that humoral mechanisms are the predominant cause of hypercalcaemia in malignancy (Stewart et al. 1980; Ralston et al. 1982, 1984a).

## II. Tumours associated with hypercalcaemia

It has been estimated that hypercalcaemia occurs in approximately 5% of all patients with cancer (Burt and Brennan 1980), but some tumours cause hypercalcaemia more frequently than others. For example, squamous carcinomas, particularly of the lung, but also of other sites such as the oesophagus, head and neck and genital tract frequently cause hypercalcaemia, as do breast cancers, myelomas and cancers of the urinary tract (Table 1). Conversely, adenocarcinomas of the large bowel, stomach cancer and small cell carcinoma of the lung, although common tumours, are seldom associated with hypercalcaemia (Bender and Hansen 1974; Fisken et al. 1980; Mundy and Martin 1982). These differences relate, not only to the frequency of bone metastases, but also to the propensity of certain tumour types to cause hypercalcaemia by releasing humoral factors which act either locally or systemically to disturb normal regulatory mechanisms of calcium homeostasis.

Many previous reviewers have restricted the term 'humoral hypercalcaemia of malignancy' to those patients with squamous or genitourinary cancers, who have few or no bone metastases and who exhibit certain biochemical features in common with primary hyperparathyroidism (Lafferty 1966; Skrabanek et al. 1980; Stewart et al. 1980; Mundy and Martin 1982; Mundy et al. 1984; Mundy 1985). Whereas these probably constitute the largest subgroup of patients with HHM, it has become apparent in recent years that humoral mechanisms contribute to the pathogenesis of hypercalcaemia in many other tumour types. In view of this, the relative importance

TABLE 1 Tumour type in 170 patients attending Glasgow Royal Infirmary with cancer-associated hypercalcaemia

| Tumour | Number | % |
|---|---|---|
| Squamous lung | 63 | 37 |
| head and neck | 6 | 3.5 |
| other | 4 | 2.3 |
| (sub total) | (73) | (42.8) |
| Bladder | 16 | 9.4 |
| Breast | 23 | 13.7 |
| Myeloma | 15 | 8.8 |
| Kidney | 6 | 3.5 |
| Lymphoma | 4 | 2.3 |
| Others* | 33 | 19.5 |
| Total | 170 | 100.0 |

* Diagnoses were: 10, lung cancer (no histology available); 2, ovarian; 1, endometrial; 2, primary liver tumours; 5, adenocarcinoma unknown primary; 3, adenocarcinoma of lung; 5, small cell carcinoma of lung; 3, gastric; 2, pancreatic.

of humoral and local osteolytic mechanisms to the pathogenesis of hypercalcaemia will be discussed in this review, according to tumour type.

## III. Pathophysiology of hypercalcaemia in haematological cancers

### A. Myeloma

Hypercalcaemia occurs in about 30% of patients with myeloma and overall, the tumour accounts for between 10 and 20% of patients with cancer-associated hypercalcaemia in clinical practice.

The hypercalcaemia of myeloma is invariably associated with osteolytic bone lesions. Biopsies of bone show evidence of increased osteoclastic resorption and depressed formation (Mundy et al. 1974a), whereas bone resorption is relatively normal at sites uninvolved by tumour (Battaille et al. 1986).

This local increase in osteoclastic activity was shown by Mundy and his colleagues to be due to the release of an osteoclast activating factor (OAF) which stimulated bone resorption *in vitro* (Mundy et al. 1974a). Although OAF was initially considered to be a single substance, current evidence suggests that it represents the sum of bone-resorptive activities associated with various lymphokines released by cells of the immune system including; interleukin-1 (Gowen et al. 1983; Dewhirst et al. 1985) and Tumour Necrosis Factors (TNF) alpha and beta (Bertolini et al. 1986). Mundy's group have suggested that the bone resorption in myeloma may principally be due to the release of TNF$\beta$ (Garrett et al. 1987).

Whilst multifocal osteoclastic bone resorption is of major pathogenic importance in the hypercalcaemia associated with this tumour, many myeloma patients with florid lytic lesions of bone do not develop hypercalcaemia. This suggests that additional factors must be of importance and indeed, the occurrence of hypercalcaemia has been shown to be related more to the degree of *renal glomerular impairment* than to the presence or extent of osteolytic lesions (Durie et al. 1981). The importance of the kidney in precipitating hypercalcaemia is emphasised by the fact that of all the haematological tumours, myeloma is unique in being associated, both with the highest incidence of hypercalcaemia and with a high incidence of renal glomerular failure due to the specific nephrotoxic effects of another tumour product — immunoglobulin light chains.

On biochemical evaluation, hypercalcaemic patients with myeloma are typically azotaemic, and as a result are hyperphosphataemic. Despite this, renal tubular phosphate reabsorption is generally reduced (Zilva and Nicholson 1973) — possibly due to the hypercalcaemia itself (Bijvoet 1977). Other PTH-like biochemical features such as elevations in NcAMP and increases in renal tubular reabsorption of calcium are generally absent (Rude et al. 1982; Van Breukelen et al. 1982; Paterson et al. 1983; Bonjour et al. 1988).

These features, in combination with the absence of systemic bone resorptive activity on bone biopsy (Battaille 1986), suggest that the hypercalcaemia in myeloma can usually be attributed to a local osteolytic mechanism.

### B. Leukaemia

Hypercalcaemia is relatively rare in leukaemia and occurs in 1 – 2% of cases (Jordan 1966). As a rcsult, the mechanisms of have been rather less well investigated than those in myeloma.

Hypercalcaemia in this situation, has invariably been associated with evidence of widespread marrow infiltration with blast cells (Jordan 1966; Gewirtz et al. 1983; Laffan 1986). Focal osteolytic lesions, such as those which occur in myeloma, are unusual (Jordan 1966). In the very few cases where bone biopsies have been performed, there has been evidence of increased osteoclastic activity and depressed bone formation, whereas biochemical assessment has with some exceptions (see below) shown depressed levels of PTH, NcAMP, 1,25-dihydroxyvitamin D and slightly decreased renal tubular reabsorption of phosphate (Gewirtz et al. 1983). Renal tubular reabsorption of calcium has not been systematically studied.

In tissue culture, leukaemic blast cells have been shown to release bone resorbing factors with characteristics similar to those of ‘OAF’ (Gewirtz et al. 1983). In other cases, ectopic production of a PTH-like substance has been implicated (Zidar et al. 1976), as has the release of adenylate cyclase stimulating factors (Gewirtz et al. 1983) and 1,25-dihydroxyvitamin D (Laffan et al. 1986).

From these observations, it is probable that many instances of hypercalcaemia associated with leukaemia are due to bone resorption mediated by factors released locally by immature blast cells (Mundy et al. 1974b; Gewirtz et al. 1983). The nature of these factors is unclear at present although lymphokines such as interleukin-1 and TNF seem likely candidates. In a few cases, humoral mechanisms of hypercalcaemia may also be operative in leukaemia, as judged by evidence of ectopic production of PTH (Zirdar et al. 1966), a PTH-related peptide (Gewirtz et al. 1983) or 1,25-dihydroxyvitamin D (Laffan et al. 1986).

## C. Lymphoma

Hypercalcaemia occurs in 2 – 3% of patients with lymphoma (Cannellos 1974; Fisken et al. 1980), although the incidence appears to be much higher in certain T-cell lymphomas (Blayney et al. 1983). Hypercalcaemia in lymphoma may occur equally in the presence (Moses and Spencer 1963; Mundy et al. 1974b; Blayney et al. 1983) or absence of focal osteolytic lesions (Moses and Spencer 1963; Singer et al. 1973; Blayney et al. 1983).

Although many lymphomas appear to cause hypercalcaemia by the local release of 'osteoclast activating factors' similar to those described in patients with myeloma (Mundy et al. 1974b), lymphoma-associated hypercalcaemia has frequently been described in the absence of focal bone lesions or marrow infiltration by the tumour (Singer et al. 1973; Schechter et al. 1982; Blayney et al. 1983; Breslau et al. 1984; Davies et al. 1985; Rosenthal et al. 1985). In such cases, the tumour appears to release systemically active bone resorbing substances; bone biopsy studies *in vivo* have showed evidence of increased osteoclastic activity in the absence of marrow infiltration (Singer et al. 1973; Grossman et al. 1981). Cell lines derived from these tumours have also been shown to release substances with potent bone resorbing activity *in vitro* (Singer et al. 1973; Mundy et al. 1974b; Grossman et al. 1981).

Biochemical evaluation of patients with lymphoma-associated hypercalcaemia has generally revealed suppressed levels of PTH, NcAMP, and $TmPO_4$ (Singer et al. 1973; Stewart et al. 1980). Serum phosphate may be raised, normal or low, depending on renal glomerular function (Zilva and Nicholson 1973; Rosenthal et al. 1985). There has been no formal assessment of renal calcium handling in this situation, but the levels of serum calcium in relation to excreted calcium in the patients described by Rosenthal et al. (1985), can be calculated to fall within, or to the left of the normal range defined by Peacock (Peacock et al. 1969), suggesting that renal tubular reabsorption of calcium is low, in keeping with a bone-resorptive mechanism of hypercalcaemia.

It has been established that circulating 1,25-dihydroxyvitamin D levels are increased in a variety of patients with lymphoma-associated hypercalcaemia. These were first noted by Breslau et al. (1984) and confirmed subsequently by the observations of Rosenthal et al. (1985) and Davies et al. (1985). Raised values of 1,25-

dihydroxyvitamin D do not appear to be confined to any particular histological type of lymphoma, having now been reported in Hodgkin's disease (Davies et al. 1985; Rosenthal et al. 1985) and non-Hodgkin's lymphomas of both B- and T-cell origin (Breslau et al. 1984; Rosenthal et al. 1985). Previously, most instances of hypercalcaemia associated with lymphoma had been attributed to the release of OAF-like substances (Mundy et al. 1974b; Grossman et al. 1981; Schechter et al. 1982), on the basis of the ability of tumour extracts to stimulate bone resorption *in vitro*. In retrospect, it is possible that this activity could have been explained by the release of 1,25-dihydroxyvitamin D — also a potent bone resorbing agent (Mundy and Martin 1982).

It is now clear that the excess circulating 1,25-dihydroxyvitamin D in these patients derives from the tumour itself. In most reported cases, there is no biochemical evidence to suggest that ectopic PTH production, or production of a PTH-like factor occurs, which in theory could increase renal synthesis of the metabolite (Breslau et al. 1984; Davies et al. 1985; Rosenthal et al. 1985). Mudde et al. (1986) have shown that tumour tissue from a patient with lymphoma-associated hypercalcaemia synthesised 1,25-dihydroxyvitamin D from 25-hydroxyvitamin D *in vitro*. Fetchick et al. (1986) have found that T-cell lymphotrophic virus type 1-transformed lymphocytes similarly possess this ability.

As is the case in sarcoidosis, where there is also evidence for extrarenal synthesis of 1,25-dihydroxyvitamin D (Singer and Adams 1987), lymphoma-associated hypercalcaemia may be exacerbated during the summer months and be made worse by ultraviolet phototherapy (Davies et al. 1985). Whilst there is good evidence to suggest that 1,25-dihydroxyvitamin D-stimulated intestinal calcium absorption contributes to the hypercalcaemia in some cases (Breslau et al. 1984) most reported patients have remained significantly hypercalcaemic in the fasting state, even after several days of anorexia, suggesting that increased bone resorption and impairment of urinary calcium excretion due to renal glomerular failure are more important factors (Rosenthal et al. 1985).

## IV. Pathophysiology of hypercalcaemia in solid tumours

### A. Breast carcinoma

Hypercalcaemia is a common complication of breast cancer, occurring in 10 – 25% of cases (Percival 1985). Although hypercalcaemia in breast carcinoma has generally been considered to be a feature of advanced osteolytic disease (Galsko and Burn 1971; Mundy and Martin 1982), we, in a retrospective study (Ralston et al. 1982) and Isales in a prospective study (Isales et al. 1987), documented hypercalcaemia (albeit mild) in 20 – 40% of unselected breast carcinoma patients without bone metastases. Despite these findings, it is probably true to say that most patients with breast carcinoma who have hypercalcaemia severe enough to merit antihypercalcaemic therapy do have local osteolytic lesions (Van Breukelen et al. 1981; Percival et al. 1985; Coleman and Reubens 1987).

Local osteolytic, rather than humoral mechanisms of hypercalcaemia have generally been thought to predominate in breast carcinoma (Galasko and Burn 1971; Mundy and Martin 1982). As is the case in myeloma, breast carcinoma cells appear to release substances which recruit and stimulate neighbouring osteoclasts to resorb bone (Galasko and Burn 1971; Galasko and Bennet 1976; Mundy and Martin 1982). Whilst there is some evidence to suggest that breast cancer cells may also resorb bone directly (Elion and Mundy, 1978), this mechanism is probably of greatest importance in advanced metastatic lesions (Galasko and Bennet 1976). At present, the identity of the osteoclast-activating mediators in breast carcinoma are not well defined but may comprise: the prostaglandins (Greaves et al. 1980) and tumour-derived growth factors (Travers et al. 1988).

Biochemical evaluation is in many cases, consistent with a non-humoral mechanism of hypercalcaemia; in Stewart's series, for example, the levels of PTH, 1,25-dihydroxyvitamin D and NcAMP were generally suppressed (Stewart et al. 1980). More recently, however, it has been recognised that humoral mechanisms may contribute to the hypercalcaemia in a proportion of cases. The first indication of this was provided by the observation that renal tubular reabsorption of calcium remained raised after correction of dehydration in occasional patients with breast cancer (Hosking et al. 1980; Ralston et al. 1984a). Subsequently, these abnormalities were shown to be prevalent in a substantial proportion of breast carcinoma patients (Kimura et al. 1985; Percival et al. 1985; Bonjour et al. 1988), as were elevations in NcAMP (Isales et al. 1987). Depending on whether raised NcAMP levels or elevations in renal tubular reabsorption of calcium are assessed, a humoral mechanism of hypercalcaemia in breast cancer appears to occur in 30 – 50% of cases (Isales et al. 1987; Bonjour et al. 1988) — even in patients with advanced osteolytic disease (Kimura et al. 1985; Percival et al. 1985).

### B. Adenocarcinoma and small cell lung carcinoma

These tumours are relatively infrequent causes of hypercalcaemia and are heterogeneous with regard to clinical and biochemical features. The extent of metastatic bone involvement is variable in adenocarcinomas but metastases are usually present in small cell lung cancer (Bender and Hansen 1974). Biochemical evaluation typically reveals suppressed levels of PTH, but variable levels of 1,25-dihydroxyvitamin D, NcAMP production (Stewart et al. 1980) and renal tubular reabsorption of calcium (Ralston et al. 1987a; Bonjour et al. 1988). These findings are consistent with a mixture of local osteolytic and humoral mechanisms of hypercalcaemia.

A case of metastatic small cell carcinoma of the lung was described by Japanese workers where hypercalcaemia was associated with the ectopic production of 1,24(R)-dihydroxyvitamin D — a metabolite with similar bone-resorptive effects to that of authentic 1,25-dihydroxyvitamin D (Shigeno et al. 1985). In this patient, the hypercalcaemia persisted even after oral calcium restriction, suggesting that its bone-resorptive effects, rather than an effect on intestinal absorption of calcium, was responsible for the hypercalcaemia (Shigeno et al. 1985). At present, this mechanism of hypercalcaemia is thought to be uncommon, although it is of interest that osteolytic sterols were previously implicated (Gordan et al. 1966) — and then discounted (Haddad et al. 1970) — as a possible mechanism of hypercalcaemia in breast cancer.

### C. Squamous, genitourinary and other solid tumours

These tumours when combined, account for the majority of cases of cancer-associated hypercalcaemia seen in clinical practice. The incidence of hypercalcaemia in individual tumour types varies however, from about 10 to 20% in squamous lung cancer (Bender and Hansen 1974; Fisken et al. 1980), to about 40% in hepatocellular carcinoma (Burt and Brennan 1980).

Although circulating levels of immunoreactive PTH are equally suppressed in both metastatic and non-metastatic subgroups of patients with cancer-associated hypercalcaemia (Riggs et al. 1971; Powell et al. 1973; Raisz et al. 1979), many other biochemical features of the syndrome point to the release of humoral mediators with end-organ effects similar to those of PTH.

Most hypercalcaemic patients with these and other solid tumours are hypophosphataemic due to a reduction in the renal tubular threshold for phosphate reabsorption (Stewart et al. 1980; Ralston et al. 1984a, b). In this respect, the syndrome is indistinguishable from primary hyperparathyroidism (Boyd and Ladenson 1984). Whilst hypercalcaemia itself has been invoked as a possible mechanism by which renal tubular reabsorption of phosphate may be inhibited in hypercalcaemic disorders (Shussler et al. 1972; Bijvoet, 1977) this is unlikely to be the sole explanation; the abnormalities of renal phosphate transport persist after hypercalcaemia has been corrected by bisphosphonate therapy (Sleeboom et al. 1983), but are promptly reversed by surgical removal of the tumour (Ralston et al. 1986a). This suggests that the tumour releases factors which have a PTH-like effect on renal phosphate handling and indeed, similar abnormalities are seen experimentally in the rat Leydig cell tumour model of HHM (Insogna et al. 1985; Rizzoli et al. 1986).

An important observation made by Stewart and his colleagues in the early 1980s was that many patients with malignant hypercalcaemia exhibited elevated nephrogenous production of cyclic AMP (Stewart et al. 1980; Rude et al. 1982). Since NcAMP levels are an index of parathyroid hormone-like activity (Broadus et al. 1977), this raised the possibility that substances with PTH-like effects on the renal tubule may have been implicated in the pathogenesis of malignancy-associated hypercalcaemia (Stewart et al. 1980).

The pattern of NcAMP excretion in normocalcaemic and hypercalcaemic cancer patients is variable; Stewart et al. (1980) initially found a clear separation between suppressed NcAMP levels in patients who may have been expected to have a local osteolytic mechanism of hypercalcaemia (i.e. breast cancer and haematological tumours associated with multiple bone metastases) and raised NcAMP levels in those where HHM was suspected (i.e. squamous and genitourinary tumours, few or no bone metastases) (Fig. 1). In similar studies however, Rude et al. (1982) found a continuous distribution of NcAMP levels in hypercalcaemic cancer patients, with no obvious pattern when patients were divided by tumour type or presence of metastatic lesions. Stewart's group have also noted raised NcAMP levels in patients with metastatic breast cancer (Isales et al. 1987). Whereas Stewart et al. (1980) have considered that raised NcAMP values are relatively specific for the syndrome of HHM, both Kukreja et al. (1980) and Van der Velden et al. (1986) have reported finding elevated NcAMP levels in many normocalcaemic cancer patients, particularly those with squamous carcinomas.

For many years, renal tubular reabsorption of calcium was thought to be depressed in patients with cancer-associated hypercalcaemia — both in patients with HHM and in those with a local osteolytic mechanism of hypercalcaemia (Stewart et al. 1980, 1982a; Mundy and Martin 1982). Evidence suggests however that, as in the case of primary hyperparathyroidism (Peacock et al. 1969), increased renal tubular reabsorption of calcium is an important aetiological factor in the pathogenesis of hypercalcaemia in HHM. Initial studies from our laboratory showed that, whilst most hypercalcaemic patients with solid tumours were indeed hypercalciuric in absolute

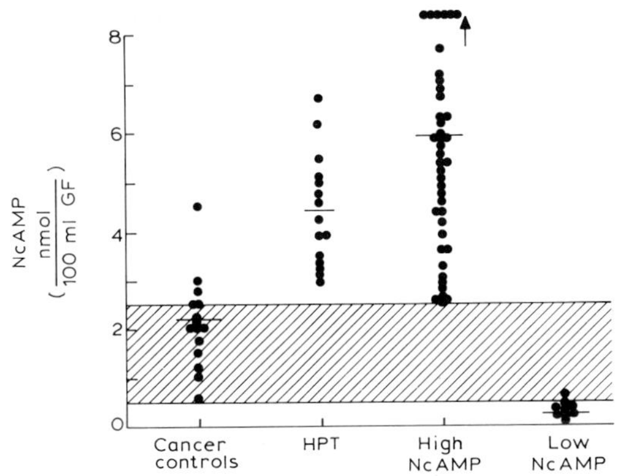


Fig. 1. Comparison of nephrogenous cyclic AMP (NcAMP) levels in cancer controls, patients with primary hyperparathyroidism (HPT) and patients with hypercalcaemia of malignancy (From Stewart et al. 1980; with kind permission from the author and publishers.) Patients in the 'low NcAMP' group had mainly breast and haematological cancers, whereas those in the 'high NcAMP' had mainly squamous and genitourinary cancers. Similar findings have been reported by other workers, although the bimodal distribution of NcAMP values in the hypercalcaemic patients and clear separation of the 'high NcAMP' group from the cancer controls, has been less clear cut.

terms, the levels of urinary calcium excretion expressed as a function of glomerular filtration rate (Peacock et al. 1969) were generally less than might have been expected for the degree of hypercalcaemia. In this respect, the renal tubular handling of calcium was indistinguishable from that in primary hyperparathyroidism (Fig. 2), suggesting that the putative humoral factors possessed a PTH-like effect on renal tubular calcium reabsorption (Ralston et al. 1984b). Similar observations have been reported by other workers (Heller and Hosking 1986) and have been extended to include many patients with breast carcinoma (Kimura et al. 1985; Percival et al. 1985; Bonjour et al. 1988).

This effect on the renal tubular reabsorption of calcium helps to explain why hypercalcaemia occurs with such high frequency in malignant disease, when compared with benign conditions associated with increased bone resorption (e.g. osteoporosis, thyrotoxicosis, immobilisation etc.). It may also explain why there is such a poor correlation between extent of osteolytic disease in malignancy and the occurrence of hypercalcaemia (Gardner et al. 1969; Ralston et al. 1982, 1984a). It is probable that normocalcaemia is preserved at the expense of hypercalciuria in most patients with

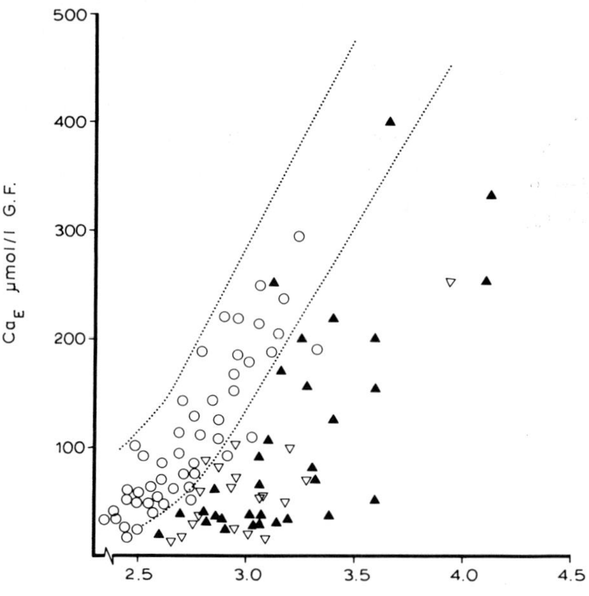


Fig. 2. Relation between serum calcium and calcium excretion (as $Ca_E$ = urine calcium/creatinine × serum creatinine) in patients with hypercalcaemia of malignancy (▲), normal controls undergoing calcium infusions (○) and patients with primary hyperparathyroidism (▽). The normal range as described by Peacock et al. (1969) is shown by the interrupted lines. The urinary excretion of calcium in hypercalcaemia of malignancy, although high in absolute terms, is depressed, relative to the degree of hypercalcaemia, indicating that renal tubular calcium is increased. Tumour type in patients with malignancy were mainly squamous bronchial cancers and genitourinary cancers. Of the three patients with breast cancer studied, two had Calcium vs. $Ca_E$ values which fell within the normal range. (Reproduced from Ralston et al. 1984; with kind permission.)

osteolytic lesions when the renal tubular threshold for calcium excretion is normal. When tubular calcium threshold is raised however, the kidney has a reduced capacity to excrete any excess calcium derived from bone resorption (Ralston et al. 1984b).

Although elevations in renal tubular reabsorption of calcium and increases in osteoclastic bone resorption are equally important in the pathogenesis of hypercalcaemia in advanced HHM, the renal tubular mechanism may predominate in the early stages of the disease; patients with surgically resectable tumours who have mild HHM often have normal bone turnover, with little evidence of increased osteoclastic activity (Ralston et al. 1986). In these patients, surgical resection of the tumour is accompanied by an acute increase in urinary calcium excretion suggesting that increased renal tubular calcium reabsorption before surgery, and its subsequent reduction after, is responsible for the maintenance and correction of hypercalcaemia (Ralston et al. 1986) (Fig. 3).

Increased renal tubular absorption of calcium may either occur as the result of a

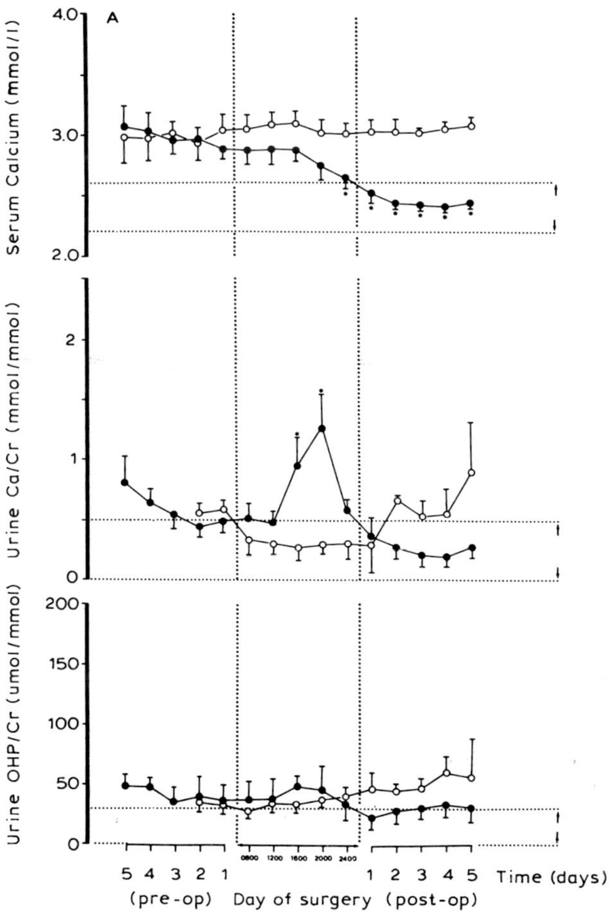

PTH-like humoral effect on the distal tubule or as the result of sodium-linked effect on the proximal tubule (Bijvoet 1977). Since non-humoral factors such as dehydration and sodium depletion primarily determine the level of proximal renal tubular calcium reabsorption, there has been some debate as to the relative importance of these, as opposed to humoral factors in the pathogenesis of raised renal tubular calcium reabsorption in cancer-associated hypercalcaemia. In a recent study, Harinck and his colleagues (Harinck et al. 1987) suggested that the high levels of renal tubular reabsorption of calcium were mainly due to the effects of sodium depletion, on the basis that the 'abnormal' renal handling of calcium could be corrected by the intravenous infusion of a sufficiently large quantity of sodium chloride.

Whilst we (Ralston et al. 1986b) and others (Heller and Hosking 1986) have also found that sodium repletion may reduce renal tubular reabsorption of calcium in this situation, a similar state of affairs is seen in patients with primary hyperparathyroi-

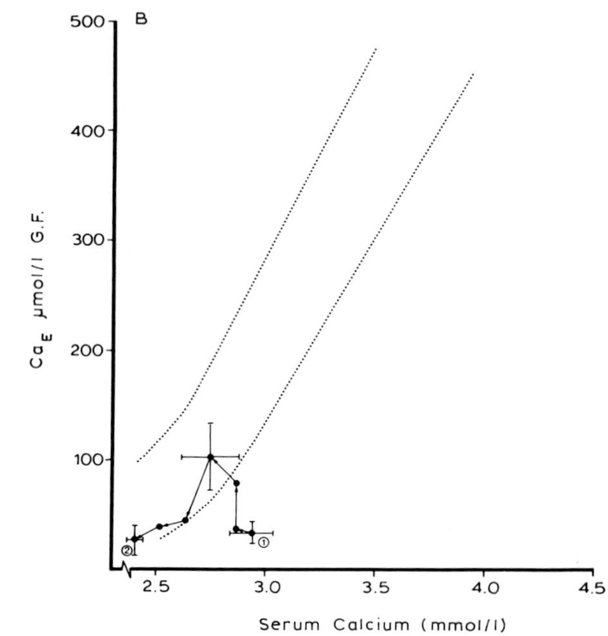


Fig. 3. Biochemical response to surgical treatment in patients with humoral hypercalcaemia of malignancy. ●, Tumour resected ($n$ = 7); ○, tumour inoperable ($n$ = 3). Values are means, bars are S.E.M. In patients where the tumour was resected, there is an acute rise in urinary calcium excretion (Ca/Cr) and a fall in serum calcium but no change in urinary hydroxyproline excretion (OHP/Cr) panel (A). In panel (B), there was a leftward shift in serum calcium vs. urinary $Ca_E$ values preoperatively (1) compared with postoperatively (2) in patients where the tumour was resected, indicating that renal tubular calcium reabsorption had fallen. Bone biopsies in these patients revealed little or no evidence of increased osteoclastic activity. These data indicate that the hypercalcaemia was mainly due to a renal tubular rather than bone-resorptive mechanism.

dism (Ralston et al. 1986b; Heller and Hosking 1986), where the stimulatory effects of PTH on distal renal tubular calcium reabsorption are well established (Peacock et al. 1969; Bijvoet et al. 1977). In our studies (Ralston et al. 1986b) and those of Heller and Hosking (1986), the renal tubular reabsorption of calcium in relation to that of sodium was identical in patients with hypercalcaemia of malignancy and primary hyperparathyroidism. Moreover, in the rat Leydig cell tumour model of HHM, increased renal tubular calcium reabsorption is also observed which cannot be attributed to the effects of sodium depletion (Rizzoli et al. 1986). These data suggest that the normalisation of renal tubular reabsorption of calcium seen by Harinck et al. (1987) was probably due to excessive natriuresis which, by its depressant effect on proximal tubular calcium reabsorption, masked a humorally-mediated increase in distal tubular reabsorption. In support of this hypothesis, Harinck et al. (1987) were also unable to find evidence of increased renal tubular reabsorption of calcium in primary hyperparathyroidism.

In addition to their effects on the renal tubule, the putative humoral mediators involved in HHM have important effects on the skeleton; accelerated osteoclastic bone resorption has long been recognised to be an important factor in the pathogenesis of HHM (Mundy and Martin 1982). Biochemically, this is reflected by hypercalciuria and hydroxyprolinuria (Stewart et al. 1980; Ralston et al. 1984a, b) and clinically by the theraputic response of the hypercalcaemia to inhibitors of bone resorption (Sleeboom et al., 1983; Harinck et al. 1987). Studies of bone histology in HHM have revealed evidence of increased osteoclastic activity in sites uninvolved by tumour (Azzopardi and Whittaker 1969; McDonnell et al. 1982; Sharp et al. 1982; Stewart et al. 1982a). These findings are of course, in keeping with the concept that bone — as well as the kidney — are target organs for the action of the putative humoral mediators of HHM. Whereas the histological appearance of bone has been likened to that of osteitis fibrosa cystica (Azzopardi and Whittaker 1969; Sharp et al. 1982), radiological signs of subperiosteal erosions are notable by their absence in HHM. In three reported cases of HHM where subperiosteal erosions have been seen, all had relatively indolent tumours (Lamberg et al. 1964; Scholz et al. 1973; Loveridge et al. 1985), suggesting that the clinical course of HHM may generally be too rapid to permit the development of such radiographic changes. Although the appearance of bone in HHM is, as stated above, superficially similar to that in hyperparathyroidism, recent quantitative bone histomorphometric studies have shown that indices of bone formation are lower in the former (McDonnell et al. 1982; Stewart et al. 1982a) (Fig. 4). This has been interpreted as representing a specific 'uncoupling' effect of the humoral mediators in HHM (Stewart et al. 1982), although since these features are particularly marked in patients with advanced tumours (Ralston et al. 1988), it is probable that immobilisation also contributes to the depressed osteoblastic activity (Ralston et al. 1988).

An important difference between HHM and primary hyperparathyroidism is in terms of the contribution of dietary calcium intake to the pathogenesis of hypercalcaemia. In the latter disorder, absorption of dietary calcium is raised due to

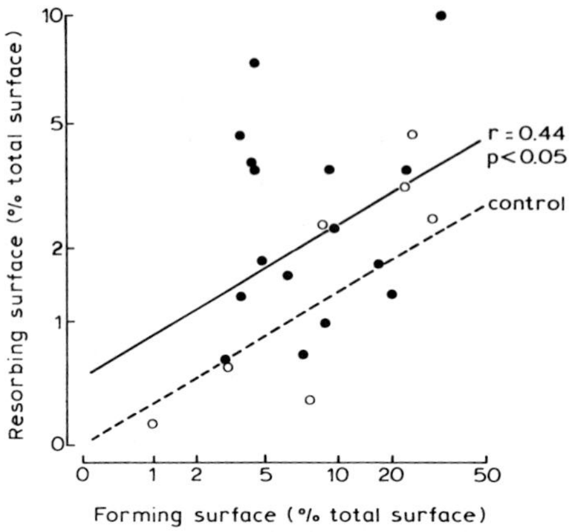


Fig. 4. Comparison of bone-forming surfaces (% osteoid) and resorbing surfaces (% surface in contact with osteoclasts) in patients with malignancy-associated hypercalcaemia and controls (patients with hyperparathyroidism, hypoparathyroidism and normals). In malignancy-associated hypercalcaemia (●, —), the forming surfaces are lower than in the control group (○, – –) for any given level of bone resorption, reflected by an upward displacement of the regression line. (From McDonnell et al., 1982; with kind permission from the authors and the publisher.)

elevated circulating levels of 1,25-dihydroxyvitamin D (Broadus et al. 1980); which result from a PTH-mediated increase in renal synthesis of 1,25-dihyroxyvitamin D (Haussler and McCain 1977).

The mean circulating levels of 1,25-dihydroxyvitamin D in cancer-associated hypercalcaemia are lower than those in primary hyperparathyroidism (Stewart et al. 1980; Ralston et al. 1984c, 1987b; Yamamoto et al. 1987). On closer analysis, however, serum 1,25-dihydroxyvitamin D concentrations in malignancy follow a bimodal distribution; levels are depressed in about 40%, detectable within the normal range in a further 40%, and raised in about 10% (Fig. 5A). Unlike primary hyperparathyroidism, intestinal absorption of calcium is generally low in malignancy (Coombes et al. 1977) and unrelated to the level of 1,25-dihydroxyvitamin D (Fig. 5B) (Ralston et al. 1987b). The lack of correlation between 1,25-dihydroxyvitamin D levels and calcium absorption may be due to the fact that, even in patients with raised 1,25-dihydroxyvitamin D levels, the intestinal effects of the D metabolite are blunted by a generalised malabsorptive process associated with the cancer (Somajyi et al. 1972).

Yamamoto et al. (1987) have reported that 'non-suppressed' 1,25-dihydroxyvitamin D levels were particularly common in renal cell carcinomas. In our studies, the finding of a *detectable* 1,25-dihydroxyvitamin D level was not confined to any particular tumour type, although levels were low in most patients with myeloma and breast carcinoma (Ralston et al. 1984c, 1987b).

The pattern of 1,25-dihydroxyvitamin D levels in malignant hypercalcaemia can be interpreted in two ways. One view, proposed by Stewart et al. (1980), is that the putative humoral mediators in HHM are functionally distinct from PTH in lacking an effect on renal 1-alpha-hydroxylase activity. An alternative interpretation which we adhere to however (Ralston et al. 1984) is that the detectable or raised 1,25-dihydroxyvitamin D levels seen in about 50% of cases are 'inappropriate' and as such, reflect a PTH-like humoral effect on 1,25-dihydroxyvitamin D synthesis. Although hypophosphataemia may elevate 1,25-dihydroxyvitamin D levels in the absence of PTH (Tanaka and DeLuca 1973), we and others have failed to find a significant relationship between serum phosphate and 1,25-dihydroxyvitamin D levels in this situation (Ralston et al. 1984c; Yamamoto et al. 1987). Since 1,25-dihydroxyvitamin D is invariably elevated in the rat Leydig cell tumour model of HHM (Insogna et al. 1984), it is possible that other factors specific to the human syndrome may contribute to the relative depression of 1,25-dihydroxyvitamin D levels in man (Horiuchi et al. 1987).

A final difference between the hypercalcaemia of malignancy and primary hyperparathyroidism is in terms of acid base balance and serum chloride levels (Lafferty 1966). Patients with humorally-mediated and local osteolytic hypercalcaemia almost invariably exhibit a hypochloraemic alkalosis whereas the chloride levels are usually normal in primary hyperparathyroidism, or in some cases raised in association with a type II renal tubular acidosis (Cohen 1987).

Clinically, these patterns may be useful in the differential diagnosis of malignant hypercalcaemia, when combined with other features such as hypoalbuminaemia and suppressed PTH levels (Boyd and Ladenson 1984). With regard to the biological effects of the humoral mediator(s) of hypercalcaemia, one can either argue that they do not share PTH-like effects on renal bicarbonate and chloride handling, or that other factors are produced by cancers which mask these effects. Since hypochloraemic alkalosis is a common finding in normocalcaemic as well as hypercalcaemic cancer patients (Boyd and Ladenson 1984), the latter view may well be correct.

## V. Proposed mediators of HHM

These are summarised in Table 2, and discussed individually below.

### A. Prostaglandins

Prostaglandins of the E series have been isolated from both serum and tumour tissue from a number of animal models of HHM (Tashjian 1975) and in some human tumours associated with the syndrome (Robertson et al. 1976; Devers et al. 1977; Josse et al. 1981). These substances are powerful stimulators of bone resorption *in vitro* (Klein and Raisz 1970) and hence have the potential to cause hypercalcaemia, but they are also present in normal tissues and in tumours which are unassociated with HHM (Greaves et al. 1980).

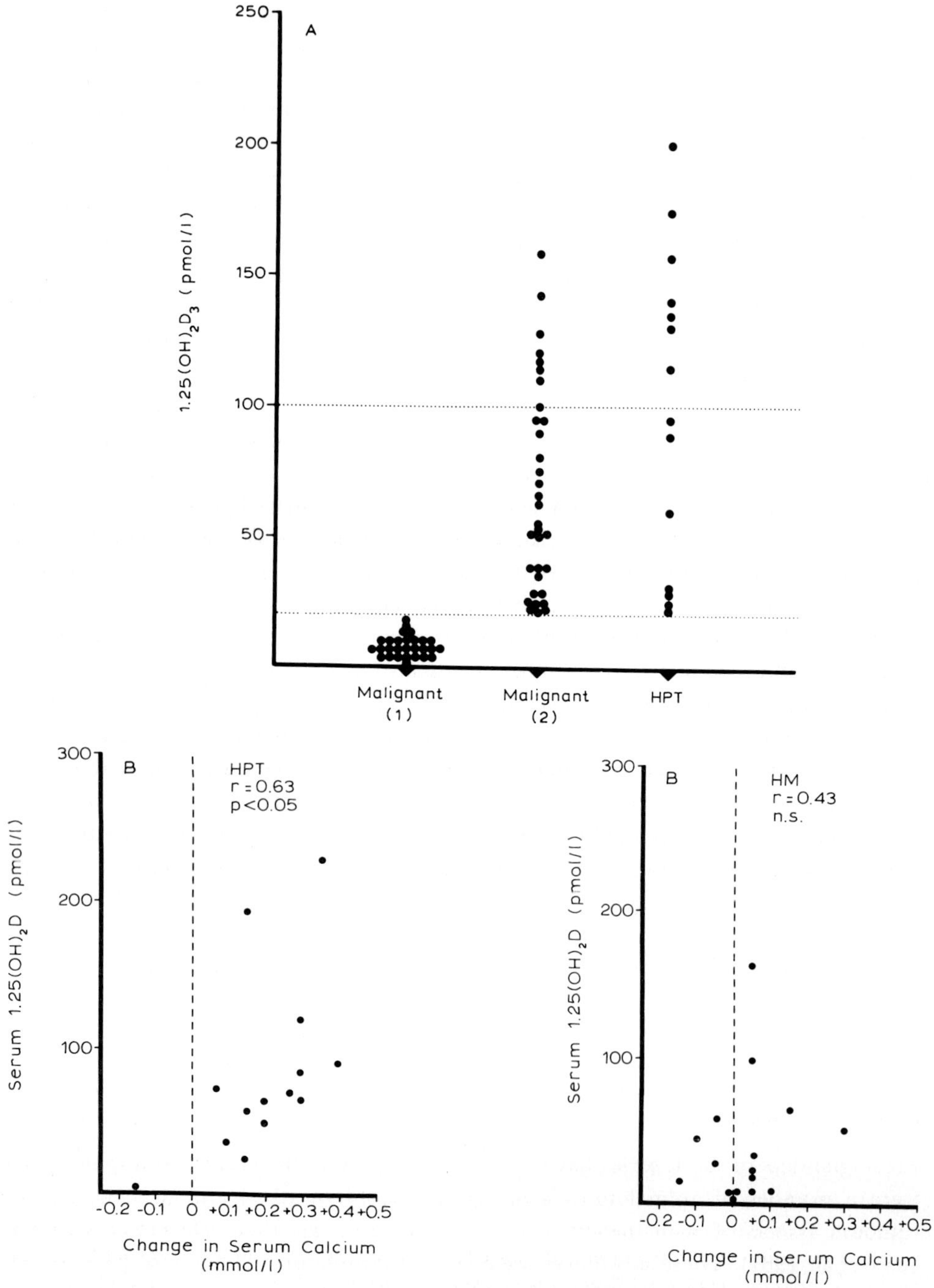


Fig. 5(A). Circulating 1,25-dihydroxyvitamin D concentrations in hypercalcaemic patients with malignancy ($n$ = 61) and primary hyperparathyroidism (HPT) ($n$ = 14). The patients with malignancy are divided into two groups: those in whom 1,25-dihydroxyvitamin D levels are depressed (group 1, $n$ = 28; 46% of cases)

The evidence that *circulating* prostaglandins are commonly involved in the pathogenesis of HHM is less than convincing. Serum levels of prostaglandin E, while elevated in many patients with malignant hypercalcaemia, are also high in many normocalcaemic cancer patients (Robertson et al. 1976; Devers et al. 1977; Brenner et al. 1982) and overall there is a poor correlation between circulating prostaglandin levels and serum calcium values (Brereton et al. 1974; Robertson et al. 1976; Devers et al. 1977; Brenner et al. 1982). Even in animal models of HHM where the tumour has been convincingly shown to release excessive amounts of prostaglandin E into the systemic circulation, serum prostaglandin E levels correlate poorly with those of serum calcium (Voelkel et al. 1975).

Although treatment with cyclo-oxygenase inhibitors has been reported to correct hypercalcaemia in a number of instances (Brereton et al. 1974; Seyberth et al. 1975), the response is often unpredictable (Brenner et al. 1982) and does not correlate with the circulating level of prostaglandin $E_2$ (Brenner et al. 1982). The above data suggest that a component of the hypercalcaemia in some cancer patients may be prostaglandin-mediated. It is probable however, that these prostaglandins are released locally by resorbing bone in response to another circulating humoral factor (Bringhurst et al. 1987) rather than systemically by the tumour. Infusions of prostaglandin E have not been consistently shown to cause hypercalcaemia in experimental animals (Beliel et al. 1973), except at extremely high doses (Franklin and Tashjian 1975). Even in the event that high concentrations of prostaglandin E were released by tumours associated with hypercalcaemia *in vivo*, the systemic bone resorptive effect would be attenuated by the rapid metabolism of this substance in the pulmonary circulation (Aangard et al. 1964) to metabolites with weak bone resorbing activity (Raisz et al. 1977).

In some tissues, the effects of prostaglandins are mediated by an adenylate cyclase-dependent mechanism (Atkins and Martin 1977). However, the patients identified by Seyberth et al. (1975) as having prostaglandin-related hypercalcaemia, did not have raised urinary cAMP excretion (Seyberth et al. 1976). The effects (if any) of prostaglandins on renal tubular reabsorption of phosphate and calcium are unknown.

---

and those in whom 1,25-dihydroxyvitamin D levels are detectable (group 2, $n$ = 26; 42% of cases, or raised ($n$ = 7, 11% of cases). Overall, 1,25-dihydroxyvitamin D levels were lower in malignancy than in HPT but there was no significant difference between those in group 2 and the HPT patients. These data would be consistent with a PTH-like effect on renal 1 alpha-hydroxylase activity in some patients. The reference range is indicated between the horizontal dotted lines. (B) Unlike primary hyperparathyroidism, the elevated 1,25-dihydroxyvitamin D levels in malignancy-associated hypercalcaemia are not accompanied by an elevation in intestinal calcium absorption. Here, the increment in serum calcium after an oral calcium load test as described by Broadus et al. (1977) is related to the serum 1,25-dihydroxyvitamin D level in hypercalcaemia of malignancy (HM) and primary hyperparathyroidism (HPT). There is a significant correlation in HPT, but none in HM. In HPT, serum calcium rose significantly (median +0.2 mmol/l), whereas there was no significant change in HM (median +0.05 mmol/l). (From Ralston et al. 1987; with kind permission.)

TABLE 2 Potential mediators of hypercalcaemia in malignancy

| Factor | Calcium elevating effect *in vivo* | Bone resorbing effect *in vitro* | PTH-like effects | Tumour(s) factor implicated in |
|---|---|---|---|---|
| Prostaglandin E | Yes (high dose) | Yes | No | Breast cancer<br>Renal cancer<br>Rabbit VX 2 carcinoma<br>Mouse HDSM-1 sarcoma |
| Prostaglandin stimulating | Unknown | Yes | No | Bladder cancer<br>Lung cancer<br>Liver cancer |
| Transforming growth factors | Yes | Yes | ?Phosphaturia | Bladder cancer<br>Breast cancer |
| PTH | Yes | Yes | Yes | Very rare |
| PTH-related peptide | Yes | Yes | Yes | Most solid tumours + 30 – 50% of breast cancers?<br>Phaeochromocytoma<br>?Leukaemia<br>Rat Leydig cell tumour<br>Canine apocrine tumour<br>Canine lymphosarcoma<br>Mouse squamous cancer |
| Interleukin-1 | Yes | Yes | No | Squamous cancer<br>?Myeloma/lymphoma<br>Leukaemia |
| Tumour necrosis factors | Yes | Yes | No | Myeloma<br>?lymphoma |
| $1{,}25(OH)_2$ D and related sterols | Yes | Yes | No | Lymphoma<br>Small cell lung cancer |

## B. Prostaglandin-stimulating factors

There is accumulating evidence to suggest that some tumours release factors which are capable of stimulating osteoclastic resorption by a mechanism which involves the local release of prostaglandins in bone.

In 1981, Minkin and his colleagues found that tissue extracts from HHM patients with hepatic, renal and bronchial tumours contained factors which stimulated bone resorption *in vitro*, by a mechanism which was blocked by pre-treating the bones with indomethacin (Minkin et al. 1981).

More detailed and extensive studies by Bringhurst and his colleagues have confirmed and extended the above observations (Bringhurst et al. 1987). In these studies, significant bone resorbing activity was found in urine and in conditioned medium from a cell line derived from a patient with HHM due to a transitional bladder carcinoma. The bone resorbing activity was inhibited by pre-treatment of the bones, but not the tumour, with indomethacin. While neither the patient's urine nor the tumour-conditioned medium contained appreciable amounts of prostaglandin E itself, both significantly enhanced prostaglandin release from the resorbing bones *in vitro*.

Initial characterisation suggested that the factor(s) responsible were macromolecules of an apparrent $M_r$ 15 000, with properties distinct from the transforming growth factors, epidermal growth factor or adenylate cyclase stimulating factors. At present, the relationship between the presence of these bone resorbing factors within the tumour and the pathogenesis of hypercalcaemia is unclear; further work will be required to look for evidence of their systemic release and to determine whether or not they have a calcium elevating effect *in vivo*.

## C. Tumour-derived growth factors

In recent years, much interest has surrounded the possible role of tumour-derived growth factors in the pathogenesis of malignancy-associated hypercalcaemia (Mundy et al. 1984; Mundy 1985a).

These are peptides produced by a variety of normal and malignant tissues, which amongst many other biological effects stimulate bone resorption *in vitro* (Ibbotson et al. 1985; Tashjian et al. 1985). In the mouse calvarial system, bone resorption stimulated by the growth factors is mediated (at least in part) by prostaglandins, whereas a prostaglandin-distinct mechanism prevails in the fetal rat long bone system (Ibbotson et al. 1985). Most interest has surrounded the role of transforming growth factor (TGF) alpha in the pathogenesis of HHM. A TGF$\alpha$-like factor which co-purified with bone resorbing activity has been isolated from the rat Leydig cell model of HHM (Ibbotson et al. 1983) and from the urine of a patient with renal cell carcinoma and HHM (Mundy et al. 1984). Further evidence that the bone-resorptive activity in this situation was indeed due to TGF$\alpha$ was the observation that it was inhibited by antibodies directed against the EGF receptor (to which TGF$\alpha$ binds) (Ibbotson et al. 1985) but not by synthetic blockers of PTH receptor binding (D'Souza et al. 1985).

Both TGF$\alpha$ and epidermal growth factor (EGF) have been shown to cause hypercalcaemia when infused into mice (Tashjian et al. 1986) and both are present in tumours associated with hypercalcaemia (Mundy 1985a; Mundy et al. 1985; Travers et al. 1988). TGF$\alpha$ has also been shown to inhibit sodium-dependent phosphate transport in renal epithelial cells *in vitro* (Pitzurki et al. 1988) suggesting that it may have a hypophosphataemic effect *in vivo*. There is no information however, on the possible effect (if any) of TGF$\alpha$ and related factors on renal tubular calcium reabsorption, NcAMP production of 1,25-dihydroxyvitamin D synthesis *in vivo*, although both EGF and TGF$\alpha$ have been reported to inhibit adenylate cyclase stimulating activity mediated by PTH- and PTH-related peptides in vitro (Bernier and Goltzman 1988).

*In vivo*, it is unclear whether TGF$\alpha$ or similar factors are released systemically in amounts sufficient to cause hypercalcaemia.

### D. Lymphokines

There are several reported cases in the Japanese literature of patients with squamous carcinomas in whom hypercalcaemia develops in association with a marked leukocytosis (Sato et al. 1986a). Cell lines derived from these tumours have been shown to contain bone resorbing activity (Sato et al. 1986a, b, 1988) and a number of other biological activities consistent with the production of: granulocyte-macrophage colony stimulating factor (GM-CSF), interleukin-1, transforming growth factors (Sato et al. 1986a, b) and adenylate cyclase stimulating factors (Sato et al. 1988).

In some of these tumours, the bone-resorptive activity co-elutes with interleukin-1 activity (Sato et al. 1986b) whereas in others, unidentified bone resorbing factors have been isolated whose effects are inhibited by indomethacin *in vitro* (Sato et al. 1986a). The accelerated bone resorption in one cell line was attributed to the combined effects of interleukin-1 and a PTH-like factor (Sato et al. 1988). The GM-CSF produced by these tumours does not possess bone resorbing activity (Sato et al. 1986a).

Both interleukin-1 and tumour necrosis factors raise plasma calcium when infused *in vivo* (Garrett et al. 1987; Sabatini et al. 1988) and both are potent stimulators of bone resorption *in vitro* (Gowen et al. 1983; Bertolini et al. 1986). If produced in sufficient amounts, either by a tumour, or by an immune response mounted against such a tumour, they might contribute to accelerated bone resorption and hypercalcaemia in HHM. However, it is unclear whether this occurs to any significant extent *in vivo*, except in the case of local osteolysis associated with haematological cancers.

### E. Vitamin D-related sterols

As has been discussed previously, 1,25-dihydroxyvitamin D is an important pathogenic factor in the hypercalcaemia associated with lymphoma (Breslau et al.

1984; Davies et al. 1985; Rosenthal et al. 1985) and may also be involved in the hypercalcaemia associated with some cases of leukaemia (Laffan et al. 1986). Production of a related sterol, 1,24(R)-dihydroxyvitamin D, has been reported in one case of hypercalcaemia associated with small cell lung carcinoma (Shigeno et al. 1985). The frequency with which this mechanism of hypercalcaemia occurs is unclear, but is probably uncommon in view of the normal or low 1,25-dihydroxyvitamin D levels which are generally observed in cancer-associated hypercalcaemia (Stewart et al. 1980; Ralston et al. 1984c). Although vitamin D-related sterols have been reportedly isolated from breast carcinomas (Gordan et al. 1966) the importance of these in the pathogenesis of hypercalcaemia and bone resorption is unclear since apparently similar phytosterols also circulate in normal subjects (Haddad et al. 1970).

The detectable 1,25-dihydroxyvitamin D levels which occur in many patients with solid-tumour hypercalcaemia (Stewart et al. 1980; Ralston et al. 1984c, 1987b; Yamamoto et al. 1987), are probably due to a stimulatory effect of PTH-like humoral mediator on renal 1-alpha-hydroxylase activity (Horiuchi et al. 1987), but are unlikely to contribute significantly to the elevation in serum calcium values (Ralston et al. 1987b).

## F. PTH

Current evidence suggests that ectopic production of PTH is seldom responsible for the occurrence of hypercalcaemia in malignancy, although ectopic production of immunoreactive, but biologically inactive PTH does occur in some normocalcaemic patients — particularly those with small cell carcinomas of the lung (Roof et al. 1971).

As discussed previously, serum immunoreactive PTH concentrations are invariably suppressed in cancer-associated hypercalcaemia when compared with patients who have primary hyperparathyroidism and an equivalent degree of hypercalcaemia (Riggs et al. 1971; Raisz et al. 1979). Although PTH may be detectable using assays with C-terminal specificity (Raisz et al. 1971; Stewart et al. 1980), this is considered to reflect release of low quantities of native PTH from the suppressed parathyroid glands rather that ectopic PTH release by the tumour (Maijer et al. 1979). In isolated cases where slightly elevated levels of PTH have been reported using N-terminal assays, the ‘ectopic PTH’ failed to dilute out in parallel with authentic PTH suggesting that the apparrent elevations in PTH were probably due to the binding of another substance to the antibody (Roof et al. 1971).

Analysis of tumour tissues from patients with HHM using PTH radioimmunoassays have, with a few exceptions (Sherwood et al. 1967), revealed similarly negative results (Powell et al. 1973; Skarabanek et al. 1980). These contrast with the apparent identification of PTH in tumours associated with HHM reported in the 1960s using complement fixation techniques (Munson et al. 1965) and more recent data which have shown positive staining for PTH in squamous carcinomas by an immunoperoxidase technique (Ilardi and Faro 1985). It is probable that the ‘ectopic

PTH' identified in these studies was due to cross-reaction of the high antibody levels with the PTH-related peptides rather than PTH itself (Martin 1988). In this respect, it has been shown that many human and animal tumours associated with the syndrome of HHM do not express messenger RNA encoding for PTH (Simpson et al. 1983).

Whilst PTH may theoretically account for many of the biochemical features of HHM, evidence in favour of the ectopic production of active PTH by tumours associated with HHM is, with a few exceptions, lacking (Sherwood et al. 1976; Zirdar et al. 1976).

### G. The PTH-related peptides

The clinical observation that nephrogenous production of cyclic AMP was commonly associated with the syndrome of HHM represented a major milestone in unravelling its pathogenesis (Stewart et al. 1980). Following Stewart's *in vivo* observations, emphasis was shifted away from the search for factors with purely bone-resorptive activity to those which also possessed adenylate cyclase stimulating activity.

In 1983, three groups reported the finding of adenylate cyclase stimulating factors in tumours associated with HHM (Rodan et al. 1983; Stewart et al. 1983; Strewler et al. 1983). Since then, similar factors have been described by two other groups (Loveridge et al. 1985; Seshadri et al. 1986). The adenylate cyclase stimulating activity associated with these tumours was due to the release of a factor or factors, which bound to the PTH receptor *in vitro*. Whilst functionally similar to PTH in this respect, their effects were not inhibited by antibodies to PTH, suggesting that they were structurally distinct from the PTH molecule. Further investigations concentrated on the isolation of these factors. Rabbani et al. (1986) isolated two adenylate cyclase stimulating peptides of similar $M_r$, 9000 and 9500, respectively, from human and rat Leydig cell tumours associated with HHM and a larger peptide of $M_r$ 28 000 from the Leydig tumour only. All three possessed calcium elevating activity as demonstrated by their ability to prevent hypocalcaemia in thyroparathyroidectomised rats *in vivo*. While the 9000 and 9500 $M_r$ species were similar to each other in terms of amino acid composition, all three were quite distinct from native PTH. A further factor with somewhat greater biological activity, and different $M_r$ (17 000) was isolated by Burtis et al. (1987) from a breast carcinoma. Again, the amino acid composition was distinct from PTH, although at this time, no sequence data was available for this factor or the factors described by Rabbani et al. (1986).

Subsequently, Moseley et al. (1987) and Suva et al. (1987) isolated a further adenylate cyclase-stimulating factor from a human squamous cell carcinoma line associated with HHM. This was purified, sequenced, cloned and expressed and named the 'parathyroid hormone-related protein' (PTHrP), on the basis of its similarity to PTH in terms of biological activity and because 8 out of the first 16 amino acids in the N-terminus were identical to those of native PTH (Moseley et al. 1987; Suva et al. 1987).

Other workers have since purified identical factors from a human breast carcinoma (Burtis et al. 1987, Stewart et al. 1987), a human renal adenocarcinoma (Strewlet et al. 1987) and a variety of other tumours associated with HHM (Ikeda et al. 1988). At least one of the adenylate cyclase stimulating factors purified by Rabbani et al. (1986) has now been cloned and appears to be identical to PTHrP (D. Goltzman, personal communication).

The similarities between the PTHrP and PTH over the first 16 N-terminal amino acids, explains why the PTHrP reproduces many of the biological effects of PTH *in vitro* and *in vivo* (Moseley et al. 1987). The poor immunogenicity of this region (Suva et al. 1987; Martin 1988) and difference between the remainder of the molecule and PTH explain why few standard PTH radioimmunoassays have been able to to detect PTHrP *in vivo*, except at low levels which dilute in a non-parallel fashion with PTH standards; presumably these results were due to weak binding of the antibody at areas of similar amino acid sequence in the N-terminal region (Moseley et al. 1987; Martin et al. 1988).

Extensive studies with recombinant and purified PTHrP have shown that it possesses all the actions necessary to reproduce the clinical and biochemical abnormalities associated with HHM *in vivo*. The 1-34 synthetic peptide is a potent hypercalcaemic agent when infused or injected into experimental animals with a potency comparable or greater than that of PTH, depending on the experimental protocol employed (Horiuchi et al. 1987; Stewart et al. 1988; Yates et al. 1988). It is similar to PTH with regard to its effect on adenylate cyclase activity in bone cells (Horiuchi et al. 1987; Kemp et al. 1987; Yates et al. 1988) and renal cells (Horiuchi et al. 1987; Yates et al. 1988), although in some systems the PTHrP seems to be slightly less active than PTH in stimulating bone-derived cell adenylate cyclase activity (Stewart et al. 1988).

PTHrP is a powerful stimulator of bone resorption, *in vivo* and *in vitro*, with a potency similar to that of PTH in most studies (Horiuchi et al. 1987; Stewart et al. 1988) and slightly less in one (Kemp et al. 1987).

The hypercalcaemia resulting from infusion or injection of PTHrP is partly due to an increase in bone resorption (Horiuchi et al. 1987), but is also associated with an increase in renal tubular reabsorption of calcium (Kemp et al. 1987; Yates et al. 1988) and increased production of 1,25-dihydroxyvitamin D (Horiuchi et al. 1987). Phosphaturia and hypophosphataemia (Horiuchi et al. 1987; Kemp et al. 1987) also occur due to enhancement of sodium-dependent phosphate transport in renal tubular cells (Strewler et al. 1987).

PTHrP levels in HHM have not yet been measured *in vivo*. There is however, much circumstantial evidence to suggest that biologically active PTHrP circulates in HHM, on the basis of the PTH-like effects on the kidney (Stewart et al. 1980; Ralston et al. 1984) and the cytochemical bioassay evidence of PTH-like activity in the serum of patients with HHM (Goltzman et al. 1981).

## VI. Conclusions

An attempt has been made to summarise the relative contribution of the various humoral factors discussed above to the pathogenesis of cancer-associated hypercalcaemia in Fig. 6. Additional discussion on the role of, and possible interactions between, these factors in HHM is dealt with below.

### A. HHM and the PTH-related peptide

There is, as yet, no radioimmunoassay sufficiently sensitive to detect PTHrP in the serum of patients with malignant hypercalcaemia. However, indirect evidence — based on the occurrence of PTH-like effects in HHM — points to a causal role in 30 – 50% of patients with breast carcinoma (Isales et al. 1987; Bonjour et al. 1988) and 80 – 90% of patients with other solid tumours (Stewart et al. 1980; Ralston et al. 1984a, b). These findings are seen less often in haematological tumours associated with hypercalcaemia, but have been documented occasionally in myeloma (Van Breukelen et al. 1981; Rude et al. 1982) and in acute leukaemia (Zirdar et al. 1976; Gewirtz et al. 1983). It should be noted that PTHrP is not only associated with HHM, but may also play an important physiological role in the skin (Meredino et al. 1986) the fetus and other situations (see Chapter 4 by Moseley and Suva, this volume). This discussion will be confined, however, to current controversies surrounding the role of PTHrP in the pathogenesis of HHM.

Raised NcAMP values have been considered to be a relatively specific marker for the syndrome of HHM (Stewart et al. 1980), but elevated levels have also been described in normocalcaemic patients with squamous tumours (Kukreja et al. 1980;

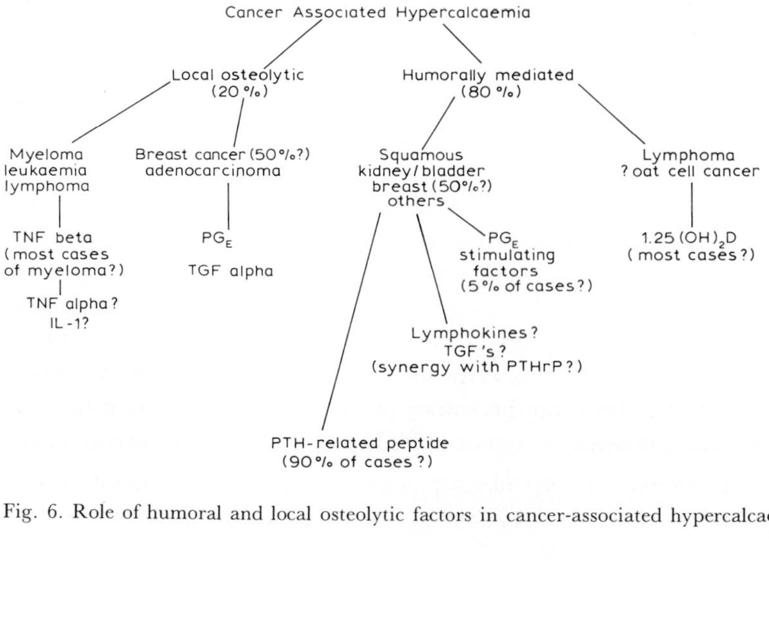


Fig. 6. Role of humoral and local osteolytic factors in cancer-associated hypercalcaemia.

Van der Velden 1983). This corresponds with the almost invariable finding of positive immunoperoxidase staining for PTHrP in squamous carcinomas and in normal skin (J. Danks, personal communication).

Normocalcaemic squamous carcinoma patients with HHM exhibit a blunted NcAMP response to PTH infusion (Naafs et al. 1986) and impaired suppression of NcAMP values to calcium infusion *in vivo* (Naafs et al. 1988). These observations suggest that tumour-derived factors (presumably PTHrP or related substances) are commonly released in normocalcaemic squamous carcinoma patients, bind to the PTH receptor, but do not behave as full agonists. Certainly, these patients do not exhibit evidence of other aspects of PTH-like activity such as phosphaturia or relative hypocalciuria (Naafs et al. 1986, 1988). These discrepancies have been explained on the basis that hypercalcaemia may only appear once the circulating levels of PTHrP reach a critical level (Martin 1988). An alternative possibility would be the release of other adenylate cyclase stimulating factors which do not cause hypercalcaemia. In this respect, it is of interest that adenylate cyclase stimulating factors have also been isolated from patients with oncogenic osteomalacia who have phosphaturia, but are normocalcaemic or even hypocalcaemic (Seshadri et al. 1985). The relationship between these substances and PTHrP remains to be established. It is possible that some tumours could release other unrelated factors such as anti-diuretic hormones, which also act on the renal tubule to increase NcAMP excretion (O'Reilly et al. 1986).

The fact that bone formation is relatively depressed in HHM when compared with primary hyperparathyroidism (McDonnel et al. 1982; Stewart et al. 1982) has also been considered to be inconsistent with a PTH-like effect on bone remodelling (Stewart et al. 1982; Mundy 1988). Although the effects of PTHrP on bone formation have not yet been fully investigated, preliminary evidence suggests that osteoblastic activity is stimulated (B. Boyce, personal communication), as is the case with PTH itself. Since tumours associated with HHM probably produce multiple bone resorbing factors, for example, TGF$\alpha$, prostaglandin stimulating factors, and Interleukin-1, it is possible that the combined effects of these and the PTHrP could cause 'uncoupling' of bone resorption and formation (Mundy 1988). An additional explanation would be a depressant effect of immobilisation on bone formation in advanced HHM (Ralston et al. 1988).

The depression of circulating 1,25-dihydroxyvitamin D levels in humans with HHM has been difficult to reconcile with the stimulatory effects of the PTHrP on 1,25-dihydroxyvitamin D production *in vivo* (Horiuchi et al. 1987) and the raised 1,25-dihydroxyvitamin D levels which occur in the rat Leydig cell tumour model of HHM (Insogna et al. 1984) — a known producer of PTHrP (Ikeda et al. 1988). Many reviewers have overlooked the fact however, that serum 1,25-dihydroxyvitamin D levels are not invariably suppressed in HHM (Ralston et al. 1984). Indeed in up to 50% of cases 1,25-dihydroxyvitamin D is clearly detectable or even raised in the serum of hypercalcaemic cancer patients (Yamamoto et al. 1987), suggesting that there is 'inappropriate' stimulation of the renal 1-alpha-hydroxylase enzyme system

(Ralston et al. 1984c, 1987a). Why some patients should have detectable 1,25-dihydroxyvitamin D when others have values which are suppressed is not known (Ralston et al. 1984c). Possible explanations include: deficiency of 25-hydroxyvitamin D, due to chronic ill health, poor diet and lack of sunlight exposure (Ralston et al. 1984c), or higher serum calcium values in HHM and a greater degree of renal impairment (Horiuchi et al. 1987). Fukomoto et al. (1988) have isolated factors from HHM-associated tumours which inhibit PTH-stimulated production of 1,25-dihydroxyvitamin D *in vitro*. It is possible that production of these factors along with PTHrP may explain the suppressed 1,25-dihydroxyvitamin D levels in some patients.

The only discrepancy between HHM and primary hyperparathyroidism which cannot readily be explained is the difference in acid base balance and serum chloride concentrations (Lafferty 1966). As yet, the effects of PTHrP on renal bicarbonate and chloride handling have not been studied, although it would be surprising if these were different from PTH, since in all other aspects, the two hormones are strikingly similar. The possibility has been raised that tumours in general, may produce substances which lead to hypochloraemic alkalosis, although there is no direct evidence to support this.

At present, this reviewer believes that the production of the PTHrP alone is sufficient to account for most cases of HHM. The following scheme is suggested as a possible way in which the syndrome may develop (Fig. 7); in the early stages, PTHrP is

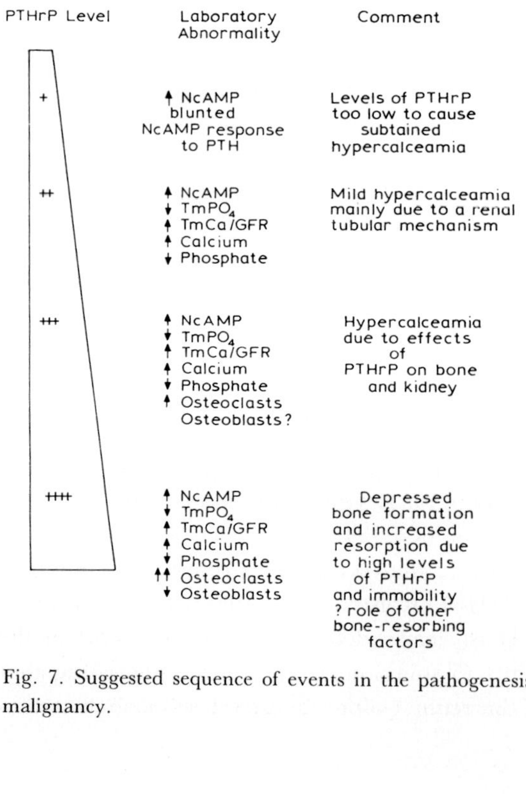


Fig. 7. Suggested sequence of events in the pathogenesis of PTHrP-related humoral hypercalcaemia of malignancy.

released at levels which activate renal adenylate cyclase activity but which are insufficient, either to cause hypercalcaemia or clinically detectable changes in renal tubular calcium and phosphate transport. Subsequently, higher circulating levels of PTHrP cause mild hypercalcaemia primarily by raising the renal tubular reabsorption of calcium (Ralston et al. 1988). Eventually, the full blown picture of humoral hypercalcaemia ensues with increased bone resorption and depressed bone formation due to synergism between high levels of PTHrP and immobilisation.

### B. HHM and vitamin D-related sterols

These factors are likely to be of greatest importance in the pathogenesis of hypercalcaemia associated with lymphomas. Until the description of elevated serum 1,25-dihydroxyvitamin D levels in patients with lymphoma-associated hypercalcaemia (Breslau et al. 1984; Davies et al. 1985; Rosenthal et al. 1985), it was thought that 'OAF'-mediated bone resorption was of major importance in the pathogenesis of hypercalcaemia in this situation. However, numerous cases of hypercalcaemia occurring in lymphoma patients without marrow infiltration or focal bone lesions have been recorded (Singer et al. 1973; Schechter et al. 1982). Since 'OAF' is thought to act locally rather than systemically, it is probable that the bone resorbing factors isolated from these tumours *in vitro* (Singer et al. 1973; Grossman et al. 1981) were in fact 1,25-dihydroxyvitamin D. This sterol may of course be equally important in the pathogenesis of hypercalcaemia in the presence of osteolytic lesions.

Serum levels of 1,25-dihydroxyvitamin D and related sterols may be raised in the absence of other evidence of PTH-like biochemical effects in isolated patients with solid tumours such as oat cell lung carcinomas (Shigeno et al. 1985) and ovarian tumours (Stewart et al. 1982). This seems to be an unusual event in clinical practice, although extensive studies of vitamin D metabolites in hypercalcaemic patients with solid tumours have not been carried out.

### C. Other humoral factors and HHM

Although PTHrP and 1,25-dihydroxyvitamin D account for the majority of instances of humorally-mediated hypercalcaemia in patients with soild tumours, a subgroup of patients may be identified who clearly have humorally-mediated hypercalcaemia (absent bone metastases; correction of hypercalcaemia after surgical cure) but who do not have elevated NcAMP levels or 1,25-dihydroxyvitamin D levels (Rude et al. 1982; Stewart et al. 1982b).

At present, most of the clinical evidence points to a role for the prostaglandin stimulating factors as mediators of hypercalcaemia in these circumstances. A subgroup of patients with HHM has been identified with absent bone metastases, elevated urinary excretion of prostaglandin metabolites, low urinary excretion of cAMP and who responded to indomethacin and aspirin therapy (Seyberth et al. 1974, 1975). Circulating prostaglandins are unlikely to be the cause of hypercalcaemia in these patients since there is no correlation between serum prostaglandin $E_2$ levels and response to indomethacin treatment (Brenner et al. 1982). While these observations may well be explained on the basis of a prostaglandin stimulating factor (Bringhurst et al. 1987), further data on the systemic release and calcium elevating activity of these substances are awaited with interest.

Other substances such as the transforming growth factors and interleukin-1 are found in tumours associated with HHM (Ibbotsen et al. 1983; Sato et al. 1987), and can cause hypercalcaemia when infused *in vivo* (Tashjian et al. 1986; Sabatini et al. 1988). They may be important as mediators of increased bone resorption and depressed bone formation in combination with the PTHrP. It is currently unclear whether these factors alone, are responsible for humorally-mediated hypercalcaemia in man.

## References


Anggard E, Sammuelsson B. Metabolism of prostaglandin $E_1$ in the guinea pig lung: The structure of two metabolites. J Biol Chem 1964;239:4097 – 4102.

Atkins D, Martin TJ. Rat osteogenic sarcoma cells: Effects of some prostaglandins, their metabolites and analogues on cyclic AMP production. Prostaglandins 1977;13:561 – 565.

Azzopardi JG, Whittaker JCS. Bronchial carcinoma and hypercalcaemia. J Clin Pathol 1969;22:718 – 724.

Battaille R, Chappard D, Alexandre C, Dessauw P, Sany J. Intrest of bone histomorphometric analysis in monoclonal gammopathy. Br J Cancer 1986;53:805 – 810.

Beliel OM, Singer FR, Coburn JW. Prostaglandins: effect on plasma calcium concentration. Prostaglandins 1973;3:237 – 241.

Bender RA Hansen H. Hypercalcemia in bronchogenic carcinoma. Ann Intern Med 1974;80:205 – 208.

Bernier SM, Goltzman D. Influence of peptides acting through the EGF receptor on the action of synthetic human PTH-like peptide of malignancy in renal and osseous cells (Abstract). J Bone Miner Res 1988:3(suppl)s67.

Bertolini DR, Nedwin GE, Brown TS, Smith DD, Mundy GR. Stimulation of bone resorption and inhibition of bone formation in vitro by human tumour necrosis factors. Nature 1986;319:576 – 578.

Bijvoet OLM. Kidney function in calcium and phosphate metabolism. In: Avioli LV and Krane SM, eds. Metabolic Bone Disease, Vol 1. New York: Academic Press, 1977;49 – 140.

Blayney DW, Jaffe ES, Fisher RI, et al. The human T-cell leukaemia/lymphoma virus, lymphoma, lytic bone lesions and hypercalcaemia. Ann Intern Med 1983;98:144 – 151.

Bonjour JP, Phillipe J, Guelpa G, et al. Bone and renal components in hypercalcaemia of malignancy and responses to a single infusion of clodronate. Bone 1988;9:123 – 130.

Boyd JC, Ladenson JH. Value of laboratory tests in the differential diagnosis of hypercalcaemia. Am J Med 1984;77:863 – 872.

Brenner DE, Harvey HA, Lipton A, Demers L. A study of prostaglandin $E_2$, parathormone and response to indomethacin in patients with hypercalcaemia of malignancy. Cancer 1982;49:556 – 561.

Brereton HD, Halushka PV, Alexandre RW, Keiser HR, DeVita VJ. Indomethacin-responsvie hypercalcemia in a patients with renal cell adenocarcinoma. N Engl J Med 1974;291:82 – 85.

Breslau NA, McGuire JL, Zerwekh JE, Frenkel EP, Pak CYC. Hypercalcemia associated with increased serum calcitriol levels in three patients with lymphoma. Ann Intern Med 1984;100:1 – 7.

Bringhurst FR, Bierer BE, Godeau F, Neyhard N, Varner V, Segre GV. Humoral hypercalcemia of malignancy: release of a prostaglandin stimulating bone resorbing factor in vitro by human transitional carcinoma cells. J Clin Invest 1986;77:456 – 464.

Broadus AE, Mahaffey JE, Barrter FC, Neer RM. Nephrogenous cyclic adenosine monophosphate as a parathyroid function test. J Clin Invest 1977;60:771 – 783.

Broadus AE, Horst RL, Lang R, Littledike ET, Rasmussen H. The importance of circulating 1,25-dihydroxyvitamin D in the pathogenesis of hypercalciuria and renal stone formation in primary hyperparathyroidism. N Engl J Med 1980;302:421 – 416.

Burt ME, Brennan MF. Incidence of hypercalcaemia in malignant neoplasm. Arch Surg 1980;115:704 – 707.

Burtis WJ, Wu T, Bunch C, Wysolmerski JJ, Insogna KL, Broadus AE. Identification of a novel 17 000 dalton PTH-like adenylate cyclase stimulating protein from a tumor associated with humoral hypercalcaemia of malignancy. J Biol Chem 1987;262:7151 – 7156.

Cannelos GP. Hypercalcaemia in malignant lymphoma and leukaemia. Ann NY Acad Si 1974;230:240 – 246.

Case Records of the Massachusetts General Hospital (Case 27401). N Engl J Med 1941;225:789 – 791.

Cohen RD. The renal tubular acidoses. In: Weatherall DJ, Ledingham JGG, Warrel DA, eds. Oxford Textbook of Medicine, 2nd edn., Vol. 2. Oxford: UK, Oxford Medical Publications, 1987.

Coleman RE, Rubens RD. 3-(amino-1,1-hydroxypropylidene) bisphosphonate (APD) for hypercalcaemia of breast cancer. Br J Cancer 1987;56:465 – 469.

Coombes RC, Ward MK, Greenberg PB, et al. Calcium metabolism in cancer: studies using calcium isotopes and immunoassays for parathyroid hormone and calcitonin. Cancer 1976;38:2111 – 2120.

Davies M, Hayes ME, Mawer EB, Lumb GA. Abnormal vitamin D metabolism in Hodgkin's lymphoma. Lancet 1985;ii:1186 – 1188.

Devers LM, Allegra JC, Harvey HA, et al. Plasma prostaglandins in patients with neoplastic disease. Cancer 1977;39:1559 – 1562.

Dewhirst FE, Stashenko PP, Mole JE, Tsurumachi T. Purification and partial sequence of human osteoclast activating factor: identity with interleukin-1 beta. J Immunol 1985;135:2562 – 2568.

Durie BGM, Salmon SE, Mundy GR. Relation of osteoclast activating factor production to the extent of metastatic bone disease in myeloma. Br J Haematol 1981;47:21 – 30.

D'Souza SM, Ibbotson KJ, Mundy GR. Failure of parathyroid hormone antagonists to inhibit in vitro bone resorbing activity produced by two animal models of the humoral hypercalcemia of malignancy. J Clin Invest 1984;74:1104 – 1107.

Elion G, Mundy GR. Direct resorption of bone by breast carcinoma cells in vitro. Nature 1978;276:726 – 728.

Fetchick DA, Bertolini DR, Sarin PS, Weintraub ST, Mundy GR, Dunn JD. Production of 1,25-dihydroxyvitamin D by human T-cell lymphotrophic virus-1 transformed lymphocytes. J Clin Invest 1986;78:592 – 596.

Fisken RA, Heath DA, Bold AM. Hypercalcaemia — a hospital survey. Q J Med 1980;196:405 – 418.

Franklin B, Tashjian AH. Intravenous infusion of prostaglandin $E_2$ raises plasma calcium concentration in the rat. Endocrinology 1975;97:240 – 243.

Fry L. Pseudohyperparathyroidism with carcinoma of the bronchus. Br Med J 1962;i:301 – 302.

Fukomato S, Matsumoto T, Yamoto H, et al. Suppression of serum 1,25 dihydroxyvitamin D in humoral hypercalcaemia of malignancy is caused by elaboration of a factor that inhibits renal 1,25 dihydroxyvitamin $D_3$ production. Endocrinology 1989;124:2057–2062.

Galasko CSB, Burn JI. Hypercalcamia in patients with advanced mammary cancer. Br Med J 1971;3:573 – 577

Galasko CSB, Bennet A. Relation of bone destruction in skeletal metastases to osteoclast activation and prostaglandins. Nature 1976;763:508 – 510.

Gardner B. The relation between serum calcium and tumour metastases. Surg Gynecol Obstet 1969;128:369 – 374.

Garret IR, Durie BJM, Nedwin GE, et al. Production of lymphotoxin — a potent bone resorbing cytokine

— by cultured myeloma cells. N Engl J Med 1987;317:562 – 532.

Gewirtz AM, Stewart AF, Vignery A, Hoffman R. Hypercalcaemia complicating acute myeloid leukaemia: a syndrome of multiple aetiologies. Br J Haematol 1983;54:133 – 141.

Goltzman D, Stewart AF, Broadus AE. Malignancy-associated hypercalcaemia: evaluation with a cytochemical bioassay for parathyroid hormone. J Clin Endocrinol Metab 1981;53:899 – 904.

Gordan GS, Cantino TJ, Erdhardt L, Hansen J, Lubich W. Osteolytic sterol in human breast cancer. Science 1965;151:1226 – 1228.

Gowen M, Wood DD, Ihrie EJ, McGuire MKB, Russell RGG. An interleukin-1 like factor stimulates bone resorption in vitro. Nature 1983;306:378 – 380.

Greaves M, Ibbotson KJ, Atkins D, Martin TJ. Prostaglandins as mediators of bone resorption in renal and breast tumors. Metabolism 1980;58:201 – 210.

Grossman B, Schechter GP, Horton JE, Pierce LP, Jaffe E, Wahl L. Hypercalcemia associated with T-cell lymphoma-leukemia. Am J Clin Pathol 1981;75:149 – 155.

Gutman A, Tyson T, Gutman E. Serum calcium, phosphate and phosphatase activity in hyperparathyroidism, Pagets disease and neoplastic disease of the bones. Arch Intern Med 1936;57:379 – 413.

Haddad JG, Courantz SJ, Avioli LV. Circulating phytosterols in normal females, lactating mothers and breast cancer patients. J Clin Endocrinol Metab 1970;30:174 – 180.

Harinck HIJ, Bijvoet OLM, Platingh AST, et al. Role of bone and kidney in tumor induced hypercalcemia and it's treatment with bisphosphonate and sodium chloride. Am J Med 1987;82:1133 – 1142.

Haussler MR, McCain TA. Basic and clinical concepts related to vitamin D metabolism and action. N Engl J Med 1977;297:974 – 982.

Hirshorn JE, Vrhovsek E, Posen S. Carcinoma of the breast associated with hypercalcemia and the presence of parathyroid hormone-like substances in the tumor. J Clin Endocrinol Metab 1979;48:2383 – 2385.

Horiuchi N, Caulfield MP, Fisher JE, et al. A similarity of synthetic peptide from human tumor to parathyroid hormone in vivo and in vitro. Science 1987;238:1566 – 1568.

Heller SR, Hosking DJ. Renal handling of calcium and sodium in metastatic and non-metastatic malignancy. Br Med J 1986;292:583 – 586.

Hosking DJ, Cowley A, Bucknall CA. Rehydration in the treatment of severe hypercalcaemia. Q J Med 1981;200:473 – 487.

Ibbotson KJ, D'Souza SM, Ng KW, et al. Tumor-derived growth factor increases bone resorption in a tumor associated with humoral hypercalcemia of malignancy. Science 1983;221:1292 – 1294.

Ibbotson KJ, D'Souza SM, Smith DD, Carpenter G, Mundy GR. EGF receptor antiserum inhibits bone resorbing activity produced by rat leydig cell tumor associated with the humoral hypercalcemia of malignancy. Endocrinology 1985;116:469 – 471.

Ikeda K, Mangin M, Dreyer B, et al. Identification of transcripts encoding a parathyroid hormone-like peptide in messenger RNA's from a variety of human and animal tumors associated with humoral hypercalcemia of malignancy. J Clin Invest 1988;81:2010 – 2014.

Ilardi CF, Faro JC. Localisation of parathyroid hormone-like substance in squamous cell carcinomas. Arch Pathol Lab Med 1985;109:752 – 755.

Insogna KL, Stewart AF, Vignery AM, et al. Biochemical and histomorphomeric characterisation of a rat model for humoral hypercalcemia of malignancy. Endocrinology 1984;114:888 – 896.

Isales C, Carcangui ML, Stewart AF, Hypercalcemia in breast carcinoma: reassessment of the mechanism. Am J Med 1987;82:1143 – 1147.

Josse RG, Wilson DR, Heersche JNM, Mills JRF, Murray TM. Hypercalcaemia with ovarian carcinoma: evidence of a pathogenic role for prostaglandins. Cancer 1981;48:1233 – 1241.

Jordan GW. Serum calcium and phosphorous abnormalities in leukemia. Am J Med 1966;41:381 – 390.

Kemp BE, Moseley JM, Rodda CP, et al. Parathyroid hormone related protein of malignancy: active synthetic fragments. Science; 238:1568 – 1570.

Kimura S, Adchi I, Yamaguchi K, et al. Stimulation of calcium reabsorption observed in advanced breast cancer patients with hypercalcemia and multiple bone metastases. Gann 1985;76:308 – 314.

Klein DC, Raisz LG. Prostaglandins: stimulation of bone resorption in tissue culture. Endocrinology 1970;80:1436 – 1440.

Kukreja SC, Shemeriak WP, Lud TE, Johnstone PA. Elevated nephrogenous 3′5′-cyclic adenosine monophosphate with normal parathyroid hormone levels in patients with lung cancer. J Clin Endocrinol Metab 1980;51:167 – 169.

Laffan MA, Talavera JG, Catovsky D. Hypercalcaemia in T-cell acute lymphoblastic leukaemia: report of two cases. J Clin Pathol 1986;39:1143 – 1146.

Lafferty FW. Pseudohyperparathyroidism. Medicine (Baltimore) 1966;45:247 – 260.

Lamberg BA, Pelkonen R, Frick MH. Hypercalcaemia in renal carcinoma: report of a case. Acta Med Scand 1964;176:187 – 194.

Loveridge N, Kent GN, Heath DA, Jones EL. Parathyroid hormone-like bioactivity in a patient with severe osteitis fibrosa cystica due to malignancy: renotropic actions of a tumour extract as assessed by cytochemical bioassay. Clin Endocrinol (Oxford) 1985;22:135 – 146.

Martin TJ, Atkins D. Biological regulators of bone resorption and their significance in cancer. Essays Med Biochem 1977;4:49 – 82.

Martin TJ. Humoral hypercalcaemia of malignancy. Bone Miner 1988;4:83 – 89.

Maijer GP, Keate JA, Hirst JG, Habener JF. Effect of plasma calcium on relative proportion of intact hormone and C-terminal fragments in parathyroid venous blood. Endocrinology 1979;104:1778 – 1784.

Mavligit GM, Cohen JL, Sherwoord LM. Ectopic production of parathyroid hormone by carcinoma of the breast. N Engl J Med 1971;285:154 – 156.

McDonnell GD, Dunstan CR, Evans RA et al. Quantitative bone histology in the hypercalcemia of malignant disease. J Clin Endocrinol Metab 1982;55:1066 – 1072.

Meredino TJ, Insogna KL, Milstone LM, Broadus AE, Stewart AF. A parathyroid hormone-like protein from cultured human keratinocytes. Science 1986;231:388 – 390.

Minkin C, Fredericks RS, Porkess S, et al. Bone resorption and humoral hypercalcaemia of malignancy: stimulation of bone resorption in vitro by tumor extracts in inhibited by prostaglandin synthetase inhibitors. J Clin Endocrinol Metab 1981;53:941 – 947.

Moseley JM, Kubota M, Diefenbach-Jagger H, et al. Parathyroid hormone-related protein purified from a human lung cancer cell line. Proc Natl Acad Sci USA 1987;84:5048 – 5052.

Moses AM, Spencer H. Hypercalcemia in patients with malignant lymphoma. Ann Intern Med 1963;59:531 – 536.

Mudde AH, Berg H vd, Breedveld FC, Nijweide PJ, Papapoulos SE, Bijvoet OLM. Lymphoma associated hypercalcemia. In vitro demonstration of 1,25-dihydroxyvitamin $D_3$ production. Calcif Tissue Int 1985;38(Suppl):s36.

Mundy GR. Pathogenesis of hypercalcemia of malignancy. Clin Endocrinol (Oxford) 1985;23:705 – 714.

Mundy GR. Hypercalcemia of malignancy revisited. J Clin Invest 1988;82:1 – 6.

Mundy GR, Martin TJ. The hypercalcemia of malignancy: pathogenesis and management. Metabolism 1982;31:1247 – 1275.

Mundy GR, Raisz LG, Cooper RA, Schechter GP, Salmon SE. Evidence for the secretion of an osteoclast activating factor in myeloma. N Engl J Med 1974a;291:1041 – 1048.

Mundy GR, Luben RA, Raisz LG, Oppenheim JJ, Buell DN. Bone-resorbing activity in supernatants from lymphoid cell lines. N Engl J Med 1974b;290:867 – 871.

Mundy GR, Ibbotson KJ, D'Souza SM, Simpson EL, Jacobs JW, Martin TJ. The hypercalcemia of cancer: clinical implications and pathogenic mechanisms. N Engl J Med 1984;310:1718 – 1726.

Mundy GR, Ibbotson KJ, D'Souza SM. Tumor products and the hypercalcemia of malignancy. J Clin Invest 1985;76:391 – 394.

Munson PL, Tashjian AH, Levine L. Evidence for parathyroid hormone in non-parathyroid tumors associated with hypercalcemia. Cancer Res 1965;25:1062 – 1067.

Naafs MAB, Fischer HRA, Mulder H, et al. End-organ resistance to PTH infusion in hypercalcaemic and normocalcaemic patients with solid tumours. Acta Endocrinol (Copenhagen) 1986;113:543 – 550.

O'Reilly, D. St J, Fraser, WD, Penney MD, Logue FC, Cowan RA, Williams BC, Walters G. Arginine blocks the action of parathyroid hormone but not vasopressin on the renal tubule in man. J Endocrinol 1986;111:501 – 506.

Peacock M, Robertson WG, Nordin BEC. Relation between serum and urinary calcium with particular reference to parathyroid activity. Lancet 1969;i:384 – 387.

Percival RC, Yates AJP, Gray RES, et al. Mechanisms of hypercalcaemia in carcinoma of the breast. Br Med J 1985;291:776 – 779.

Papapoulos SE, Hendy GN, Tomlinson S, Lewin JG, O'Riordan JLH. Clearance of endogenous parathyroid hormone in normal and uraemic man. Clin Endocrinol (Oxford) 1977;7:211 – 225.

Paterson AD, Kanis JA, Cameron EC, et al. The use of dichloromethylene diphosphonate for the treatment of hypercalcaemia in multiple myeloma. Br J Haematol 1983;54:121 – 132.

Pitzurki L, Rizzoli R, Bonjour JP. Effect of synthetic parathyroid hormone-related peptide (PTHrP 1 34) on cAMP production and sodium-dependent phosphate transport (NaPiT) in renal epithelial cells: modulation by transforming growth factor alpha (Abstract). J Bone Miner Res 1988;3(Suppl):s72.

Powell D, Singer FR, Murray TM, Minkin C, Potts JT. Non-parathyroid humoral hypercalcaemia in patients with neoplastic diseases. N Engl J Med 1973;289:176 – 181.

Rabbani SA, Mitchell J, Roy DR, Kremer R, Bennet HPJ, Goltzman D. Purification of peptides with parathyroid hormone-like bioactivities from human and rat malignancies associated with hypercalcemia. Endocrinology 1986;118:1200 – 1210.

Raisz LG, Dietrich JW, Simmonds HA, Seyberth HW, Hubbard W, Oates JA. Effect of prostaglandin endoperoxidases and metabolites on bone resorption in vitro. Nature 1977;267:532 – 534.

Raisz LG, Chaitanaya HY, Bockman RS, Bower BF. Comparison of commercially available immunoassays in differential diagnosis of hypercalcemia due to primary hyperparathyroidism or malignancy. Ann Intern Med 1979;91:739 – 740.

Ralston SH, Fogelman I, Gardner MD, Boyle IT. Hypercalcaemia and metastatic bone disease: is there a causal link? Lancet 1982;i:903 – 905.

Ralston SH, Fogelman I, Gardner MD, Boyle IT. Relative contribution of humoral and metastatic factors to the pathogenesis of hypercalcaemia in malignancy. Br Med J 1984a;288:1405 – 1408.

Ralston SH, Fogelman I, Gardner MD, Dryburgh FJ, Cowan RA, Boyle IT. Hypercalcaemia of malignancy: evidence for a non-PTH humoral agent with an effect on renal tubular calcium handling. Clin Sci 1984b;66:187 – 191.

Ralston SH, Cowan RA, Robertson AG, Gardner MD, Boyle IT. Circulating vitamin D metabolites and hypercalcaemia of malignancy. Acta Endocrinol (Copenhagen) 1984c;106:556 – 563.

Ralston SH, Boyce BF, Cowan RA, Gardner MD, Dryburgh FJ, Boyle IT. Humoral hypercalcaemia of malignancy: metabolic and histomorphometric studies during surgical treatment of the primary tumour. Q J Med 1986a;227:325 – 335.

Ralston SH, Gardner MD, Dryburgh FJ, Cowan RA, Boyle IT. Influence of urinary sodium excretion on the clinical assessment of renal tubular calcium reabsorption in hypercalcaemic man. J Clin Pathol 1986b;39:641 – 646.

Ralston SH, Cowan RA, Gardner MD, Fraser WD, Marshall E, Boyle IT. Comparison of intestinal calcium absorption and circulating 1,25-dihydroxyvitamin D levels in malignancy-associated hypercalcaemia and primary hyperparathyroidism. Clin Endocrinol (Oxford) 1987a;26:281 – 291.

Ralston SH, Gardner MD, Jenkins AS, McKillop JH, Boyle IT. Malignancy-associated hypercalcaemia: relationship between mechanisms of hypercalcaemia and response to antihypercalcaemic therapy. Bone Miner 1987b;2:227 – 242.

Ralston SH, Boyce BF, Cowan RA, Gardner MD, Fraser WD, Boyle, IT. Contrasting mechanisms of hypercalcaemia in early and advanced humoral hypercalcaemia of malignancy. Ann Intern Med 1989;4:103–111.

Riggs BL, Arnaud CD, Reynolds JC, Smith LH. Immunologic differentiation of primary hyperparathyroidism from hyperparathyroidism due to non-parathyroid cancer. J Clin Invest 1971;50:2079 – 2083.

Rizzoli R, Caverzasio J, Fleisch H, Bonjour JP. Parathyroid hormone-like changes in renal calcium and phosphate reabsorption induced by Leydig cell tumour in thyroparathyroidectomized rats. Endocrinology 1986;119:1004 – 1009.

Robertson RP, Baylink DJ, Metz SA, Cummings KB. Plasma prostaglandins in patients with cancer with and without hypercalcemia. J Clin Endocrinol Metab 1976;43:1330 – 1335.

Rodan SB, Insogna KL, Vignery, A et al. Factors associated with humoral hypercalcemia of malignancy stimulate adenylate cyclase in osteoblastic cells. J Clin Invest 1983;72:1151 – 1515.

Roof B, Carpenter B, Fink J, Gordan GS. Some thoughts on the nature of ectopic parathyroid hormones. Am J Med 1971;50:686 – 691.

Rosenthal N, Insogna KL, Godsall JW, Smaldone L, Waldron JA, Stewart AF. Elevations in circulating 1,25-dihydroxyvitamin D in three patients with lymphoma associated hypercalcemia. J Clin Endocrinol Metab 1985;60:29 – 33.

Rude RK, Sharp CF, Fredericks RS, et al. Urinary and nephrogenous cyclic 3′,5′adenosine monophosphate in the hypercalcemia of malignancy. J Clin Endocrinol Metab 1981;52:765 – 771.

Sabatini M, Boyce BF, Aufdemorte T, Bonewald L, Mundy GR. Infusions of recombinant interleukin 1 alpha and beta cause hypercalcemia in normal mice. Proc Natl Acad Sci USA 1988;85:5235 – 5239.

Sato K, Mimura H, Han DC, et al. Production of bone resorbing activity and colony stimulating activity in vivo and in vitro by a human squamous cell carcinoma associated with hypercalcemia and leukocytosis. J Clin Invest 1986a;78:145 – 154.

Sato K, Fuji Y, Kasono K, Shizume K. Production of interleukin-1 alpha-like activity and colony stimulating activity by clonal squamous cell carcinomas derived from patients with hypercalcaemia and leukocytosis. In: Cohn DV, Martin TJ and Meunier PJ, eds. Calcium Regulation and Bone Metabolism: Basic and Clinical Aspects, Vol 9. Amsterdam: Elsevier, 1986b;149 – 154.

Sato K, Fuji Y, Kasonok, et al. Production of interleukin-1$\alpha$ and a parathyroid hormone-like factor by a squamous cell carcinoma of the oesophagus (EC-GI) derived from a patient with hypercalcemia. J Clin Endocrinol Metab 1988;67:593 – 601.

Seshadri MS, Mason RS, Cornish CJ, Pryke AM, Posen S. Humoral hypercalcaemia of malignancy: report of two further patients with biochemical studies on tumour extracts. Clin Sci 1986;71:261 – 269.

Schechter GP, Jaffe ES, Grossman J, Horton JE, Whitcombe CC. Malignant lymphoma with hypercalcemia. N Engl J Med 1982;306:995.

Scholz DA, Riggs BL, Purnell DC, Goldsmith RS, Arnaud CD. Ectopic hyperparathyroidism with renal calculi and subperiosteal bone resorption. Mayo Clin Proc 1973;48:124 – 126.

Schussler GC, Verso MA, Nemoto T. Phosphaturia in hypercalcemic breast cancer patients. J Clin Endocrinol Metab 1972;35:497 – 504.

Seyberth HW, Segre GV, Morgan JL, Sweetman BJ, Potts JT, Oates JA. Prostaglandins as mediators of hypercalcemia associated with certain types of cancer. N Engl J Med 1975;273:1278 – 1283.

Seyberth HW, Segre GV, Hamet P, Sweetman BJ, Potts JT, Oates JA. Characterisation of the group of patients with hypercalcemia of cancer who respond to treatment with prostaglandin synthesis inhibitors. Trans Assoc Am Phys 1976;89:92 – 105.

Sharp CF, Rude RK, Terry R, Singer FR. Abnormal bone and parathyroid histology in cancer patients with pseudohyperparathyroidism. Cancer 1982;49:1449 – 1455.

Sherwood LM, O'Riordan JLH, Aurbach GD, Potts JT. Production of parathyroid hormone by non-parathyroid tumors. J Clin Endocrinol 1967;27:140 – 146.

Shigeno C, Yamamoto I, Dokoh S, et al. Identification of 1,24(R)-dihydroxyvitamin $D_3$-like bone-resorbing lipid in a patient with cancer-associated hypercalcemia. J Clin Endocrinol Metab 1985;61:761 – 768.

Simpson EL, Mundy GR, D'Souza SM, Ibbotson KJ, Bockman R, Jacobs JW. Absence of parathyroid hormone messenger RNA in non-parathyroid tumor associated with hypercalcemia. N Engl J Med 1983;309:325 – 330.

Singer FR, Adams JS. Abnormal calcium homeostasis in sarcoidosis. N Engl J Med 1986;315:755 – 757.

Singer FR, Powell D, Minkin C, Bethune JE, Brickman A, Coburn JW. Hypercalcaemia in reticulum cell sarcoma without hyperparathyroidism or skeletal metastases. Ann Intern Med 1973;78:365 – 369.

Skrabanek P, McPartlin D, Powell DM. Tumour hypercalcemia and ectopic hyperparathyroidism. Medicine (Baltimore) 1980;59:262 – 282.

Sleeboom HP, Bijvoet OLM, Van Oosteroom AT, Gleed JH, O'Riordan JLH. Comparison of intravenous (3-amino-1-hydroxypropylidene)-1,1bisphosphonate and volume repletion in tumour-induced hypercalcaemia. Lancet 1983,ii:239 – 243.

Somayaji BN, Nelson RS, McGregor RF. Small intestinal function in malignant neoplasia. Cancer 1972;29:1215 – 1222.

Stewart AF, Horst R, Deftos LJ, Lang R, Broadus AE. Biochemical evaluation of patients with cancer-associated hypercalcemia: evidence for humoral and non-humoral subgroups. N Engl J Med 1980;303:1377 – 1383.

Stewart AF, Vignery A, Silvergate A, et al. Quantitative bone histomorphmetry in humoral hypercalcemia of malignancy: uncoupling of bone cell activity. J Clin Endocrinol Metab 1982a;55:219 – 227.

Stewart AF, Romero R, Schwartz PE, Kohorn EI, Broadus AE. Hypercalcemia associated with gynecological malignancies. Cancer 1982b;49:3289 – 3294.

Stewart AF, Insogna KL, Golzman D, Broadus AE. Identification of adenylate cyclase stimulating activity in extracts of tumor associated with humoral hypercalcemia of malignancy. Proc Natl Acad Sci 1983;80:1454 – 1458.

Stewart AF, Wu T, Goumas D, Burtis WJ, Broadus AE. N-terminal amino acid sequence of two novel tumor derived adenylate cyclase stimulating proteins: identification of parathyroid hormone-like and parathyroid hormone-unlike domains. Biochem Biophys Res Commun 1987;146:672 – 678.

Stewart AF, Mangin M, Wu T, et al. Synthetic parathyroid hormone-like protein stimulates bone resorption and causes hypercalcemia in rats. J Clin Invest 1988;81:596 – 600.

Strewler GJ, Williams RD, Nissenson RA. Human renal carcinoma cells produce hypercalcemia in the nude mouse and a novel protein recognized by parathyroid hormone receptors. J Clin Invest 1983;71:769 – 774.

Strewler GJ, Stern PH, Jacobs JW, et al. Parathyroid hormone-like protein from renal carcinoma cells: structural and functional homology with parathyroid hormone. J Clin Invest 1987;80:1803 – 1807.

Suva LJ, Winslow GA, Moseley JM, et al. A parathyroid hormone related protein implicated in malignant hypercalcemia: cloning and expression. Science 1987;237:893 – 896.

Sztern M, Barkan A, Rakowsky E, Shainkin Kestenbaum R, Marilus R, Blum I. Hypercalcemia in carcinoma of the breast without evidence of bone destruction. Cancer 1981;48:2383 – 2385.

Tanaka Y, Deluca HF. The control of 25-hydroxyvitamin D metabolism by inorganic phosphate. Arch Biochem Biophys 1973;154:566 – 570.

Tashjian AH. Tumor humors and the hypercalcemia of cancer. N Engl J Med 1975;293:1317 – 1318.

Tashjian AH, Voelkel EF, Lazzaro M, et al. Alpha and Beta human transforming growth factors stimulate prostaglandin production and bone resorption in cultured mouse calvariae. Proc Natl Acad Sci USA 1985;82:4535 – 4538.

Tashjian AH, Voelkel EF, Lloyd W, Derynck R, Winkler ME, Levine L. Actions of growth factors on plasma calcium. J Clin Invest 1986;78:1405 – 1409.

Travers MT, Barret Lee PJ, Berger U, et al. Growth factor expression in normal, benign and malignant breast tissue. Br Med J 1988;296:1621 – 1624.

Van Breukelen FJM, Bijvoet OLM, Frijlink WB, Sleeboom HP, Mulder H, Van Oosterom AT. Efficacy of aminohydroxypropylidene bisphosphonate in hypercalcaemia: observations on regulation of serum calcium. Calcif Tissue Int 1982;34:321 – 327.

Van der Velden PC, Naafs MAB, Fischer HRA, et al. The urinary excretion of cyclic AMP in patients with malignant tumours. Neth J Med 1983;26:10 – 17.

Voelkel EF, Tashjian AH, Franklin R, Wasserman E, Levine L. Hypercalcemia and tumour prostaglandins: the VX-2 carcinoma model in the rabbit. Metabolism 1975;24:973 – 986.

Wills MR, Gill JR, Barrter FC. The inter-relationships of calcium and sodium excretion. Clin Sci

1979;37:621 – 630.

Yamamoto I, Kitamura N, Aoki J, et al. Circulating 1,25-dihydroxyvitamin D concentrations in patients with renal cell carcinoma hypercalcemia are rarely suppressed. J Clin Endocrinol Metab 1987;64:175 – 179.

Yates AJP, Gutierrez GE, Smoles P, et al. Effects of a synthetic peptide of a parathyroid hormone-related protein on calcium homeostasis, renal tubular calcium reabsorption and bone metabolism in vivo and in vitro. J Clin Invest 1988;81:932 – 938.

Zilva JF, Nicholson JP. Plasma phosphate and potassium levels in the hypercalcaemia of malignancy. J Clin Endocrinol Metab 1973;36:1019 – 1026.

Zirdar BL, Shadduck RK, Winkelstein A, Ziegler Z, Hawker CD. Acute myeloblastic leukemia and hypercalcemia: a case of probable ectopic PTH production. N Engl J Med 1976;295:692 – 694.

Zondek P, Peitow H, Siebert W. Die beteitung der calcium bestimmung im blut fur die diagnose der niereninsuffizienz. Z. Klin Med 1924;99:129 – 138.

*Bone and Mineral Research/7*
*Johan N.M. Heersche and John A. Kanis, editors*



# Isolation, biochemistry and molecular biology of the PTH-related protein of malignant hypercalcemia

JANE M. MOSELEY AND LARRY J. SUVA

*Department of Medicine, University of Melbourne, and St. Vincent's Institute of Medical Research, St. Vincent's Hospital, Fitzroy, Victoria 3065, Australia*

## I. Introduction

The recent isolation, sequencing, cloning and characterization of the gene for a novel parathyroid hormone-like protein has provided an exciting culmination to the search for the mediator of the parathyroid hormone-like features of humoral hypercalcemia of malignancy (HHM) (Moseley et al. 1987; Strewler et al. 1987; Suva et al. 1987; Mangin et al. 1988a; Thiede et al. 1988). HHM is the term coined by Martin and Atkins (1979) to describe the syndrome in patients with certain cancers, exhibiting many of the characteristic symptoms of hyperparathyroidism, but with normal levels of immunoreactive parathyroid hormone (PTH), and little or no evidence of bony metastases. In the absence of secondary lesions, removal of the tumor results in restoration of normocalcemia, suggesting that the tumors (commonly of squamous origin) produce a factor or factors responsible for the observed effects. Like PTH, the responsible agent apparently acts upon the kidney to reduce calcium excretion as well as to increase cyclic AMP (cAMP) and phosphorus excretion in a manner similar to the manifestations of hyperparathyroidism.

The parathyroid hormone-related protein, (PTHrP*) exhibits sufficient N-terminal sequence homology to PTH to account for its similar actions via the PTH receptor and these actions of PTHrP have also now been confirmed with biologically active synthetic peptides. It is however the product of a distinct gene which probably originally

* Also referred to in the literature as hHHF, hHCF, hACSF or PLP.

arose as the result of duplication of the *PTH* gene.

Although HHM and hyperparathyroidism share many biochemical features, there are several distinguishing characteristics in the manifestations of these two syndromes (Stewart et al. 1980; Rude et al. 1981). Firstly, renal bicarbonate wasting seen in hyperparathyroidism is not a feature of HHM and secondly, as well as increased osteoclastic resorption there is a reduced rate of bone formation seen in HHM. In contrast, in hyperparathyroidism, the normal relationship between bone formation and bone loss is retained. It is possible that there are several as yet undefined ways in which the actions of the two hormones differ. Also the interaction of PTHrP with other humoral tumor factors such as transforming growth factors and tumor necrosis factors, all of which have been implicated in bone metabolism (Raisz et al. 1980; Gowen et al. 1983; Ibbotson et al. 1983, 1985; Tashjian et al. 1978, 1985; Bertolini et al. 1986; Gutierrez et al. 1987), may be relevant in producing the distinctive features of HHM which differ from hyperparathyroidism (Mundy and Martin 1982; Mundy et al., 1985; Martin and Mundy 1987; Martin 1988; Mundy 1988).

## II. Background

The pathophysiology and clinical aspects of HHM are dealt with in detail elsewhere in this volume but a brief historical summary of the events leading up to the isolation of PTHrP is pertinent here.

It was Albright in 1941 who originally ascribed malignancy-associated hypercalcemia, first described in the 1920s (Zondek et al. 1923), to the ectopic production of PTH by the tumors involved. With the advent of radioimmunoassays for PTH, elevated levels of immunoreactive PTH were found either in tumor extracts or in serum, in some cases of bronchogenic carcinoma (Berson and Yalow 1966; Sherwood et al. 1967; Buckle et al. 1970; Melick et al. 1972). The ectopic PTH hypothesis was soon thrown into dispute by reports which showed that the elevated levels of circulating immunoreactive PTH in a number of patients with malignancy-associated hypercalcemia did not assay parallel to the standard curve (Roof et al. 1971; Benson et al. 1974; Riggs et al. 1971), nor were the levels as high as those generally observed in hyperparathyroidism. At the time it was concluded that these observations were due to the inadequacies of the assays then in use.

A comprehensive study by Powell (1973) presented observations on 11 patients with undetectable serum immunoreactive PTH levels but whose tumor extracts caused active calcium resorption from bone *in vitro*. Furthermore, Atkins et al. (1977) studying a group of renal cortical carcinoma patients found that 9 out of 13 extracts from these tumors could cause resorption in mouse calvaria *in vitro*. Again immunoreactive PTH was undetectable. Further evidence that the PTH-like tumor product was not PTH then followed with the development of more sensitive bioassays for PTH in the late 1970s.

More detailed clinical studies at this time (Kukreja et al. 1980; Stewart et al. 1980; Rude et al. 1981) provided a better understanding of the biochemical picture of HHM and it became clear that the manifestations of the disease were mediated via the PTH receptor in bone and kidney (Mundy and Martin 1982). Stewart et al. (1983) demonstrated that extracts of tumors from patients with HHM were able to stimulate adenylate cyclase in a PTH responsive renal cortical membrane assay and also to stimulate glucose-6-phosphate dehydrogenase, using a sensitive cytochemical bioassay for PTH in the same kidney preparation. This assay could also detect increased circulating bioactivity in patients with HHM in which immunoreactive PTH was undetectable (Goltzmann et al. 1981). Similarly, Rodan et al. (1983) showed that tumor extracts of rat and human origin could stimulate adenylate cyclase in PTH-responsive osteoblast cells, and that there was a good correlation between stimulation of cAMP and bone resorption in culture and the association of the tumor with HHM *in vivo*. In all of these assays, PTH competitive antagonists could block activity but preincubation with PTH antibodies did not neutralize the responses observed. Furthermore, mRNA for PTH could not be detected in these tumors (Simpson et al. 1983).

It is now clear from the sequence of PTHrP, that PTH antibodies exhibiting N-terminal epitopes might weakly cross-react with PTHrP, which could explain the observed anomalies of the radioimmunoassay results. Furthermore, it is also likely that the immunohistochemical studies which detected PTH in tumors from patients with HHM (Ilardi and Faro 1975; Mayes et al. 1984) were incorrectly interpreted due to cross-reactivity of the antibodies with PTHrP at the high concentrations of the PTH antibody used. The characteristic features of HHM have therefore never convincingly been demonstrated to be due to ectopic production of authentic PTH.

Thus began the task to purify and sequence the active agent. PTH-like biological activity was soon to be described in experimental animal models of HHM, in cell cultures established from them and in cell cultures established from human tumors (Rodan et al. 1983; Strewler et al. 1983; Gkonos et al. 1984; Rosol et al. 1987; Ikeda et al. 1988c; Rosol and Capen 1988a), all of which, it was anticipated, would produce sufficient protein for purification. Several groups reported the purification of the active protein to a single band of apparent homogeneity on gels (Rabbani et al. 1986; Burtis et al. 1987; Nissenson et al. 1987b) and active materials with $M_r$ ranging from 3000 to 28 000 were described. Sequence was finally obtained (Moseley et al. 1987; Suva et al. 1987) from protein purified from conditioned medium produced by a human lung cancer cell line. Subsequently, two other groups obtained similar N-terminal sequences from material purified from a human lung, a breast and a renal cell carcinoma respectively (Stewart et al. 1987b; Strewler et al. 1987).

### III. Purification, cloning and sequence determination

Purification and cloning of PTHrP was first achieved from conditioned medium produced by a lung cancer cell line (BEN) originally derived from a patient with squamous cell carcinoma of the lung associated with hypercalcemia (Ellison et al. 1975). Crucial to the purification process was the sensitive biological assay in the PTH-responsive clonal osteogenic sarcoma cell line UMR 106-01 (Forrest et al. 1985; Kubota et al. 1986). Conditioned medium from BEN cells at dilutions as great as 1 in 100 produced a response in this assay, indicating the production of large quantities of PTH-like material by these cells. The adenylate cyclase response could be blocked by PTH antagonists but was not abolished by preincubation with PTH antibodies. Furthermore, Northern blots of mRNA from BEN cells could not demonstrate the presence of mRNA for PTH (Moseley et al. 1987).

Sufficient purified material for sequence analysis was obtained from large batches of serum-free conditioned medium processed according to the schedule in Fig. 1; biological activity was monitored at all stages. This schedule is essentially the same as that described in Moseley et al. (1987) with some changes in the types of HPLC columns employed.

Fresh conditioned medium was acidified to pH 4.8 and loaded onto an ion-exchange medium (SP Sephadex), which was subsequently packed into a column and eluted in a salt gradient of 0.1 – 1.0 M sodium chloride in acetate buffer. Biological activity was eluted at 0.4 – 0.6 M sodium chloride, collected, desalted and concentrated by HPLC on a $C_{18}$ Bondapak guard column in 0.1% trifluoracetic acid in acetonitrile. Three further sequential HPLC steps were necessary to achieve pure material. All three were carried out using the same high resolution analytical Bakerbond $C_{18}$ column in 0.1% trifluoracetic acid in a gradient of acetonitrile, increasing the time of execution of the gradient and thus the slope, for each run.

The first of the Bakerbond HPLC steps (HPLC 1: Fig. 1) resolved two major regions of protein (peak A and peak B) coinciding with biological activity, which by gel analysis were seen to comprise components ranging in molecular mass from 16 – 25 kDa. Peak B (16 – 20 kDa) was taken on to the final purification since this represented the material of greatest specific activity at this stage of the purification. When this material was resolved and eluted from polyacrylamide gels the biological activity coincided with a protein of 16 – 18 kDa.

Peak B material was resolved by a second HPLC step (HPLC 2: Fig. 1) and the active fractions pooled and subjected to a final separation (HPLC 3: Fig. 1). Final purification steps revealed biological activity coinciding with a single silver stained band on gels of 17 kDa. and the peak fraction from HPLC 3 (Fig. 1) was subjected to microsequencing and tryptic peptide analysis. A sequence of 50 amino acids, including an overlapping tryptic peptide located at residues 68 – 78, was obtained on 30 pmol of material, confirming previous N-terminal sequence carried out on material eluted from gels. cDNA cloning confirmed the amino acid sequence obtained by direct

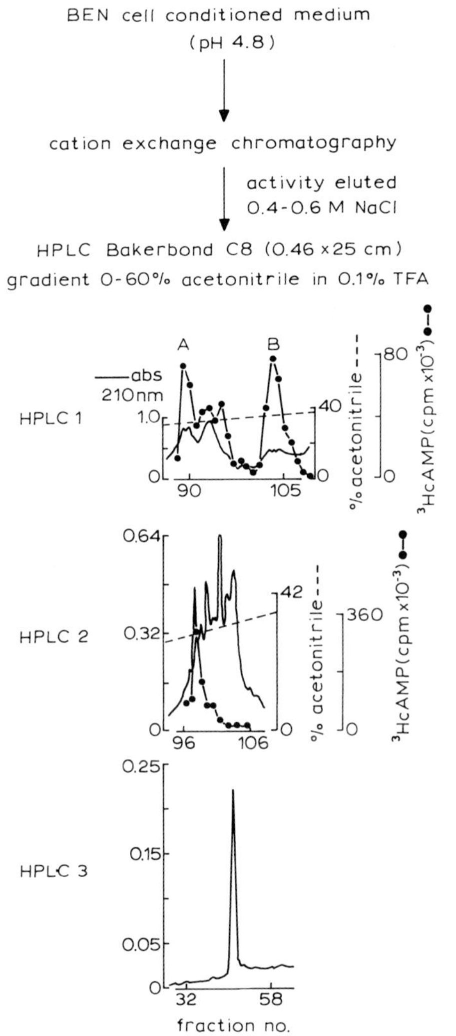


Fig. 1. Purification schedule for the purification of PTHrP from a human cancer cell line (BEN) conditioned medium (For details see text).

microsequencing as well as the remaining undetermined sequence of the purified protein.

A cDNA library was prepared from BEN cells using λgt10 as vector, and $10^6$ clones were generated. $2.5 \times 10^5$ clones were screened using a mixture of two 72-mer synthetic oligonucleotide probes, the sequences of which were based on early sequence information of the the first 24 amino acid residues. The first oligonucleotide sequence was based on common codon usage tables and the second on the codon usage preferred in human PTH. Six positive clones were identified encoding full length translated sequences corresponding to a mature protein of 141 amino acids and of molecular weight approximately 16.5 kDa, including a 36 amino acid prepro-sequence.

The N-terminal sequence of the mature 141 amino acid protein shows considerable homology with PTH (Fig. 2). Eight of the first 13 amino acids are identical, thus providing an immediate explanation for its ability to act via the PTH receptor as well as for its reactivity with some PTH antibodies. Although negligible further homology is apparent, the properties of the amino acids constituting the prepro-sequence are reminiscent of PTH. This sequence contains a hydrophobic core of amino acids surrounded by charged residues, characteristic of a secretory protein. Possible cleavage sites at glycine −8 or serine −6 would leave a short pro-sequence which could be cleaved during the secretory process.

The sequence of mature PTHrP predicted by the cDNA, is 57 amino acids longer than mature PTH and contains a sequence of many basic residues between amino acids 87 and 108. These basic amino acids are followed by a unique sequence of 33 residues, and it is possible that this peptide may be cleaved at the basic residues and released into the circulation shortly after secretion, leaving a primary circulating form of PTHrP of between approximately 86 – 108 amino acids in length. Consistent with this hypothesis is the presence of potential amidation signals, within the basic sequence, suggestive of post-translational processing. As yet, no function has been ascribed to the C-terminal peptide, should any exist. It is possible that it may simply represent a processing product similar to the C-peptide of insulin.

Limited N-terminal sequence data has now also been obtained from material purified from a breast carcinoma, a pulmonary carcinoma and a renal carcinoma cell line, using similar procedures as those described above (Stewart et al. 1987b; Strewler et al. 1987). Protein in conditioned medium from the renal carcinoma cell line was bound onto controlled pore glass beads, eluted from them and then processed by ion-exchange and HPLC. Acid-urea extracts were made of the solid tumors of breast and lung and then processed by ethanol/sodium chloride precipitation and sequential HPLC.

```
                          -20                   -10                   1                10
hPTH            M I P A K D M A K V M I V M L A I C F L T K S D G K S V K K R S V S E I Q L M H N
PTHrP M Q R R L V Q Q W S V A V F L L S Y A V P S C G R S V E G L S R R L K R A V S E H Q L L H D

                    20                  30                  40                  50
hPTH  L G K H L N S M E R V E W L R K K L Q D V H N F V A L G A P L A P R D A G S Q R P R K K E D
PTHrP K G K S I Q D L R R R F F L H H L I A E I H T A E I R A T S E V S P N S K P S P N T K N H P

          60                  70                  80                  90                  100
hPTH  N V L V E S H E K S L G E A D K A D V D N L T K A K S Q
PTHrP V R F G S D D E G R Y L T Q E T N K V E T Y K E Q P L K T P G K K K K G K P G K R K E Q E K

              110                 120                 130                 140
PTHrP K K R R T R S A W L D S G V T G S G L E G D H L S D T S T T S L E L D S R R H
```

Fig. 2. Amino acid sequence of prepro-PTHrP. Sequence of hPTHrP compared with the sequence of human PTH. Homology is indicated by the boxes.

Several species of biologically active molecules were purified ranging in molecular mass from 3 to 9 kDa from the renal cells; 7 – 9 kDa from the pulmonary carcinoma and 17 kDa from the breast carcinoma. Since all the N-terminal sequences are identical, it is assumed that the smaller species are breakdown or processing products of the larger protein. Breakdown may have taken place during the purification procedure, but as yet the range of secretory and metabolized products generated by any of the model systems studied *in vitro* or *in vivo* has not been elucidated. The 25 kDa material, peak A (Fig. 1; Moseley et al. 1987) has not been fully characterized at this time and the exact nature of this relative to the 141 amino acid cloned sequence is unknown. However, as will be seen in subsequent sections the full length genetically expressed material (Hammonds et al. 1988) has an apparent molecular mass of approximately 25 kDa suggesting that the 17 – 18 kDa proteins are either not full length or have lost some post-translational modification.

Using probes based on the N-terminal sequences obtained, Mangin et al. (1988a) have cloned PTHrP cDNA from a renal cell carcinoma and verified the 141 amino acid sequence of PTHrP from BEN cells. This again supports the view that the small fragments are generated from a larger common parent protein. Thiede et al. (1988) cloned PTHrP cDNA from a renal cell carcinoma cell line (786-0) and found an identical coding sequence with the exception that it lacked the last two C-terminal residues. Mangin et al. (1988b) however have reported another cDNA clone which encodes a protein of 166 amino acids and which is identical apart from the additional sequence. All three groups have reported clones with divergent 5′- and 3′-untranslated regions (UTR) as well as the existence of multiple forms of mRNA encoding PTHrP (Ikeda et al. 1988a, b; Mangin et al. 1988b; Suva et al. 1988, 1989; Thiede et al. 1988). The characterization and possible significance of these observations will be discussed later in this chapter when the molecular biology of PTHrP is addressed specifically.

## IV. Biological potency and actions of purified PTHrP

### A. In PTH responsive systems

Purified PTHrP has not been obtained in sufficiently large quantities to allow extensive investigations of its biological actions. Sufficient studies have been undertaken to enable assessments of its potency as well as to demonstrate PTH-like actions in bone and kidney assays, compatible with its role as the mediator of the PTH-like actions of HHM.

The 18 kDa material of Moseley et al. (1987) was found to be approximately six times more potent than bovine PTH (bPTH) 1-34, both in its stimulation of cAMP production in osteogenic sarcoma cells, UMR 106-01, and its stimulation of plasminogen activator in the same cells. However, the 17 kDa protein of Burtis et al. (1987) was approximately one third as potent as bPTH 1-34 using the same assay in

ROS 17/2.8 cells. The use of autopsy material from which the protein was purified may have resulted in some loss of activity in this case.

Partially purified proteins from a rat tumor, with molecular mass ranging from 8500 to 28 000 (Rabbani et al. 1986), had a potency of approximately 1.5% of that of PTH. However, these authors were able to show that the purified product could prevent hypercalcemia in thyroparathyroidectomized rats as well as to stimulate urinary cAMP production. It is likely that the active material in this study, was heavily contaminated with unrelated protein.

The 6 kDa protein from a human renal cell line (Strewler et al. 1987) was less effective than PTH 1-34 on bone resorption but had an estimated potency similar to that of bPTH 1-34 in stimulating cAMP production in osteogenic sarcoma cells. It was however, 20-fold less potent in the canine renal membrane adenylate cyclase assay (Strewler et al. 1987). The relative insensitivity of this latter assay has been noted previously in respect of the relative potencies of PTH and PTHrP preparations (Nissenson et al. 1985; Stewart et al. 1987a).

Iodinated 6 kDa material could bind to renal membranes and could be competed for equally well by equivalent amounts of either PTH or unlabelled 6 kDa protein, suggesting that they bind to the same receptor. The purified proteins of Rabbani (1986) and Strewler (1987) could also mimic PTH in inhibiting sodium-dependent phosphate transport in opossum kidney OK cells, an effect apparently mediated by cAMP (Caverzasio et al. 1986).

Due to the small amounts of material purified, most estimates of potency have been approximate and it is not yet clear if discrepancies in the biological potencies of the purified proteins are due to intrinsic properties of the different length proteins purified, incorrect assessments of purity, degradation during purification or in the receptor coupling abilities of the proteins in the assay systems employed (Nissenson et al. 1985; Stewart et al. 1987a). It will be seen in subsequent sections that there have also been discrepancies, particularly *in vitro*, in the potencies of the synthetic peptides in the various assays and even between different laboratories using similar assays.

### B. In non-PTH responsive systems

A unique action of PTHrP, of presumed physiological relevance in normal physiology, is its action on the placental transfer of calcium from mother to fetus. In experiments using an isolated perfused placental model from parathyroidectomized sheep fetuses, neither PTH nor vitamin D metabolites influence placental transfer of calcium nor can they restore the calcium gradient which is lost by parathyroidectomy (Care et al. 1985). Both sheep placenta and fetal parathyroids have been shown to contain PTHrP, distinguishable from PTH by its immunological and chromatographic behavior (Kubota et al. 1987) and purified 18 kDa PTHrP from BEN cells can restore the calcium gradient in the perfused placental model (Rodda et al. 1988). PTHrP 1-34, however, is inactive in this system consistent with the lack of effect of PTH and suggesting that it is not the N-terminal region of PTHrP which is responsible for this activity.

This finding reveals for the first time a mechanism whereby calcium is made available to the developing fetal skeleton (Rodda et al. 1988) and provides a putative physiological role for PTHrP in fetal development. Thiede and Rodan (1988) have demonstrated that mRNA for PTHrP is expressed in lactating rat mammary tissue and that the expression of PTHrP is increased under the influence of suckling by the litter. This observation adds further support for a role of PTHrP in calcium regulation at early stages of development and may also provide a clue to the reason for PTHrP expression by some breast carcinomata.

## V. Biological actions of synthetic peptides of PTHrP in vitro

At the time of writing it is a little over 18 months since the sequence of PTHrP was determined. Synthesis of peptides and studies of its actions are thus at an early stage and most of the data available on the actions of these peptides are at best preliminary. Much more detailed work, both with synthetic peptides and genetically expressed full length protein (Hammonds et al. 1988) must be carried out in order to define the precise mode of action of PTHrP and its role in HHM.

Our decision to synthesize PTHrP 1-34 was based firstly, on the assumption that like PTH itself, the biological activity is likely to be contained in the first 34 residues; and secondly, on the fact that some purified biologically active species had $M_r$ as low as 3000. The data accumulated so far and outlined below confirm that PTHrP possesses the intrinsic ability to reproduce the major components of the HHM syndrome and probably does so in the main by its actions via the PTH receptor.

### A. Actions in bone and kidney assays

Studies with synthetic PTHrP 1-34 have in general confirmed initial observations made using tumor extracts and purified material. Assays using rat osteoblast-like cells (UMR106-01) or chick renal membranes (Kemp et al. 1987) indicated that PTHrP 1-34 was 3 – 4 times more potent than PTH 1-34 in stimulating cAMP production (Fig. 3), in contrast to the 6-fold more active purified protein from BEN cells (Moseley et al. 1987). Four groups using ROS 17/2.8 cells found PTHrP 1-34 and PTH 1-34 to be equipotent (Horiuchi et al. 1987; Rodan et al. 1988; Stewart et al. 1988; Shigeno et al. 1988) and two of them (Horiuchi et al. 1987; Stewart et al. 1988) that PTHrP 1-34 was less potent in canine or bovine renal membrane assays, confirming observations with the purified protein (Strewler et al. 1987).

Equal potencies of PTHrP 1-34 and PTH 1-34 have been reported in the adenylate cyclase assay in UMR 106 cells; in renal cyclase assays using rat or rabbit kidney membranes (Yates et al. 1988) or cultured kidney cells from opossum (Rabbani et al.

1988) and on glucose-6-phosphate in the distal convoluted tubule of the guinea pig (Nakai et al. 1988). The similar potencies of PTHrP and PTH in these assays suggests there may either be a species specific difference in breakdown of PTHrP or that there is reduced coupling ability of PTHrP in the renal membrane assays of Stewart et al. (1988) and Horiuchi et al. (1987).

Pronounced effects of PTHrP 1-34 on cAMP and calcium excretion have been demonstrated in an isolated perfused rat kidney model (Ebeling et al. 1988). These workers found similar effects of PTHrP 1-34 and PTH 1-34 on phosphate excretion but that the cAMP response of PTHrP was much greater which is consistent with *in vivo* observations of Horiuchi et al. (1987).

### B. Actions in bone resorption assays in vitro

Whilst it is clear that PTHrP 1-34 does stimulate bone resorption *in vitro,* conflicting reports have emerged as to its potency in bone resorption assays. Kemp et al. (1987) found that PTHrP 1-34, which was 3 – 4 times more potent than bPTH 1-34 in

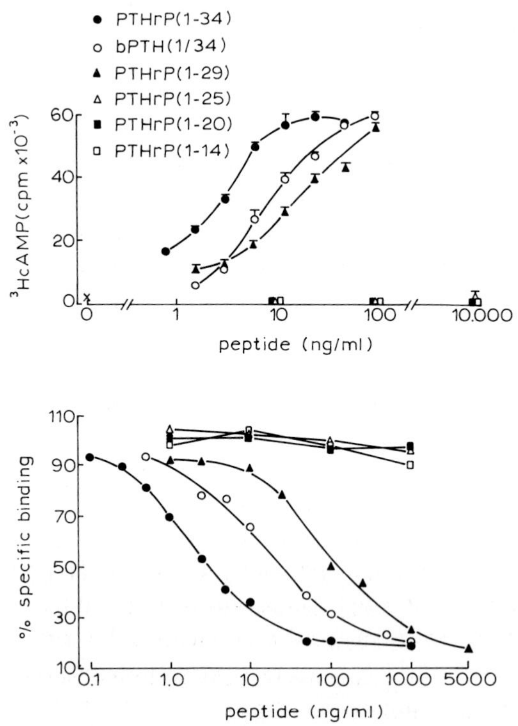


Fig. 3. Biological activity of PTHrP peptides. Upper panel: activation of adenylate cyclase in intact UMR106-01 cells by PTHrP peptides. Lower panel: binding of $^{125}$I-labelled PTHrP 1-34 and competition by PTHrP peptides. PTHrP 1-34 was labelled as previously described for calcitonin (Findlay et al. 1980).

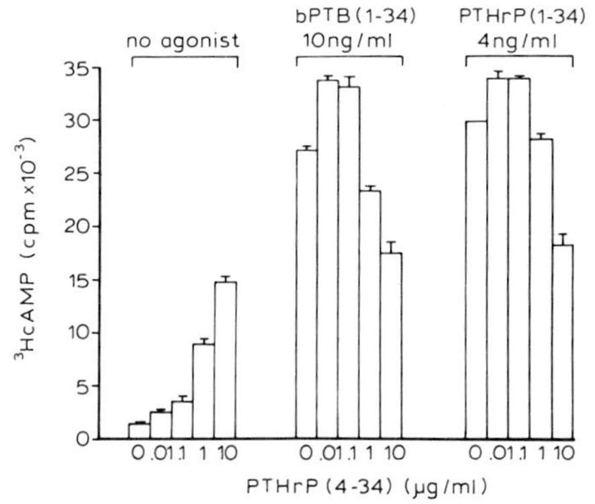


Fig. 4. Antagonist actions of PTHrP 4-34 in the intact cell assay for adenylate cyclase in UMR 106-06 cells. The dose response to PTHrP 4-34 shows partial agonist activity. In the presence of doses of bPTH 1-34 and PTHrP 1-34, matched for equivalent responses, effects were additive at the lower doses but at higher doses of the PTHrP 4-34 equivalent antagonism of bPTH 1-34 and PTHrP 1-34 are seen. Points are means ± S.E.M. of triplicate estimations.

stimulating cAMP in UMR106-01 cells, was only 6% as effective as PTH 1-34 in inhibiting bone resorption in the fetal long bone assay of Raisz. The possibility of increased degradation of PTHrP in these assays was addressed and concluded not to be contributory. Similar results were reports by Lorenzo et al. (1988) in newborn mouse calvaria. Two other groups however, have reported equipotent effects in the fetal long bone assay (Stewart et al. 1988; Yates et al. 1988).

Although PTHrP clearly does increase bone resorption, the reasons for the discrepancies in these assays are puzzling, but may reflect different degradation fates of the two peptides in each of the assays. It may also be relevant that preliminary work of Lowik et al. (1988) suggests that PTHrP 1-34 may be more effective than PTH 1-34 in bone resorption assays in which osteoclast induction can be observed. However, recent work (Rosol and Capen 1988b; Thompson et al. 1988), indicates that whilst PTHrP does stimulate osteoclast recruitment, PTH is equally effective in their assays.

### C. Actions on post-receptor activation events

Investigation of the PTH-like actions believed to be further along the cAMP-induced activation pathways add support to the action of PTHrP being via the PTH receptor. Rodan et al. (1988) demonstrated identical effects of dexamethasone on the similar growth inhibitory responses induced by PTH 1-34 and PTHrP 1-34. Both peptides also suppressed alkaline phosphatase activity, implying that the same pathways are involved. Furthermore, the same relative potencies of the two peptides on adenylate cyclase and plasminogen activator have been observed in UMR 106-01 cells (Kemp et al. 1987).

Similar responses of PTHrP and PTH have also been reported on sodium-dependent phosphate transport in renal epithelial cells (Strewler et al. 1987; Pizurki et al. 1988; Sartori et al. 1988; Stewart et al. 1988) confirming the observations with purified PTHrP.

A number of other workers have shown essentially equipotent actions of PTHrP 1-34 and PTH 1-34 in various other assays for PTH, for example, on calcium accumulation in UMR 106-01 cells (Civitelli et al. 1988; Donahue et al. 1988; Lowik et al. 1988). Although the responses were small, it is interesting that Lowik and Donahue's results suggest that the time course of the responses to PTHrP and PTH differed. Many of the responses of the two peptides can be easily understood by actions through the PTH receptor eliciting identical post-receptor activation. However, these latter results suggest that the peptides may also act by distinctive means.

## D. Structure activity studies

Investigation of the structure activity relationships of PTHrP peptides shorter than the first 34 amino acids has indicated a strong similarity between the regions of PTH and PTHrP involved in activation and binding. Kemp et al. (1987) showed that PTHrP 1-29 had a potency of approximately 10% of PTHrP 1-34 and that peptides of less than 25 amino acids in length had no activity at all in UMR 106-01 cells (Fig. 3), emphasizing the importance of residues 25 – 30 in activation despite lack of homology with PTH in this region.

The ability of these peptides to compete for binding of $^{125}$I-labelled PTHrP 1-34 to UMR 106-01 cells also correlated with their ability to activate adenylate cyclase (Fig. 3). These observations are essentially the same as those of Tregear et al. (1973) with PTH peptides of similar length, and again stress the functionally-related structural similarities between PTH and PTHrP.

Like PTH, PTHrP peptides with N-terminal deletions have agonist actions in PTH assays. PTHrP 4-34 retains partial agonist activity in adenylate cyclase assays and it also equally antagonizes the actions of doses of PTH and PTHrP matched for equivalent responses (Fig. 4). Unlike PTH 7-34, [Tyr$^{34}$]PTHrP 7-34 retains some weak agonist activity. It has been shown to be eight times more potent than PTH 7-34 in inhibiting PTH-stimulated cAMP production in ROS 17/2.8 cells, even though most of the homologous region is absent (McKee et al. 1988). These findings allow for the possibility that more potent antagonists to PTH receptor-mediated action might be designed incorporating the regions of PTHrP not homologous with PTH.

PTHrP 3-34 has also been synthesized (Rabbani et al. 1988; Shigeno et al. 1988) and was found to be a partial agonist and produce equivalent inhibition of both PTHrP 1-34 and PTH 1-34 stimulated adenylate cyclase activity. It was not however, effective in stimulating cAMP excretion in thyroparathyroidectomized (TPTX) rats except at very high concentrations when a marked effect on urinary phosphate excretion was seen. These data suggest that not only are N-terminal amino acids important for the potent effects of PTHrP on cAMP but also that important interactions with the PTH receptor are in regions not homologous with PTH, again confirming the observations of Kemp et al. (1987).

### E. Binding and receptor studies

The lack of methionine residues in the active sequence of PTHrP has provided us with a much more amenable ligand than native PTH for iodination without loss of biological activity and precluding the need to design more stable analogues. Several investigators have synthesized PTHrP 1-34 with an additional tyrosine at the carboxy terminus (Jueppner et al. 1988; McKee et al. 1988; Nissenson et al. 1988; Orloff et al. 1988; Stewart et al. 1988) although iodination of the histidine residues is also possible without loss of biological activity (P. Smith and J.M. Moseley 1988, unpublished observations).

All the binding studies carried out so far confirm those of Strewler et al. (1987) with the purified protein and support the view that PTHrP and PTH bind to the same receptor. A good correlation between binding and adenylate cyclase activation has been observed (Horiuchi et al. 1987; and Fig. 3) and PTHrP or PTH will compete with either labelled ligand using [Tyr$^{36}$]PTHrP 1-36 or [Nle$^{8}$,$^{18}$Tyr$^{36}$]PTH. Further, affinity crosslinking with either of these iodinated ligands results in a crosslinked complex of $M_r$ 80 000 in ROS 17/2.8 cells (Jueppner et al. 1988; Shigeno et al. 1988) and 85 000 in canine renal membranes and UMR106 cells (Nissenson et al. 1987a). Finally, preincubation of cells with PTHrP or PTH brings about down regulation with respect to binding of the alternative ligand (Jueppner et al. 1988). These data indicate that the actions of PTHrP are via authentic PTH receptors, although the possibility of specific receptors or some action through specific additional receptor components cannot be eliminated. The situation could be analogous to that for insulin and the insulin-like growth factor I which exhibit only 40% homology but bind freely to each other's receptors.

Reduced binding and adenylate cyclase activation in some renal membrane assays has led to the suggestion that either the renal receptor for PTH is different from the bone receptor or that PTHrP occupation of the renal receptor results in less efficient coupling of adenylate cyclase than with PTH. As discussed in a previous section, the reduced potency of PTHrP in these systems may be a degradation artefact due to the crude membrane systems employed. However, these observations *in vitro* are not generally supported by *in vivo* studies (see Section VI) and there is clearly a need for studies comparing full length proteins, in which activation and binding can be observed at the same time under similar conditions. The structure activity studies of Kemp et al. (1987) suggest that as in PTH, PTHrP residues 14-34 have a function in binding and coupling. Since only three residues are shared by PTH and PTHrP in the region of amino acids 14-34 this could indeed confer a different coupling capability on the two proteins, perhaps even to different, as yet undefined activation events.

## VI. Actions of synthetic PTHrP 1-34 in vivo

The potent hypercalcemic effect of PTHrP *in vivo* leaves little doubt that PTHrP can stimulate bone resorption in addition to its potent effect on renal calcium handling. Perfusion of PTHrP into TPTX rats, either acutely or chronically, results in hypercalcemia, reduced calcium excretion, reduced serum phosphate and increased urinary cAMP and phosphate (Horiuchi et al. 1987; Rizzoli et al. 1988; Thompson et al. 1988; Yates et al. 1988). A hypercalcemic effect of PTHrP 1-34, 6 – 10 times more potent than that to PTH was demonstrated in TPTX rats (Horiuchi et al. 1987) in addition to more potent effects on renal excretion of phosphate and cAMP. These observations are consistent with the *in vitro* effects observed by Ebeling et al. (1988) and indicate a potent effect of PTHrP on renal function. Equipotent effects of the two peptides on renal function in intact rats have, however, been reported (Yates et al. 1988).

In Horiuchi's studies, hypercalcemia was accompanied by reduced serum phosphate and increased serum 1,25-dihydroxyvitamin $D_3$. The latter effect is of particular interest in view of the inconsistent finding of raised serum levels of 1,25-dihydroxyvitamin $D_3$ in HHM patients (Stewart et al. 1981; Yamamoto et al. 1987), although it is commonly elevated in animal models of HHM (Gkonos et al. 1984; Strewler et al. 1986). It has been suggested that 1,25-dihydroxyvitamin $D_3$ levels may be depressed later in the course of HHM by prolonged hypercalcemia or by compromised renal function.

Horiuchi et al. (1987) also studied the contribution of the kidney to the hypercalcemic response in TPTX rats which were also nephrectomized and fed a low calcium diet. In these animals, an equipotent effect of PTHrP 1-34 and PTH 1-34 was observed on serum calcium, in contrast to the greater response observed in animals with intact kidneys. This suggests a prime role of the kidney in the hypercalcemic response to PTHrP.

Chronic treatment of intact rats with PTHrP 1-34 has been shown to cause a substantial hypercalcemia which returned to normal on withdrawal of the peptide (Stewart et al. 1988). A dose-dependent hypercalcemic response to PTHrP 1-34, equivalent to that seen for PTH 1-34 was reported by Yates et al. (1988) who also observed that chronic treatment of intact mice with PTHrP caused a greater sustained hypercalcemia than that of PTH 1-34. Histomorphometric observations on the bones of these mice showed essentially similar effects of the two peptides on parameters of osteoclastic activity. In another study in which athymic mice were chronically perfused with PTHrP 1-34 for 7 days, increases in serum calcium and phosphate and urinary phosphate as well as a reduction in urinary calcium, similar to the effects of PTH, were observed (Rosol and Capen, 1988b). Furthermore, increased numbers of tartrate-resistant acid phosphatase positive osteoclasts, as well as both larger osteoclasts and osteoblasts were found in the bones of these mice indicating effects on both bone formation and resorption. Chronically perfused PTHrP or PTH into nephrectomized TPTX animals have also been seen to be equally effective in the induction of osteoclasts (Thompson et al. 1988).

In summary of these early studies of PTHrP action, it is clear that PTHrP can mimic PTH in all the systems investigated and that it can thus probably reproduce the essential features of HHM in the absence of other tumor factors, by its action via the PTH receptor. The data reviewed suggest that the most relevant initial action of PTHrP may be that on the kidney, and that it is this action which is responsible for the initial hypercalcemic response. PTHrP clearly can resorb bone and has been shown to stimulate an increase in osteoclast and osteoblast numbers. Thus, it seems likely that it must at least contribute to the gross effects on bone observed in the later stages of the syndrome, allowing for the probability that other tumor factors are also implicated.

The potent effects of PTHrP on the kidney *in vivo* points to either a possible higher affinity of PTHrP to the renal PTH receptor and/or more effective coupling to activation pathways. These effects are also in direct contrast to some of the *in vitro* studies with PTHrP which have been discussed earlier. It is possible that there may be interactions between specific PTHrP activated pathways or components of them which are not all functional in the *in vitro* assays. We have seen that non-homologous regions of PTHrP are involved in binding and activation, giving plenty of scope for the recruitment of additional mechanisms to express the distinctive effects of the two hormones and even to the possibility of the involvement of different receptor components.

Since most studies have been carried out on short biologically active peptides we must reserve our speculation until more detailed *in vitro* and *in vivo* studies have been carried out with the full length protein to establish whether the regions of the molecule beyond the first 34 amino acids contribute to the distinctive features of HHM.

## VII. Actions of recombinant PTHrP

Preliminary studies in our laboratory with recombinant PTHrP 1-141 (Hammonds et al. 1988), have shown that it is equipotent on a molar basis with PTHrP 1-34 in its ability to stimulate adenylate cyclase in UMR106-01 cells. PTHrP 1-141 is also equipotent with PTHrP 1-34 both in the bone resorption assay in fetal rat long bones (L.G. Raisz, personal communication), and in production of hypercalcemia and hypophosphatemia when infused into nude mice (S.C. Kukreja, personal communication).

These early studies suggest that the recombinant material can reproduce the PTH-like effects of the synthetic 1-34 peptide. Non PTH-like responses have yet to be addressed, and these will be of particular interest with regard to the actions of PTHrP on placental calcium transport.

In view of the likelihood that most tumors produce tumor factors which themselves directly or indirectly influence bone resorption, the relevance of such factors in the full expression of the HHM syndrome must also be considered.

## VIII. Interaction of PTHrP with other tumor factors

Many of the extracts and purified preparations of PTH-like activity from HHM-associated tumors have also been reported to exhibit transforming growth factor alpha (TGF-$\alpha$) activity and in some cases both activities co-purified through several purification stages (D'Souza et al. 1983; Insogna et al. 1987; Klein et al. 1987; Rosol et al. 1987). It now seems likely that the TGF activity was a contaminant rather than being an intrinsic property of PTHrP. In at least one case of a pancreatic tumor associated with HHM, purification separated these activities out to a large extent (Akatsu et al. 1988). These observations point to the probability that many tumors producing PTHrP also secrete growth factors such as TGF-$\alpha$, and EGF, all of which are potent resorbers of bone (Raisz et al. 1980; Ibbotson et al. 1983; Ibbotson et al. 1985; Tashjian et al. 1985). Certainly neither D'Souza et al. (1984) nor Klein et al. (1987) could inhibit the *in vitro* bone resorbing activity in their tumor extracts with PTH antagonists, suggesting that the bone resorption resulted largely from activity other than the PTH-like actions of PTHrP. The co-production of these factors could therefore result in actions and interactions which contribute to the distinctive features of the HHM syndrome (Mundy and Martin 1982; Mundy et al. 1985; Mundy 1988).

As yet there is no clear evidence for the direct involvement of bone resorbing cytokines such as tumor necrosis factors TNF-$\alpha$ and TNF-$\beta$ or interleukin-1 (IL-1) in the pathogenesis of HHM. Cytokine activity has been demonstrated in cells of solid tumor origin (Nimberg et al. 1978), and they are commonly produced by circulating cells in cancer patients. It is possible that their production may be influenced by PTHrP and other tumor factors thereby contributing to the effects on bone resorption (Garret et al. 1987). Synergistic actions of IL-1 and cAMP stimulated bone resorption have also been demonstrated, stressing the relevance of such possible interactions (Dewhirst et al. 1987) and there is increasing evidence that there are interactions between the effects of PTH and growth factors on bone cells (Gutierrez et al. 1987; Centrella et al. 1988). Preliminary work of Lorenzo et al. (1988) has demonstrated stimulation of the release of IL-1 from mouse calvaria by PTHrP and the possible influence of EGF and TGFs on PTHrP action has been addressed (Bernier et al. 1988). Clearly this is a particular area for future investigation that may help resolve the question of the contribution of PTHrP to bone resorption in HHM and also explain the other anomalies in the characteristic features of PTH receptor-mediated HHM and hyperparathyroidism.

## IX. Immunological studies with antibodies to synthetic PTHrP peptides

Although the region of greatest homology with PTH is located in the first 13 amino acids of PTHrP, the first 10 appear to be the most antigenic, whilst the same region of PTH is notoriously poor. Theoretical antigenicity analysis (Welling et al. 1985;

Kemp et al. 1987) supports this observation, although detection of raised levels of PTH in patients with HHM using the early radioimmunoassays (RIA) could, however, be explained by recognition of a common N-terminal epitope.

With the availability of synthetic PTHrP peptides came many attempts to raise antibodies which could be used for characterization and localization studies, as well as to establish RIAs to detect and monitor PTHrP in patients with HHM.

As predicted by Welling, antibodies raised against PTHrP peptides have demonstrated largely N-terminal specificity, even to the extent that removal of the first three amino acids has abolished recognition. They have shown little or no cross-reactivity with PTH either in RIA (Fig. 5) or at higher concentrations used in histochemical analysis or to block biological activity (Moseley et al. 1987: Danks et al. 1989). These PTHrP antisera specifically block PTHrP stimulation of cAMP in UMR106-01 cells and renal membranes (Burtis et al. 1988; Rodda et al. 1988), and can reduce hypercalcemia in the nude mouse model of HHM (Kukreja et al. 1988). The latter observation adds weight to the proposal that the cause of the hypercalcemia in HHM is the result of PTHrP action. Furthermore, these antibodies will bind specifically to PTHrP but not PTH on Western blots. Several RIAs have been described which can detect as little as 1 pmol of peptide (Moseley et al. 1987; Burtis et al. 1988) but attempts to measure PTHrP in patients' sera have been largely unsuccessful or inconsistent due to inhibiting serum factors. It is generally agreed that a two-site assay is required, using more specific monoclonal antibodies possibly in conjunction with a higher affinity polyclonal antibody than has yet been generated.

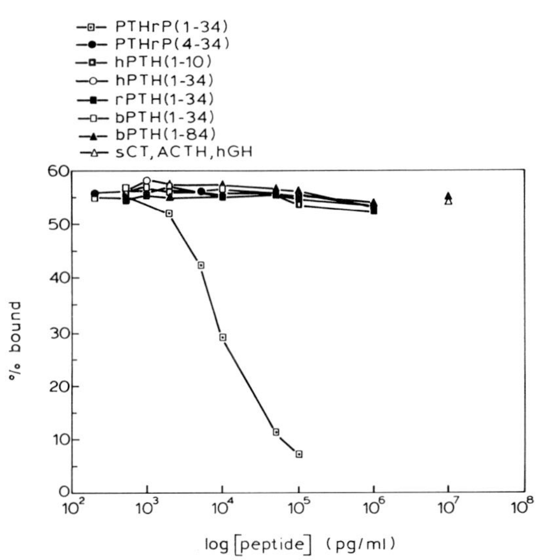


Fig. 5. Radioimmunoassay of PTHrP and PTH peptides. Anti-PTHrP 1-16 antibody does not cross-react with PTH peptides, with PTHrP 4-34 nor with unrelated peptides.

The antibodies which are currently available have been used most productively in the immunohistochemical localization of PTHrP (Danks et al. 1989; Hayman et al. 1989). Using immunoperoxidase procedures, 100% of squamous cell carcinomata from normocalcemic patients stained positive for PTHrP (Fig. 6). Basal cell tumors were all negative. Of a series of adenocarcinomata, only one of breast origin was positive. A significant proportion of breast tumors have been associated with PTH-like symptoms (Powles et al. 1976) and therefore are likely to produce PTHrP. It should be noted that PTHrP from a breast carcinoma has been purified and partially sequenced (Stewart et al. 1987) and mRNA for PTHrP has been detected in lactating rat mammary tissue (Thiede and Rodan 1988) suggesting a normal role for PTHrP in breast tissue. Thus, it is also highly possible that there could be increased expression in a cancer. Other tumors associated with HHM which have been shown to stain positively for PTHrP are, for example, renal cortical carcinomata, canine anal sac tumors (Danks et al. 1988; T.J. Rosol and J.A. Danks, personal communication) and a percentage of HTLV-1 positive tumors (J.M. Moseley and M. Horton, unpublished data). Messenger RNA for PTHrP has also been identified in HTLV-1 positive cells (Motokura et al. 1988).

This immunohistochemical approach may have diagnostic value particularly since the squamous cell carcinomata contain PTHrP at a stage when patients are normocalcemic and presumably normal homeostatic mechanisms are functioning adequately. It cannot be excluded however that in some cases secretion does not occur.

The localization of PTHrP in normal skin and specifically in the spinous keratinocytes has confirmed the finding of Merendino et al. (1986) who described production of PTH-like activity, which was not authentic PTH in conditioned medium of cultured foreskin cells. None of the basal, parabasal, granular or cornified layers of the skin stain for PTHrP but the inner root sheath of the hair follicle is positive (Fig. 6). The spinous keratinocyte or acanthocyte is considered to be the main differentiating feature of squamous cell carcinomata and this finding is therefore consistent with the detection of PTHrP in 100% of squamous carcinomata so far investigated.

The role of PTHrP in skin is unclear, skin fibroblasts respond to PTHrP (Wu et al. 1987) and one may speculate on its possible autocrine and paracrine roles in the regulation of local calcium fluxes, on vitamin D metabolism or in skin cell differentiation as suggested by the recent studies of Holick et al. (1988).

## X. The human PTHrP gene

The isolation of cDNA clones encoding PTHrP from a human lung cancer cell line (Suva et al. 1987) and from two human renal cell carcinoma cell lines (Mangin et al. 1988a, b; Thiede et al. 1988) has shown that they contain essentially the same PTHrP coding sequence. However, further analysis revealed that these clones contain divergent 5′- and 3′-untranslated regions (UTR), suggesting that alternatively spliced

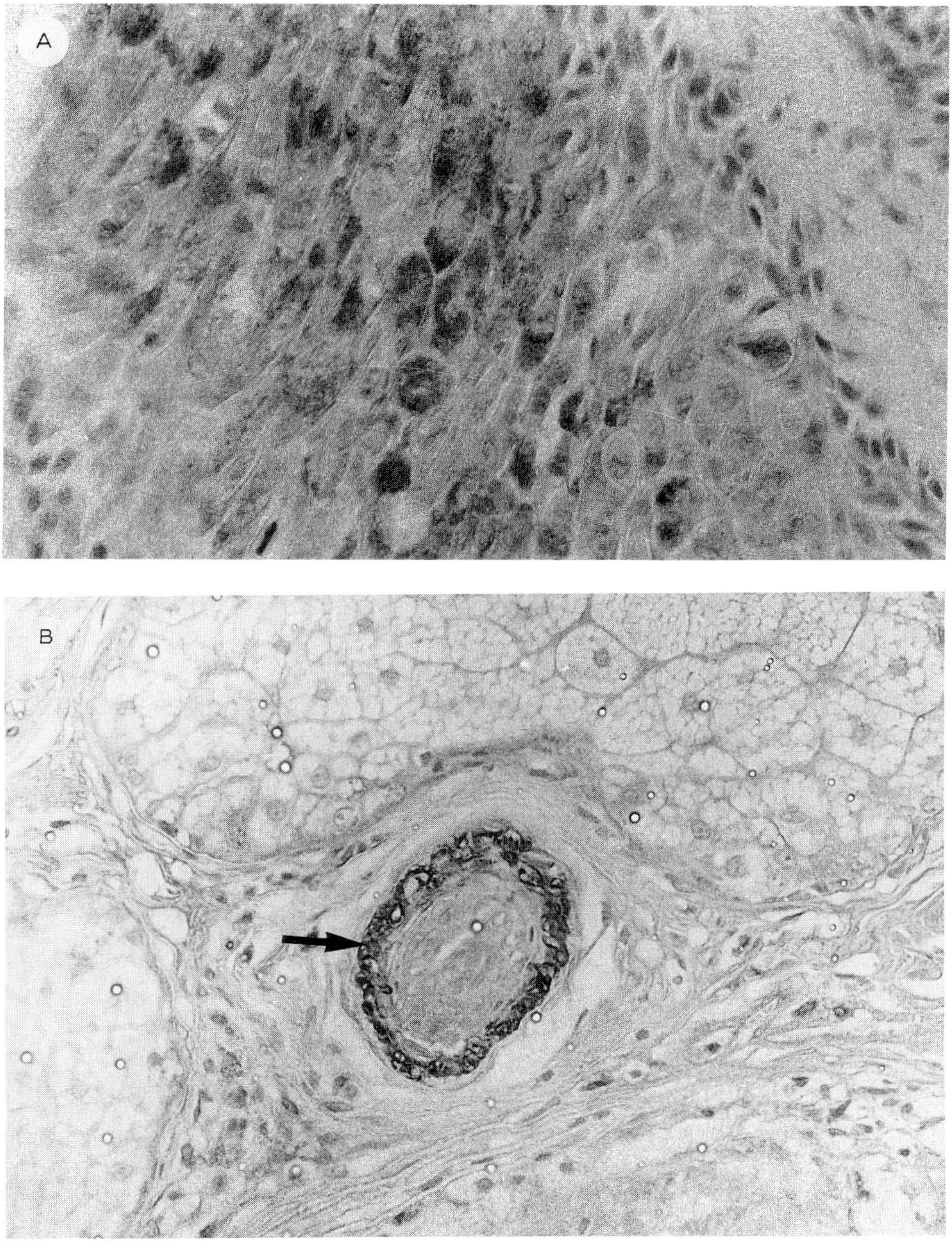


Fig. 6. Immunocytochemical localization of PTHrP. (A) Squamous cell carcinoma of the anus, showing PTHrP staining of the cytoplasm of tumor cells which have squamous differentiation ( × 190). (B) Inner root sheath of hair follicle in normal skin, seen in cross-section (arrow). Cells of sebaceous glands also seen in the photomicrograph, do not stain positive for PTHrP ( × 166). Methods are described in Danks et al. (1989). PTHrP 1-34 antibody was used at a dilution of 1/20. Controls carried out with non-immune rabbit serum and after pre-absorption with PTHrP 1-34 were negative.

mRNAs produce multiple cDNA species that encode the same protein. The isolation of alternate cDNA species encoding this new hormone suggests that the isolation and characterization of the human PTHrP gene is essential for our understanding of PTHrP action.

## A. Isolation and sequencing of the human PTHrP gene

Approximately 5 × $10^5$ plaques from a human genomic library were screened using a nick translated 1103 bp *Xho*I fragment of a PTHrP cDNA clone that corresponds to the entire coding region of PTHrP (Suva et al. 1987).

The two positive clones which were isolated were re-screened using two oligonucleotides, one based on the 5′-UTR of PTHrP cDNA clone pBRF61 and the other on the 3′-coding region, corresponding to residues Serine 14 to Histidine 25 of PTHrP (Suva et al. 1987). Specific hybridization suggested that the genomic fragment contained only the 5′ end of the gene. Within this 15 kb genomic region, a 2.1 kb *Bam*HI-*Sal*I fragment, located at the 3′ end of the genomic DNA insert was identified as containing the 5′ end of the *PTHrP* gene (Fig. 7). This upstream region of the gene should contain the sequence elements that regulate gene expression.

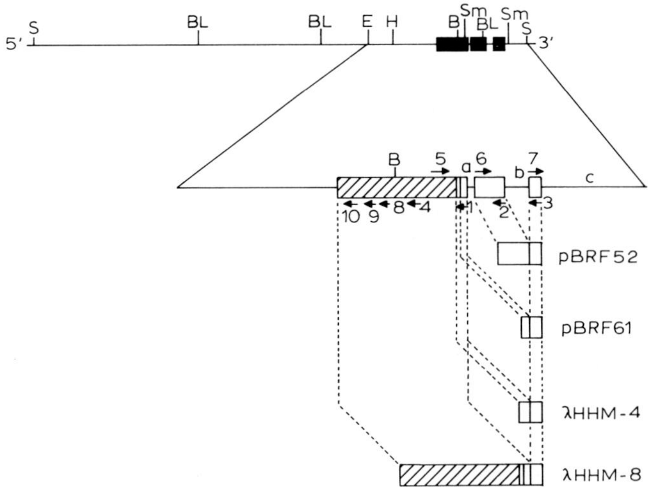


Fig. 7. Structure of the 5′ region of the *PTHrP* gene.4.I. Restriction map showing relevant sites is indicated at the top; restriction sites are indicated by: B, *Bam*HI; BL, *Bal*I; E, *Eco*RI; H, *Hin*dIII; Sal, *Sal*I; S, *Sma*I. The positions of the exons (boxed regions) in the 5′-terminal region are illustrated below, along with the potential alternate splicing mechanism, that results in the variable 5′-UTRs of PTHrP cDNA. mRNA species produced are shown and correspond to cDNA clones pBRF52, pBRF61 (Suva et al. 1987), λHHM-4 and λHHM-8 (Mangin et al. 1988a, b). Shaded region represents the 5′-UTR extension of λHHM-8 beyond pBRF61 and λHHM-4. The sequencing oligonucleotides numbered 1 through 10 are shown in the relative positions around the intron-exon boundaries. Arrows indicate the direction of sequence extension. The position of the introns are indicated by a, b and c (single unbroken line).

The nucleotide sequence (Fig. 8) of the human genomic clone was determined by conventional dideoxy sequencing of genomic fragments (Sanger et al. 1980). The location of the exons in the 5′ end of the *PTHrP* gene were determined by comparing the genomic sequence with that of PTHrP cDNA clones pBRF61 and pBRF52 (Suva et al. 1987). The intron-exon structure of the *PTHrP* gene has obvious homology with the human *PTH* gene (Vasicek et al. 1983). For example, the position of the intron-

```
-1610  aaaggatgggttagactcccgaccatgagtgaaaagggccgtgtgcgtgctccaggagtgtcggtcccccctctgcaattcaaaag
-1525  ggggatctctcctgtgcgcgggtttttgggaccggctccagatgtctcccagcgagttctgaaacagcaaaaagtgcaatttag
                       C
-1440  atatgaaatctggaaCTGTTTTTGTTCTTCTAAGCAAAAGATCTCCCTCTCTCTAGCCGATGCTCCCCACTCAGTTCATCCCGGG
                                                                      ***
-1355  AATGGGCCAGGGAGGAAGGTTCTCATGCATCGCCCCGAGCTGCCAGGCGACCTTCGGGCTCCTTAAATTCACAGGCCAACAGCCC
-1270  GCGTCCTCTCCGCGCAGGCTCCCGGTTGCCCGCGGTCCCCGGCCCAGCTCCTTGGCCTCCTCCTCGTCGGTCCGCCCCTGGTGGT
-1185  CTTGGCGCCCGCTCGTCCAGCTCGGCGCGCCGGGGACCGCCGGCTGCCCGGGGCAGTCCGCACGCCCTCGGGGATCTCGGCTCCC
                                                       G   C            GG    C        C
-1100  GGATCCGCCGCGCCGGCAGGAGCCGGCCGGGCCTGGAGGGAGCAAGCGGATCGCCACGCCCCCGGCACGGATGGGCGACAGGGCC
                                  ***           C       C
-1015  GGGCTCCGGGGTGGGGCTCGGCAGAGCTCCTGACAGCTCCGGGGTCGGCAGCGGGGAGGGGGGAGCTCCGCCGCTCGCCGCTCAT
                                                     C G          C
- 930  TCCCGGCTCGGGGCTCCCCTCCACTCGCTCGGGCGGCGCGGGGCCCGTTGCGCCGCCCGTCGCGCCCCCGCCCCCCGCGCGCCCG
                   T C    TCGCT                                                 CCG
- 845  CCCGCCAGCCCGCCCGTGCCCGCTTCGCCCCGCGCGCGTTCCTAGGGCGCCACCTCTTTGCGACTAGCTCACTTCTAGCAGGTTT
                                                             CC                     CCCG
- 760  GCCTCGGAGCGTGTGAACATTCCTCCGCTCGGTTTTCAACTCGCCTCCAACCTGCGGCCCGGCCAGCATGTCTCCGCCCGTGAAG
                           CC        ***             GCC
- 675  CGGGCTCGCCTCCCTGGCTCCGGCTGCCACTAACGACCCGCCCTCGCCCGACCTGGCCCTCCTGATCGACGACACACGCACTTGA
- 590  AACTTGTTCTCAGGGTGTGTGGAATCAACTTTCCGGAAGCAACCAGCCCACCAGAGGAGgtagacagacagctatgtatatatat
- 505  gtgggtttcgctacaagtggctctggaacgaaagGGCCTGGTTCGCAAAGAAGCTGACTTCAGAGGGGGAAACTTTCTTCTTTTA
- 420  GGAGGCGGTTAGCCCTGTTCCACGAACCCAGGAGAACTGCTGGCCAGATTAATTAGACATTGCTATGGGAGACGTGTAAACACAC
- 335  TACTTATCATTGATGCATATATAAAACCATTTTATTTTCGCTATTATTTCAGAGGAAGCGCCTCTGATTTGTTTCTTTTTTCCCT
- 250  TTTTGCTCTTTCTGGCTGTGTGGTTTGGAGAAAGCACAGTTGGAGTAGCCGGTTGCTAAATAAgtaagtgctgagaggctccaga
- 165  gaaatttttttcttttcaacttgggagatgcccttgatgttgaagaggcttttgagagcgggctaaaaagggggagcggagta
                                                                                   -1 M  Q
-  80  gtgcggggagatggagagtcctgactgacacctcgggtcccattcccttctgttgcagGTCCCGAGCGCGAGCGGAGACGATGCA
         R  R  L  V  Q  Q  W  S  V  A  V  F  L  L  S  Y  A  V  P  S  C  G  R  S  V  E  G  L
+   6  GCGGAGACTGGTTCAGCAGTGGAGCGTCGCGGTGTTCCTGCTGAGCTACGCGGTGCCCTCCTGCGGGCGCTCGGTGGAGGGTCTC
       S  R  R  L
+  91  AGCCGCCGCCTgtaagtcccccatcctccccagggcgccgggttggggaggccagggggaggggctgccaagctgggatgctgcc
+ 176  gaggcgttgcagcggtcaccgatcgtccttgcccgggttagggagagggaccatcccgcatacctgccgggcctgagccgttctc
+ 261  aaacctggcaggagaactggttgatcttcaaccggagacaggcaagagagagactttatgtgtgtttccataagagggagctttc
+ 356  acagaatctcttctagggaaagatccttgcctcta
```

Fig. 8. Nucleotide sequence of the 5′ region of the *PTHrP* gene. The nucleotides are numbered ( – 1610 to – 1) from the start ATG codon (A = + 1). The positions of the exons are represented in upper case, the introns in lower case and the potential TATA sequences are boxed, putative promoter region A at – 1558 bp and promoter B at – 514 bp, the mRNA cap site from promoter B is at – 493 bp. The transcriptional start site, A′, is located in the region 100 bp upstream of mRNA cap sites indicated by triangles at – 646 bp and – 616 bp. The position of the upstream ATGs are underlined and the in-frame stop codons are indicated with stars. Sp-1 binding site and its inverted repeat are indicated by dots. The bases given as superscripts represent the differences between λHHM-8 (Mangin et al. 1988) and the genomic sequence.

exon junction at the 3′ end of exon 2 (Fig. 8) is exactly the same as seen in the *PTH* gene, where the prepro-sequence is separated by an intron from the lysine (– 2)/arginine (– 1) doublet (Vasicek et al. 1983). Withing the 5′ end of the human *PTHrP* gene are 3 exons separated by 2 introns (Fig. 7). This region of the gene comprises, in order, exon 1a (approximately 900 bp), intron A (60 bp), exon 1b (283 bp), intron B (165 bp), exon 2 (123 bp) and intron C. Interestingly, intron B interrupts the cDNA sequence 22 bp upstream of the initiating ATG and corresponds exactly to the point of divergence between cDNA clones pBRF52 and pBRF61 (Suva et al. 1987). The exon sequence in the human *PTHrP* gene are identical to those described in BEN cells and the sequences surrounding the intron-exon boundaries, believed to be involved in splicing, agree with those proposed by Mount (1982).

### B. Expression of recombinant PTHrP

Recombinant PTHrP of variable chain length has been expressed in bacteria and shown to have a biological activity that is similar to synthetic PTHrP peptides (Hammonds et al. 1988).

Expression of biologically active PTHrP was achieved by the construction of a plasmid that encoded a fusion protein of full length PTHrP 1-141. The vector was prepared from a plasmid containing the *trp* promoter and the medium LE fusion protein. Construction involved inserting an oligonucleotide coding for the 5′ end of PTHrP 1-141, up to *Sau*3AI internal site, and a 444 bp *Sau*3AI-*Nsi*I fragment of PTHrP cDNA (Suva et al. 1987), behind the bacterial *trp* LE sequence that was separated from the PTHrP sequence by a methionine residue. This construct, along with similar plasmids coding for shorter PTHrP analogs, was transformed into *E. coli* resulting in high level, intracellular expression of recombinant PTHrP. Since PTHrP lacks internal methionine residues, fusion proteins can be specifically cleaved by cyanogen bromide. This approach allows the production, by recombinant DNA methods, of altered forms of PTHrP that will be useful in addressing the questions regarding the alternate processing of PTHrP in a variety of systems.

### C. Characterization of the human PTHrP gene

The genomic region upstream of the transcription start sites should contain the promoter elements and enhancer elements required for the regulation of gene expression (Maniatis et al. 1987). Promoters are DNA sequences that are usually located upstream, within 100 bp, of the transcription start site and direct the accurate and efficient initiation of transcription by RNA polymerase II (Breatnach and Chambon 1981). Enhancers are DNA sequences that increase the rate, but not the accuracy, of transcription from promoters and are often found $>100$ bp upstream of the transcriptional start site (Dierks et al. 1983; Everett et al. 1983). These sequences are modular in nature, consist of short arrays of recognition elements and interact with specific transcription factors. A number of both positive and negative regulatory elements that function in both specific cell types or in response to specific inducers have been identified.

The region of the human *PTHrP* gene, upstream of the translation initiation codon, contains three transcriptional start sites. One potential regulatory domain, containing a consensus TATA motif, is located in intron A, – 22 bp upstream of the putative exon 1b cap site. Initiation of transcription in this putative promoter region (B) (Fig. 8) would produce mRNA transcripts equivalent to cDNA clones pBRF52 (Suva et al. 1987) and 10B5 (Thiede et al. 1988). The position of the exon 1b cap site has been determined by Thiede et al. (1988), who analyzed cDNA clones from a human renal carcinoma cell line (786-0) and found by sequence analysis and primer extension only a single species of 5′ untranslated sequence for PTHrP mRNA. The exact position of the exon 1b cap site has been confirmed by our own S1 nuclease mapping and primer extension studies, that have localized the 5′ end of PTHrP mRNA fron BEN cells (Fig. 8). This mRNA would be initiated 15 – 17 bp downstream of promoter B, in agreement with genomic sequence information. The nucleotide sequence of the 5′-UTR of 786-0 mRNA is identical to the sequence of pBRF52.

Isolation of divergent cDNA clones suggests that another regulatory domain is located some distance upstream of the exon 1a cap site. Initiation of transcription in this region will generate mRNA species corresponding to PTHrP cDNA clones pBRF50 and pBRF61 (Suva et al. 1987,1988). Support for the existence of this putative regulatory region comes from Mangin and colleagues (1988a) who identified a cDNA clone (λHHM-8) from a renal carcinoma cell line (SKRC-1) that is identical to pBRF50 and pBRF61, but extended 826 bp upstream. The extended sequence of λHHM-8 is virtually identical to the genomic sequence (Fig. 8) and suggests that pBRF61 is identical to λHHM-8. Possibly, pBRF61 could have been foreshortened due to some cDNA cloning artefact.

The 5′-UTR of λHHM-8 is unusually long. In eukaryotic mRNAs, approximately 70% contain fewer than 80 nucleotides in their 5′-UTR (Kozak 1984). However, if λHHM-8 represents a mRNA species that is the result of an upstream initiation event, the sequences defining the position of the putative upstream promoter (A) (Fig. 8) will be located 5′ of the end of λHHM-8. No typical TATA box (Breatnach and Chambon 1981) is located in this region, but it is possible that the CAAAAA sequence (Corden et al. 1980), could function as promoter A (Fig. 8). In addition, another motif resembling the TATA sequence, TAGA, is found in this region. Such modified TATA sequences have been associated with multiple initiations (Bucher and Trifinov 1986). This upstream region also contains the enhancer sequence GCAAT, that has been shown to have similar activity to the consensus CCAAT sequence (Hatomochi et al. 1988). Initiation of transcription in this region would generate an mRNA transcript corresponding to λHHM-8 (Mangin et al. 1988a).

However, should pBRF61 represent a mRNA species corresponding to an alternate transcriptional start, and not a shortened cloning artefact, the sequences defining the upstream promoter should be localized within 100 bp of the 5′ end of pBRF51 (Fig. 8). No consensus TATA sequence is found in this region and no other apparent consensus regulatory motifs. There are however, many GC box motifs in this region, including six repeats of the inverted Sp-1 binding site sequence (Dynan and Tjian 1985).

Mangin et al. (1988b) reported the characterization of another PTHrP cDNA clone (λHHM-4), which contains divergent coding and 3′-UTRs and a 5′-UTR of similar length to pBRF61. This clone is of particular interest for the identification of the alternate transcriptional start site (A′, Fig. 8) since the 5′-untranslated sequence of λHHM-4 is 45 bp longer than pBRF61 and 805 bp shorter than λHHM-8, suggesting that pBRF61 and λ-HHM4 represent mRNA species that correspond to alternate transcriptional initiation. Their identification supports the notion that the unusually long 5′-untranslated region of λHHM-8 may be due to an additional upstream transcription start site.

This idea has been supported by the primer extension localization of multiple transcription initiation sites, in BEN cell mRNA, that correspond to pBRF61 and λHHM-4 mRNA. The pBRF61 start site is located upstream of the end of pBRF61 cDNA (Fig. 8) with another transcriptional start corresponding to λHHM-4 located at −646 bp or −645 bp (Fig. 8), suggesting that pBRF61 and λHHM-4 represent mRNA species that are produced by multiple transcription initiations in the region corresponding to promoter A′ (Fig. 8). Initiation in the region far upstream of these sites, which is absent in BEN cells, results in the production of higher molecular weight mRNAs, perhaps corresponding to λHHM-8. Far upstream initiation is possibly due to the presence of weak consensus promoter sequences in this region.

Nucleotide sequence analysis, of the promoter region 100 bp upstream of these mapped transcriptional start sites (A′, Fig. 8), does not reveal any consensus promoter or enhancer sequences. McKnight and Kingsbury (1982) have shown that TATA boxes determine the start of transcription and that genes lacking consensus TATA sequences often have multiple transcriptional start sites and a high GC content. An increasing number of eukaryotic genes have been shown to lack these upstream regulatory sequences, including hamster 3-hydroxyl-3-methylglutaryl-CoA reductase (Reynolds et al. 1984), human epidermal growth factor receptor (Ishii et al. 1985), human hypoxanthine-guanine phosphoribosyltransferase (Patel et al. 1986) and mouse and human osteonectin (McVey et al. 1988; Young et al. 1989). As with these other mammalian genes, the human *PTHrP* gene has multiple transcriptional start sites and is highly GC rich.

Primer extension studies support the idea that production of PTHrP mRNA species, containing divergent 5′-untranslated regions, occurs by initiation of transcription from three separate transcriptional start sites. Northern gel analysis, using specific 5′- and 3′-UTR oligonucleotides, has demonstrated that two promoter regions are functioning in BEN cells (Suva et al. 1989). In addition, Northern gel analysis of BEN cell RNA using oligonucleotide probes based on the far 5′-UTR of λHHM-8 have been unable to detect the presence of this mRNA. These data again support the existence of multiple transcriptional start sites and suggest that multiple PTHrP mRNA species are produced by initiation from distinct promoter regions. It is likely that another transcriptional start site, located further 5′, is responsible for the production of higher molecular weight mRNA species corresponding to λHHM-8 (Mangin et al. 1988a), but which is undetectable in BEN cells.

## D. Alternative splicing of the human PTHrP gene

There is at present no data available regarding the regulation of *PTHrP* gene expression, so the existence of multiple initiation sites is fascinating. Leff et al. (1986) have suggested that the alternative splicing of a single gene may serve as a potential mechanism for developmental and tissue-specific gene expression. Multiple promoter regions may confer tissue specificity on *PTHrP* gene expression, perhaps analogous to the expression of the mouse-α-amylase gene (Hägenbuchle et al. 1981; Young et al. 1981).

cDNA cloning data suggests that the alternate splicing of the human *PTHrP* gene is possibly even more complex. PTHrP mRNA species have been reported that correspond to initiation from separate promoter regions (Suva et al. 1989) and to alternate mRNA splicing at the 3′ end (Mangin et al. 1988a; Thiede et al. 1988). As there is no sequence information available regarding the 3′ end of the human *PTHrP* gene, the evidence for alternate splicing in this region comes only from these cDNA cloning studies.

Thiede et al. (1988) have shown that 3′-alternate *PTHrP* mRNA splicing occurs and suggest the presence of multiple intron-exon junctions at the 3′ end which allow splicing to occur. This proposed intron interrupts the PTHrP mRNA at Arginine 139, 9 bp upstream of the termination codon of 1-141 *PTHrP* (Suva et al. 1987). Genomic sequence information (D. Goltzman, personal communication) would suggest that the additional intron occurs after the exon coding for the longer PTHrP molecule. Further, Mangin et al. (1988b) describe a cDNA clone that encodes a longer PTHrP molecule of 173 amino acids, with a divergent C-terminus from amino acids 142-173. The existence of such complex genes, that produce multiple mRNA species with different 5′ and 3′ ends, are rare, but have been reported. Setzer et al. (1982) described the mouse dihydrofolate reductase (DHFR) gene that produces multiple mRNA species by initiation from distinct non-consensus promoters and alternate splicing.

The complex nature of *PTHrP* gene expression is supported by the Northern blot analysis of Mangin et al. (1988a, b) which shows multiple transcripts of PTHrP mRNA, which is similar to our earlier work (Suva et al. 1987). This complex pattern of PTHrP gene expression has been shown in a variety of normal tissues. Multiple PTHrP mRNA species were detected in keratinocytes, fetal liver, brain, parathyroid, adrenal cortex, medulla and stomach mucosa (Ikeda et al. 1988a, b). This work has been extended to include the detection of PTHrP mRNA species in a variety of human and animal tumors thought to be associated with HHM (Ikeda et al. 1988a, b). In the case of the human *PTHrP* gene, the existence of multiple potential tissue specific promoters and alternative splicing events presents a complex picture of gene expression.

## E. Chromosomal localization of the human PTHrP gene

The probable evolutionary relationship between PTH and PTHrP is supported by the conservation of intron-exon boundaries in both genes and by their similar biological actions. This idea is further supported by the localization of the human *PTHrP* gene to the short arm of chromosome 12, sub-bands 12p11.1 to 12p12.2 (Mangin et al. 1988a; Suva et al. 1989; Fig. 9). Point localization of the human PTHrP gene in this region was achieved by chromosomal *in situ* hybridization over good quality prophasic chromosome 12 (Fig. 9).

The localization of the human *PTH* gene to chromosome 11, band 11p15, (Mannens et al. 1987; Fig. 9) supports the concept that the genes for PTH and PTHrP have a common evolutionary origin via the duplication of the two chromosomes. Human chromosomes 11 and 12 are of similar size, centromere index and banding pattern and are thought to have a common origin, perhaps in tetraploidy (Comings 1972). Thus, the human *PTH* and human *PTHrP* genes join a number of pairs of related genes that are located on the evolutionarily related chromosomes 11 and 12.

In view of recent experiments demonstrating an important physiological role for PTHrP in fetal calcium transport (Rodda et al. 1988), it is intriguing to speculate on the role of PTHrP in the evolution of calcium regulation. If PTHrP is the fetal equivalent of PTH, then it is possible that it is the common ancestral gene, not PTH. The resolution of this question awaits the identification of the PTHrP gene in lower species.

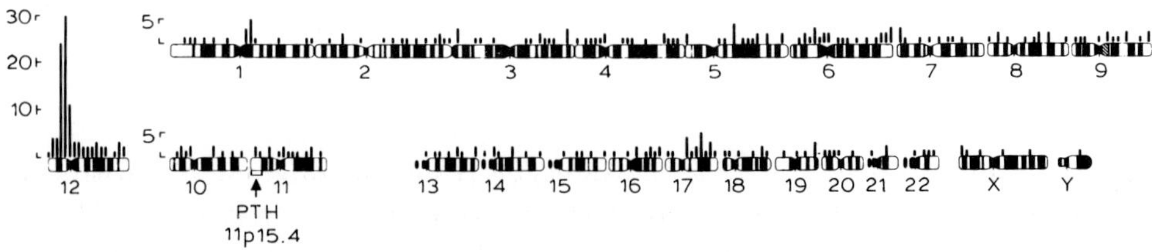


Fig. 9. Chromosomal localization of *PTHrP* gene. Score of grains over all chromosomes showing a peak of 30 grains over sub-band 12p11.2 with a background of no more than 5 grains over the other chromosomes. The location on chromosome 11 of the gene coding for *PTH*, band 11p15, is also shown. The low peak of grains over the long arm of chromosome 17 is seen on most of our *in situ* hybridization slides (Board et al. 1988) and is regarded as an artefact.

## XI. Summary

This chapter has reviewed an exciting period of research in which PTHrP has been identified, cloned and sequenced. Its potential physiological actions and precise contribution to the syndrome of HHM are now the subject of intense investigation. The availability of cDNA probes will allow detailed studies of the tissue localization of PTHrP and functional studies of gene expression will enable the identification of factors involved in the regulation of PTHrP production both in normal physiology and disease.

## Acknowledgements

Research by these authors is supported by The National Health and Medical Research Council of Australia, The Anti-Cancer Council of Victoria and Genentech Inc. The authors wish to thank C.P. Rodda, J.A. Danks and P.R. Ebeling for inclusion of some of their unpublished data and Professor T.J. Martin for his support and guidance in the preparation of the manuscript and in whose laboratory the authors' work is carried out.

## References

Akatsu T, Nagata N, Kugai N, et al. On the activities of parathyroid hormone-like factor and transforming growth factors in extracts of pancreatic cancer associated with humoral hypercalcemia of malignancy. Acta Endocrinol 1988;118:232 – 238.

Albright F. Case records of the Massachusetts General Hospital (Case 27401). New Engl J Med 1941;225:789 – 791.

Atkins D, Ibbotson KJ, Hillier K, Hunt NH, Hammonds JC, Martin TJ. Secretion of prostaglandins as bone-resorbing agents by renal cortical carcinoma in culture. Br J Cancer 1977;36:601 – 607.

Benson RC, Riggs BL, Pickard BM, Arnaud CD. Immunoreactive forms of circulating parathyroid hormone in primary and ectopic hyperparathyroidism. J Clin Invest 1974;54:175 – 181.

Bernier SM, Goltzman D. Influence of peptides acting through the EGF receptor on the action of synthetic parathyroid hormone-like peptide of malignancy in renal and osseous cells in vitro. J Bone Miner Res 1988;3:(Suppl 1):A3.

Berson SA, Yalow RS. Parathyroid hormone in plasma in adenomatous hyperparathyroidism, uremia and bronchogenic sarcoma. Science 1966;154:907 – 909.

Bertolini DR, Medwin GE, Bringham TS, Smith DD, Mundy GR. Stimulation of bone resorption and inhibition of bone formation in vitro by human tumor necrosis factors. Nature 1986;319:516 – 518.

Breatnach R, Chambon P. Organization and expression of eukaryotic split genes coding for proteins. Ann Rev Biochem 1981;50:349 – 383.

Board PG, Webb GC, McKee J, Ichinose A. Localisation of the coagulation factor XIIIA subunit gene (F13A) to human chromosome bands 6p24-p25. Cytogenet Cell Genet 1988;48:25 – 27.

Buckle RM, McMillan M, Mallison C. Ectopic secretion of parathyroid hormone by a renal adenocarcinoma in a patient with hypercalcemia. Br Med J 1970;IV:724 – 726.

Burtis WJ, Wu J, Bunch CM, et al. Identification of a novel 17,000-dalton parathyroid hormone-like adenylate cyclase-stimulating protein from a tumor associated with humoral hypercalcemia of malignancy. J Biol Chem 1987;262:7151 – 7156.

Burtis WJ, Brasy TC, Wu TL, Mitnick M, Weir EC, Insogna KL, Ikeda K, Stewart AF. Immunologic studies of humoral hypercalcemia of malignancy using antisera to synthetic HHM(1 – 36). J Bone Miner Res 1988;3(Suppl 1):A5.

Care AD, Caple IW, Pickard DW. The role of the parathyroid and thyroid glands on calcium homeostasis in the ovine fetus. In: Jones CT and Nathaniels P, eds. The Physiological Development of the Fetus and Newborn. Academic Press, 1985;135 – 140.

Caverzasio J, Rizzoli R, Bonjour J-P. Sodium dependent phosphate transport inhibited by parathyroid hormone and cyclic AMP stimulation in an oppossum kidney cell line. J Biol Chem 1986;261:3233 – 3232.

Centrtella M, McCarthy TL, Canalius E. Parathyroid hormone modulates transforming growth factor $\beta$ activity and binding in osteoblast-enriched cell cultures from fetal rat parietal bone. Proc Natl Acad Sci USA 1988;83:5889 – 5893.

Civitelli A, Martin TJ, Hruska KA, Avioli LV. Parathyroid hormone-related peptide (PTHrP) transiently increases intracellular calcium in UMR 106-01 osteoblastic cells. J Bone Miner Res 1988;3(Suppl 1):A14.

Comings DE. Evidence for ancient tetraploidy and conservation of linkage groups in mammalian chromosomes. Nature 1972;238:455 – 457.

Corden J, Wasylyk B, Buchwalder A, et al. Promoter sequences of eukaryotic protein-coding genes. Science 1980;209:1406 – 1414.

Danks JA, Ebeling PR, Hayman J, et al. Parathyroid hormone-related protein of cancer: Immunohistochemical localization in cancers and in normal skin. J Bone Miner Res 1989 (In press).

Dewhirst FE, Ago JM, Peros WJ, Stashenko P. Synergism between parathyroid hormone and interleukin 1 in stimulating bone resorption in organ culture. J Bone Miner Res 1987;2:127 – 134.

Dierks P, van Ooyen A, Cochran M, et al. Three regions upstream from the cap site are required for efficient and accurate transcription of the rabbit beta-globin gene in mouse 3T6 cells. Cell 1983;32:695 – 706.

Donahue AJ, Fryer FJ, Heath H, III. Synthetic fragment 1-37 of human parathyroid hormone-related peptide (PTHrP) increases ionized calcium in ROS/17.2 cells. J Bone Miner Res 1988;3(Suppl 1):A156.

D'Souza SM, Ibbotson KJ, Smith DD, Mundy GR. Co-purification of a transforming growth factor (TGF) with bone resorbing activity in the Walker rat carcinosarcoma: a mechanism for humoral hypercalcemia of malignancy (HHM). Calcif Tissue Int 1983;35:A658.

D'Souza SM, Ibbotson KJ, Mundy GR. Failure of parathyroid hormone antagonists to inhibit in vitro bone resorbing activity produced by two animal models of humoral hypercalcemia of malignancy. J Clin Invest 1984;74:1104 – 1107.

Dynan WS, and Tjian R, Control of eurkaryotic messenger RNA synthesis by sequence-specific DNA-binding proteins. Nature 1985;316:774 – 778.

Ebeling PR, Adam WR, Moseley JM, Martin TJ. Actions of parathyroid hormone-related protein on the isolated rat kidney. J Endocrinol 1988;12:45 – 50.

Ellison M, Woodhouse D, Hillyard CJ, Dowsett M, Coombes RC, Gilby ED. Immunoreactive calcitonin production by human lung cancer cells in culture. Br J Cancer 1975;32:373 – 379.

Everett RD, Baty D, Chambon P. The repeated GC-rich motifs upstream from the TATA box are important elements of the SV40 early promoter. Nucl Acid Res 1983;11:2447 – 2484.

Findlay DMF, DeLuise M, Michelangeli VP, Ellison M, Martin TJ. Properties of a calcitonin receptor and adenylate cyclase in BEN cells, a human cancer cell line. Cancer Res 1980;40:1311 – 1317.

Forrest SM, Ng KW, Findlay DMF, et al. Characterization of an osteoblast-like clonal cell line which responds to both parathyroid hormone and calcitonin. Calcif Tissue Int 1985;37:51 – 56.

Garret IR, Durie BGM, Nedwin GE, et al. Production of lymphotoxin, a bone resorbing cytokine, by cultured human myeloma cells. New Engl J Med 1987;317:526 – 532.

Gkonos PJ, Hayes T, Burtis W, et al. Squamous carcinoma model of humoral hypercalcemia of malignancy. Endocrinology 1984;115:2384 – 2390.

Goltzman D, Stewart AF, Broadus AE. Malignancy-associated hypercalcemia evaluation with a cytochemical bioassay for parathyroid hormone. J Clin Endocrinol Metab 1981;53:899 – 905.

Gowen M, Wood DW, Ihrie EJ, McGuire MB, Russell RGG. An interleukin 1-like factor stimulates bone resorption in vitro. Nature 1983;306:378 – 380.

Graves BJ, Johnson PF, McKnight SL. Homologous recognition of a promoter domain common to the MSV LTR and the HSV tk gene. Cell 1986;44:565 – 576.

Greenberg PB, Martin TJ, Sutcliffe HS. Synthesis and release of parathyroid hormone by a renal carcinoma in cell culture. Clin Sci Mol Med 1973;45:183 – 187.

Gutierrez GE, Mundy GR, Derynck R, Hewlett EL, Katz MS. Inhibition of parathyroid responsive adenylate cyclase in clonal osteoblast-like cells by transforming growth factor alpha and epidermal growth factor. J Biol Chem 1987;262:15845 – 15850.

Hägenbuchle O, Tosi M, Schibler U, et al. Mouse liver and salivary gland $\alpha$-amylase mRNA differ only in their 5′-untranslated sequences. Nature 1981;289:643 – 646.

Hammonds RG, Winslow G, Wood WI. Expression of full length PTH-related protein in E. Coli. Calcif Tissue Int 1988;42(Suppl A):164.

Hatamochi A, Golumbek PT, Van Schaftingen E, de Crombrugghe BA. CCAAT DNA binding factor consisting of two different components that are both required for DNA binding. J Biol Chem 1988;263:5940 – 5947.

Hayman JA, Danks JA, Ebeling PR, Moseley JM, Kemp BE, Martin TJ. Expression of parathyroid hormone-related protein in normal skin and in tumors of skin and skin appendages. J Path 1989;158:293 – 296.

Horiuchi N, Caulfield MP, Fisher JE, et al. Similarity of synthetic peptide from human tumor to parathyroid hormone in vivo and in vitro. Science 1987;238:1566 – 1568.

Holick MF, Nussbaum S, Persons KS. PTH-like humoral hypercalcemia factor of malignancy may be an epidermal differentiation factor; Synthetic hHHF(1 – 14)$NH_2$ inhibits proliferation and induces terminal differentiation of cultured human keratinocytes. J Bone Miner Res 1988;3(Suppl.1):A582.

Ibbotson KJ, D'Souza SM, Ng KW, et al. Tumor derived growth factor increased bone resorption, in a tumor associated with humoral hypercalcemia of malignancy. Science 1983;221:1292 – 1294.

Ibbotson KJ, Twardzik DR, D'Souza SM, Hargreaves WR, Todaro GJ, Mundy GR. Stimulation of bone resorption in vitro by synthetic transforming growth factor-alpha. Science 1985;228:1007 – 1008.

Ikeda K, Mangin M, Dreyer BE, et al. Identification of transcripts encoding a parathyroid hormone-like peptide in messenger RNAs from a variety of human and animal tumors associated with humoral hypercalcemia of malignancy. J Clin Invest 1988a;81:2010 – 2014.

Ikeda K, Weir E, Mangin M, Brown E, Broadus AE. Tissue-specific and developmental expression of mRNAs encoding a PTH-like peptide. J Bone Miner Res 1988b;3(Suppl.1):A578.

Ikeda K, Matsumoto T, Fukumoto S, et al. A hypercalcemic nude rat model that completely mimics human syndrome of humoral hypercalcemia of malignancy. Calcif Tissue Int. 1988c;43:97 – 102.

Ilardi CF, Faro JC, Localization of parathyroid hormone-like substance in squamous cell carcinoma. Arch Path Lab Med 1975;109:752 – 755.

Insogna KL, Weir EC, Wu T, Stewart AF, Broadus AE, Burtis WJ, Centrella M. Co-purification of transforming growth factor beta-like activity with PTH-like and bone resorbing activities from a tumor associated with humoral hypercalcemia of malignancy. Endocrinology 1987;120:2183 – 2185.

Ishii S, Xu Y-H, Stratton RH, Roe BA, Merlino GT, Pastan, I. Characterization and sequence of the promoter region of the human epidermal growth factor receptor gene. Proc Natl Acad Sci USA 1985;82:4920 – 4924.

Jueppner H, Abou-Samra AB, Uneno S, Gu WX, Potts JT, Segre GV. The parathyroid hormone-like peptide associated with humoral hypercalcemia of malignancy and parathyroid hormone bind to the same receptor on the plasma membrane of ROS 17/2.8 cells. J Biol Chem 1988;263:8557 – 8568.

Karin M, Haslinger A, Holtgreve H, et al. Characterization of DNA sequences through which cadmium and glucocorticoid hormones induce metallothionein-$II_A$ gene. Nature 1984;308:513 – 519.

Kemp BE, Moseley JM, Rodda CP, et al. Parathyroid hormone-related protein of malignancy: Active synthetic fragments. Science 1987;238:1568 – 1570.

Kozak M. Comparison of initiation of protein synthesis in procaryotes, eukaryotes and organelles. Micro Rev 1983;47:1 – 45.

Kozak M. Compilation and analysis of sequences upstream from the translational start site in eukaryotic mRNAs. Nucl Acids Res 1984;12:857 – 871.

Klein RF, Strewler GJ, Leung SC, Nissenson RA. Parathyroid hormone-like adenylate cyclase-stimulating activity from a human carcinoma associated with bone-resorbing activity. Endocrinology 1987;120:504 – 511.

Kubota M, Ng KW, Murase J, et al. Efficacy and specificity of human parathyroid hormone analogues or antagonists in intact clonal osteogenic sarcoma cells. J Endocrinol 1986;108:261 – 265.

Kubota M, Moseley JM, Rodda CP, Heath J Caple IW, Martin TJ. In: Cohn DV, Martin TJ, Meunier PJ, eds. Calcium Regulation and Bone Metabolism. Amsterdam: Excerpta Medica, 1987;718.

Kukreja SC, Shermerdiak WP, Lad TE, Johnson PA. Elevated nephrogenous cyclic AMP with normal serum parathyroid hormone levels in patients with lung cancer. J Clin Endocrinol Metab 1980;51:167 – 169.

Kukreja SC, Schavin DH, Wimbuscus S, et al. Antibodies to parathyroid hormone-related protein lower serum calcium in athymic mouse models of malignancy associated hypercalcemia due to human tumors. J Clin Invest 1988;82:1798 – 1802.

Leff SE, Rosenfeld MG, Evans RM. Complex transcriptional units: Diversity in gene expression by alternative RNA processing. Ann Rev Biochem 1986;55:1091 – 1117.

Lorenzo J, Sousa S, Kemp BE, Martin TJ. Comparison of parathyroid hormone related peptide(1 – 34) of malignancy and bovine parathyroid hormone (1 – 34) on bone resorption and the release of interleukin-1-like activity in 4 – 5 day newborn mouse calvaria cultures. J Bone Miner Res 1988;3(Suppl 1):A618.

Lowik C, Pluijm G vd, Most W, et al. Differences in bone resorbing responses of synthetic PTH-like protein (1 – 34) compared to PTH might be due to different effects on intracellular calcium in osteoblasts. J Bone Miner Res 1988;3(Suppl 1):A152.

Mangin M, Webb AC, Dreyer BE, et al. Identification of a cDNA encoding a parathyroid hormone-like peptide from a human tumor associated with humoral hypercalcemia of malignancy. Proc Natl Acad Sci USA 1988a;85:597 – 601.

Mangin M, Ikeda K, Dreyer BE, Milstone L, Broadus AE. Two distinct tumor-derived parathyroid hormone-like peptides result from alternative ribonucleic acid processing. Mol Endocrinol 1988b;2:1049 – 1055.

Maniatis T, Fristch EF, Sanbrook J. Regulation of inducible and tissue-specific gene expression. Science 1987;236:1237 – 1244.

Mannens M, Slater RM, Heyting C, et al. Regional localization of DNA probed on the short arm of chromosome 11 using anirdia-Wilms' tumor associated deletions. Hum Genet 1987;75:180 – 187.

Martin TJ. Humoral hypercalcemia of malignancy. Bone Miner 1988;4:83 – 89.

Martin TJ, Atkins D. Biochemical regulators of bone resorption and their significance in in cancer. Essays Med Biochem 1979;4:49 – 82.

Martin TJ, Mundy GR. Hypercalcemia of malignancy. In: Martin TJ, Raisz LG, eds. Clinical Endocrinology of Calcium Metabolism. New York: Marcel Dekker, 1987;171 – 199.

Mayes LC, Kasselberg AG, Rolott JS, Lukens JN. Hypercalcemia associated with immunoreactive parathyroid hormone in a malignant rhabdoid tumor of the kidney (Rhabdoid Wilm's Tumor). Cancer 1984;54:882 – 884.

McKee RL, Goldman ME, Caulfield MP, et al. The 7-34 fragment of human hypercalcemia factor is a partial agonist/antagonist for parathyroid stimulated cAMP production. Endocrinology 1988;122:3008 – 3010.

McKnight SL, Kingsbury R. Transcriptional control signals of eukaryotic protein-coding gene. Science 1982;217:316 – 324.

Melick RA, Martin TJ, Hicks RA. Parathyroid hormone production and malignancy. Br Med J 1972;2:204 – 206.

McVey JH, Nomura S, Kelly P, Mason IJ, Hogan BLM. Characterization of the mouse SPARC/Osteonectin gene Intron.exon arrangement of an unusual promoter region. J Biol Chem 1988;263:11111 – 11116.

Merendino TJ, Insogna KL, Milstone LM, Broadus AE, Stewart AF. A parathyroid hormone-like protein from cultured human keratinocytes. Science 1986;231:388 – 390.

Miyata T, Yasunoga T, Nishida T. Nucleotide sequence divergence and functional constraint in mRNA evolution. Proc Natl Acad Sci USA 1980;77:7328 – 7332.

Moseley JM, Kubota M, Diefenbach-Jagger H, et al. Parathyroid hormone-related protein purified from a human lung cancer cell line. Proc Natl Acad Sci USA 1987;84:5048 – 5052.

Motokura T, Fukumoto S, Takahashi S, et al. Expression of parathyroid hormone-related protein in a human T cell lymphotrophic virus type 1-infected T cell line. Biochem Biophys Res Commun 1988;154:1182 – 1188.

Mount SM. A catalogue of splice junction sequences. Nucl Acids Res 1982;10:459 – 472.

Mueller PP, Hinnebusch AG. Multiple upstream AUG codons mediate translational control of GCN4. Cell 1986;45:201 – 207.

Mundy GR. Hypercalcemia of malignancy revisited. J Clin Invest 1988;82:1 – 6.

Mundy GR, Martin TJ. The hypercalcemia of malignancy: pathogenesis and treatment. Metabolism 1982;31:1247 – 1277.

Mundy GR, Ibbotson KJ, D'Souza SM. Tumor products and the hypercalcemia of malignancy. J Clin Invest 1985;76:391 – 394.

Myers RM, Tilly K, Maniatis T. Fine structure genetic analysis of a $\beta$-globin promoter. Science 1986;232:613 – 618.

Nagamini Y, Reich E. Gene expression and cAMP. Proc Natl Acad Sci USA 1985;82:4606 – 4610.

Nakai M, Fukase M, Sakaguchi K, et al. Human parathyroid hormone-related protein fragment (1-34) had glucose-6-phosphate dehydrogenase activity on distal convoluted tubules in cytochemical bioassay. Biochem Biophys Res Commun 1988;154:146 – 150.

Negrini M, Silini E, Zozak C, Tsujimoto Y, Croce CM. Molecular analysis of mbcl-2: Structure and expression of the murine gene homologous to the human gene involved in follicular lymphoma. Cell 1987;49:455 – 463.

Nimberg RB, Humphries DE, Lloyd WA et al. Isolation of a bone resorptive factor from human cancer ascites fluid. Cancer Res 1978;38:1983 – 1989.

Nissenson RA, Strewler GJ, Williams RD, Leung SC. Activation of the parathyroid hormone receptor adenylate cyclase in osteosarcoma cells by a human renal carcinoma factor. Cancer Res 1985;45:5358 – 5368.

Nissenson RA, Diep D, Strewler GJ. Synthetic amino terminal peptides of parathyroid and of tumor-derived PTH-like protein bind to a common receptor in bone and kidney. J Bone Miner Res 1988;3(Suppl 1):A19.

Nissenson RA, Karpf D, Bambino T, et al. Covalent labeling of a high-affinity, guanyl nucleotide-sensitive parathyroid hormone receptor in canine renal cortex. Biochemistry 1987a;26:1874 – 1878.

Nissenson RA, Leung S, Diep D, Williams RD, Strewler GJ. Purification of low molecular weight forms of tumor-derived parathyroid hormone-like protein. J Bone Miner Res 1987b;2(Suppl 1):A388.

Orloff JJ, Wu T, Brady T, Stewart AF. Binding of synthetic 1-36 humoral hypercalcemia of malignancy peptide to human renal membranes. J Bone Miner Res 1988;3(Suppl 1):A6.

Patel PI, Framson PE, Caskey CT, Chinault AC. Fine structure of the human hypoxanthine phosphoribosyltransferase gene. Mol Cell Biol 1986;6:393 – 403.

Pizurki L, Rizzolo R, Moseley JM, Martin TJ, Caversazio J, Bonjour J-P. Effect of synthetic tumoral parathyroid hormone related peptide on cAMP production and sodium-dependent phosphate transport in cultured renal epithelial cells. Am J Physiol 1988;255:957 – 961.

Powell D, Singer FR, Murray TM, Minkin C, Potts JT. non-parathyroid humoral hypercalcemia in patients with neoplastic disease. New Engl J Med 1973;289:176 – 181.

Powles TJ, Dowsett M, Easty DM, Easty GC, Neville AM. Breast cancer osteolysis. bone metastases and antiosteolytic effect of aspirin. Lancet 1976;1:608 – 610.

Rabbani SA, Mitchell J, Roy DR, Kremer R, Bennett HPJ, Goltzmann D. Purification of peptides with parathyroid hormone-like bioactivity from human and rat malignancies associated with humoral hypercalcemia. Endocrinology 1986;118:1200 – 1210.

Rabbani SA, Roy DR, Hendy GN, Goltzman D. Role of the $NH_2$-terminus in the bioactivity of synthetic parathyroid hormone-like peptide of malignancy in vivo and in vitro. J Bone Miner Res 1988;3(Suppl 1):A4.

Raisz LG, Simmons HA, Sandberg AL, Canalis E. Direct stimulation of bone resorption by epidermal growth factor. Endocrinology 1980;107:270 – 278.

Riggs BL, Arnaud CD, Reynolds JC, Smith LH. Immunological differentiation of primary hyperparathyroidism from hyperparathyroidism due to non-parathyroid cancer. J Clin Invest 1971;50:2079 – 2083.

Reynolds GA, Basu SK, Osborne TF, et al. HMG CoA reductase: A negatively regulated gene with unusual promoter and 5′ untranslated regions. Cell 1984;38:275:285.

Rizzoli R, Caverzasio J, Moseley JM, Martin TJ, Vadas L, Bonjour J-P. Synthetic tumoral parathyroid hormone-related peptide stimulates renal tubular reabsorption of calcium. J Bone Miner Res 1988;3(Suppl 1):A13.

Rodan SB, Insogna KL, Vignery AM-C, et al. Factors associated with humoral hypercalcemia of malignancy stimulate adenylate cyclase in osteoblastic cells. J Clin Invest 1983;72:1511 – 1515.

Rodan SB, Noda M, Wesolowski G, Rosenblatt M, Rodan GA. Comparison of postreceptor effects of 1-34 human hypercalcemic factor and 1-34 human parathyroid hormone in rat osteosarcoma cells. J Clin Invest 1988;81:924 – 927.

Rodda CP, Kubota M, Heath JA, et al. Evidence for a novel parathyroid hormone-related protein in fetal lamb parathyroid glands and sheep placenta: Comparisons with a similar protein implicated in humoral hypercalcemia of malignancy. J Endocrinol 1988;117:261 – 271.

Roof BS, Carpenter B, Fink DJ, Gordan GS. Some thoughts on the nature of ectopic parathyroid hormones. Am J Med 1971;50:686 – 691.

Rosol TJ, Capen CC. Effects of infusion of human parathyroid hormone related protein (1-40) PTHrP on serum and urine calcium and phosphorus and bone histomorphometry in athymic mice. J Bone Miner Res 1988a;3(Suppl 1):A12.

Rosol TJ, Capen CC. Inhibition of in vitro bone resorption by parathyroid hormone receptor antagonist in the canine adenocarcinoma model of humoral hypercalcemia of malignancy. Endocrinology 1988b;122:2098 – 2102.

Rosol TJ, Capen CC, Brooks CL. Bone and kidney adenylate cyclase-stimulating activity produced by a hypercalcemia canine adenocarcinoma line (CAC-8) maintained in nude mice. Cancer Res 1987;47:690 – 695.

Rude RK, Sharp CF Jr, Fredericks RS, et al. Urinary and nephrogenous adenosine 3′5′-monophosphate in the hypercalcemia of malignancy. J Clin Invest 1981;52:765 – 771.

Sanger F, Coulson PR, Barrel BG, Smith AJH, Roc BA. Cloning in single stranded bacteriophage as an aid to rapid DNA sequencing. J Mol Biol 1980;143:161 – 178.

Sartori L, Weir EC, Stewart AF, et al. Synthetic and partially purified adenylate cyclase stimulating proteins from tumors associated with humoral hypercalcemia of malignancy inhibit phosphate transport in a PTH-responsive renal cell line. J Clin Endocrinol Metab 1988;66:459 – 461.

Setzer DR, McGrogan M, Schimke RT. Nucleotide sequences surrounding multiple polyadenylation sites in the mouse dihydrofolate reductase gene. J Biol Chem 1982;257:5143 – 5147.

Sherwood LM, O'Riordan JLH, Aurbach GD. Production of parathyroid hormone by non-parathyroid tumors. J Clin Endocrinol Metab 1967;27:140 – 146.

Shigeno C, Hiraki Y, Westerberg DP, Potts JT Jr, Segre GV. Photoaffinity labeling of parathyroid hormone receptors in clonal rat osteosarcoma cells. J Biol Chem 1988;263:3864 – 3871.

Simpson EL, Mundy GR, D'Souza SM, Ibbotson KJ, Bockman R Jacobs JW. Absence of parathyroid hormone messenger RNA in non-parathyroid tumors associated with hypercalcemia. New Engl J Med 1983;309:325 – 330.

Stewart AF, Horst R, Deftos LJ, Cadman EC, Lang R, Broadus AE. Biochemical evaluation of patients with cancer-associated hypercalcemia. Evidence for humoral and non-humoral groups. New Engl J Med 1980;303:1377 – 1381.

Stewart AF, Vignery A, Silvergate A, et al. Quantitative bone histomorphometry in humoral hypercalcemia of malignancy: uncoupling of bone cell activity. J Clin Endocrinol Metab 1981;55:219 – 227.

Stewart AF, Insogna KL, Goltzman D, Broadus AE. Identification of adenylate cyclase-stimulating activity and cytochemical glucose-6-phosphate dehydrogenase stimulating activity in extracts of tumors from patients with humoral hypercalcemia of malignancy. Proc Natl Acad Sci USA 1983;80:1454 – 1458.

Stewart AF, Insogna KL, Burtis WJ, et al. Frequency and partial characterization of adenylate cyclase-stimulating activity in tumors associated with humoral hypercalcemia of malignancy. J Bone Miner Res 1986;1:267 – 276.

Stewart AF, Mangin M, Wu T, et al. Synthetic human parathyroid hormone-like protein stimulates bone resorption and causes hypercalcemia rats. J Clin Invest 1988;81:596 – 600.

Stewart AF, Wu T, Burtis WJ, Weir EC, Broadus AE, Insogna KL. The relative potency of a human tumor-derived PTH-like adenylate cyclase stimulating preparation in three bioassays. J Bone Miner Res 1987a;2:37 – 43.

Stewart AF, Wu T, Goumas D, Burtis WJ, Broadus AE. N-terminal amino-acid sequence of two novel tumor-derived adenylate cyclase-stimulating proteins: Identification of parathyroid hormone-like and unlike domains. Biochem Biophys Res Commun 1987b:146:672 – 678.

Strewler GJ, Williams RD, Nissenson RA. Human renal carcinoma cells produce hypercalcemia in the nude mouse and a novel protein recognised by parathyroid hormone receptors. J Clin Invest 1983;71:769 – 774.

Strewler GJ, Stern PH, Jacobs JW, et al. Parathyroid hormone-like protein from human renal carcinoma cells. Structural and functional homology with parathyroid hormone. J Clin Invest 1987;80:1803 – 1807.

Strewler GK, Wronski TJ, Halloran BP, et al. Pathogenesis of hypercalcemia in nude mice bearing a human renal carcinoma. Endocrinology 1986;119:303 – 310.

Suva LJ, Winslow GA, Wettehall REH, et al. A parathyroid hormone-related protein implicated in malignant hypercalcemia: Cloning and expression. Science 1987;237:893 – 896.

Suva LJ, Mather KA, Ng KW, et al. Genomic structure of the promoter and 5′-untranslated region of the gene encoding parathyroid hormone-related protein. J Bone Miner Res 1988;3(Suppl 1):A580.

Suva LJ, Mather LA, Gillespie MT, et al. Structure of the 5′ flanking region of the gene encoding human parathyroid hormone-related protein (hPTHrP). Gene 1989;77:95 – 105.

Tashjian AH, Levine L. Epidermal growth factor stimulates prostaglandins and bone resorption in cultured mouse calvaria. Biochem Biophys Res Commun 1978;85:966 – 975.

Tashjian AH, Voelkel EF, Lazzaro M. $\alpha$ and $\beta$ human transforming growth factors stimulate prostaglandin production and bone resorption in cultured mouse calvaria. Proc Natl Acad Sci USA 1985;82:4635 – 4538.

Thiede MA, Rodan GA. Expression of a calcium-mobilizing parathyroid hormone-like peptide in lactating mammary tissue. Science 1988;242:278 – 280.

Thiede MA, Strewler RA, Nissenson RA, Rosenblatt M, Rodan GA. Human renal carcinoma expresses two messages encoding a parathyroid hormone like peptide: Evidence for the alternate splicing of a single copy gene. Proc Natl Acad Sci USA 1988;85:4605 – 4600.

Thompson DD, Seedor JG, Fisher J, Rosenblatt M, Rodan GA. Direct action of the human hypercalcemic factor on bone in thyroparathyroidectomised rats. Proc Natl Acad Sci USA 1988;85:5673 – 5677.

Tregear GW, Van Reitschotten J, Greene E, et al. Bovine parathyroid hormone: Minimum chain length of synthetic peptide required for biological activity. Endocrinology 1973;93:1349 – 1353.

Vasicek TJ, McDevitt BE, Freeman MW, et al. Nucleotide sequence of the human parathyroid hormone gene. Proc Natl Acad Sci USA 1983;80:2127 – 2131.

Weir EC, Norrdin RW, Matus RE, et al. Humoral hypercalcemia of malignancy in canine lymphosarcoma. Endocrinology 1988;122:602 – 608.

Welling GW, Wejser WJ, Van der Zee R, Welling-Webster S. Production of sequential antigenic regions in proteins. FEBS Lett 1985;188:215 – 219.

Wu T, Insogna KL, Hough LM, Milstone L, Stewart AF. Skin derived fibroblasts respond to human parathyroid hormone-like adenylate cyclase-stimulating proteins. J Clin Endocrinol Metab 1987;65:105 – 109.

Yaffe D, Nudel U, Mayer Y, Neuman S. Highly conserved sequences in the 3′ untranslated regions of mRNAs coding for homologous proteins in distantly related species. Nucl Acids Res 1985;13:3723 – 3737.

Yamamoto I, Kitamura N, Aoki J, et al. Circulating 1,25-dihydroxyvitamin D concentrations in patients with renal cell carcinoma-associated hypercalcemia are rarely suppressed. J Clin Endocrinol Metab 1987;64:175 – 179.

Yates AJP, Gutierrez GE, Smoleus P, et al. Effects of a synthetic peptide of a parathyroid hormone-related protein on calcium homeostasis, renal tubular calcium reabsorption and bone metabolism in vivo and in vitro in rodents. J Clin Invest 1988;81:932 – 938.

Young MF, Findlay DM, Dominguez P, et al. Osteonectin promoter: Primary sequence and S1 sensitive structure associated with potential regulatory activity. J Biol Chem 1989;264:450 – 456.

Young RA, Hägenbuchle O, Schibler V. A single mouse $\alpha$-amylase gene specifies two different tissue-specific mRNAs. Cell 1981;23:451 – 458.

Zernick J, Stover ML, Thiede MA, Rodan GA, Rowe DW. Isolation and characterization of a genomic clone corresponding to the promoter of the gene for rat bone alkaline phosphatase. J Bone Miner Res 1988;3(Suppl 1):A555.

Zhou H. Leaver DD, Moseley JM, Kemp BE, Ebeling PR, Martin TJ. Actions of parathyroid hormone-related protein on the rat kidney in vivo. J Endocrinol 1989;122:129 – 132.

Zondek H, Petrow H, Siebert W. Die bedeutung der calcium-bestimmering im blute fur die Sdiagnose der niereninsuffizientz. Z Klin Med 1923;99:129 – 132.

*Bone and Mineral Research/7*
*Johan N.M. Heersche and John A. Kanis, editors*



# Osteogenesis imperfecta

David W. Rowe

*Department of Pediatrics, University of Connecticut Health Center, Farmington, CT 06032, U.S.A.*

## I. Introduction

Astonishing advances have been made in understanding the fundamental basis of osteogenesis imperfecta (OI). In a span of 15 years, research has progressed from the initial discovery of an abnormality in type I collagen associated with lethal OI [1] to the generation of OI in a transgenic mouse [2]. The principles derived from this research will serve as a paradigm for many other heritable orders of connective tissue involving other collagen genes as well as noncollagenous structural genes. We understand in some detail the various types of mutations within the collagen gene that compromise structural and other functions of tissues rich in type I collagen. This same set of principles can be applied to diseases of cartilage, blood vessels and to some degree, basement membrane. The study of OI has not only provided radically new and powerful molecular techniques for genetic diagnosis, but has also paved the way for new therapeutic strategies.

Thus, the primary objective of this chapter is to show how biochemical, molecular, and genetic concepts have shaped our current understanding of OI and to suggest new areas of research. Emphasis will be placed on explanations for the extreme heterogeneity of clinical expression of the disease, which in most cases, result from mutations within the two genes that code for type I collagen.

## II. Connective tissue biology

In the following, the major biochemical and molecular aspects of collagen structure and formation will be reviewed with specific attention to how these principles relate to understanding the pathophysiological basis of OI.

## A. Major and minor protein constituents of connective tissue

Type I collagen is the primary collagenous constituent of skin, bone, and ligament and is the collagen type most frequently abnormal in OI. Because it is the most ubiquitous collagen in nature, it was the first one to be described at the biochemical and molecular level. Subsequently, at least 12 other collagen types have been described [3]. Some of the collagens seem to be tissue-specific, such as type II (cartilage and vitreous humor), type III (visceral tissues), and type IV (basement membrane). As more collagen types were discovered, they were grouped according to their biochemical and physical properties, such as fibrillar or interrupted collagens and short-chained or extra long fiber collagens (Fig. 1A). The uninterrupted fibrillar collagen (types I, II, III, V and XI) can be recognized as banded structures in tissue sections. The collagens have the *in vitro* property of self-aggregation into fibrils. Type IV was the first identified long chain collagen. This group of collagens have an interrupted helix, do not form banded structures in tissue section and do not self-aggregate *in vitro*. Type VII is the longest collagen in this group and co-localizes with the anchoring fibrils. The smaller interrupted collagen, types IX and XII, have three discontinuous helical domains and a covalently linked glycosaminoglycan linked to the N-terminal interrupting sequence

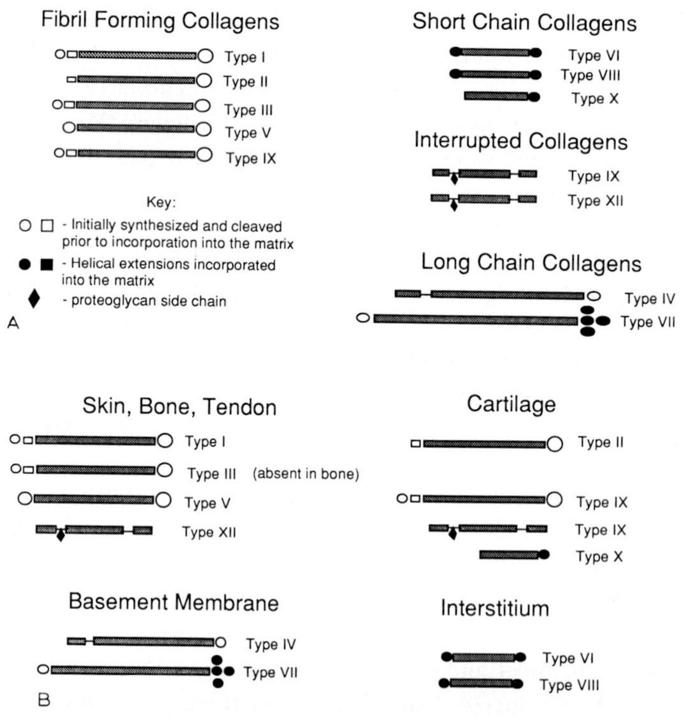


Fig. 1. Collagen types grouped by their physical- (A) or tissue- (B) associated features. The schematic for the collagen types are modified from Burgeson [3].

[4, 5]. The short chain collagens (types VI, VIII and X) have an uninterrupted triple helical conformation.

This bewildering array of different collagens, along with other extracellular matrix proteins, are combined in various proportions to yield connective tissue with a wide variety of physical properties. Appreciating how these combinations produce the observed physical features will be essential for understanding the pathophysiological basis of OI. The biochemical classification described above does not convey the interactive process that exists between various collagen types to produce the physical properties of a specific tissue. A classification that this author finds more functional groups the minor collagens in association with the three major connective tissue types, i.e. fibrillar, cartilagenous and interstitial/basement membrane (Fig. 1B). The fibrous connective tissues are composed of collagen types I, III, V, and XII, while the cartilagenous connective tissue include collagen types II, XI, IX and X [6]. The importance of the association between the minor collagens and their major types with a specific tissue has been further strengthened by the observation of co-localization and interchain crosslinks between type III and type V with type I collagen [7] and type XI with type II collagen [8]. It is assumed, because of the biochemical similarity between type IX and type XII collagen, that crosslinks between type I and type XII collagen also exist. Type IX and XII collagen appear to lie on the surface of the major collagen fibril [9] and the glycosaminoglycan side chain that protrudes from the molecule may provide a means for the complex to interact with the other matrix components [10, 11]. Interspersed within both major connective tissue types is a fine meshwork composed of type VI and VIII collagen. Although these collagens do not appear to be covalently linked to the major collagens, they are intimately associated and may provide a means for interactions with noncollagenous or cellular components. The interaction of the noncollagenous proteins such as fibronectin, hexibrachion and proteoglycans plus tissue-specific extracellular matrix proteins such as osteocalcin or osteopontin in bone provide further tissue heterogeneity [12]. Finally, since the connective tissue matrix needs to be continually renewed and remodelled, there must be communication between the matrix and the cells that determine its synthesis. This appears to occur through interaction of the extracellular matrix proteins with cell membrane proteins, termed integrins, which in turn modulate the synthetic activity of the cells [13].

Figure 2 portrays a fanciful schema for the assembly of the extracellular matrix in fibrous and cartilagenous tissue. It begins with the production of the major collagen type (I or II) followed by incorporation within the fiber of varying amounts of a second fibrillar collagen type (V or XI) which may modify the character of the fiber in as yet an unappreciated manner. The surface of the collagen microfibrils of each connective tissue is decorated with type IX or XII collagen. This may modulate the size of the collagen fiber and have the potential to enhance its interaction with other extracellular matrix proteins. The collagen fibers can also interact directly with proteoglycans and noncollagenous protein specific to a connective tissue to further modify that tissue. In

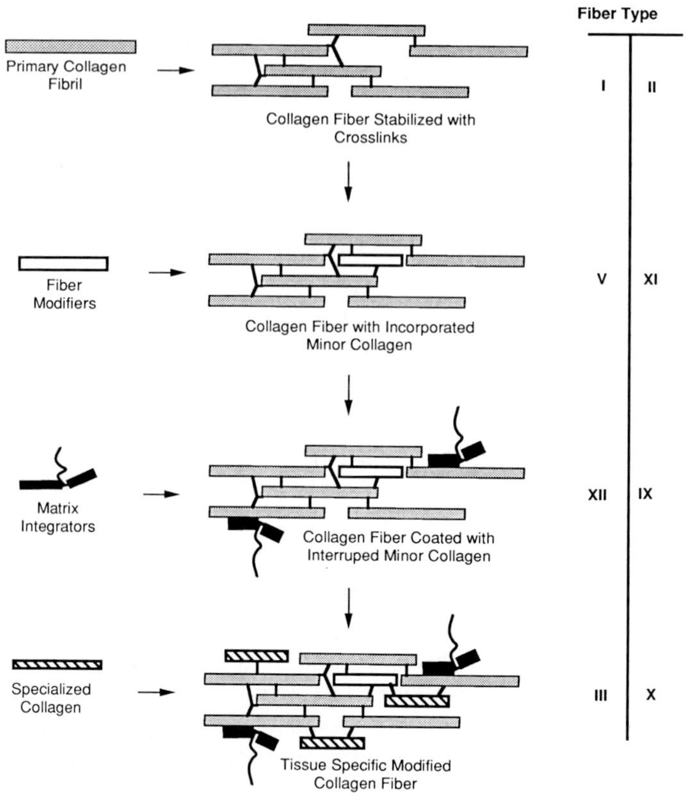


Fig. 2. Interaction of various collagen types with the major collagen of fibrous or cartilage tissue.

exceptionally specialized tissues, a second modifying collagen is added to the fiber. For example, connective tissue exposed to excessive ambient tissues such as the viscera or fetal skin (but interestingly not bone), have an increased content of type III collagen. In the calcifying hypertrophic cartilage, type X collagen is added to the extracellular matrix.

Thus, the extracellular matrix of any tissue can be envisioned as an alloy consisting of the major collagen type which is modified by the relative content of minor collagens and noncollagenous proteins. This complex set of interactions may underlie the fact that certain mutations of type I collagen have their primary effect on bone but little effect on other tissues rich in type I collagen, whereas other mutations of type I have a pronounced effect on ligament and no effect on bone. The complex nature of the matrix may also be responsible for genetic heterogeneity (same phenotype caused by mutations of different genes) of the connective tissue disorders. For example, most forms of OI have been shown to have mutations in type I collagen genes; however, this finding is not universal and probably suggests that mutations in other matrix genes (type V, XII) could be involved. The fact that only a few mutations of type I collagen have been found in the Ehlers-Danlos and Marfan's syndrome (disorders which show involvement of tissues rich in type I collagen) suggests that proteins associated with type I collagen are likely to be responsible.

### B. Organization of collagen in mature connective tissue

Although the final understanding of the connective tissue diseases will require knowledge of the complex molecular interactions discussed above, at present we can analyze the structure and function of collagen only as an isolated molecule. Even at this level however, information regarding the properties of the molecule may provide valuable insight into the pathophysiology of OI.

Type I collagen, as it is found in mature tissues, is a rod-like structure consisting of three chains, each of approximately 1000 amino acids in length [14]. The molecule is a heterotrimer composed of two $\alpha1(I)$ and one $\alpha2(I)$ chain. These chains are arranged in a triple helical structure because the repetitive gly-X-Y triplet extends uninterrupted throughout the length of each chain. Collagen is not synthesized in this form but as procollagen containing noncollagenous globular domains at both the *N*- and C-termini. These procollagen extensions appear to keep the molecule in a soluble form prior to secretion into the extracellular matrix. It is only after the extensions are removed by specific N- and C-propetidases that the helical domain precipitates and begins to form the microfibril with other collagen molecules [15].

The formation of the collagen fibril is essential to the strength of collagen in tissue. Collagen fibrils are composed of collagen molecules arranged in a specific quarter stagger that is determined by charge distribution along the surface of the molecule [16]. The specific alignment of the collagen molecules in the fibril is important for subsequent growth of the normal collagen fiber and formation of intermolecular crosslinks from adjacent lysine residues [17, 18]. Collagen fibrils generated *in vitro* from molecules obtained from cultured lethal OI fibroblasts produce a pattern of kinked collagen fibrils and an arborized network of interacting fibers unlike the expected linear array of fibrils [19]. It is likely that such an arborization would yield a structure incapable of resisting high tensile loads.

The kinking of the collagen fibril is the result of a mutation which interrupts the gly-X-Y triplet within the helical domain [20]. Amino acid deletions, insertions, or a first position glycine substitution of the gly-X-Y triplet are all sufficient to disrupt the tight helical conformation which in turn lead to a fibril with improper alignment [21]. The effects of these changes include: (1) a collagen fibril with altered crosslinkage and reduced strength [22]; (2) a distorted collagen helix with increased susceptibility to proteases such as chymotrypsin and pepsin *in vitro* and presumably similar sensitivity to tissue proteases *in vivo* [23, 24]; (3) reduced cellular secretion of those molecules lacking the normal helical conformation [25]. It is also likely that the abnormal collagen fibril does not form the appropriate interactions with other collagen types and other non-collagenous matrix protein [26]. The net effect is reduced accumulation of collagen in the extracellular matrix (reduced secretion and enhanced degradation). Those fibrils which do assemble have reduced structural integrity and do not form the normal interaction with the other extracellular components.

It should be apparent that fibrils composed of normal molecules will be compromised once abnormal molecules are incorporated into the growing fibril. Since every fibril will contain abnormal molecules, all fibrils will be affected and the phenotype will be inherited as a dominant trait [27]. Dominant mutations are observed when an abnormal protein compromises the function of the protein coded by the normal allele. In contrast, mutations of enzymes are inherited as recessive traits because there is sufficient function from the remaining normal allele. For collagen, the strength of the dominant trait and thus the severity of the disease is, in part, related to the quantity of abnormal protein that is incorporated into the extracellular matrix and the type of the disruption in the helical domain. Mutations inflicting the most severe clinical consequences are those which disrupt the C-terminal domain of helix, yet remain sufficiently stable to be exported from the cell. Those least likely to cause severe disease are mutations which reduce the synthesis of an otherwise normal collagen molecule. Such mutations are dominantly inherited but are relatively mild because the collagen that does accumulate in the extracellular matrix is not compromised by an abnormal collagen.

The size of the insertion or deletion within the helix does not appear to be a major determinant of helix disruption because the disease severity is no more severe than that caused by a first position glycine substitution of the gly-X-Y triplet. Instead there appears to be a correlation between the severity of the clinical phenotype and the position of the mutation along the collagen helix: the more C-terminal the location of the mutation the more severe the disease [28]. The reason for this observation relates to the way in which the molecule is formed. The procollagen molecule initially assembles through the interaction of sequences within the C-terminal propeptide and subsequently generates the helix in a C-terminal to N-terminal direction [29]. Until the mutation is encountered helix formation is normal, but once the interacting chains are placed out of register the remainder of the helical domain is defective. Thus, the more C-terminal the mutation the greater the extent of the collagen molecule that is compromised.

### C. Transcription and splicing of collagen mRNA

The genes that code for the two type I collagen $\alpha$ chains are present as single copy genes located on the 17th and 7th chromosomes [30, 31]. Although no longer the largest recognized gene, they are still among the most complex with regards to the number of exons. For the $\alpha$1(I) collagen gene (COL1A1), there are 51 exons distributed over an 18 kb domain [32], whereas the $\alpha$2(I) gene (COL1A2) contains 52 exons distributed over a distance of 40 kb [33]. The structural organization of the type I collagen genes is similar for all the fibrillar collagen: the first five exons code for the procollagen domain, the 6th exon includes the procollagen cleavage site and initiates the helical domain. The next 42 exons are composed of units of 45, 54, 99, 108 or 162 bases coding for 5, 6, 11, 12 or 18 gly-X-Y triplets. Since the helical exons code for discrete gly-X-Y units, deletion of an exon removes a triplet unit but does not alter the reading frame of the remainder of the collagen gene sequence. The terminal 3 exons code for the C-terminal propeptidase site and the procollagen assembly domain.

The transcriptional control elements within the type I collagen molecule regulate the amount of collagen synthesized and thus are candidates for mutations which would affect the amount of collagen entering the extracellular matrix. For example, DNA sequences that respond to general transcription signals such as the TATA box, CAAT box, SP1 and NF1 binding sequence are located within the first 500 bp of the body of the gene [34, 35]. It is also becoming clear that there are transcriptional enhancers that are active in cultured fibroblasts located within the first intron of the gene [36 – 38]. Mutations within elements of this type would be expected to result in reduced collagen production (null mutation) from the affected allele in all the type I collagen-producing cells. Null mutations of collagen have been observed in experimental situations such as chemical [39, 40] or retroviral mutagenesis [41], but a naturally occurring mutation that results from inactivation of a transcription control region has not been observed [42].

Sequences within the transcriptional control domains which act in a tissue-specific manner may account for mutations of type I collagen that are limited to a specific connective tissue. In regard to bone, a number of unrelated studies suggest that transcriptional control of type I collagen in bone cells differs from that of other type I collagen-producing cells: (1) 1,25-dihydroxyvitamin D has an inhibitory effect on collagen synthesis in bone cells but not fibroblastic or periosteal cells [43]. Since 1,25-vitamin D receptors are present in both cells, the bone-specific response to 1,25-dihydroxyvitamin D indicates that the gene is regulated in bone cells differently from the regulation in fibroblasts. This element has been mapped to sequences 1.6 kb upstream of the gene [43]. (2) There is evidence that bone cells contain factors which are able to interact with an enhancer element located approximately 3 kb upstream of the transcription start site [44]. A similar element is not expressed in fibroblasts. (3) The MOV-13 mouse resulted from an experimentally-induced inactivation of the $\alpha 1$(I) allele by a murine retrovirus. The insertion occurred in the first intron and inactivated the gene presumably by interrupting the function of the enhancer located in that region [45]. When the animal is bred to homozygosity, a lethal phenotype results from the total failure of type I production at approximately 8 – 9 days of development. Cultured fibroblasts from this cell line fail to synthesize the $\alpha 1$(I) chain and yet readily utilize an exogenously introduced normal $\alpha 1$(I) collagen gene [46, 47]. However, when tooth rudiments from the MOV-13 mouse are allowed to develop, type I collagen is produced [48]. These data suggest that transcription of the type I collagen gene in the MOV-13 mouse is effectively inhibited in fibroblastic cells, but not in odontoblasts nor presumably, bone cells. In both cell types there may exist transcriptional factors sufficient to overcome the inhibitory effect of the inserted retrovirus.

After the collagen mRNA is transcribed from the gene, it undergoes a number of processing steps before it can be transported to the cytoplasm. These steps include capping the 5′ end, removal of 50-51 introns and addition of the polyadenylation sequence at the 3′ end of the mRNA. The process of splicing any eukaryotic message involves the interaction of specific sequences within the RNA to be spliced (consensus splice sequence). A number of distinct, small nuclear ribonuclear proteins (snRNPs) as well as small uridine-rich nuclear RNAs (U-snRNAs) are also involved. A complex of snRNP and U-snRNA bind to consensus donor and acceptor sequences located at the junctions between the intron and exon and in a processive manner cleaves the intron and joins the exons. A third sequence, located approximately 30 bases 5′ of the acceptor site is the branch point sequence and serves as an essential intermediate step in the formation of the spliced mRNA [49, 50].

The hybridization affinity of the consensus splicing signals to their corresponding U-snRNA is one of the major determinants for selection of the proper donor and acceptor sequence within the unspliced RNA [51]. A number of studies suggest that the process begins with a protein complex containing U5-snRNA that binds to a polypyrimidine rich tract (acceptor site) of the mRNA. The intron is then scanned for the most proximal donor site which is determined by the hybridization strength between the consensus donor site and U1-snRNA. A third element within the intron, the branch point, also participates in this process. At that point cleavage of the donor site occurs, and a lariat is formed between the 5′ end of the intron and the branch point sequence. Subsequently, the acceptor site is cleaved and the two ends of the exons rejoined. Other aspects inherent in the sequence of the RNA that control where splicing occurs include the size of the intron sequence [52], sequences that are contained within the adjacent exons [53], and secondary structure within the mRNA [54]. It is also likely that there are factors extrinsic to the RNA which can modulate the splicing choices made by the cell and account for tissue-specific splicing of certain proteins [55]. Although alternative splicing of type I collagen has not been observed, it is found frequently in other extracellular matrix proteins [56 – 58]. In the case of mutations of a splice size within the collagen gene, alternative splicing may be another reason for tissue heterogeneity type I collagen expression.

When a mutation occurs that alters the normal splicing reaction, the splicing process selects alternative splice choices. In many cases the choices can be explained by selection of a secondary consensus splice site with a greater hybridization than the mutated authentic site [59]. Thus, the mutations in the consensus donor sequence will lead to selection of alternative donor site sequences upstream of the authentic donor either within the exon or at the next upstream authentic donor site. Similarly, mutations within a cryptic donor site, located in either an exon or an intron, can generate a new donor site with an affinity stronger than the authentic site and thus lead to splicing to a new position within the RNA [60, 61]. Mutations of globin mRNA associated with $\alpha$ and $\beta$ thalassemia attest to the wide variety of alternatives in splicing one can observe from a single mutation within either an intron or an exon [62].

In terms of disease severity, the consequence of altered splicing depends on the relative proportion of the altered spliced products: severity will be high when inframe splice products are produced, but will be mild if most of the spliced RNA is out of frame. Exon skipping of collagen mRNA almost always results in an inframe spliced RNA and produces a collagen protein with a deletion within the helix [63]. To date, most of the splicing defects described are exon skips because they were initially uncovered in patients with severe OI who also demonstrated a population of shortened $\alpha$ chains. Another example of an inframe splicing mutation was found in an infant with lethal OI where a mutation within an intron activated a cryptic donor site that produced a spliced RNA containing 75 bases of intron sequence [64]. Since the retained bases did not contain a stop codon and did not disrupt the reading frame, the protein product was a helix domain disrupted with 25 nontriple helical amino acids.

In contrast, when splicing results in an RNA with an altered reading frame, the normal triple helix is not synthesized. RNA that is read out of frame will usually generate numerous stop codons well before the authentic stop codon is reached. By a process that is still poorly understood, RNAs which are either out of frame or contain premature stop sites are recognized by the cell and do not reach the cytoplasm for translation. The net effect is a reduction of mature RNA that reaches the cytoplasm; the mutant allele becomes null. This type of mutation is analogous to $\beta$-thalassemias which contain low amounts of the $\beta$-globin mRNA because the underlying spliced mutation generates an out-of-frame mRNA, little of which reaches the cytoplasm for translation [65 – 67]. These thalassemias are characterized by low synthesis of $\beta$-globin, low cytoplasmic content of the abnormally spliced mRNA and by the accumulation of the abnormal RNA within the nucleus. There appears to be a similar pattern for mild forms of OI, that is low synthesis of a normal collagen [68], low $\alpha1(I)$ mRNA in the cytoplasm [69], and an accumulation of the RNA within the nucleus [70]. The difference between thalassemia and OI is that a disease phenotype is usually visible when only one collagen allele is null, while both globin alleles need to be affected to be symptomatic. In fact, the severity of mild OI may be so mild as to be unsuspected or passed off as a family trait that does not attract medical attention. In such cases the level of underproduction of normal RNA from the mutant allele may not be complete since there still may be some splicing that results from the authentic but altered consensus site. It should be clear that when a fraction of the spliced products from the mutant allele is a shortened or extended but translatable RNA, the severity may increase. Stated another way, it is better to synthesize no RNA than to produce an RNA that codes for an $\alpha$ chain which disrupts the helical domain.

Another mechanism of heterogeneity of expression of mutations affecting collagen expression may be variations in the manner that various cell types (fibroblasts vs. osteoblasts) handle an altered authentic splice site. Osteoblasts may select one set of splice alternatives while skin and tendon fibroblasts select another. Known examples of tissue-specific splicing of other multiexon mRNA such as fibronectin and elastin raise the possibility that a similar process might become evident when a cryptic site can successfully compete with an authentic splice site weakened by a mutation. Because the selection of a splicing site is dependent on hybridization between the consensus site and the U-snRNA, it might be anticipated that various potential splice sites would be affected by the temperature of the cell which would be significantly different in the skin and aorta. Thus, a mutation which alters a donor site may still use the impaired donor site generating a normal mRNA in one tissue but select an upstream donor site that produced a skipped exon in another tissue. The relative distribution of the two mRNA populations would eventually determine the severity of the underlying disease and in which tissues that mutation was expressed.

### D. Translation and chain assembly of procollagen

After the fully spliced RNA is transported to the cytoplasm, it interacts with ribosomes on the rough ER where the initial pro$\alpha$ chains are synthesized. The quantity of pro$\alpha$ chains that are eventually produced is a function of the quantity of RNA present to be translated and the rate at which translation occurs. The steady state level of RNA is influenced by the rate of transcription of the gene and the rate of degradation of the mature mRNA. Regulation of transcription was described above. Regulation of degradation may, in fact, be an important component in the determination of total collagen synthesis. There is evidence of certain hormones and growth factors affecting the mRNA half-life of other genes [71] and there is similar evidence for collagen [72]. It has been suspected for a number of years that the highly conserved nontranslated domain at the 5′-end of the collagen mRNA might have an effect on the efficiency at which the message is translated. This conserved region has the potential to form a stem loop in both the $\alpha$1(I) and $\alpha$2(I) chains and the preliminary deletion studies suggested that it may exert a negative translational effect [73]. However, more detailed studies of this phenomenon have failed to confirm this observation [74]. It would not be surprising for certain cell types to contain translational control factors that might facilitate collagen synthesis in one setting and impede it in another. For example, in the embryonic chick cartilage there is ample mRNA for type I collagen present although it is not translated into protein [75]. It should be anticipated that mutations which enhance the rate of collagen mRNA degradation or prevent its translation would behave as a null mutation producing a mild clinical phenotype.

After the pro$\alpha$ chains are synthesized, they enter the Golgi apparatus where hydroxylation of specific proline and lysines occurs. Regulation of the degree of hydroxylation does not appear to be related to the amount of hydroxylating enzyme present but rather the state of helix formation of molecule [76]. The enzymes only act on pro$\alpha$ chains prior to their incorporation into the triple helical conformation. This accounts for the excessive post-translational modification of the collagen chains that are incorporated into a molecule that is slow to assemble due to a disruption within the helical domain [77]. As peptide chain synthesis and hydroxylation are progressing, chain assembly is initiated. The process begins by interaction of sequences contained within the C-terminal propeptide of both pro$\alpha$ chains. The associated chains are stabilized by the formation of interchain disulfide bonds and subsequently helix assembly occurs spontaneously in a C-terminal to a N-terminal direction. The importance of the chain assembly sequence was illustrated by a frameshift mutation that preceded this region in the pro$\alpha$2(I) gene [78]. The resulting protein product was not incorporated into the collagen molecule even though the body of the helical domain was normal. This is another example of a null mutation of a collagen allele which, in the heterozygous state, was mild.

The completely formed procollagen molecule is secreted from the cell in a process that is not well understood. Molecules that form an unstable helix are secreted inefficiently and undergo degradation intracellularly [25]. The more efficient the process of preventing the mutant collagen molecule from reaching the extracellular matrix, the less severe will be the clinical trait. Tissue differences in this process may be another factor that accounts for the heterogeneity of this disease.

Once secreted from the cell, N- and C-terminal procollagen peptidases cleave the procollagen peptide extensions, allowing the body of the molecule to form the microfibril [79]. Failure to cleave the N-propeptide is associated with Ehlers-Danlos VII syndrome which is characterized by severe joint laxity but no bone disease [80, 81]. It has become apparent that proper alignment of the pro$\alpha$ chains at the site of enzyme cleavage is required for the process to occur efficiently [82]. Whereas most of the cases of EDS VII result from mutation within the cleavage site, cases have been found where the mutation lies well within the helical domain. The net clinical effect is an overlap syndrome with elements of EDS VII and OI [83]. The rate or extent of removal of the procollagen propeptides may play a role in the size of the collagen microfibril providing another step in the production of tissue-specific modulation of the extracellular matrix which might be susceptible for mutagenesis. Another potential role for the N- and C-terminal propeptides may be regulation of collagen synthesis, either at the translation or transcriptional level. High affinity receptors for these peptides have been demonstrated which appear to down-regulate the synthesis of type I collagen when occupied by the N- or C-terminal propeptide [84]. These findings probably explain the excessive synthesis for type I collagen that has been reported in EDS VII because of failure to generate the N-terminal propeptide [85].

Normal fibril formation is also required for lysyl oxidase to initiate crosslink formation [86] while normal alignment of the fibrils is necessary for the appropriate intermolecular reactions to proceed [87]. Normal fibrils may also be required for deposition of hydroxyapatite crystals [88].

## III. Biochemical and molecular techniques used to study OI

The following is not designed to be an exhaustive discussion of all methodologies employed but rather to give an overview with examples of their use to further our understanding of this disease.

### A. Biochemical analysis of matrix proteins

Most of the studies of collagen synthesis in OI have been carried out in cultured fibroblasts derived from skin or ligament, rather than cultured bone cells. Although these studies have revealed important information regarding the structure of the procollagen molecule as it is synthesized by the cultured cells, it should be kept in mind that this system may not reveal the consequences of these mutations on the interaction of collagen with noncollagenous components of bone. The proteins synthesized by the cultured cells are isotopically labelled for analysis of the chain within SDS polyacrylamide gels. The pro$\alpha$ chains can be examined by this method and usually show bands derived from the intact pro$\alpha$ chains as well as partial conversion products (pN and pC collagen bands). Less complex analysis of mutations within the helical domain can be obtained by enzymatic removal of the propeptides with controlled pepsin digestion followed by delayed-reduced SDS gel electrophoresis. The pattern of normal cells are $\alpha 1(\mathrm{I})$ and $\alpha 2(\mathrm{I})$ chains present in a 2:1 ratio with type III and V collagen separated as minor collagen bands. If there is underproduction of an otherwise normal type I collagen, then the relative ratio between type III collagen band and the type I collagen bands is increased. If the helical domain contains a deletion, then a population of $\alpha$ chains of smaller size can be detected. Since the type I collagen helical domain lacks cysteine, substitution of first position glycine residues with this amino acid is detected as a disulfide dimer of two chains. Finer mapping of insertions or deletions to a specific region of the chain is usually done on cyanogen bromide (CNBr) fragments that can be separated on SDS gels.

A biochemical marker for abnormal helix formation is excessive post-translational modification of the collagen chains. The process of prolyl and lysyl hydroxylation and glycosylation can only occur on chains that have not yet become incorporated into a tightly wound helix. In the case of a mutation within the helix that slows rate of helix assembly, excessive hydroxylation of lysine residues and over-glycosylation of the resulting hydroxylysine residues N-terminal to the mutation results. These post-translational changes are readily detectable at the biochemical level by an alteration of the chain mobility by SDS acrylamide gel electrophoresis [89]. The length of the molecule that is excessively modified is proportional to the position of the mutation: the more C-terminal the mutation the greater the length of molecule that becomes over-hydroxylated. This phenomenon has been effectively used by Byers and his co-workers [90] to localize the approximate location of mutations that destabilize the collagen helix. By cleaving the procollagen molecule into smaller peptide fragments with

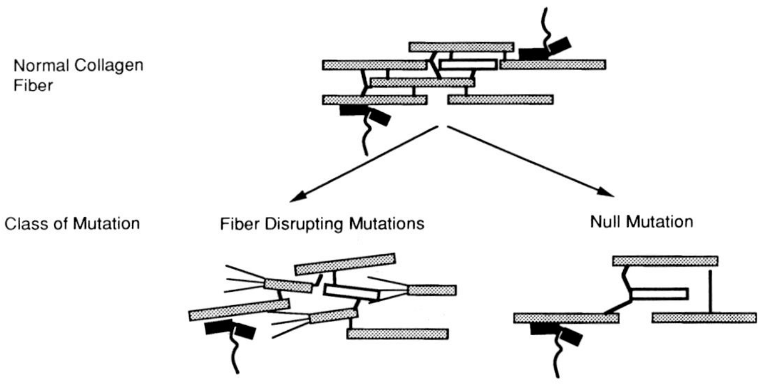


| | | |
|---|---|---|
| DELETIONS | Partial intronic gene deletion with loss of a few exons from the expressed mRNA | Complete gene deletion or loss of transcription elements |
| POINT MUTATION WITHIN AN EXON | First position gly of the Gly-X-Y triplet | Generation of a stop codon within an exon |
| POINT MUTATION WITHIN AN INTRON | Inactivation of a splice site leading to exon skipping or activation of cryptic splice site with a retained inframe intron segment | Inactivation of splice site with retension of an out of frame intron segment |

Fig. 3. Distinctly different mechanisms for abnormal connective tissue in osteogenesis imperfecta. The fiber disrupting mutation produces a disorganized connective tissue matrix. The null mutation produces less collagen with smaller fiber diameter but the matrix is otherwise normal. The broad categories of molecular disorders which can produce these types of connective tissue changes are listed below the diagram.

cyanogen bromide, fragments that are N-terminal of the mutation show a delay in their rate of migration, whereas those which are C-terminal of the mutation migrate at a normal rate. By carrying out the analysis in a two-dimensional SDS gel in which the first direction separates the $\alpha$ chains and the second direction separates CNBr peptides, a characteristic upward deflection of the peptides with delayed migration is observed. Identifying those CNBr peptides that do and do not show delayed migration can map the mutation to a specific CNBr peptide.

The effect of a helix disrupting mutation on the structural integrity of the helical domain is inferred by a change in the melting temperature ($t_m$) of the molecule. The thermal denaturation curve determines the temperature at which the collagen helix becomes susceptible to controlled proteolytic digestion [91]. Normal collagen fibers have a $t_m$ of 41°C while that of a mutant molecule may range from 34 to 37°. There is a rough correlation between the disease severity, length of helix disruption and the lowered melting temperature [92] of the collagen molecule from individual cases of OI.

## B. DNA LINKAGE

Mutation analysis of the COL1A1 and COL1A2 gene by Southern blot hybridization only rarely detects the disease-causing base change, although this approach has been very powerful in uncovering gene deletions or insertions [93]. Despite the insensitivity for finding point mutation, Southern analysis has had a prominent role in identifying mutant genes through genetic linkage studies of polymorphic DNA within a specific family pedigree. The concept of genetic linkage, although inherently very simple, is often misunderstood. In principle, one is trying to demonstrate that inheritance of a specific allele is always associated with the disease phenotype. If the molecular marker is physically close to the mutant allele, it is highly unlikely that the two loci will be separated by crossover that normally occurs during meiosis. As a result the molecular marker will always segregate with the clinical phenotype and can be used as a predictor for inheritance of the mutant allele. It is important to remember that the marker itself is not the mutation that causes the disease phenotype but always appears with the mutant allele because of their physical proximity. In most cases the molecular marker is an endonuclease restriction site DNA polymorphism which is found in a significant percentage of the normal population and can be demonstrated to be transmitted within any given family in a Mendelian dominant pattern.

Because there is crossover between homologous chromosomes during meiosis, there is the possibility that any polymorphic marker which originally was on the same chromosome as the allele causing the phenotypic disorder, is no longer associated with the abnormal phenotype. The likelihood that the crossing-over event could occur between the marker and the disease is proportional to the distance between the two of them. The log score is the geneticist measure of the likelihood that there is linkage between a polymorphic marker and the observed phenotype. By examining a large pedigree, the log score provides a statistical measure for the likelihood that there is close association between the marker and the trait.

There are two general uses of linkage for predicting whether an individual is carrying the gene for the suspected phenotype. In the first case the linkage polymorphism is so close to the candidate gene that crossing over is very unlikely to dissociate the polymorphic marker from the mutation-bearing locus. This application is used when a candidate gene is already known, and one is trying to associate a given phenotype to that candidate locus. In practice, linkage of a polymorphic marker located within a candidate can be used to score directly for the mutant allele. For example, prediction of affected or unaffected offspring within a family known to have type IV OI can be based DNA polymorphisms close to or within the COL1A1 and COL1A2 genes [94 – 96]. Milder forms of OI have been shown to be the results of mutations within either the COL1A1 and COL1A2 genes in the majority of cases; however, in a minority, linkage to these genes was excluded, indicating that mutations of matrix genes other than type I collagen can have the same clinical mild phenotype [97]. This is an example of genetic heterogeneity.

From a research perspective, genetic linkage is invaluable. Before a detailed study to define the precise mutation within a complex collagen gene is initiated, it is important to know that the mutation is present within that gene. Thus, linkage studies need to be first carried out to show or exclude linkage to a specific candidate gene. For example, analysis of the type II collagen gene in certain forms of Ehlers-Danlos syndrome can be avoided, since there are linkage studies showing that the type II gene has been excluded as a candidate gene for these disorders [98].

The second and now more common application is linkage of an inherited phenotype to a polymorphic site within a DNA fragment that is known to exist as a single copy on one specific chromosome [99]. In this case, no candidate gene for the phenotype is known. DNA blots from the entire pedigree are repetitively hybridized with a battery of anonymous probes derived from fragments scattered throughout the entire human genome to find those fragments which have a high log score (low frequency) of crossover with the observed phenotype. This type of linkage has been used to localize diseases such as Huntington's chorea [100] and cystic fibrosis [101] to specific domains of a chromosome; however they do not identify the primary gene. The closer the polymorphic site is to the candidate gene the less likely the crossover (higher log score) and the more useful the polymorphic site for diagnostic purposes.

As with linkage to a polymorphic site within a candidate gene, linkage through an anonymous probe can be used for prenatal diagnosis and for investigation of genetic heterogeneity of a specific trait. However, the most exciting value of these probes is a chromosomal entry point to begin a 'walk or jump' strategy toward the candidate gene [102, 103]. In most cases the distance of the linked polymorphic site to a candidate gene is 1 – 5 centimorgans (approximately 1 – 5 million bases), a distance that precludes reaching that site by standard DNA sequencing methods. New strategies for cloning large segments of DNA in yeast or jumping along a chromosome from a given entry point should eventually yield the candidate gene causing the mutant phenotype [104, 105]. This strategy will be important to define those families with forms of heritable bone disease including OI which fail to link to the type I collagen gene as well as other common connective tissue disorders such as Ehlers-Danlos syndrome, Marfan's syndrome and achondroplasia.

### C. Mutation localization and identification

Once there is evidence (biochemical or genetic) that a mutation is present within a collagen gene, then studies designed to define the precise base change underlying the mutation can be initiated. Because it is still not practical to DNA sequence the entire collagen gene from both alleles, it is necessary to localize the mutation to a small region of the gene. A number of strategies have now evolved for mutation localization that are based on the fact that it is easier to find and localize a mutation within a large gene by analysis of the protein or RNA than the gene directly. (1) Mapping an amino acid change to a specific CNBr fragment was described above. (2) Analysis of the collagen mRNA directly by hybridization techniques that are capable of detecting an insertion or deletion that would result from errors of splicing or point mutation within the coding sequences. These localization strategies have been based on protection of the test RNA by a radiolabelled cDNA [106] or cRNA probe from enzymatic [107] or chemical cleavage [108]. Other methods protect the test RNA with a nonradiolabelled cDNA [109, 110]. (3) Analysis of cDNA transcribed from the test RNA by standard reverse transcription followed by amplification of the transcript with the polymerase chain reaction (PCR, see below) [111]. DNA fragments produced in this fashion can be analyzed by hybridization techniques mentioned above or by subtle differences in denaturation temperature between the normal and mutant allele [112]. It can also be used for DNA sequencing.

After the mutation has been localized to a segment of protein or mRNA, a fragment of DNA is produced by PCR amplification of a specific region of genomic DNA [113]. No longer is it necessary to create a DNA library from a specific patient for screening

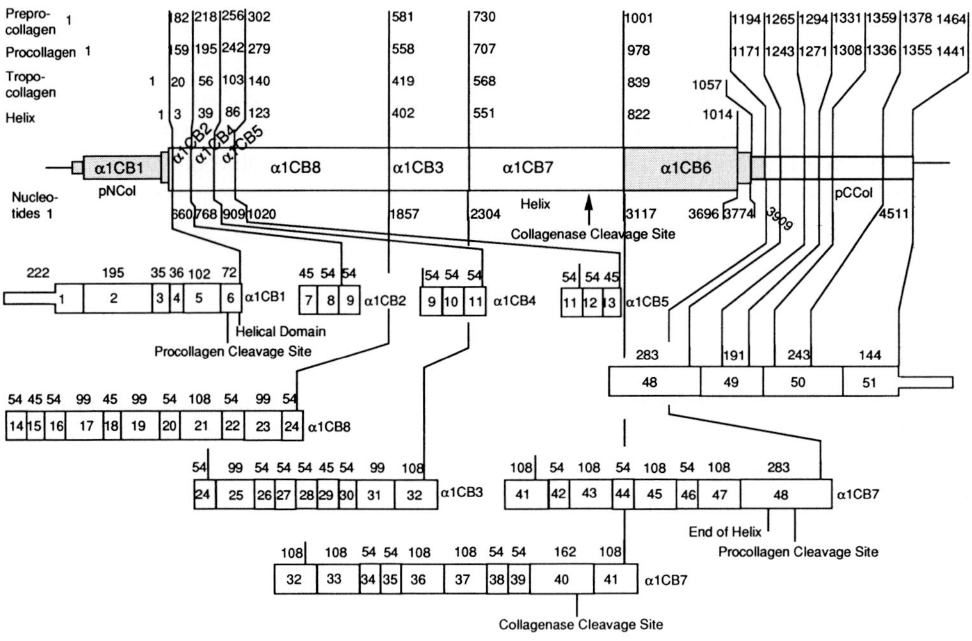


Fig. 4. Map of the α1(I) protein and mRNA. The central figure depicts the collagen protein. Above the figure are given the codon number based on starting the numbering from the prepropeptide, procollagen, telopeptide or the helix. Beneath the figure is the nucleotide number of the mRNA starting from the transcription start site. The numbers are the first position of the CNBr peptides. The α1CB1 peptide includes the signal peptide, pN collagen propeptide, telopeptide and the first two amino acids of the helical domain. The α1CB6 peptide contains the C-terminal portion of the helix, the telopeptide and a small portion of the pC collagen propeptide. The exons which code for each CB peptide are aligned beneath the collagen diagram. The map allows the alignment of protein and mRNA localization data so that a focused PCR strategy can be directed at finding the mutation within the mRNA or gene.

and identification of plaques containing the gene fragments. This rather laborious technique has been rapidly replaced by the PCR in which a small segment of DNA can be amplified in vitro without the need of constructing a genomic library. Using synthetic oligonucleotides (19 – 25 bases) that flank the region of interest as hybridization primers, a series of repetitive denaturing and polymerization steps will exponentially amplify the included DNA sequence. The product can be visualized in gels and the DNA can be sequenced directly or cloned to identify both alleles. This approach has been applied both to genomic DNA and to cDNA and it now provides a rapid method of correlating specific mutations of the collagen gene to the spectrum of disease severity in OI. Figures 4 and 5 show the relationship of the collagen CB peptides with their corresponding exons. Coordination of protein and mRNA data is essential for a directed DNA sequencing strategy designed to identify a mutation within the COL1A1 and COL1A2 genes.

### D. Transgenic animals

One of the major uncertainties in mutation identification of any heritable trait including mutations of collagen is definitive proof that the disease-causing base change has been identified. The ability to introduce mutations into mice and observe a phenotype that is similar to the disease that occurred in humans is the geneticist's equivalent of Koch's postulates. Fortunately for many of the mutations of the collagen gene, the phenotype is strongly dominant so that the effect of the mutant gene can

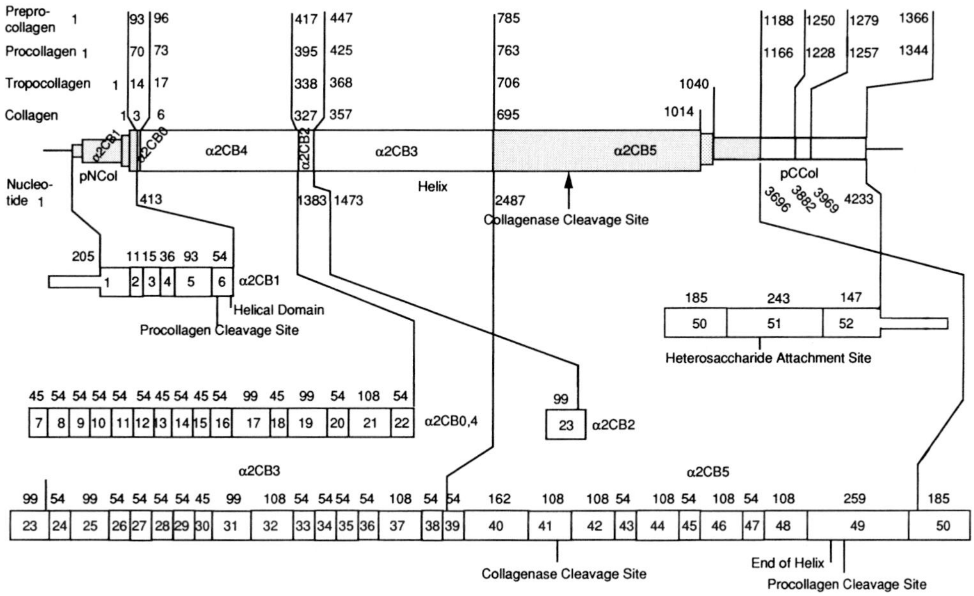


Fig. 5. Map of the α2(I) protein and mRNA. See Fig. 4 for the description of the map.

override the background of two normal alleles. Thus mutations associated with the lethal OI phenotype in humans also causes a lethal bone disease in mice, even when the RNA produced from the transgene represents only 10% of the total collagen RNA [2].

Unfortunately, this approach is not valuable when analyzing null mutations of a structural gene or mutations of an enzymatic activity because the function of endogenous gene is not disrupted. Two recent developments in transgenic animal technology should overcome this problem. (1) Transgenic animals can be produced from embryonic stem (ES) cell. These cells can be maintained *in vitro* in an undifferentiated state. When introduced back into a blastula of another mouse strain, a chimeric offspring is produced. If the mouse is chimeric in the germline, then a transgenic mouse strain can be developed. The ES cells can be transfected *in vitro* and selected for the presence of the transgene so that the resulting transgenic mouse will carry the desired transgene [114]. (2) It has now become feasible to target a specific sequence within the entire mammalian genome by homologous recombination which can occur during mitosis in tissue culture [115]. The insertion vector is constructed to contain sequences that flank the region to be mutagenized. In many cases the mutation is designed to disrupt the normal coding sequence such that if homologous recombination occurs, the endogenous gene will become null. Since the desired recombination is a relatively rare event and many undesired recombinations also occur, the success of this approach depends on a selection strategy that only identifies those cells in which the endogenous gene is targeted. When these two techniques are combined it will be possible to produce a chimeric animal bearing an inactivate endogenous gene. By developing a transgenic strain of mice from the chimera, it will be possible to assess the effect of the null allele when present in the heterozygous and homozygous state [116].

## IV. The clinical spectrum of heritable bone disease

OI, the most obvious form of heritable bone disease, was originally classified as congenital or tarda based primarily on clinical severity. This classification has given way to a more detailed nosology based on a more detailed clinical description and inheritance pattern. The classifications that was originally proposed by Silence [117] had four categories (OI type I, II, III, and IV) has been further subclassified by Silence and others, based primarily on clinical considerations [118]. It is likely that these organizational schemes will be modified further as the molecular basis for the clinical features are more fully appreciated. In the following discussion the various forms of heritable bone disease will be listed in order of their decreasing severity rather than following the arbitrary numerical system proposed originally by Silence.

### A. Neonatal lethal OI (Silence type II)

This is the most severe form of the disease in which multiple fractures are sustained during gestation causing the characteristic short and deformed limbs and beaded appearance of the extremities and ribs. Within this form of the disease a spectrum exists from infants whose bone disease is so severe that cerebral trauma or dismemberment occurs during delivery to other infants who survived for a few months after birth. This heterogeneity has now been subgrouped into five types based primarily on their X-ray appearance [119]. The most severe shows marked shortening of the limbs, impaired craniofacial ossification and prominent beading of ribs. The least severe form demonstrates long slender osteopenic bones with multiple fractures and metaphyseal flaring. It appears that those infants with the least severe bone disease have the longest post-natal life, but in all cases these infants eventually succumb to respiratory insufficiency secondary to muscle weakness.

It was from studying fibroblast cell lines derived from such infants that an appreciation of the integrity of the triple helical domain of the type I collagen molecule became apparent. In the majority of cases that have been studied, a common underlying theme is a mutation within the $\alpha1(I)$ or occasionally the $\alpha2(I)$ collagen gene that disrupts the stability of the triple helical molecule [120]. The consequences of this mutation is a collagen molecule that is kinked and forms poorly aligned fibrils, is defective in the quantity and type of crosslinked collagen fibers, is poorly secreted into the extracellular matrix and is susceptible to tissue proteases. Presumably a balance between these four factors, and probably others, ultimately determines the severity of the disease. Mutations that destabilize the C-terminal region of helix appear to have the most severe clinical consequence because the large stretch of collagen helix N-terminal to the mutation is disrupted. There is a rough correlation between the position of the mutation, the degree of helical instability as judged by thermal denaturation and the clinical severity. Another important determinant is the quantity of abnormal product that eventually accumulates in the extracellular matrix. Studies of transgenic mice carrying a mutant $\alpha1(I)$ allele show that as little as 10% of the total $\alpha1(I)$ RNA from the mutant allele is necessary to induce the lethal phenotype [2].

At least five distinctly different types of mutations within the type I collagen gene have now been associated with the lethal phenotype. (1) The first mutation that was described was partial gene deletion within COL1A1 that excised three exons to generate an inframe but shortened $\alpha1(I)$ mRNA [121, 122]. The result was two populations of protein, one that was normal and one that contained a shortened $\alpha1(I)$ chain [120]. Subsequently, similar deletions within the $\alpha2(I)$ chain have also been associated with the lethal phenotype [123]. (2) A gene duplication placing extra exons within the helical domain of the pro$\alpha2(I)$ chain has been observed [124]. (3) Probably most common are point mutations of first position glycines within the gly-X-Y codon. Initially cysteine substitutions for glycines (G $\rightarrow$ T transversion of the GGX codon) were uncovered primarily because of the ease of detecting intrahelical cysteines by

SDS acrylamide gels [125, 126]. Subsequently, arginine mutations have been uncovered because of the charged differences in a CNBr peptide when arginine [127, 128] or aspartate [129] is substituted for glycine. (4) An error in RNA splicing due to a mutation in a splice acceptor site which results in a skipped exon within the midhelical domain of the $\alpha 2(I)$ mRNA has now been demonstrated in one case of lethal OI [61]. It is likely that exon skipping is a common feature of many forms of OI and the range of mutations found to date reflect more the means of patient ascertainment rather than the frequency of the mutation. (5) Another consequence of an abnormality of RNA splicing is the result of a point mutation within an intron which activated a cryptic donor site that extended the upstream exon by another 75 bases [64]. Because these bases did not contain a stop codon, the resulting exon coded for a protein with 25 random and nonhelical amino acids.

In the majority of cases lethal OI appears to represent a sporadic new mutation rather than a recessive trait as was previously thought. However, there is one example of an apparently normal parent who expresses the same mutation (gly → cys) in her cultured fibroblasts as did the affected infants [130]. This is an extremely difficult case to rectify with our current understanding of the pathogenesis of OI. Other cases of recurrence of OI within a pedigree can be explained as germ cell mosaicism of either parent [131]. Presumably a spontaneous somatic mutation arose within the germ cell line so that a proportion of the sperm or ova could transmit the mutation.

Because of these exceptions, families with one child with lethal OI need to be counselled that there is a finite risk of recurrence. Currently, prenatal diagnosis has relied on detection of deformed limbs by ultrasound between the 16th and 20th week of gestation [132]. However, with the advent of the PCR it will be possible to detect at a much earlier stage whether or not a fetus is carrying the same mutation as the first affected sibling [133].

### B. Progressively deforming or severe nonlethal OI (Silence type III)

This form of the disease fills the spectrum of severity from infants with some of the characteristics of the lethal disease to those with moderate deformity and some degree of ambulation. Usually these infants are severely affected at birth with multiple fractures and deformity and it may not be obvious that they will survive the perinatal period. Their early growth and development is markedly delayed with severe hypotonia that prevents good head control and other neuromuscular milestones. They have a characteristic facial appearance of a triangular facies with frontal bossing, extensive moulding of the frontal and occipital bones, micrognathia, and a sunset appearance of the eyes. The sclerae have either a blue or gray color and the teeth may show evidence of dentinogenesis imperfecta (DI). The growth retardation is aggravated by the severe bowing, fractures and scoliosis as the children attempt to stand and ambulate. The X-ray appearance of the long bones are characterized by thin shafts that are severely bowed with metaphyseal flaring while in older children cystic changes in the metaphysis may develop. Wormian bones of the skull and scoliosis are other common radiological features.

It is often difficult to predict from the deformities at birth whether or not a child will have all the features of this form of OI. Children with severe fractures and bowing at birth who receive optimal orthopedic care may well straighten the bones and eventually ambulate [134]. Aggressive rodding of the extremities [135] or fixation of the spine [136] during mid to late childhood in the patient may preserve skeletal function, although in some infants whose bone mass is so severely reduced such a procedure may not be helpful. These children may have 50 – 100 fractures during their childhood years but the fracture frequency tends to diminish as they approach early adulthood. However, the progressive nature of the disease can lead to cardiovascular complications secondary to the scoliosis. Subtle compression of the medullary centers due to eventration of the base of the skull and foramen magnum can lead to a communicating hydroencephalus, cortical atrophy, motor and sensory loss of the extremities, and sudden death [137]. These individuals are also particularly prone to cerebral trauma from auto accidents, falls from a wheelchair, or assaults.

The underlying molecular defect in this disease has been surprisingly resistant to characterization. The structural mutations within the helical domain have been suggested from biochemical studies but were difficult to prove. Although mutations of type I collagen are still likely to frequently underlie this form of OI, it is likely that mutation of other extracellular matrix molecules may be found. A case resulting from a glycine substitution within an $\alpha2(I)$ chain has been demonstrated [138]. The best characterized and most unusual case of type III OI resulted from a frameshift mutation within the C-terminal propeptide of the $\alpha2(I)$ chain [78]. Since the mutation blocked incorporation of the $\alpha2(I)$ chain into the molecule [139], the homozygous infant failed to produce any $\alpha2(I)$ chains. The result was the formation of $\alpha1(I)$ trimer molecules which do not have the structural properties of heterotrimer molecules [140]. This case has been very instructive to understand the role of the C-terminal propeptide in chain assembly and importance of $\alpha2(I)$ chain to helical stability.

Although it is likely that many of the mutations in this group of disorders are new sporadic events, multiple affected siblings definitely occur in this group and thus a conservative 25% recurrence risk should be counselled. Prenatal diagnosis based on radiological criteria is effective [141]. With the improved methods for defining mutations of the collagen and other matrix genes, it will be possible to distinguish between sporadic and recessive inheritance of the mutation. It is in this group of families that definitive genetic counseling based on precise molecular testing is required.

### C. Dominantly inherited OI (Silence type I and type IV)

The separation of two types of dominantly inherited OI into type I or type IV has been based on scleral color, degree of deformity, and the presence or absence of DI. In any individual family there are often features which defy classification into one or the other group when the discriminator is eye color or degree of deformity. Characteristically, those individuals classed as type IV have white sclera, moderate short stature, moderate limb deformity, and may have DI. Those individuals categorized as type I have blue sclera, minimal deformity and short stature and may or may not have DI. These children may be born with no deformities or fractures and only start to show fractures during infancy at times of changing clothes or with minor falls when the child first ambulates. It is the parent of this infant who is frequently a suspect for child abuse and in whom ruling out OI can be difficult if blue sclerae and deformity are not present [142]. Children that present at birth with fractures and deformity generally straighten their limbs with bracing. Multiple fractures with moderate deformity can be seen upon ambulation and rodding is generally helpful in preventing progression of deformity while maintaining ambulation during these years. Once puberty is reached further fractures tend to diminish. However, as these individuals approach the post-menopausal period, fractures occur along with the development of premature osteoporosis [143]. Radiographs of the bones in mild cases may appear normal but bone densitometry studies at all ages clearly show significant osteopenia [144].

The application of genetic linkage studies have been particularly useful in this form of the OI. Prior to defining the precise localization of a mutation, it can give information as to which collagen gene harbors the underlying mutation and if the disease carrying allele has been inherited in fetal tissue. A collaborative study of dominantly inherited OI has shown that more than 90% of cases have linkage to either the COL1A1 or COL1A2 gene [145]. There is no particular phenotypic trait between those individuals who have a mutation in either gene. Of particular interest are to 5 – 10% of families where linkage to type I collagen cannot be demonstrated [97]. This finding underlines the importance of the other constituents of connective tissue to normal bone.

Two fundamentally different molecular abnormalities account for these two types of OI. The first is a mutation that affects the structure of the helical domain. The types of mutation are similar to those found in lethal OI except that the location of the mutations are more N-terminal and more frequently located within the $\alpha2(I)$ chain. Besides the first positioned glycine substitutions [146], gene deletions and exon skips [147], mutations of a non-first position glycine residues of the $\alpha1(I)$ chain have been found [148, 149]. Presumably the disease in this case was mild because the mutation had a minimal disruptive effect on the helix [150]. Other mechanisms which might weaken collagen fibers include an alteration of the charge distribution along the helix which affects fibril formation, substitutions of lysine or histidine residues involved in interchain crosslinks and substitutions of in third position (hydroxy)prolines that contribute to the overall thermal stability of the triple helix. The unifying concept in all of these dominantly inherited forms is that there is production of an abnormal collagen chain which in some way alters the stability of collagen fibrils with the remainder of the extracellular matrix. Analysis of a large number of patients with this form of OI will be required to fully appreciate the susceptibility of the collagen helical domain to mutation.

The second major category of mutations underlying dominantly inherited OI are null mutations of the $\alpha1(I)$ chain. This has been more frequently associated with type I OI, although patients with mild to moderate bone deformity (type IV) have this type of mutation. If the allele is completely inactive, the collagen that is produced is normal but is reduced by 50% of normal total collagen synthesis. Since there is an absolute requirement for two $\alpha1(I)$ chains to be present in a type I collagen molecule, the rate of $\alpha1(I)$ chain synthesis determines total type I collagen production. Half of the $\alpha2(I)$ chains remain unincorporated into the collagen molecule [68]. Unlike the situation when an $\alpha2(I)$ allele is null and the resulting $\alpha1(I)$ trimer accumulates in the matrix, an abnormal collagen $\alpha2(I)$ trimer molecule is not produced because it is unstable at physiological temperatures [151].

Defined molecular causes for a null $\alpha1(I)$ collagen allele include a frameshift mutation in the C-terminal propeptide in humans [152] and a retroviral insertion into the first intron in the MOV-13 mouse [41]. Abnormalities of splicing that leave an out of frame intron within the transcript are likely to be a common cause for a null allele. Consistent with this hypothesis is the finding of $\alpha1(I)$ to $\alpha2(I)$ mRNA ratio of 1:1 rather than the expected 2:1 ratio [69]. Unlike the ratio found in total cellular RNA or RNA extracted from the cytoplasmic compartment, the $\alpha1(I)$ to $\alpha2(I)$ ratio in the nuclear compartment is 3 – 4:1. This difference in ratios suggests an accumulation of the unprocessed RNA within the nucleus [70]. RNase protection clearly demonstrates the presence of a species of $\alpha1(I)$ mRNA which is not completely protected by $\alpha1(I)$ cDNA suggesting the presence of an unspliced intron [109]. This abnormal mRNA species is only found in the nuclear compartment further supporting the concept that the unspliced RNA does not enter the cytoplasm and thus does not lead to synthesis of an abnormal collagen chain [67]. Because an error of splicing often results in a number of alternatively spliced products, a high degree of complexity can be anticipated depending on the quantity of product which is out of frame and null, and the quantity which is in frame but codes for a helix-disrupting deletion or insertion.

## D. Overlap syndromes

Clinicians have noticed that a few individuals with bone fragility have features of Marfan's syndrome (MS) or of Ehlers-Danlos syndrome (EDS) [153]. The best characterized patient is one with severe joint laxity characteristic of EDS type VII who had affected family members with bone fractures. Molecular studies revealed a deletion of exon 11 within the $\alpha2(I)$ mRNA which is C-terminal to the N-terminal procollagen peptidase cleavage site [154]. The probable explanation for the overlapping clinical features is that mild bone disease resulted from helical disruption near the N-terminal location of the molecule. The features of EDS resulted from impaired cleavage of the procollagen peptidase site secondary to misalignment of that region of the molecule. No explanation for overlap with the MS is apparent, particularly because linkage studies have not shown that MS results from mutations within the type I collagen gene.

### E. Heritable osteoporosis

Although osteoporosis is usually viewed as a consequence of nongenetic factors such as hormonal status and lifestyle of the individual, there is increasing evidence that environmental factors can interact with genetic factors to predispose or protect an individual to osteoporosis. Genetic factors such as sex and race have long been recognized as important contributors to the onset of bone disease. Studies have shown that bone mass of children can be correlated with the mid-parental bone mass, again demonstrating the polygenic control of bone mass [155]. To date, there are no adequately designed studies to answer the question of the importance of heritable factors that predispose to the onset of bone disease. Sufficiently large pedigrees demonstrating vertical inheritance of osteoporosis are yet to be assembled. The difficulty in identifying pedigrees relates to the insidious nature of the disease, the confounding effect of environmental factors and a method to quantitate asymptomatic loss of bone mass. With the application of accurate densitometric methods of bone mass measurement and appropriate population bone mass standards for adults and children, it may be possible to develop pedigrees that could be used for genetic linkage to the type I collagen, other extracellular matrix genes and anonymous DNA probes.

The importance of identifying an 'osteoporosis gene' in early childhood is the potential for adopting a lifestyle that maximizes bone accretion during the adolescent and early adulthood years when bone mass is optimal. Such a strategy would have the possibility for prolonging bone mass during the period of gradual decline prior to menopause and would forewarn individuals at risk to maintain sex hormones after the menopause to minimize subsequent bone loss.

## V. Future directions

Advances in OI research has presaged development in all aspects of heritable disorders of connective tissue. The rapid advance in diagnostic methods now open the possibility for greatly improved genetic counseling and therapies tailored for the specific mutation. Having familiarity with these exciting developments is especially important for the clinicians who must deal with an OI family and share with them the disappointment of recurring fractures. The physician is obliged to stay current with the advances to provide hope that new developments may have a positive impact on their disease.

### A. Improved methods for diagnosis of OI

It is likely that OI will be reclassified based on the nature of the underlying molecular mutation, the type of collagen fiber that is produced or the loss of certain interactions with other components of the extracellular matrix. These new molecular methods will permit a method for rapid diagnosis and give us a conceptual framework to understand the disease. It is entirely feasible that all patients with the disease will be characterized at the molecular level such that any questions of subsequent prenatal diagnosis can be answered definitively with molecular tools. This will have immediate benefit to families with a prior affected individual, and will not be useful for the sporadic case. The greatest impact of identifying mutations causing heritable bone disease may be in the field of osteoporosis. Of particular diagnostic challenge will be defining sporadic cases of OI or osteoporosis that represent a genetic compound [156], i.e. patients who inherit one mutation from each parent located in a separate matrix gene or in a different region of the same gene.

### B. Medical therapy

To date, there is no proven therapeutic intervention to increase the bone mass associated with OI. The diminution of fracture frequency as one enters puberty suggests that sex hormones might play a role in decreasing fracture frequency. Fluoride therapy, which appears to be able to enhance bone mass in post-menopausal osteoporotic women, has had limited trials in OI with inconclusive results [157]. Growth hormone, another agent which can increase bone mass, has yet to be shown to be effective in OI or osteoporosis. Part of the difficulty contributing to interpreting results of various medical regimens may be the heterogeneity of the study population. If the treatment population consists of a mixture of patients with structural mutations within the helical domain and others are null mutations, mixed results might be anticipated. Augmentation of bone mass when the collagen is inherently flawed is less likely to have a positive outcome than when the only collagen produced comes from the remaining normal allele.

### C. Animal models

The ability to introduce mutant transgenes into mice allows the generation of colonies of animals all with a similar disease. This experimental model provides a means for evaluating various therapeutic intervention such as stimulation of bone collagen production when the underlying mutation is a mild structural mutation versus a null allele. One of the more exciting possibilities that can be evaluated in homogeneous mouse populations will be strategies of somatic gene therapy. An example of this possibility is the experimentally induced null allele of the MOV-13. Cultured cells from homozygous mice fail to synthesize procollagen. Upon transfection of the cells with a complete human $\alpha1(I)$ allele procollagen production was restored [46, 47]. A similar experiment was successful when a human $\alpha2(I)$ collagen transgene was transfected into $\alpha2(I)$ deficient hepatic cells [158].

More demanding will be somatic gene therapy of the intact animal. Strategies for introducing exogenous genes into somatic cells with retroviruses [159, 160] or through specific cellular receptors are now in progress. In most cases a therapy for introducing a normal allele into somatic cells will be most beneficial for an enzyme disorder with a deficient enzyme activity or for a structural protein with a null mutation [161]. In the case of most collagen disease in which the structural mutation is compromising normal alleles, it will be necessary to specifically inactivate the abnormal allele. Targeting of vectors to specific genes is still in its infancy but strategies are now being developed that may make this an eventual possibility.

## References


1 Pentinnen RP, Lichtenstein JR, Martin GR, McKusick VA. Abnormal collagen metabolism in cultured cells in osteogenesis imperfecta. Proc Natl Acad Sci USA 1975;72:586 – 589.

2 Stacey A, Bateman J, Choi T, Mascara T, Cole W, Jaenisch R. Perinatal lethal osteogenesis imperfecta in transgenic mice bearing an engineered mutant pro$\alpha$1(I) collagen gene. Nature 1988;332: 131 – 136.

3 Burgeson RE. New collagens, new concepts. Ann Rev Cell Biol 1988;4:551 – 577.

4 Bruckner P, Mendler M, Steinmann B, Huber S, Winterhalter KH. The structure of human collagen type IX and its organization in fetal and infant cartilage fibirls. J Biol Chem 1988;263:16911 – 16917.

5 McCormick D, Van Der Rest M, Goodship J, Lozano G, Ninomiya Y, Olsen BR. Structure of the glycosaminoglycan domain in the type IX collagen-proteoglycan. Proc Natl Acad Sci USA 1987;84: 4044 – 4048.

6 Mendler M, Eich-Bender SG, Vaughan L, Winterhalter KH, Bruckner P. Cartilage contains mixed fibrils of collagen types II, IX, and XI. J Cell Biol 1989;108:191 – 197.

7 Birk DE, Fitch JM, Babiarz JP, Linsenmayer TF. Collagen type I and type VA are present in the same fibril in the avian corneal stroma. J Cell Biol 1988;106:999 – 1008.

8 Van der Rest M, Mayne R. Type IX collagen proteoglycan from cartilage is covalently cross-linked to type II collagen. J Biol Chem 1988;263:1615 – 1618.

9 Vaughan L, Mendler M, Huber S, Bruckner P, Winterhalter KH, Irwin MI, Mayner R. D-periodic distribution of collagen type IX along cartilage fibrils. J Cell Biol 1988;106:991 – 997.

10 Muller-Glauser W, Humbel B, Glatt M, Strauli P, Winterhalter KH, Bruckner P. On the role of type IX collagen in the extracellular matrix of cartilage: Type IX collagen is localized to intersections of collagen fibrils. J Cell Biol 1986;102:1931 – 1939.

11 Wotton SF, Duance VC, Fryer PR. Type IX collagen: A possible function in articular cartilage. FEBS Lett 1988;234:79 – 82.

12 Cidadao AJ. Interactions between fibronectin, glycosaminoglycans and native collagen fibrils: An EM study in artificial three-dimensional extracellular matrices. Eur J Cell Biol 1989;48:303 – 312.

13 Hynes RO, Marcantonio EE, Stepp MA, Urry LA, Yee GH. Integrin heterodimer and receptor complexity in avian and mammalian cells. J Cell Biol 1989;109:409 – 420.

14 Kuhn K. The classical collagens: Types I, II and III. In: Mayne R, Burgeson, R: eds. Structure and Function of Collagen Types. New York: Academic Press, 1987;1 – 42.

15 Miyahra M, Hayashi K, Berger J, Tanzawa K, Njieha SK, Trelstaad RL, Prockop DJ. Formation of collagen fibrils by enzymic cleavage of precursors of type I collagen in vitro. J Biol Chem 1984;259: 9891 – 9898.

16 Gelman RA, Poppke DC, Piez KA. Collagen fibril formation in vitro. J Biol Chem 1979;254: 11741 – 11745.

17 Brodsky B, Eikenberry E. Supramolecular collagen assemblies. Ann NY Acad Sci 1985;460:73 – 84.

18 Kadler KE, Hojima Y, Prockop DJ. Assembly of type I collagen fibrils de novo. Between 37 and 41°C the process is limited by micro-unfolding of monomers. J Biol Chem 1988;263:10517 – 10523.

19 Vogel BE, Doelz R, Kadler KE, Hojima Y, Engel J, Prockop DJ. A substitution of cysteine for glycine 748 of the $\alpha1$ chain produces a kink at this site in the procollagen I molecule and an altered pN-proteinase cleavage site over 225 nm away. J Biol Chem 1988;263:19249 – 1925.

20 Traub W, Steinmann B. Structural study of a mutant type I collagen form a patient with lethal osteogenesis imperfecta containing an intramolecular disulfide fone in the triple helical domain. FEBS Lett 1986;198:213 – 216.

21 Baker AT, Ramshaw JAM, Chan D, Cole WG, Bateman JF. Changes in collagen stability and folding in lethal perinatal osteogenesis imperfecta. The effect of $\alpha1$(I)-chain glycine-to-arginine substitutions. Biochem J 1989;261:253 – 257.

22 Petrovic OM, Miller J. An unusual pattern of peptide-bound lysine metabolism in collagen from an infant with perinatal osteogenesis imperfecta. J Clin Invest 1984;73:1569 – 1575.

23 Bonadio J, Holbrook KA, Gelinas RE, Jacob J, Byers PH. Altered triple helical structure of type I procollagen in lethal perinatal osteogenesis imperfecta. J Biol Chem 1985;260:1734 – 1742.

24 Constantinou CD, Vogel BE, Jeffrey JJ Prockop DJ. The A and B fragments of normal type I procollagen have a similar thermal stability to proteinase digestion but are selectively destabilized by structural mutations. Eur J Biochem 1987;163:247 – 251.

25 Barsh GS, Byers PH. Reduced secretion of structurally abnormal type I procollagen in a form of osteogenesis imperfecta. Proc Natl Acad Sci USA 1981;78:5142 – 5147.

26 Nogami H, Oohira A. Defective association between collagen fibrils and proteoglycans in fragile bone of osteogenesis imperfecta Clin Orthop Rel Res 1988;232:284 – 291.

27 Prockop DJ. Osteogenesis imperfecta: phenotypic heterogeneity, protein suicide, short and long collagen. Am J Hum Gen 1984;36:499 – 505.

28 Byers PH, Bonadio JF. The molecular basis of clinical heterogeneity in osteogenesis imperfecta: mutations in type I collagen genes have different effects on collagen processing. In: Lloyd JK, Scriver CR, eds. Genetic and Metabolic Diseases in Pediatrics. London: Butterworth International Medical Reviews, 1985;56 – 90.

29 Yamada Y, Kuhn K, de Crombrugghe B. A conserved nucleotide sequence, coding for a segment of the C-propeptide is found at the same location in different collagen genes. Nucl Acid Res 1983;11: 2733 – 2744.

30 Junien C, Weil D, Myers JC, Van Cong N, Chu ML, Foubert TC, Gross MS, Prockop DJ, Kaplan JC, Ramirez F. Assignment of the human pro$\alpha2$(I) collagen structural gene (COLIA2) to chromosome 7 by molecular hybridization. Am J Hum Gen 1982;34:381 – 387.

31 Retief E, Parker MI, Retief AE. Regional chromosome mapping of human collagen genes $\alpha2$(I) and $\alpha1$(I) (COLIA2 and COLIA1). Hum Genet 1985;69:304 – 308.

32 D'Alessio M, Bernard M, Pretorious PJ, De Wet W, Ramirez F. Complete nucleotide sequence of the region encompassing the first twenty-five exons of the human pro$\alpha1$(I) collagen gene (COL1A1). Gene 1988;67:105 – 115.

33 De Wet W, Bernard M, Benson-Chanda V, Chu M-L, Dickson L, Weil D, Ramirez F. Organization of the human pro$\alpha2$(I) collagen gene. J Biol Chem 1987;262:16032 – 16036.

34 Hatamochi A, Paterson B, de Crombrugghe B. Differential binding of CCAAT DNA binding factor to the promoters of the mouse $\alpha2$(I) and $\alpha1$(III) collagen genes J Biol Chem 1986;261:11310 – 11314.

35 Rossi P, Karsenty G, Roberts AB, Roche NS, Sporn MD, de Crombrugghe, B. A nuclear factor 1 binding site mediates the transcriptional activation of a type I collagen promoter by transforming growth factor-$\beta$. Cell 1988;52:405 – 414.

36 Rossi P, de Crombrugghe B. Identification of a cell-specific transcriptional enhancer in the first intron of the mouse $\alpha2$(I) collagen gene. Proc Natl Acad Sci 1987;84:5590 – 5594.

37 Rossouw CMS, Vergeer WP, du Plooy SJ, Bernard MP, Ramirez F, de Wet WJ. DNA sequences in the first intron of the human pro$\alpha1$(I) collagen gene enhance transcription. J Biol Chem 1987;262:15151 – 15157.

38 Bornstein P, McKay J, Liska DJ, Apone S, Devarayalu S. Interactions between the promoter and

first intron are involved in transcriptional control of $\alpha$1(I) collagen gene expression. Mol Cell Biol 1988;8:4851 – 4857.

39 Marsilio E, Sobel ME, Smith BD. Absence of procollagen $\alpha$2(I) mRNA in chemically transformed rat liver epithelial cells. J Biol Chem 1984;259:1401 – 1404.

40 Parker MI, Smith AA, Gevers W. Absence of $\alpha$2(I) procollagen synthesis in a clone of SV40-transformed WI-38 human fibroblasts. J Biol Chem 1989;264:7147 – 7152.

41 Harbers K, Khehn M, Delius, H, Jaenisch R. Insertion of retrovirus into the first intron of the $\alpha$1(I) collagen gene leads to embryonic lethal mutation in mice. Proc Natl Acad Sci USA 1984;81: 1504 – 1508.

42 Karsenty G, Golumbek P, De Crombrugghe B. Point mutations and small substitution mutations in three different upstream elements inhibit the activity of the mouse $\alpha$2(I) collagen promoter. J Biol Chem 1988;263:13909 – 13915.

43 Lichtler A, Stover ML, Angilly J, Kream B, Rowe DW. Isolation and characterization of the rat $\alpha$1(I) collagen promoter. Regulation by 1,25-dihydroxyvitamin D. J Biol Chem 1989;264:3072 – 3077.

44 Pavlin D, Lichtler A, Angilly J, Kream BE, Rowe DW. Domains within the rat $\alpha$1(I) collagen promoter that mediate its basal expression and regulation by 1,25-dihydroxyvitamin D3 in bone (Abstract) ICCRH/ASBMR Joint Meeting, Quebec, Canada, September 9 – 14, 1989.

45 Hartung S, Jaenisch R, Briendl LM. Retrovirus insertion inactivates mouse $\alpha$1(I) collagen gene by blocking initiation of transcription. Nature 1986;320:365 – 367.

46 Schnieke A, Dziadek M, Bateman J, Mascara T, Harbers K, Gelianas R, Jaenisch R. Introduction of the human pro$\alpha$1(I) collagen gene into pro$\alpha$1(I)-deficient Mov-13 mouse cells leads to formation of functional mouse-human hybrid type I collagen. Proc Natl Acad Sci USA 1987;84:764 – 768.

47 Stacey A, Mulligan R, Jaenisch R. Rescue of Type I collagen-deficient phenotype by retroviral vector-mediated transfer of human pro$\alpha$1(I) collagen gene into mov-13 cells. J Virol 1987;61:2549 – 2554.

48 Kratochwil K, Von der Mark K, Kollar EJ, Jaenisch R, Mooslehner K, Schwarz M, Haase K, Gmachl I, Harbers K. Retrovirus-induced insertional mutation in Mov13 mice affects collagen I expression in a tissue-specific manner. Cell 1989;57:807 – 816.

49 Aebi M, Weissmann C. Precision and orderliness in splicing. TIG 1987;3:102 – 107.

50 Burke JM. Molecular genetics of group I introns: RNA structures and protein factors required for splicing — A review. Gene 1988;73:273 – 294.

51 Weber S, Aebi M. In vitro splicing of mRNA precursors: 5′ cleavage site can be predicted from the interaction between the 5′ splice region and the 5′-terminus of U1 snRNA. Nucl Acid Res 1988;16:471 – 486.

52 Hawkins JD. A survey on intron and exon lengths. Nucl Acid Res 1988;16:9893 – 9908.

53 Trumbull-Ross AD, Else AJ, Eperon IC. The dependence of splicing efficiency on the length of 3′ exon. Nucl Acid Res 1988;16:395 – 411.

54 Eperon LP, Graham IR, Griffiths AD, Eperon IC. Effects of RNA secondary structure on alternative splicing of pre-mRNA: Is folding limited to a region behind the transcribing RNA polymerase? Cell 1988;54:393 – 401.

55 Barone MV, Henchcliffe C, Baralle FE, Paolella G. Cell type specific trans-acting factors are involved in alternative splicing of human fibronectin pre-mRNA. EMBO J 1989;8:1079 – 1085.

56 Oyama F, Murata Y, Suganuma N, Kimura T, Titani K, Sekiguchi K. Patterns of alternative splicing of fibronectin pre-mRNA in human adult and fetal tissues. Biochemistry 1989;28:1428 – 1434.

57 Gulcher JR, Nies DE, Marton LS, Stefansson K. An alternatively spliced region of the human hexabrachion contains a repeat of potential N-glycosylation sites. Proc Natl Acad Sci USA 1989;86: 1588 – 1592.

58 Yeh H, Anderson N, Ornstein-Goldstein N, Bashir MM, Rosenbloom JC, Abrams W, Indik Z, Yoon K, Parks W, Mecham R, Rosenbloom J. Structure of the bovine elastin gene and SI nuclease analysis of alternative splicing of elastin mRNA in the bovine nuchal ligament. Biochemistry 1989;28: 2365 – 2370.

59 Aebi M, Hornig H, Weissmann C. Alternative splice sites when mutation of consensus 5′ cleavage site in eukaryotic pro-mRNA splicing is determined by the overall 5′ splice region, not by the conserved 5′ GU. Cell 1987;50:237 – 246.

60 Vidaud M, Gattoni R, Stevenin J, Vidaud D, Amselem S, Chibani J, Rosa J, Goossens MA. 5′ splice-region G-C mutation in exon 1 of the human B-globin gene inhibits pre-mRNA splicing: a mechanism for B + – thalassemia. Proc Natl Acad Sci USA 1989;86:1041 – 1045.

61 Weil D, D'Alessio M, Ramirez F, De Wet W, Cole WG, Chan D, Bateman JF. A base substitution in the exon of a collagen gene causes alternative splicing and generates a structurally abnormal polypeptide in a patient with Ehlers-Danlos syndrome type VII. EMBO J 1989;8:1705 – 1710.

62 Orkin SH, Kazazian HH Jr, Antonarakis SE, Goff SC, Boehm CD, Sexton JP, Waber PG, Giardina PJ. Linkage of $\beta$-thalassaemia mutations $\beta$-globin gene polymorphisms with DNA polymorphisms in human $\beta$-globin gene cluster. Nature 1982a;296:627 – 631.

63 Tromp G, Prockop DJ. Single base mutation in the pro$\alpha$2(I) collagen gene that causes efficient splicing of the RNA from exon 27 to exon 29 and synthesis of a shortened but in-frame pro$\alpha$2(I) chain. Proc Natl Acad Sci USA 1988;85:5254 – 5258.

64 Brufsky A, Shapiro J, Stover ML, Rowe DW. Lethal osteogenesis imperfecta resulting from expression of an unspliced intron within the $\alpha$1(I) mRNA (submitted).

65 Maquat LE, Kinniburgh AJ. A $\beta$-thalassemic $\beta$-globin RNA that is labile in bone marrow cells is relatively stable in HeLa cells. Nucl Acid Res 1985;13:2855 – 2867.

66 Fukumaki Y, Ghosh PK, Benz EJ, Reddy BV, Lebowitz P, Forget G, Weissman SM. Abnormally spliced messenger RNA in erythroid cells from patients with $\beta^+$ thalassemia and monkey cells expressing a cloned $\beta^+$ thalassemic gene. Cell 1982;28:585 – 593.

67 Atweh GF, Brickner HE, Zhu X-X, Kazazian HH, Jr, Forget BG. New amber mutation in a $\beta$-thalassemic gene with nonmeasurable levels of mutant messenger RNA in vivo. J Clin Invest 1988;82:557 – 561.

68 Barsh GS, David KE, Byers PH. Type I osteogenesis imperfecta: A nonfunctional allele for pro$\alpha$1(I) chains of type I procollagen. Proc Natl Acad Sci 1982;79:3838 – 3842.

69 Rowe DW, Shapiro JR, Poirier M, Schlesinger S. Diminished type I collagen synthesis and reduced $\alpha$1(I) collagen mRNA in cultured fibroblasts from patients with dominantly inherited (type I) osteogenesis imperfecta. J Clin Invest 1985;71:689 – 697.

70 Genovese C, Rowe D. Analysis of cytoplasmic and nuclear messenger RNA in fibroblasts from patients with type I osteogenesis imperfecta. Methods Enzymol 1987;145:223 – 235.

71 Rodgers JR, Johnson ML, Rosen JM. Measurement of mRNA concentration and mRNA half-life as a function of hormonal treatment. Methods Enzymol 1985;109:572 – 593.

72 Rowe LB, Schwarz RI. Role of procollagen mRNA levels in controlling the rate of procollagen synthesis. Mol Cell Biol 1983;3:241 – 249.

73 Yamada Y, Mudryj M, De Crombrugghe B. A uniquely conserved regulatory signal is found around the translation initiation site in three different collagen genes. J Biol Chem 1983;258:14914 – 14919.

74 Bornstein P, McKay J, Devarayalu S, Cook SC. A highly conserved, 5′ untranslated, inverted repeat sequence is ineffective in translational control of the $\alpha$1(I) collagen gene. Nucl Acids Res 1988;16:9721 – 9736.

75 Bennett VD, Weiss IM, Adams SL. Cartilage-specific 5′ end of chick $\alpha$2(I) collagen mRNAs. J Biol Chem 1989;264:8402 – 8409.

76 Kivirikko KK, Myllya R. Post-translational enzymes in the biosynthesis of collagen: intracellular enzymes. Methods Enzymol 1982;82A:245 – 304.

77 Bateman JF, Chan D, Mascara T, Rogers JG, Cole WG. Collagen defects in lethal perinatal osteogenesis imperfecta. Biochem J 1986;240:699 – 708.

78 Pihlajaniemi T, Dickson LA, Pope FM, Korhonen VR, Nicholls A, Prockop DJ, Myers JC. Osteogenesis imperfecta: cloning of a pro$\alpha$2(I) collagen gene with a frameshift mutation. J Biol Chem 1984;259:12941 – 12944.

79 Peltonen L, Halila R, Ryhanen L. Enzymes converting procollagens to collagens. J Cell Biochem 1985;28:15 – 21.

80 Steinmann B, Tuderman L, Peltonen L, Martin GR, McKusick VA, Prockop DJ. Evidence for a structural mutation of procollagen type I in a patient with the Ehlers-Danlos Syndrome Type VII. J Biol Chem 1980;285:8887 – 8893.

81 Eyre DR, Shapiro FD, Aldridge JF. A heterozygous collagen defect in a variant of the Ehlers-Danlos syndrome type VII. Evidence for a deleted amino-telopeptide domain in the pro-$\alpha$2(I) chain. J Biol Chem 1985;260:11211 – 11329.

82 Dombrowski KE, Prockop DJ. Cleavage of type I and type II procollagens by type I/II procollagen N-proteinase. Correlation of kinetic constants with the predicted conformations of procollagen substrates. J Biol Chem 1988;263:16545 – 16552.

83 Sippola M, Kaffe S, Prockop DJ. A heterozygous defect for structurally altered pro-$\alpha$2 chain of type I procollagen in a mild variant of osteogenesis imperfecta. The altered structure decreases the thermal stability of procollagen and makes it resistant to procollagen N-proteinase. J Biol Chem 1986;259:14094 – 14100.

84 Wu CH, Donovan CB, Wu GY. Evidence for pretranslational regulation of collagen synthesis by procollagen propeptides. J Biol Chem 1986;261:10482 – 10484.

85 Lichtenstein JR, Martin GR, Kohn L, Byers PH, McKusick VA. Defect in conversion of procollagen to collagen in a form of Ehlers-Danlos syndrome. Science 1973;182:298 – 300.

86 Cronlund AL, Smith BD, Kagan HM. Binding of lysyl oxidase to fibrils of type I collagen. Conn Tissue Res 1985;14:109 – 119.

87 Eyre DR, Oguchi H. The hydroxypyridinium crosslinks of skeletal collagens: their measurement, properties and a proposed pathway of formation. Biochem Biophys Res Commun 1980;92:403 – 410.

88 Fisher LW, Eanes ED, Denholm LJ, Heywood BR, Termine JD. Two bovine models of osteogenesis imperfecta exhibit decreased apatite crystal size. Calcif Tissue Int 1987;40:282 – 285.

89 Bonadio J, Byers PH. Subtle structural alterations in the chains of Type I procollagen produce osteogenesis inperfecta type II. Nature 1985;316:363 – 366.

90 Cohn DH, Byers PH. Osteogenesis imperfecta and other inherited disorders of the structure and synthesis of type-I collagen — models for the analysis of mutations that result in inherited chondrodysplasias. Path Immunopath Res 1988;7:132 – 138.

91 Bonadio J, Holbrook KA, Gelinas RE, Jacob J, Byers PH. Altered triple helical structure of type I procollagen in lethal perinatal osteogenesis imperfecta. J Biol Chem 1985;260:1734 – 1742.

92 Rao VH, Steinmann B, De Wet W, Hollister DW. Decreased thermal denaturation temperature of osteogenesis imperfecta mutant collagen is independent of post-translational overmodifications of lysine and hydroxylysine. J Biol Chem 1989;264:1793 – 1798.

93 Chu ML, Williams CJ, Pepe G, Hirsch JL, Prockop DJ, Ramirez F. Internal deletion in a collagen gene in perinatal lethal form of osteogenesis imperfecta. Nature 1983;304:78 – 80.

94 Tsipouras P, Myers JC, Ramirez F, Prockop D. RFLP associated with the pro$\alpha$2(I) gene of human type I procollagen. J Clin Invest 1983;72:1262 – 1267.

95 Sykes B, Ogilvie D, Wordsworth P, Anderson J, Jones N. Osteogenesis imperfecta is linked to both type I collagen structural genes. Lancet 1986;2:69 – 72.

96 Falk CT, Schwartz RD, Ramirez F, Tsipouras P. Use of molecular haplotypes specific for the human pro$\alpha$2(I) collagen gene in linkage analysis of the mild autosomal dominant forms of osteogenesis imperfecta. Am J Hum Gen 1986;38:269 – 279.

97 Aitchison K, Ogilvie D, Honeyman M, Thompson E, Sykes B. Homozygous osteogenesis imperfecta unlinked to collagen I genes. Hum Genet 1988;78:233 – 236.

98 Wordsworth P, Ogilvie D, Smith R, Sykes B. Exclusion of the $\alpha$1(II) collagen structural gene as the mutant locus in type II Ehlers-Danlos syndrome. Ann Rheum Dis 1985;44:431 – 433.

99 Donis-Keller H, et al. A genetic linkage map of the human genome. Cell 1987;51:319 – 337.

100 Zehetner G, Wasmuth JJ, Gusella J, Lehrach H, Frischauf A-M. Construction of a NotI linking

library and isolation of new markers close to the Huntington disease gene. Nucl Acids Res 1988;16: 9185 – 9188.

101 Collins FS, Drumm ML, Cole JL, Lockwood WK, Vande Woude GF, Iannuzzi MC. Construction of a general human chromosome jumping library, with application to cystic fibrosis. Science 1987;235:1046 – 1049.

102 Smith CL, Lawrance SK, Gillespie GA, Cantor CR, Weissman SM, Collins FS. Strategies for mapping and cloning macroregions of mammalian genomes. Methods Enzymol 1987;151:461 – 489.

103 McKusick VA. Mapping and sequencing the human genome. N Engl J Med 1989;320:910 – 915.

104 Coulson A, Waterston R, Kiff J, Sulston J, Kohara Y. Genome linking with yeast artificial chromosomes. Nature 1988;335:184 – 186.

105 Porteous DJ. Chromosome mediated gene transfer: a functional assay for complex loci and an aid to human genome mapping. TIG 1987;3:177 – 182.

106 Atweh GF, Baserga SJ, Brickner HE. Detecting small mutations in expressed genes by a combination of S1 nuclease and RNase A. Nucl Acids Res 1988;16:8709 – 8709.

107 Marini JC, Grange DK, Gottesman GS, Lewis MB, Koeplin DA. Osteogenesis imperfecta type IV. Detection of a point mutation in one $\alpha$1(I) collagen allele (COL1A1) by RNA, RNA hybrid analysis. J Biol Chem 1989;264:11893 – 11900.

108 Cotton RGH, Rodrigues NR, Campbell RD. Reactivity of cytosine and thymine in single-based pair mismatches with hydroxylamine and osmium tetroxide and its application to the study of mutations. Proc Natl Acad Sci 1988;85:4397 – 4401.

109 Genovese C, Brufsky A, Shapiro J, Rowe, D. Detection of mutations in human type I collagen mRNA in osteogenesis imperfecta by indirect RNase protection. J Biol Chem 1989;264:9632 – 9637.

110 de Wet W, Sippola M, Tromp G, Prockop D, Chu ML, Ramirez F. Use of R-loop mapping for the assessment of human collagen mutations. J Biol Chem 1986;261:3857 – 3862.

111 Patterson E, Smiley E, Bonadio J. RNA sequence analysis of a perinatal lethal osteogenesis imperfecta mutation. J Biol Chem 1989;264:10083 – 10087.

112 Latham T, Smith FI. Detection of single-base mutations in DNA molecules using the solution melting method. DNA 1989;8:223 – 231.

113 Mihovilovic M, Lee JE. An efficient method for sequencing PCR amplified DNA. BioTechniques 1989;7:14 – 16.

114 Doetschman T, Gregg RG, Maeda N, Hooper ML, Melton DW, Thompson S, Smithies O. Targetted correction of a mutant HPRT gene in mouse embryonic stem cells. Nature 1987;330:576 – 578.

115 Capecchi MR. Altering the genome by homologous recombination. Science 1989;244:1288 – 1292.

116 Joyner AL, Skarnes WC, Rossant J. Production of a mutation in mouse En-2 gene by homologous recombination in embryonic stem cells. Nature 1989;38:153 – 156.

117 Silence D. Osteogenesis Imperfecta: an expanding panorama of variants. Clin Orthop 1981;159: 11 – 25.

118 Silence DO, Barlow KK, Garber AP, Hall JG, Rimon DL. Osteogenesis imperfecta type II delineation of the phenotype with reference to genetic heterogeneity. Am J Med Genet 1984;17:407 – 423.

119 Byers PH, Tspiouras P, Bonadio JF, Starman BJ, Schwarz RC. Perinatal lethal osteogenesis imperfecta (OI type II): A biochemically heterogeneous disorder usually due to new mutations in the genes for type I collagen. Am J Hum Genet 1988;42:237 – 248.

120 Williams CJ, Prockop DJ. Synthesis and processing of a type I procollagen containing shortened pro $\alpha$1(I) chains by fibroblasts from a patient with osteogenesis imperfecta. J Biol Chem 1983;258: 5915 – 5921.

121 Chu ML, Williams CJ, Pepe G, Hirsch JL, Prockop DJ, Ramirez F. Internal deletion in a collagen gene in perinatal lethal form of osteogenesis imperfecta. Nature 1984;304:78 – 80.

122 Barsh GS, Roush CL, Bonadio J, Byers PH, Gelinas RE. Intron-mediated recombination may cause a deletion in an $\alpha$1(I) collagen chain in a lethal form of osteogenesis imperfecta. Proc Natl Acad Sci USA 1985;82:2870 – 2874.

123 Willing MC, Cohn DH, Starman B, Holbrook KA, Greenberg CR, Byers PH. Heterozygosity for a large deletion in the $\alpha2$(I) collagen gene has a dramatic effect on type I collagen secretion and produces perinatal lethal osteogenesis imperfecta. J Biol Chem 1988;263:8398 – 8404.

124 Byers PH, Starman BJ, Cohn DH, Horwitz AL. A novel mutation causes a perinatal lethal form of osteogenesis imperfecta: an insertion in one $\alpha1$(I) collagen allele (COL1A1). J Biol Chem 1988;263:7855 – 7861.

125 Cohn DH, Byers PH, Steinmann B, Gelinas PE. Lethal osteogenesis imperfecta resulting from a single nucleotide change in one human pro$\alpha1$(I) collagen allele. Proc Natl Acad Sci 1986;83:6045 – 6047.

126 Vogel BE, Minor RR, Freund M, Prockop DJ. A point mutation in a type-I procollagen gene converts glycine-748 to the $\alpha1$ chain to cysteine and destabilized the triple helix in a lethal variant of osteogenesis imperfecta. J Biol Chem 1987;262:4737 – 4744.

127 Bateman JF, Chan D, Walker ID, Rogers JG, Cole WG. Lethal perinatal osteogenesis imperfecta due to the substitution of arginine for glycine at residue 391 of the $\alpha1$(I) chain of type I collagen. J Biol Chem 1987;262:7021 – 7027.

128 Bateman JF, Lamande SR, Dahl H-H, Chan D, Cole WG. Substitution of arginine for glycine 664 in the collagen $\alpha1$(I) chain in lethal perinatal osteogenesis imperfecta. Demonstration of the peptide defect by in vitro expression of the mutant cDNA. J Biol Chem 1988;263:11627 – 11630.

129 Baldwin CT, Constantinou CD, Dumars KW, Prockop DJ. A single base mutation that converts glycine 907 of the $\alpha2$(I) chain of type I procollagen to aspartate in a lethal variant of osteogenesis imperfecta. The single amino acid substitution near the carboxyl terminus destabilizes the whole triple helix. J Biol Chem 1989;26:3002 – 3006.

130 Constantinou CD Nielsen KB, Prockop DJ. A lethal variant of osteogenesis imperfecta has a single base mutation that substitutes cysteine for glycine 904 of the $\alpha1$(I) chain of type I procollagen. The asymptomatic mother has an unidentified mutation producing an overmodified and unstable type I procollagen. J Clin Invest 1989;83:574 – 584.

131 Cohn DH, Starman BJ, Blumberg B, Byers PH. Detection of germinal mosaicism for a mutation in a type I collagen gene (COL1A1) indicates that a small number of cells is irrevocably allocated to the germline early in human development (submitted).

132 Milsom I, Mattison LA, Dahler-Nilsson I. Antenatal diagnosis of osteogenesis imperfecta by real time ultrasound: two case reports. Br J Radiat 1982;55:310 – 312.

133 Orkin SH. Genetic diagnosis by DNA analysis: progress through amplification. N Engl J Med 1987;317:1023 – 1025.

134 Binder H, Hawks L, Graybill G, Gerber NL, Weintrab JC. Osteogenesis imperfecta: rehabilitation approach with infants and young children. Arch Phys Med Rehab 1984;65:537 – 541.

135 Ryoppy S, Alberty A, Kaitila I. Early semiclosed intramedullary stabilization in osteogenesis imperfecta J Ped Ortho 1987;7:139 – 144.

136 Hanscom DA, Bloom BA. The spine in osteogenesis imperfecta. Orthop Clin NA 1988;19:449 – 459.

137 Tsipouras P, Barbas G, Mathews WS. Neurologic correlates of osteogenesis imperfecta. Arch Neur 1986;43:150 – 152.

138 Tenni R, Cetta G, Dyne K, Rossi A, Quacci D, Lenzi L, Castellani AA. Type I procollagen in the severe non-lethal form of osteogenesis imperfecta. Defective pro$\alpha1$(I) chains in a patient with abnormal proteoglycan metabolism and mineral deposits in the dermis. Hum Genet 1988;79:245 – 250.

139 Deak SA, Nicholls FM, Pope FM, Prockop DJ. The molecular defect in a nonlethal variant of osteogenesis imperfecta. Synthesis of proa$\alpha2$(I) chains which are not incorporated into trimers of type I procollagen. J Biol Chem 1983;258:15192 – 15197.

140 Deak SB, van der Rest M, Prockop DJ. Altered helical structure of a homotrimer of $\alpha1$(I) chains synthesized by fibroblasts from a variant of osteogenesis imperfecta. Col Rel Res 1985;5:305 – 313.

141 Robinson LP, Worthen NJ, Lachman RS, Adomian GE, Rimoin DL. Prenatal diagnosis of osteogenesis imperfecta type III. Prenat Diag 1987;7:7 – 15.

142 Taitz LD. Child abuse and osteogenesis imperfecta. Br Med J 1987;295:1082 – 1083.
143 Paterson CR, McAllion S, Stellman JL. Osteogenesis imperfecta after the menopause. N Engl J Med 1984;310:1694 – 1696.
144 Kurtz D, Moorish K, Shapiro JR. Vertebral bone mineral content in osteogenesis imperfecta. Calcif Tissue Int 1985;37:14 – 18.
145 Wallis G, Beighton P, Boyd C, Mathew CG. Mutations linked to the pro$\alpha$2(I) collagen gene are responsible for several cases of osteogenesis imperfecta type I. J Med Genet 1986;23:411 – 416.
146 Wenstrup RJ, Cohn DH, Cohen T, Byers PH. Arginine for glycine substitution in the triple-helical domain of the products of one $\alpha$2(I) collagen allele (COL1A2) produces the osteogenesis imperfecta type IV phenotype. J Biol Chem 1988;263:7734 – 7740.
147 Byers PH, Shapiro JR, Rowe DW, David KE, Holbrook KA. Abnormal $\alpha$2 chain in type I collagen from a patient with a form of osteogenesis imperfecta. J Clin Invest 1983;71:689 – 697.
148 Steinmann B, Nicholls A, Pope FM. Clinical variability of osteogenesis imperfecta reflecting molecular heterogeneity: cysteine substitutions in the $\alpha$1(I) collagen chain producing lethal and mild forms. J Biol Chem 1986;261:8958 – 8964.
149 de Vries WN, de Wet WJ. The molecular defect in an autosomal dominant form of osteogenesis imperfecta. Synthesis of type I procollagen containing cysteine in the triple-helical domain of pro$\alpha$1(I) chains. J Biol Chem 1986;261:9056 – 9064.
150 Wenstrup RJ, Hunter AGW, Byers PH. Osteogenesis imperfecta type IV: evidence of abnormal triple helical structure of type I collagen. Hum Genet 1986;74:47 – 53.
151 Tkocz C, Kuhn K. The formation of triple-helical collagen molecules from $\alpha$1 or $\alpha$2 polypeptide chains. Eur J Biochem 1969;7:454 – 462.
152 Bateman JF, Lamande SR, Dahl H-HM, Chan D, Mascara T, Cole WG. A frameshift mutation results in a truncated nonfunctional carboxyl-terminal pro$\alpha$1(I) propeptide of type I collagen in osteogenesis imperfecta. J Biol Chem 1989;264:10960 – 10964.
153 Biering A, Iverson T. Osteogenesis imperfecta associated with Ehlers-Danlos Syndrome. Acta Paed 1955;44:279 – 286.
154 Kuivaniemi H, Sabol C, Tromp G, Sippola-Thiele M, Prockop DJ. A 19-base pair deletion in the pro$\alpha$2(I) gene of type I procollagen that cause in-frame RNA splicing from exon 10 to exon 12 in a proband with atypical osteogenesis imperfecta and in his asymptomatic mother. J Biol Chem 1988;263:11407 – 11413.
155 Seeman E, Hopper JL, Bach LA, Cooper ME, Parkinson E, McKay J, Jerums G. Reduced bone mass in daughters of women with osteoporosis. N Engl J Med 1989;320:554 – 558.
156 de Wet WJ, Pihlajaniemi T, Myers JC, Kelly TE, Prockop DJ. Synthesis of a shortened pro$\alpha$2(I) chain and decreased synthesis of pro$\alpha$2(I) chains in a proband with osteogenesis imperfecta. J Biol Chem 1983;258:7721 – 7728.
157 Gertner J, Baron R, Vigery A, Lasng R. Cyclical therapy of osteogenesis imperfecta with fluoride and 25 hydroxyvitamin D. (Abstract) Calcif Tissue Int 1980;3:62.
158 Lee S-T, Smith BD, Greenspan DS. J Biol Chem 1988;263:13141.
159 Miller AD, Bender MA, Harris EAS, Kaleko M, Gelinas RE. Design of retrovirus vectors for transfer and expression of the human $\beta$-globin gene. J Virol 1988;62:4337 – 4345.
160 Miyanohara A, Sharkey MF, Witztum JL, Steinberg D, Friedmann T. Efficient expression of retroviral vector-transduced human low density lipoprotein (LDL) receptor in LDL receptor-deficient rabbit fibroblasts in vitro. Proc Natl Acad Sci 1988;85:6538 – 6542.
161 Peng H, Armentano D, MacKenzie-Graham L, Shen R-F, Darlington G, Ledley FD, Woo SLC. Retroviral-mediated gene transfer and expression of human phenylalanine hydroxylase in primary mouse hepatocytes. Proc Natl Acad Sci 1988;85:8146 – 8150.

*Bone and Mineral Research/7*
*Johan N.M. Heersche and John A. Kanis, editors*



# Osteogenic stem cells in the bone marrow

A.J. FRIEDENSTEIN

*Immunomorphological Laboratory, The Gamaleya Institute for Epidemiology and Microbiology, Academy of Medical Sciences of the USSR, Gamaleya Str 18, Moscow D-98, USSR*

## 1. Introduction

Bone has the important homeostatic function of participating in physiological processes which regulate the level of calcium in the extracellular fluid. In the adult, most of the metabolic activity of the skeleton is in the form of remodelling, in which osteoclastic bone resorption and osteoblastic bone formation are coupled. This process continues throughout the entire life-span of an individual. Bone turnover requires continuous generation of osteoclasts and osteoblasts. Osteoclasts are known to be of hemopoietic cell lineage and are recruited from hemopoietic stem cells. The earliest osteoprogenitor cells well-characterised in adult mammals are preosteoblasts. However, according to autoradiographic studies (Owen 1970), maintenance of the osteogenic cell populations is dependent on less differentiated percursors which remain unidentified due to the lack of reliable markers for osteogenic lineage cells. Osteogenic cells belong to the family of mechanocytes (fibroblasts) (Willmer 1964), their main distinctive feature being synthesis of types I, II and III collagen. Mechanocytes are components of many organs, and the types of collagen they synthesize have organ-specific differences. Unfortunately, these signs of mechanocyte diversity become unreliable when the cells are cultured *in vitro* and cannot be used as markers of genetic diversity of mechanocyte precursors. With regard to non-collagenous extracellular matrix proteins, including those characteristic of the bone matrix, it still remains unclear which of these will turn out to be useful for determining the hierarchy of precursor cells of the osteogenic lineage.

Under normal steady-state conditions the bone turnover rate is slow. It may speed up considerably, for example, during callus formation, which proves that osteogenic tissue in the adult is capable of extensive bone production. The cellular background of this capability awaits further clarification. It is not clear, for example, whether bone tissue in the adult contains a sufficient pool of precursors which are not self-maintaining and which are gradually spent throughout the life-span or whether bone also contains a population of self-renewing stem cells. The same questions apply to other mechanocyte lineages. The issue is of great interest in view of the intriguing possibility that common stem cells exist for all mechanocytes in the adult. With respect to osteoprogenitor cells, all those hypothetical possibilities are rather important because of the presence of determined osteogenic precursors (DOPC) in the skeleton and of inducible osteogenic precursors (IOPC) in extraskeletal cell populations (Friedenstein 1973, 1976).

The presence of osteoprogenitor cells in bone marrow has recently received much attention. Bone marrow is highly osteogenic when engrafted heterotopically and contains both osteogenic and hemopoietic precursors. Interestingly, hemopoietic marrow needs to be closely associated with bone tissue and is considerably less effective outside the bone than within (Ascenzi 1976). This is illustrated by the observation that ectopic ossicles formed from IOPC become populated by hemopoietic cells. This also indicates that bone tissue forms a suitable hemopoietic microenvironment (HME) (Tavassoli and Friedenstein 1983). The question why bone marrow, being the central organ of hemopoiesis and immunity, is encased in bone appears teleological. Nonetheless, it is precisely this question that stimulates interest in the proliferative and differentiative properties of marrow stromal cells, in the interactions between osteogenic and hemopoetic cell lineages and in the possible role of bone tissue in hemopoiesis.

The discussion to follow deals mainly with bone marrow clonogenic stromal cells (CFUf), which are the osteogenic precursors and possibly the osteogenic stem cells.

## II. Marrow heterotopic transplantation

It has been known for more than a hundred years that bone is formed when marrow plugs are transplanted heterotopically. This does not necessarily prove, however, that marrow includes osteoprogenitor cells, since osteogenic cells may enter from outside. Direct proof of osteogenic potential of marrow cells was provided by Petrakova et al. (1963) and Friedenstein et al. (1966), who demonstrated that single-cell marrow suspensions form mineralized bone when transplanted in diffusion chambers and in organ culture (Luria et al. 1987, 1988). When transplanted in an open-cell system, plugs and single-cell suspensions form heterotopic bone marrow organs. Their development, which mimics the sequential stages of intramembranous ossification in the embryo, begins with reticular cell proliferation, followed by differentiation of osteoblasts and formation of osteoid. Subsequent penetration of capillaries, mineralization of extracellular bone matrix and bone remodelling is accompanied by the development of medullary spaces populated by hemopoietic cells. By day 30, bone organs with a medullary cavity occupied by marrow are formed (Fig. 1) (Danis 1957; Tavassoli and Crosby 1968; Friedenstein et al. 1982). In mice, such ossicles stay present for up to 2 years, producing mature cells and committed precursors of all hemopoietic lineages as well as hemopoietic stem cells (Schofield et al. 1987).

Effective hemopoiesis has been shown to be the product of an interplay between hemopoietic stem cells and their supporting stroma, which provides a favorable HME for sustained and regulated proliferation and differentiation of stem cells (Tavassoli and Friedenstein 1983). The occurrence of hemopoiesis inside heterotopic ossicles suggests the presence of stromal cells which are capable of establishing a hemopoietic microenvironment. When marrow from $Sl/Sl^d$ mice was transplanted into normal hosts, the marrow in the ossicle showed abnormalities characteristic of the $Sl/Sl^d$ mutation, indicating that the HME operative in the donor was transferred to the heterotopic bone marrow organ (Fried et al. 1973; Eble et al. 1977). With allogeneic marrow transplantation, no ossicle formation takes place. During the first 2 weeks however, syngeneic and allogeneic grafts are similar morphologically, and bone trabeculae and intertrabecular spaces occupied by reticular tissue develop in both. After a period of 3 weeks, resorption of bone and reticular tissue takes place in allogeneic grafts. Thus, the development of heterotopic bone marrow organs requires engraftment of the transplanted marrow, which requires immunological compatibility with the host. This is not to say that engraftment of all the transplanted marrow cells is required: Only those cells which serve as progenitors for the cell lineages which retain donor origin in heterotopic bone marrow organs have to survive.

According to chromosome analysis, the hemopoietic cells (including stem cells) in long-term heterotopic bone marrow organs are of recipient, not of donor origin (Friedenstein et al. 1968). Hence, heterotopic ossicle formation can be used as a model for testing lineage relationships between the osteogenic and the hemopoietic marrow cells. When ossicles are established by grafting semi-syngeneic marrow into $F_1$

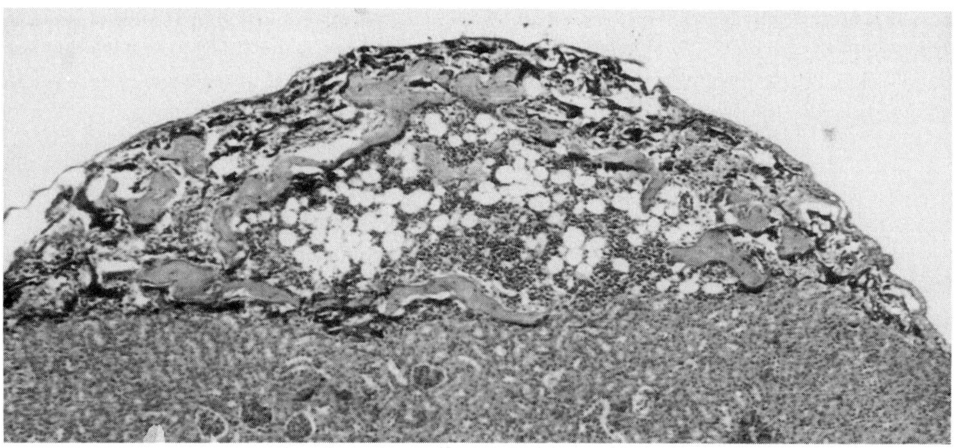

Fig. 1. Heterotopic 45-day-old transplant initiated by $6 \times 10^5$ marrow cells.

hybrids, they turn out to be populated with $F_1$ hemopoietic cells that immunologically mismatch with the initial donor line. However, when the ossicles remained in $F_1$ hybrids for more than a year, their marrow was still capable of forming ossicles when regrafted into the initial donor line (Friedenstein et al. 1968). This proves that this heterotopic marrow is a mixed structure, containing osteogenic and HME-transferring cells of donor origin and hemopoietic cells belonging to the host (Fig. 2). It has also been demonstrated that the osteogenic cells of host origin are not recruited in ossicles in addition to the osteogenic cells transplanted from the donor (Fig. 3) (Friedenstein and Kuralesowa 1971).

The above conclusions are further supported by results of heterotopic grafting of marrow from radiochimeras. The hemopoietic cells in whole-body lethally irradiated mice reconstituted with marrow, spleen or embryonic liver cells are known to be of the donor origin (Micklem and Loutit 1966). Formation of ossicles by heterotopic grafting of marrow from radiochimeras is independent of the source of cells used for restoration of radiochimeras, and only depends on how well the host matches by transplantation antigens with the irradiated chimera, not with the donor of

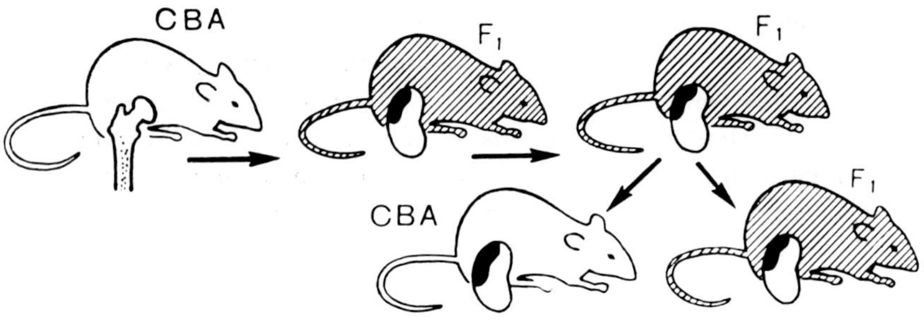


Fig. 2. Schematic semisyngeneic heterotopic bone marrow transplantation into $F_1$ host with subsequent serial retransplantation every 1.5 – 3 months. The second regrafting was accomplished by simultaneous test transplantation into the line of the initial donor.

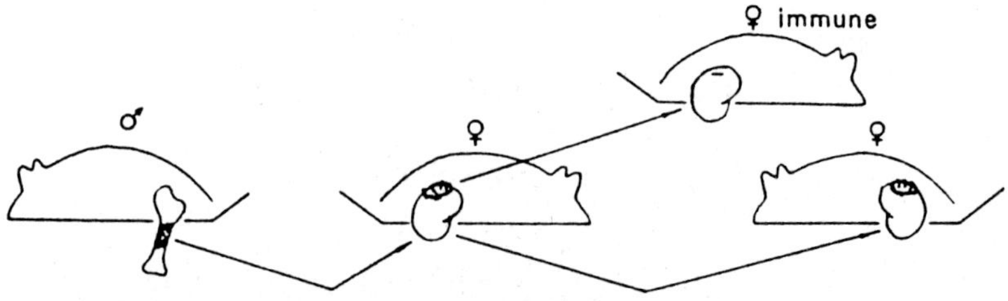


Fig. 3. Schematic of semisyngeneic heterotopic transplantation of bone marrow from male donor into non-immunized $F_1$ female, with subsequent test transplantation into non-immunized and preimmunized $F_1$ female.

hemopoietic cells used for restoration (Fig. 4) (Friedenstein and Kuralesova 1971). These results indicate that in radiochimeras the osteogenic and the HME-transferring cells are of recipient origin, while the hemopoietic cells are of donor origin. Thus, there is no evidence for a common stem cell that gives rise to marrow DOPC and to hemopoietic cells.

## III. An in vitro colony assay for clonogenic precursors of marrow stromal fibroblasts

Cells of hemopoietic and lymphoid tissues are easily disaggregated by light mechanical treatment into single-cell suspensions and can be used for *in vitro* cloning of stromal fibroblasts (Friedenstein et al. 1970, Wilson et al. 1974). The colony-forming fibroblasts (CFUf) *in vitro* are proliferative adherent cells that occur at low frequencies in hemopoietic and lymphoid cell populations. When cell suspensions obtained from marrow, spleen, thymus and lymph nodes of adult mice, rats, guinea pigs, rabbits, dogs, hamsters and humans are cultured, the CFUf form discrete fibroblast colonies (Friedenstein et al. 1970, 1974b, 1976, 1978; Friedenstein and Lalikina 1973; Friedenstein and Luria 1980; Luria 1977). In 24-h cultures of murine marrows cells, the CFUf can be recognised as separate spread fibroblasts adherent to the surface of the culture vessel. Already on day 3 – 4 they form foci consisting of several fibroblasts. After 5 days, the number of CFUf-derived colonies remains stable, many of them increasing in size and by day 10 some colonies reach 0.5 – 0.8 cm in diameter and comprise several thousand fibroblasts (Fig. 5).

In marrow cell cultures in medium supplemented with 20% serum, CFUf colony formation does not require additional growth factors, provided that the explantation density of marrow cells is around $5 \times 10^4$ per $cm^2$. At higher densities of explanted marrow cells, the fibroblasts tend to grow as a monolayer, while at lower densities the

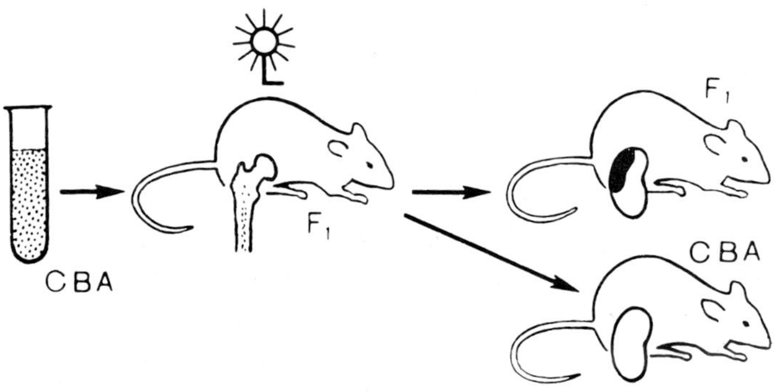


Fig. 4. Schematic of transplantation of bone marrow obtained from radiochimeras and grafted into both lines participating in producing radiochimeras.

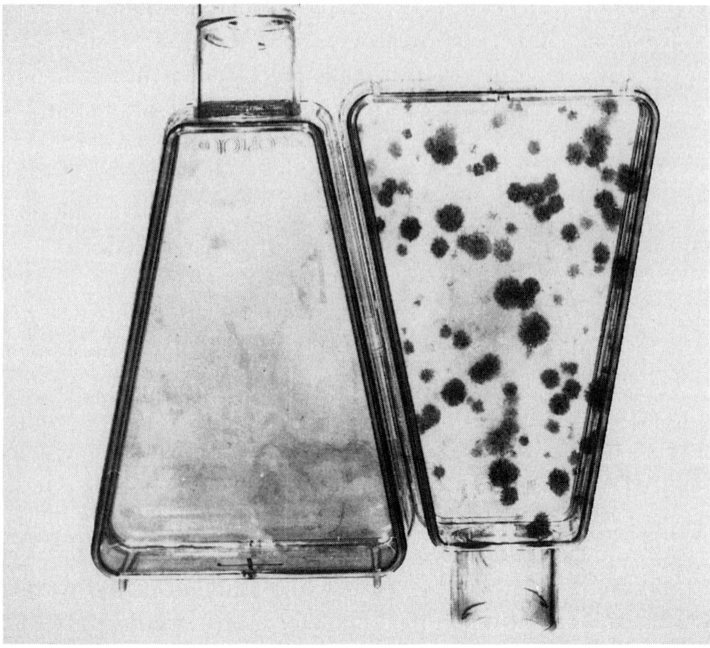

Fig. 5. CFUf colony formation from of 7 × $10^5$ mouse marrow cells. Left: 5-day culture; right: 10-day culture.

colony forming efficiency (CFEf) decreases. The fibroblasts in CFUf-derived colonies synthesize type I and III collagen and fibronectin, are acid-phosphatase positive and have a low non-specific esterase activity (in cultures of murine, rat, hamster and human marrow cells they are also alkaline-phosphatase positive). They do not synthesize factor VIII-associated antigen, and lack FC and C receptors and the antigenic markers characteristic of macrophages and hemopoietic cells (Wilson et al. 1974; Castro-Malaspina et al. 1980; Latzinik et al. 1980; Bently et al. 1982; Friedenstein et al. 1982, 1990; Piersma et al. 1985). At present, synthesis of collagen type I and III remains the main positive marker for identification of fibroblasts in the marrow cell cultures (Fig. 6).

The first monoclonal antibody specifically recognising marrow fibroblasts seems to be R-4-A-9 and was raised by immunisation of rats with a clonal marrow preadipocyte line $H^{1/A}$ (Akasaka et al. 1987). R-4-A-9 recognises a cell surface antigen characteristic of H-1 cells, and binds to marrow fibroblasts localised between vascular sinuses and to the walls of the sinuses, but shows no reactivity with the walls of blood vessels in the marrow. In the spleen, R-4-A-9 reacted with cells of the splenic cords of the red pulp. One can expect that by using monoclonal antibodies our knowledge of antigens by which stromal fibroblasts of various hemopoietic organs differ will increase, and that it will be possible to use antigen-specific markers to study the diversity of marrow CFUf. Different CFUf colonies contain fibroblasts of different shapes and densities. Usually, they consist of monolayers, but in large colonies they multilayer, particularly in the center of the colonies. Most colonies consist of fibroblasts only, but some colonies include adipocytes or have a mineralised extracellular matrix (Howlett et al. 1985). The colonies may also include large cells with giant polyploid nuclei. At present, there is no indication that differences in morphology of fibroblasts can be regarded as markers of CFUf diversity. About 2 – 5% of colonies consist of squamous fibroblasts; such colonies are small and loose. CFUf colonies may also include some macrophages and myeloid cells. Their number differs depending on the origin of explanted marrow cells (in guinea pig marrow cultures the number is low, in mouse marrow cultures it is higher), on the medium composition and on the explantation density of marrow cells. Cells plated at densities below $10^4$ per $cm^2$ develop fibroblast colonies containing hardly any cells of other types.

In 10 – 12-day cultures, the number of fibroblasts per colony may vary from 50 to $15 \times 10^3$, indicating that within that period of cultivation the CFUf descendents undergo from 6 to 14 population doublings. Whether this is a result of the initial heterogeneity of CFUf or should be explained by stochastic reasons remains unknown. If cultivation lasts for more than 2 weeks, the diversity of colonies by size and content of proliferating cells becomes more pronounced. By that time some colonies (less than 10% of the total) are composed of several thousands of fibroblasts and their proliverative pool exceeds 30%. The remaining colonies appear to grow much slower and have a proliferative pool of less than 7%. The mitotic cycle mean time (T) for CFUf-derived fibroblasts is about 20 h. The proliferative pool in the colonies, determined by [$^3$H]thymidine incorporation depends on the CFUf colony size and the age of the culture (Friedenstein 1973). In 4 – 5-day colonies consisting of less than 30 cells it is close to 100%, while in large 7 and 12 day colonies the proliferative pool makes up 85 and 65%, respectively (Luria et al. 1977).

Fibroblast colonies in these cultures represent cell clones. According to chromosome analysis in mixed cultures of marrow cells from male and female guinea pigs, male and female rabbits and CBA and $T_6T_6$ mice, karyotypes within individual colonies were identical (Friedenstein et al. 1987, 1990; Latzinic et al. 1986). There is, however, the possibility that some colonies originated from non-disaggregated stromal fragments preserved in the marrow suspensions. If the number of such fragments in the original dispersed cell population had been found to be comparable with the number of CFUf, the similarity of the karotypes within the colonies in mixed cultures would not prove the clonal nature of CFUf colonies. However, the concentration of stromal aggregates in marrow suspensions was less than 1% of the number of fibroblast colonies. Consequently, the conformity of karyotypes within colonies in mixed cultures proved that CFUf-derived fibroblast colonies are cell clones (Friedenstein et al. 1987).

After a 72-h course of *in vivo* [$^3$H]thymidine administration, 15% and 2% of CFUf in marrow cultures of 6- and 14-day-old guinea pigs, respectively, were labelled, while in mature guinea pigs no CFUf were labelled (Epichima and Latzinik 1976). Thus

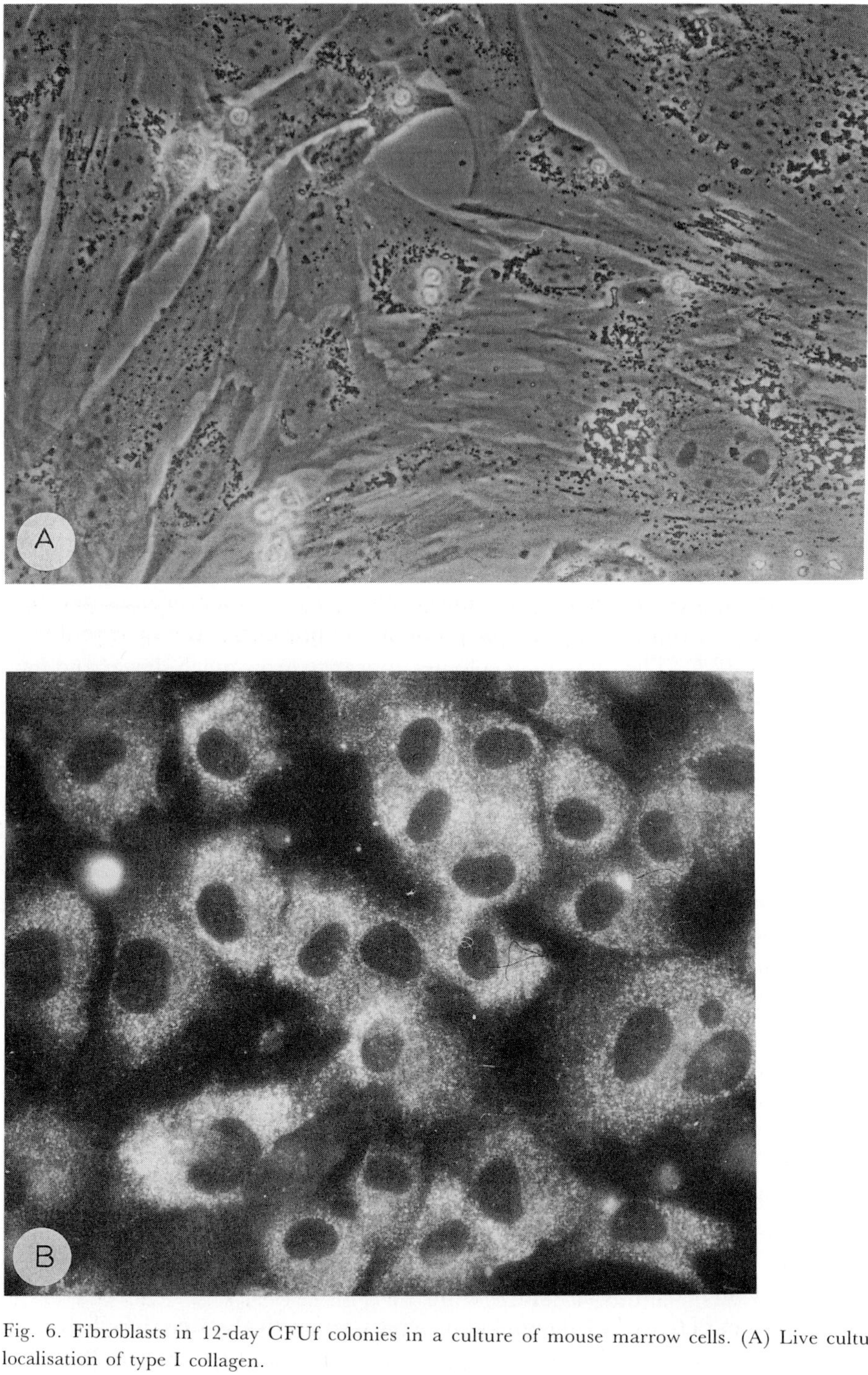


Fig. 6. Fibroblasts in 12-day CFUf colonies in a culture of mouse marrow cells. (A) Live culture; (B) localisation of type I collagen.

most guinea pig CFUf *in situ* are outside the cycle, presumably arrested in $G_0$. This also seems to be the case for human CFUf (Kaneko et al. 1982).

Once attached in culture, the CFUf enter S-phase between 28 and 60 h after explantation (Keilis-Borok et al. 1972). CFUf colony formation depends on two factors: on $G_0$-arrested CFUf to be stimulated to enter S-phase and on proliferation of the fibroblasts comprising the CFUf colonies. These two events are likely to involve different growth-stimulating factors. The standard CFUf colony assay is performed in cultures with high (15 – 20%) serum content. Such a culture medium contains a mixture of competence and progression factors and stimulates growth in various cultured fibroblast populations, including cultured marrow fibroblasts (Friedenstein et al. 1974). To assay individual growth-stimulating factors one would normally use medium with a low serum content or serum-free medium, to be able to detect the stimulating activity of the factor in question. In cultures of murine or human marrow cells in medium with 1% serum medium or in serum-free medium, the activity of PDGF, GM-CSF, hydrocortisone, IL-1, and IL-3 was tested. Only PDGF and IL-3 increased the CFEf to the level seen in cultures with a high serum content (Hirata et al. 1985; McIntyre and Bjornson 1986, Wang and Wolf 1987). However, even when the culture medium contained 20% serum a decrease in the $O_2$ concentration increased CFEf (Gupta et al. 1987). This indicates that even with 20% serum in the culture media the maximum CFEf is not reached, i.e. not all explanted CFUf form colonies.

In media containing 20% serum, the efficiency of CFUf colony formation depends, first and foremost, on the explantation density of marrow cells. In murine and human marrow cultures, the CFEf is 50 times lower at an explantation density of $2 \times 10^4$ marrow cells per $cm^2$ than at explantation density of $4 \times 10^5$ (Fig. 7) (Friedenstein 1990). A very high density of marrow cells in cultures used for CFUf colony assay can be reached if low density marrow cultures are supplemented with irradiated feeder marrow cells (Friedenstein et al. 1976; Latzinik et al. 1986). In such feeder supplemented cultures, the CFEf remains constant and is independent of the number of explanted live marrow cells, i.e. each of the explanted CFUf forms a colony. On the other hand, in feeder-non-supplemented cultures, these fibroblasts remain either nondividing cells (45%) or form 2 – 6 cell colonies (40%) (Friedenstein 1990). Irradiated feeder cells derived from marrow or spleen have colony-stimulating activity, while those derived from thymus and lymph nodes and blood leucocytes have not. Isolated platelets also have colony-stimulating activity (Fig. 8). Feeder cells and platelets do not replace serum growth factors. Furthermore, the feeder effect is highest in medium containing 20% serum (Friedenstein 1990). Whether megakaryocytes and platelets improve culture conditions for CFUf by secreting growth-stimulating factors remains to be clarified. PDGF is unlikely to be the factor in question since addition of PDGF to culture medium with 20% serum does not increase CFEf (Hirata et al. 1985; McIntyre and Bjornson 1986; Wang and Wolf 1987). It seems likely, however, that some factor associated with the hemopoietic lineage cells triggers the progression of CFUf from $G_0$ into S-phase, while the subsequent proliferation of CFUf *in vitro* is probably stimulated by serum growth factors. Under standard CFUf culture conditions, triggering of CFUf into the cycle is probably induced by marrow cells accompanying CFUf.

The number of stromal colonies detected by the CFUf colony assay is dependent on the mode of cell disaggregation in preparing marrow cell suspensions. In trypsin-disaggregated marrow cell suspensions of mice and guinea pigs, the CFUf concentration is higher than in suspensions prepared by mechanical disaggregation. The differences largely depend on inactivation of a considerable number of CFUf by mechanical treatment of the marrow (Fig. 7) (Latzinik et al. 1981; Friedenstein et al. 1982).

Fibroblast differentiation in CFUf colonies can be affected by various factors. For instance, hydrocortisone enhances the alkaline phosphatase activity in rabbit CFUf colonies and increases the number of adipocytes in human CFUf colonies (McIntyre and Bjornson 1986; Owen et al. 1987). The intercellular matrix produced by fibroblasts in CFUf colonies also depends on colony-stimulating factors.

CFUf colonies synthesize types I and III collagen and fibronectin when in liquid cultures with serum-supplemented medium. In addition to this, they synthesize type IV collagen and laminin when cultured in methyl-cellulose and plasma in the presence of conditioned medium from PHA-stimulated leucocytes (Lim et al. 1986). The dif-

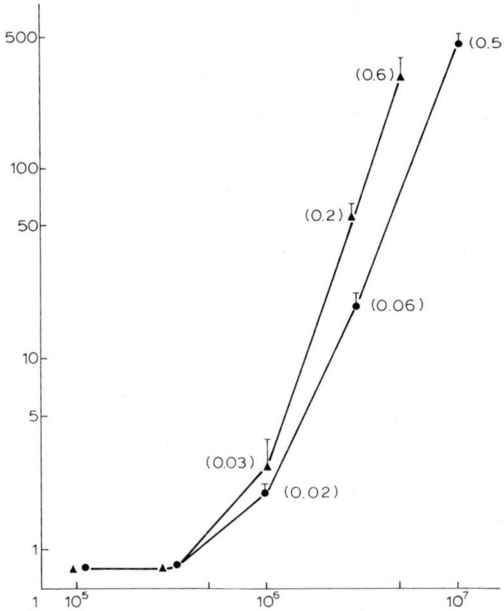


Fig. 7. Dependence of colony-forming efficiency on explantation densities of marrow cells. Marrow cells disaggregated by trypsinization (▲) or by mechanical treatment (●) and explanted in 25 $cm^2$ culture flasks. Ordinate: number of CFUf colonies per flask; abscissa: number of marrow cells explanted.

ferences could be explained by different CFUf proliferating under the different culture conditions. It could also be that the same CFUf generate different descendants depending on the growth factors used to induce CFUf colony formation. The last possibility seems more probable since the number of colonies formed in both colony assay systems are similar.

The origin of CFUf in heterotopic marrow and in radiochimeras was determined according to the donor or host origin of the fibroblasts in CFUf-derived colonies (Friedenstein et al. 1978). $T^6$ chromosomes and sex chromosomes were used as

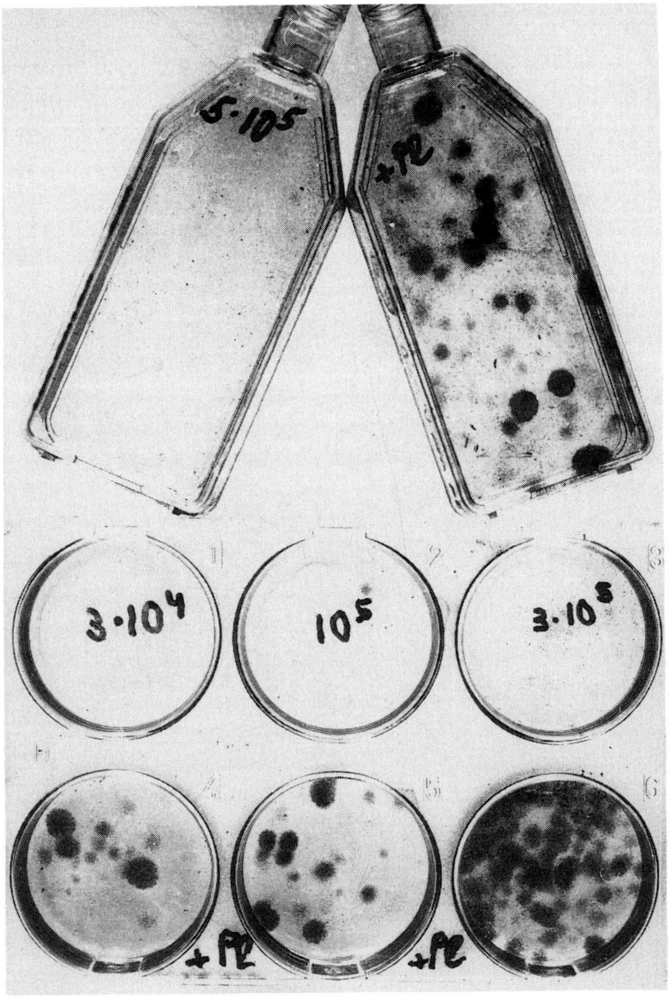


Fig. 8. Colony-stimulating activity of platelets. 10-day cultures of indicated numbers of mouse marrow cells. Non-adherent marrow cells were decanted at 2 h after explantation and platelets were added to half of the cultures.

markers for mouse and guinea pig cells, respectively. The CFUf derived from 2.5 – 8 month heterotopic bone marrow organs in mice were found to be solely of donor origin, while those derived from the marrow of radiochimeras were of recipient origin (Fig. 9). This agrees with the results of the experiments testing the origin of the DOPC and the HME-transferring cells using heterotopic grafting (Figs. 2 – 4), and is another indication that CFUf are of non-hemopoietic cell lineage.

## IV. Proliferative properties and osteogenic potency of marrow CFUf

The results of heterotopic marrow grafting experiments and chromosome typing of fibroblasts in CFUf-derived colonies have provided evidence that marrow stromal mechanocytes do not belong to the hemopoietic cell lineage. Heterotopic grafting exposes osteogenic precusors, while the CFUf colony assay detects clonogenic cells. These two tests seem to address different aspects of the same category of stromal cells. This was further supported by experiments in which cells in chicken-quail limb bud

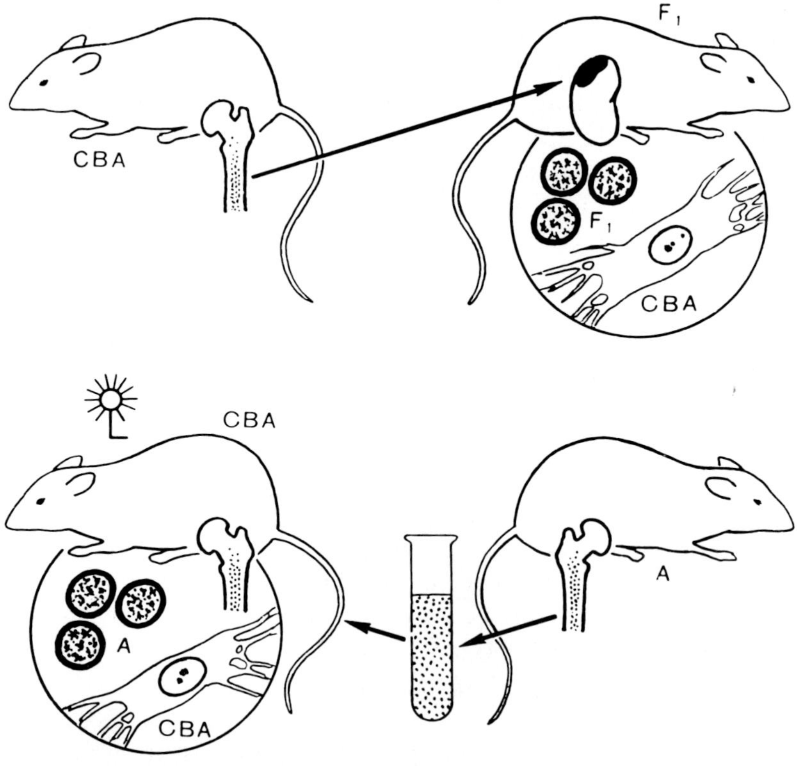


Fig. 9. Origin of hemopoietic cells in heterotopic ossicles and in bone marrow of radiochimeras as determined by chromosome typing.

heterotopic grafts were typed. Using inter-species differences in heterochromatin structure, Le Douarin et al. (1975) demonstrated that both osteogenic and marrow reticular cells were the donor cells, while endothelial cells, despite being part of the marrow stroma, were of host origin. Thus, in heterotopic transplants, CFUf, DOPC and reticular osteogenic cells derived from marrow all originate from donor tissue.

### A. Multicolony-derived cultures of marrow fibroblasts

Pure stromal fibroblast cultures can be obtained by passaging multiple CFUf colonies from primary cultures of human, rabbit, guinea pig, rat and hamster marrow, spleen and thymus cells. This produces multicolony-derived fibroblast cultures consisting of the descendants of multiple CFUf. Passaging does not require any additional growth factors besides those present in serum and can be continued for over 25 passages. Beginning with the second passage, the cultures are free from detectable non-fibroblast cells. To get murine stromal fibroblast cultures not contaminated with macrophages, the latter have to be eliminated by repeated treatment of the cultures with carrageenin or with anti-macrophage antibodies and complement (Latzinik et al. 1986, 1981). Human stromal fibroblast cultures of marrow, spleen and thymus origin have similar morphological features and synthesize types I and III collagen and fibronectin. They are highly adhesive cells, do not ingest latex beads or reduce tetrazolium, stain to varying degrees for alkaline and acid phosphatase activity (depending on species and organ of origin), stain positive with alpha naphthylacetate esterase and PAS, do not stain with myeloperoxidase or the T-lymphocyte specific monoclonal antibodies MI and MI20, and lack factor VIII-associated antigen and FC and C receptors (Friedenstein and Luria 1980; Lee et al. 1987). Cultured marrow fibroblasts remain diploid at least until the 20th passage. In rabbit bone marrow fibroblast cultures, 75.2% of metaphases have a diploid set of chromosomes; aneuploid cells (24.8%) are mostly hypodiploid cells and are probably artefactual and the result of damage during the process of analysis. The content of hyperdiploid cells (0.95%) does not exceed the level of spontaneous mutation, while the frequency of chromatid and mixed deletions (1%) corresponds to the level of spontaneous chromosome mutations for mammalian cells (Miskarova et al. 1970).

Multicolony-derived fibroblast cultures derived from marow cells from guinea pig heterotopic ossicles were of donor origin, while those derived from femoral marrow cells from the hosts bearing the ossicles were of host origin (Friedenstein et al. 1978). This confirms that CFUf do not migrate from one hemopoietic organ to another. In most of the studies with primary (non-passaged) cultures of marrow stromal cells from murine and human radiochimeras, the fibroblasts were found to be exclusively recipient cells, indicating that marrow CFUf injected intraveneously do not settle in the marrow of the irradiated host and do not proliferate there (Friedenstein et al. 1978; Wilson et al. 1978; Golde et al. 1980; Bentley et al. 1982; Hollings et al. 1984; Lennon and Micklem 1986). However, a donor origin of fibroblasts in such cultures has also been reported (Marshall et al. 1980; Keating et al. 1982; Piersma et al. 1983). The conflicting results are probably caused by difficulties with the identification of fibroblasts in the mixed stromal cell populations present in primary marrow cultures.

The upper limit of the number of CFUf initiating a multicolony-derived fibroblast strain is calculated from the CFEf value and the number of explanted marrow cells. This number is the base for estimating the mean number of population doublings in the course of cell passaging. For rabbit marrow fibroblast cultures, 18 passages represent at least 20 population doublings, which is an indication of the high proliferative potential of the initial CFUf (Fig. 10) (Friedenstein et al. 1987).

When transplanted in diffusion chambers, guinea pig and rabbit marrow fibroblast cultures can form bone or both bone and cartilage (Friedenstein et al. 1970, 1987; Ashton et al. 1982). Bone formation occurred in almost every diffusion chamber, provided it was inoculated with the total cell harvest from a first passage-culture initiated by at least 25 CFUf. This means that at least 4% of the CFUf are DOPC. To observe bone formation by fibroblasts of later passages, it was sufficient to transplant only a part of the total cell harvest. It is thus possible to calculate the lower limit of the number of osteogenic units the strain contains at each passage, providing that bone formation signifies that at least one osteogenic precursor unit had been transplanted in the chamber. The number of osteogenic units increased in parallel with the number of fibroblasts in the course of consecutive passages. After the tenth passage, the

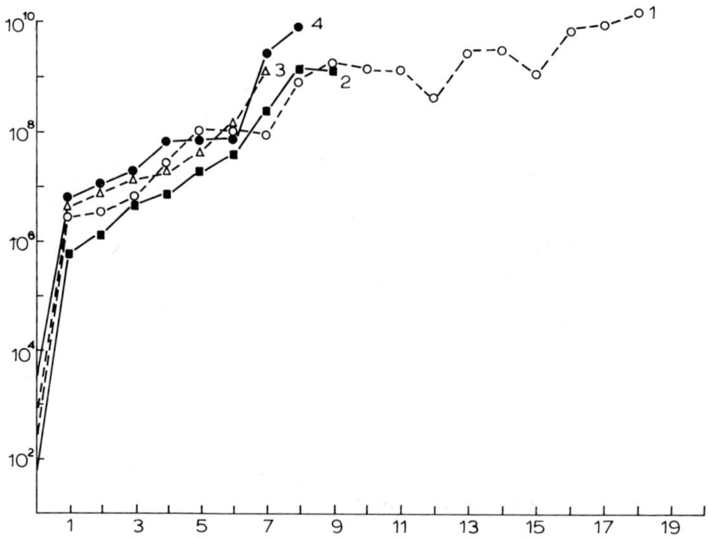


Fig. 10. Cell numbers in sequential passages of multicolony-derived marrow fibroblast cultures. 1: Culture initiated by explantation of $3 \times 10^4$ marrow cells (37 CFUf); 2: culture initiated by explantation of $10^5$ marrow cells (175 CFUf); 3: culture initiated by explantation of $10^6$ marrow cells (300 CFUf): 4: culture initiated by explantation of $10^7$ marrow cells (3000 CFUf). Ordinate: number of fibroblasts in the cell harvest; abscissa: number of passages.

number of osteogenic units was several hundred times greater than the number of the initiating CFUf, which proves that the osteogenic precursors proliferate intensively in marrow fibroblast cultures. When passaged marrow fibroblasts are transplanted in diffusion chambers, the number of osteogenic units transplanted probably exceeds one osteogenic unit. The results, therefore, indicate only the lower limit of the number of osteogenic units present. The amount of bone tissue formed in diffusion chambers by the *in vitro* descendants of the marrow CFUf proved surprisingly large. Cells derived from the CFUf contained in a 0.5 g pelvic bone fragment were capable of forming 30 kg of bone (dry weight) (Friedenstein et al. 1987).

### B. Single colony derived cultures of marrow fibroblasts

Large colonies in rabbit marrow primary cultures (making up about 30% of all CFUf colonies) contain $10^3 - 10^4$ fibroblasts. Their initial CFUf are capable of extensive proliferation and go through no less than 17 population doublings when the colonies are subcultured individually. When transplanted in diffusion chambers, 20% of single colony-derived cultures form bone, cartilage and reticular-like tissue; 20% form bone only and 27% form reticular-like tissue only (Friedenstein et al. 1987) (Fig. 11). The term 'reticular-like' is used for cells that, by morphological criteria, were non-osteogenic. CFUf are thus heterogeneous and include at least three categories of clonogenic stromal cells: those which can be regarded as multipotential precursors of bone, cartilage and reticular-like cells (CFUb,c,r), committed osteogenic precursors (CFUb) and committed reticular-like cell precusors (CFUr).

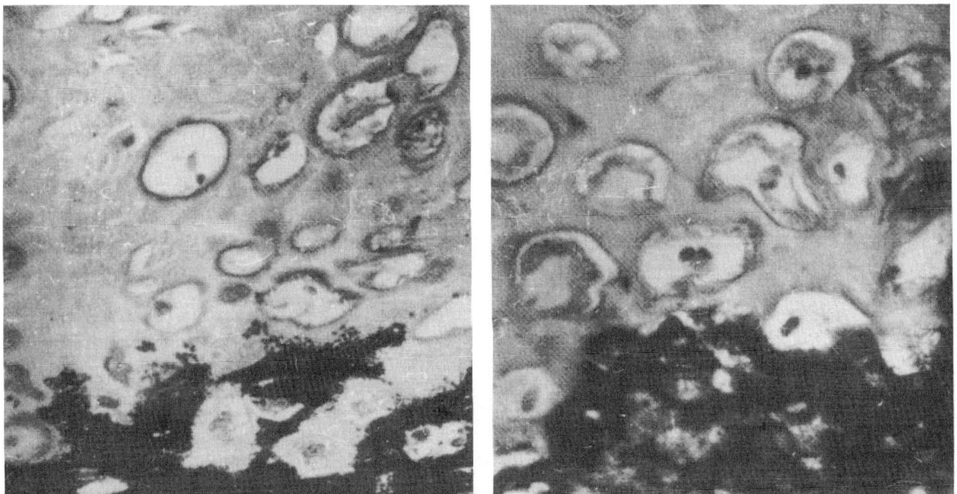

Fig. 11. Bone and cartilage formation by single colony-derived marrow fibroblasts transplanted in a diffusion chamber. (left) von Kossa-haematoxylin; (right) Gomory reaction for alkaline phosphatase.

### V. The ability of marrow fibroblasts to transfer the HME in vivo and to establish a HME in vitro

Heterotopic grafting of multicolony-derived rabbit marrow fibroblast cultures results in the formation of bone marrow organs (Friedenstein et al. 1974a). The results are basically the same as those obtained with heterotopic transplantation of marrow fragments, indicating that marrow CFUf (or at least some marrow CFUf) are HME-transferring cells. Heterotopic transplantation of single CFUf colonies from primary cultures of murine marrow cells resulted in the formation of ossicles with marrow cavities containing hemopoietic cells in 10% of the transplants (Friedenstein 1980) (Fig. 12). Thus, at least some category of marrow fibroblasts is able to transfer the HME. These cells, or their *in vivo* descendants, either secrete hemopoietic growth factors themselves or attract cells which produce these factors. Marrow fibroblasts have been shown to secrete a broad spectrum of hemopoietic growth factors *in vitro,* including M-CSF, G-CSF, GM-CSF, BFUf and Mix-colony-CSF (Gordon et al. 1981, 1987; Greenberg et al. 1981; Bagby et al. 1983; Brockbank and Van Peer 1983; Brondy et al. 1986; Lovhang et al. 1986; Munker et al. 1986; Zucali et al. 1986, 1987). They elaborate growth factors either constitutively or after stimulation by endotoxin, IL-1 or TNF. IL-1 stimulates the dose-dependent release of GM-CSF, which may be the mechanism by which monocytes and stromal marrow fibroblasts regulate cellular growth and differentiation in the HME (Lee et al. 1981). However, hemopoietic growth factors are produced by a variety of cell types, including T-lymphocytes (Bagby et al. 1981) and endothelial cells (Qusenberry and Gimbrone 1980).

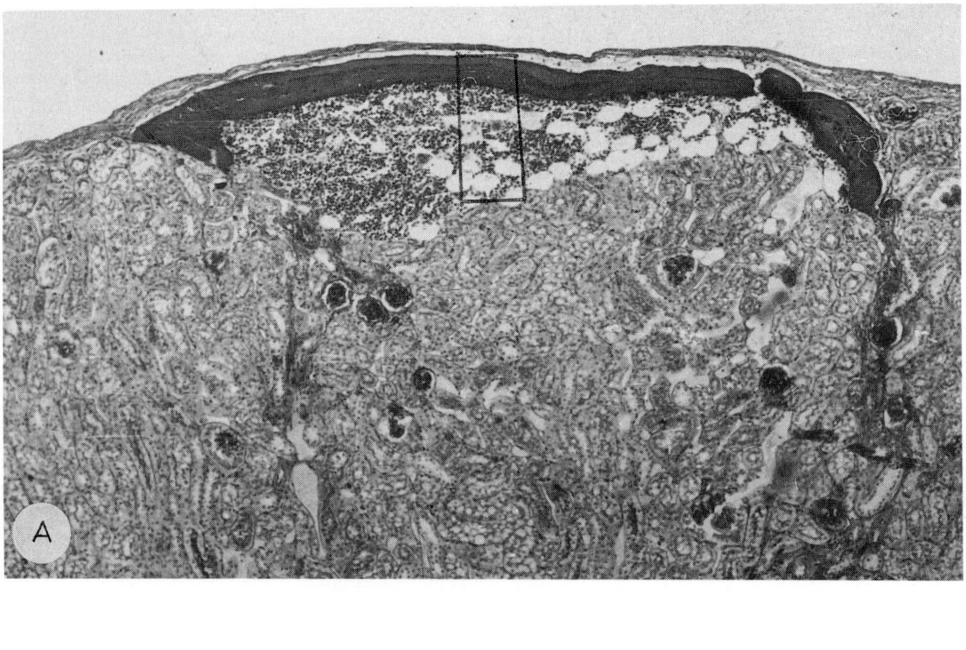

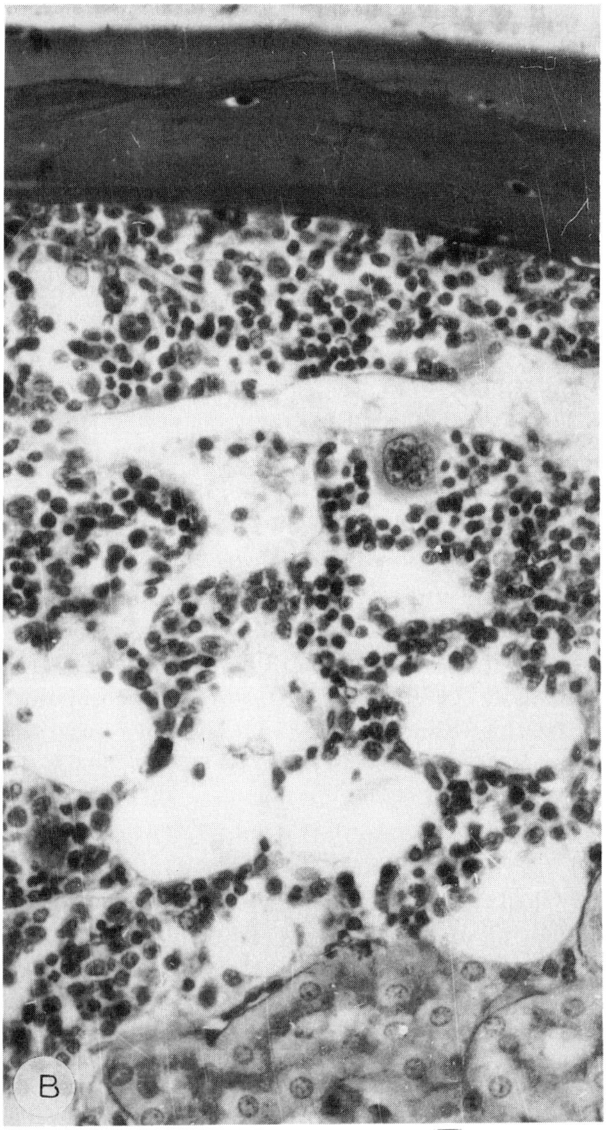

Fig. 12. Ossicle formed by heterotopic transplantation of a single CFUf colony from a mouse marrow culture.

Convincing evidence of microenvironmental competence of marrow fibroblasts was obtained when they were tested in the systems for long-term maintenance of hemopoiesis *in vitro*. The original system (Dexter and Lajtha 1977) required a stromal underlayer composed of adherent marrow cells, including macrophages, fibroblasts, adipocytes and, possibly, endothelial cells. Identification of the exact cellular composition of the underlayer, especially with respect to the type of HME-competent cells, turned out to be difficult. Assumptions were made with respect to many cell types, including adipocytes, endothelial cells and macrophages, but not with respect to fibroblasts: overgrowth by fibroblasts was for a long time associated with termination of hemopoiesis *in vitro*. Marrow fibroblasts were rehabilitated as HME-competent cells, however, as a result of the experiments of Brockbank et al. (1986). They showed that multi-colony-derived cultures of murine marrow fibroblasts, deprived of macrophages and endothelium, supported hemopoiesis when seeded with marrow suspensions depleted of stromal cells. Thus, cultured marrow fibroblasts release hemopoietic growth factors and are capable of presenting them in a proper way to support hemopoiesis, which proves that they are HME-competent cells.

## VI. Changes in the number of CFUf in situ

The number of CFUf in the bone marrow is influenced by a variety of factors. In guinea pigs, bleeding results in a 2.5-fold increase in their numbers after 2 h (Friedenstein et al. 1974b). This, of course, does not mean that stromal cells are sensitive to erythropoietin: their response might be induced by activated erythropoietin-dependent marrow cells. The content of marrow CFUf also changes drastically after mechanical trauma of the medullary cavity (curettage), a procedure known to induce osteogenesis in the marrow. In the curettaged mouse femur, 11 days after curettage, the number of CFUf had increased 5 times while in the contralateral femur the number had increased by 4 times (Wilson et al. 1974). In the curettaged guinea pig tibia, the CFUf content started to increase between days 1 and 7. On day 20 the number of CFUf in the curettaged marrow cavity and in the contralateral tibia had increased 2.5-fold (Gerasimov and Chailakhyan 1978). These results agree with the results of radioautographic studies showing that partial depopulation of the medullary cavity stimulates proliferation of stromal cells in undamaged areas of the marrow (Meyer-Hammer et al. 1971). The mechanisms underlying the systemic response of the stromal cells remain unclear.

Noticeable changes in the content of marrow CFUf are also caused by whole-body and local irradiation. The radiosensitivity of murine and guinea pig CFUf, as determined by inhibition of colony formation following *in vitro* irradiation (Kusmenko et al. 1972; Friedenstein et al. 1981), is similar to that of human bone marrow CFUf (Hendry and Lord 1983). The development of secondary bone marrow aplasia after local exposure to high doses of radiation (Knospe et al. 1966) and the inability of marrow of irradiated donors to form heterotopic ossicles when grafted during the first month after irradation (Friedenstein and Kuralesova 1971; Chamberlain et al. 1974) also demonstrate that radiation damages the marrow stroma and its osteogenic cells.

The dynamics of the changes in CFUf content after whole-body irradiation of mice with 1.5 Gy are shown in Fig. 13. The changes observed after irradiation of guinea

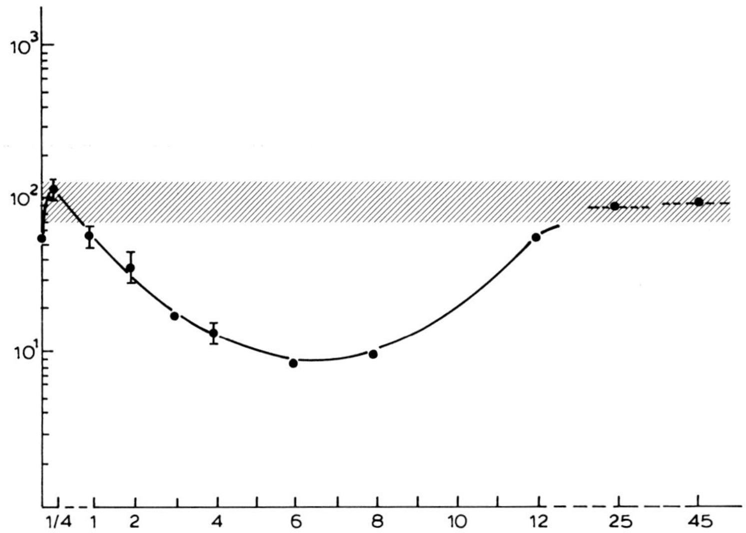


Fig. 13. CFUf per femur for bone marrow from mice irradiated with 1.5 Gy. Ordinate: CFUf content for irradiated mice (log of percentage) as compared with normal mice; abscissa: days after irradiation.

pigs with 4.0 Gy are similar (Friedenstein et al. 1976, 1981). The decrease in CFUf number immediately after irradiation agrees with CFUf survival observed after irradiation of marrow *in vitro*. The temporary sharp increase in the number of CFUf after 6 h is probably the result of repair of sublethal damage characteristic of resting CFUf (Epichina and Latzinic 1976). Regeneration of CFUf is characterised by a marked secondary loss and post-irradiation lag and dip, lasting 6 days, followed by return to normal or subnormal values by about the 25th day. In human patients conditioned for marrow transplantation and engrafted with marrow cells, the number of CFUf during the first 3 weeks is significantly lower than that before transplantation, while the proportion of CFUf in S-phase is increased during the early period after transplantation. Within 6 weeks the number of CFUf returns to normal (Wan-Ming et al. 1986).

After local irradiation of the tibia of guinea pigs with 4 Gy, post-irradiation aplasia reaches maximal values by the 3rd to the 5th day (Fig. 14). Thereafter, the number of bone marrow cells rapidly increases, reaching normal values by the 14th to the 20th day. The time course of the change in the number of CFUf is different. Irradiation damages about 85% of the CFUf, and their number continues to decrease up to day 3. During the next 3 months the number of CFUf gradually increases to levels slightly below normal (Fig. 14). The degree of regeneration of the marrow cells is always greater than that of the CFUf. After local irradiation with 20 Gy, the dynamics of the restoration of hemopoietic marrow cells are similar to those observed after irradiation with 4 Gy up to the 20th day. During this recovery, CFUf are almost completely ab-

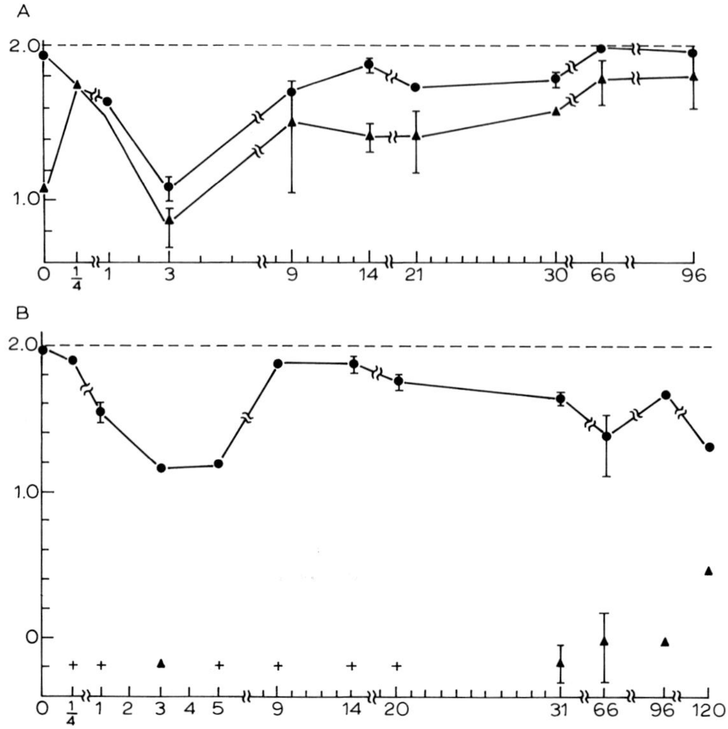


Fig. 14. CFUf content in tibial bone marrow of guinea pigs after local irradiation. Ordinate: proportion of nucleated cells (●) and CFUf (▲) in irradiated tibia (log of percentage) as compared with the non-irradiated tibia of the same donors. Abscissa: days after irradiation. (A) Irradiation with 4 Gy; (B) irradiation with 20 Gy.

sent (Fig. 14). After 3 weeks, however, secondary aplasia of the bone marrow gradually develops. The number of CFUf in this period does not exceed 1 – 3% of the normal values, i.e. is close to zero.

Thus, the marrow HME *in vivo* remains functionally active for several weeks after radiation doses of 20 Gy and supports hemopoiesis by repopulating hemopoietic stem cells (Knospie et al. 1966, 1968). Stromal fibroblasts are quite long lived, i.e. they are slowly renewing cells, and very little cell proliferation is required to maintain the reticular stroma. The same applies to the osteogenic marrow cells and to maintenance of bone tissue. This also appears to be the case *in vitro,* since stromal cells that have reached confluency in long-term marrow cultures survive for relatively long periods of time and have a very low proliferative activity. Therefore, radiation doses that result in inhibition of all proliferation and new DNA synthesis have little effect on the HME. The same is true for stromal cells in murine long-term marrow cultures (mainly fibroblasts and macrophages) which were shown to survive extremely high doses of *in vitro* irradiation and to continue to release hemopoietic growth factors (Gualtieri 1987).

After *in vitro* exposure to 500 Gy, the cells constitutively produced predominantly M-CSF. After stimulation with endotoxin, a significant increase in production of other hemopoietic growth factors, including multilineage growth factor, was observed. Adherent stromal cells in murine marrow cultures also showed no evidence of substantial cell death during a 6-week period after irradiation with 100 Gy, and maintained HME-supportive functions when irradiated up to at least 50 Gy (Zuckerman et al. 1986).

Thus, two different functions of stromal fibroblasts can be distinguished with regard to their role as osteogenic precursors and HME-competent cells: (1) bone formation and transfer of the HME with heterotopic grafting, for which proliferative stromal precursors (CFUf) are required and (2) the release and presentation of hemopoietic growth factors by non-proliferating stromal cells. After local irradiation, or whole-body irradiation followed by injection of marrow cells, the hemopoietic cells can quickly regenerate, mainly by repopulation with hemopoietic progenitor cells. Conversely, the CFUf regenerate slowly, relying only on local cells. These differences confirm that the hemopoietic cells and the stromal cells belong to different lineages.

## VII. Inducible osteogenic precursor cells (IOPC)

DOPC are not the only early osteogenic precursors present in adult mammals. Ectopic bone formation can start outside the skeleton, a result of the presence of inducible osteogenic precursor cells (Friedenstein et al. 1973). Ossification foci in various organs of humans and other mammals are no great rarity. Far more important, however, is that two experimental procedures, implantation of decalcified bone matrix (Urist 1965) and transplantation of transitional epithelium of the urinary tract (Huggins 1932) both induce ectopic osteogenesis with high frequency. The osteogenic activity of the bone matrix depends on bone morphogenetic protein (BMP) which induces the development of cartilage followed by bone formation (Urist et al. 1984), while that of the transitional epithelium depends on an unidentified inducing factor secreted by epithelial cells. The latter became evident when transitional epithelium was transplanted into millipore diffusion chambers: epithelium grew within the chambers, while bone tissue was formed on the outer surface of the chambers (Friedenstein 1962).

When transitional epithelium is grafted, epithelial bands and cysts develop and aggregates of stacked connective tissue cells appear in the connective tissue nearby the epithelium. By day 8, osteoblasts differentiate among these cells, and by day 10 the first bony trabeculae are formed. Later on, the epithelial cysts become encased by the bone tissue. Cartilage does not develop at all initially, but small cartilage foci may appear at later times in sites away from the epithelium (Friedenstein 1968). Subsequently, the ectopic ossicles become populated by hemopoietic cells, and by 25 – 30 days the ossicles induced by epithelium contain marrow. The same applies for ectopic bone marrow organs induced by the transitional epithelium of the renal pelvis following ligation of the renal artery (Sacerdotti and Frattin 1902; Maximov 1906; Bridges and Pritchard 1958; Friedenstein 1968).

When spleen, thymus and peritoneal fluid cells are transplanted in diffusion chambers together with transitional epithelium or decalcified bone matrix, bone is formed inside the chambers (Friedenstein et al. 1966, 1968, 1972). This means that IOPC competent to both osteogenic inductors are present in these cell populations. When induced by decalcified bone matrix, both cartilage and bone are formed in the diffusion chambers, whereas induction with transitional epithelium results in formation of bone tissue only. It is not known whether this is due to heterogeneity of IOPC, some of them being inducible by BMP and others by the transitional epithelium, or whether the descendants of the same IOPC develop differently depending on the inductor which triggers their development.

Spleen, thymus and peritoneal fluid cells possess CFUf which form fibroblast colonies *in vitro* (Friedenstein et al. 1974b). Multicolony-derived cultures of spleen, thymus and peritoneal fluid fibroblasts are nonosteogenic when tested by transplantation in diffusion chambers. However, they form bone and cartilage, or bone only, when transplanted together with bone matrix or with transitional epithelium (Friedenstein et al. 1970, 1973). Thus, the clonogenic mechanocyte precursors of thymus and spleen origin, in distinction from those of marrow origin, are IOPC and not DOPC.

Upon induction by transitional epithelium, the osteogenic cells are recruited from IOPC. Whether inductor-independent self-maintaining osteogenic precursors, equivalent to DOPS, are also induced remains to be clarified. The ectopic ossicles induced by autotransplantation of bladder epithelium persist for a long time (not less than a year) and remain in close contact with the epithelium. When allogeneic epithelium is used as the inductor, immunological resorption of the epithelium starts before marrow has developed inside the ossicle. This results in gradual disappearance of the induced bone, despite the fact that the bone is composed of recipient cells and contains a thick layer of osteoblasts and preosteoblasts at the time of epithelium resorption. By conditioning the recipient, immunological resorption of allogeneic epithelium can be delayed until marrow is formed in the ossicle. This may abolish the disappearance of bone and marrow when the epithelium is later resorbed (Keilis-Borok et al. 1982). The marrow from ectopic ossicles induced in the renal pelvis by transitional epithelium also contains CFUf with osteogenic properties similar to those of skeletal DOPC: they give rise to fibroblast cultures which, after several passages *in vitro,* retain osteogenic properties when retransplanted *in vivo* (Friedenstein and Luria 1980).

Thus, the early stages of bone formation induced by transitional epithelium seem to be dependent on IOPC-derived osteogenic cells. However, when the ectopic ossicles acquire HME-competent stroma and become populated by marrow cells, they aquire determined self-maintaining osteogenic precursors similar to the IOPC present in the skeletal marrow. The origin of the DOPC in the induced ectopic ossicles has not been determined. Up to now, there is no experimental proof that they are descendants of the same IOPC from which the initial osteogenic cell population was recruited. The possibility that the DOPC in the marrow of induced ectopic ossicles originate from CFUf which circulate in the blood stream can not be excluded.

Peripheral blood cells have been shown to form bone when transplanted in diffusion chambers together with transitional epithelium (Friedenstein and Lalykina 1970), suggesting that IOPC circulate in blood. The circulation of fibroblast precursors was demonstrated by A.A. Maximov in his last work with plasma clot cultures of blood cells (Maximov 1928). Maximov's results were confirmed by Luria et al. (1971, 1989), who showed that blood contains circulating CFUf which have the ability to form colonies of fibroblasts which synthesize type I collagen, form collagen fibers and lack factor VIII-associated antigen (Fig. 15). Blood-derived cultured guinea pig fibroblasts were found to form bone when transplanted in diffusion chambers together with the transitional epithelium (Friedenstein and Luria 1980). It remains unknown from where the CFUf migrate into blood, where they settle (if they really do) and why CFUf are not detectable in the blood of some mammals, including humans.

## VIII. Conclusion

The CFUf are clonogenic stromal precursors of the osteogenic and reticular marrow stromal cells. Some CFUf are multipotent progenitors of bone and cartilage and have the properties of stem cells of skeletogenic cell lineage. Under steady-state conditions they are outside the cycle and have a sufficiently high proliferative potential to ensure production of differentiated osteogenic tissue cells throughout the entire life-span.

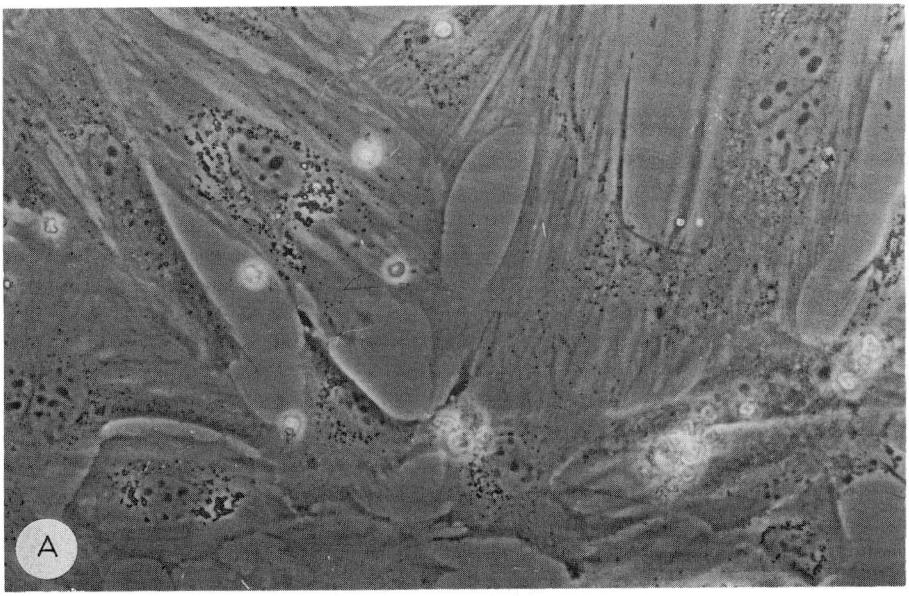

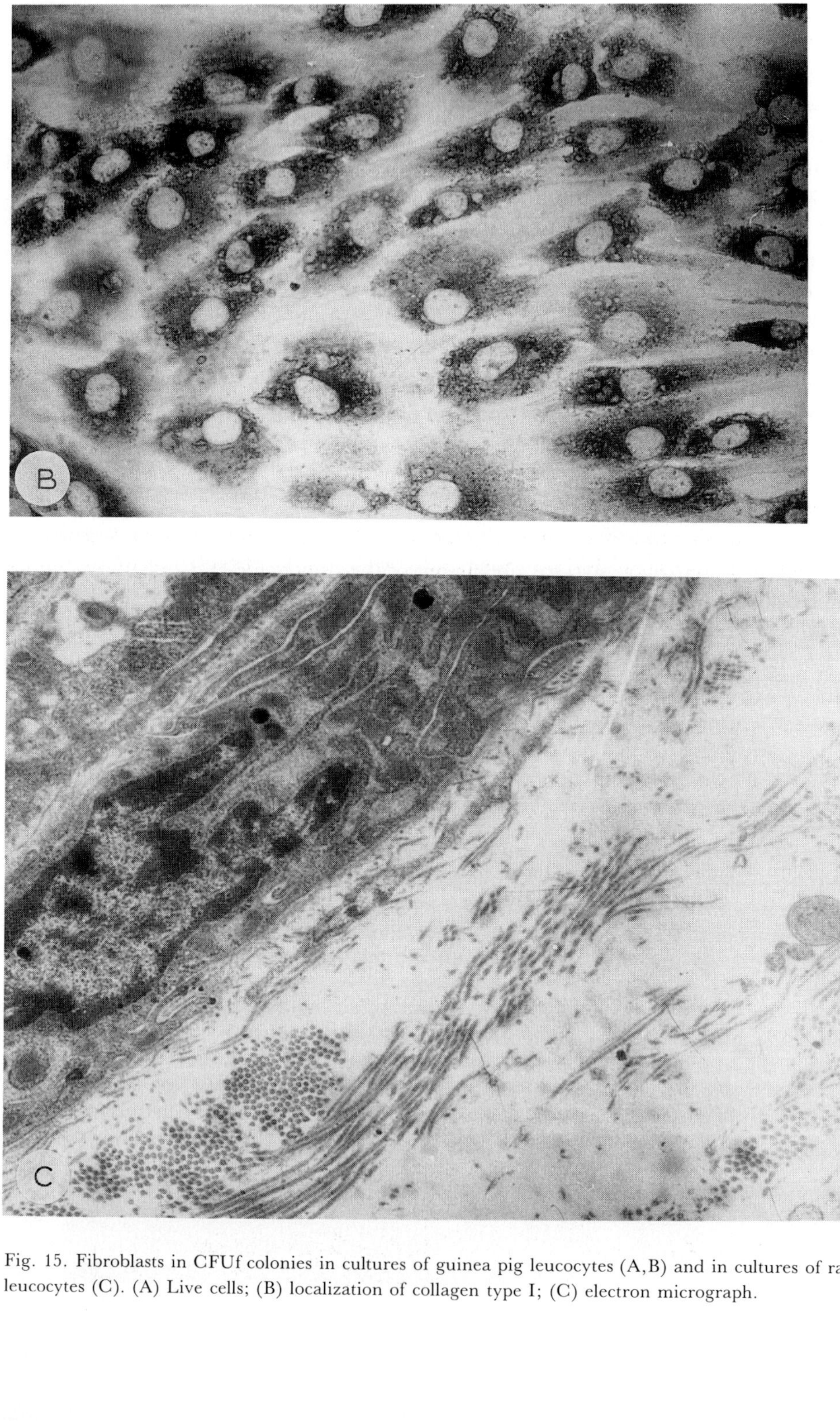


Fig. 15. Fibroblasts in CFUf colonies in cultures of guinea pig leucocytes (A,B) and in cultures of rabbit leucocytes (C). (A) Live cells; (B) localization of collagen type I; (C) electron micrograph.

CFUf are a heterogeneous cell population, comprising precursors of different standing in the hierarchy of stromal cells, i.e. multipotent skeletogenic CFUf, committed osteogenic CFUf, and committed reticular CFUf. It seems likely that osteogenic and reticular cell CFUf are of the same stromal cell lineage, assuming that reticular cells and all CFUf in single CFUf-derived heterotopic ossicles are of donor origin. This was proven for ossicles formed by engraftment of pooled CFUf, but the origin of the CFUf present in single CFUf derived ossicles remains to be ascertained.

Cell renewal in osteogenic and reticular tissues is very slow, although the number of clonogenic precursor cells in these tissues appears to be comparatively high. CFUf (50% of which are osteogenic precursor cells) comprise no less than 10% of marrow reticular cells, but this value may prove to be much higher in view of the observation that every viable reticular cell in disaggregated marrow suspensions appears to be clonogenic. Therefore, most reticular marrow cells may turn out to be CFUf.

Stromal mechanocytes of bone marrow and marrow CFUf are genetically independent of hemopoietic cells. The same applies to spleen and thymus CFUf, which are IOPC. The genetic relationship of IOPC circulating in blood with hemopoietic cells remains to be determined.

Stromal reticular cells are important for the HME, and there is total dependence of hemopoietic cells on intimate stromal cell contact. Stromal cells synthesize hemopoietic growth factors, and it is suggested that they are retained by binding to stromal cell extracellular matrix (Gordon et al. 1987). Stromal cells synthesize proteoglycans, including heparan sulfate, chondroitin sulfate and glucuronic acid. It was shown that growth factors bind to heparan sulphate, and can be presented in that form to hemopoietic cells (Roberts et al. 1988). The extracellular matrix of bone also contains various proteoglycans (Termine 1988) which may sequester growth factors and modulate their biological actions through complex modes of release and presentation to responding cells. Hauschka et al. (1988) suggested to call the cellular interaction with bone matrix-adsorbed factors ‘matricrine’, as distinct from endocrine, paracrine and autocrine routes of growth factor stimulation. The release by osteoclasts of active transforming growth factor $\beta$ (TGF-$\beta$) from bone matrix has been demonstrated (Pfeilschifter et al. 1986).

Hemopoietic growth factors have not yet been identified in bone extracellular matrix. The reason for this may be that hemopoietic cells were not used as target cells when these bone-derived growth factors were tested. Going back to the question of why marrow is locally associated with bone, one possibility is that bone extracellular matrix serves as a storage depot for local hemopoietic growth factors secreted by reticular cells. If so, this should make the endosteal bone surface a suitable place for hemopoiesis and give physiological grounds for genetic relations between the lineage of osteogenic cells and marrow stromal system (Owen 1985; Owen and Friedenstein 1988).

## References

Akasaka Y, Fujimoto J, Hato J, Watanabe Y, Harigaya K. Production of monoclonal antibody to a clonal bone marrow preadipocite line (H-1/A). Exp Hematol 1987;15:610 – 618.

Ascenzi A. Physiological relationship and pathological interferences between bone tissue and marrow. In: Bourne JH, ed. The Biochemistry and Physiology of Bone, Vol IV. New York: Academic Press, 1976;403 – 444.

Ashton BA, Allen TD, Howlett CR, Eagleson CC, Hattori A, Owen M. Formation of bone and cartilage by marrow stromal cells in diffusion chambers in vivo. Clin Orthop 1980;151:294 – 306.

Bagby JC, Rigas VD, Bennett RH, Vanderbark AA, Garewal HS. Interaction of lactoferrin, monocytes, and T-lymphocyte subsets in the regulation of steady-state granulopoiesis in vitro. J Clin Invest 1981;68:56 – 63.

Bagby JC, McCall F, Layman DL. Regulation of colony-stimulating activity production: interaction of fibroblasts, mononuclear phagocyctes and lactoferrin. J Clin Invest 1983;71:340 – 347.

Bentley SA, Knutsen T, Whangpeng J. The origin of the hemopoietic microenviroment in continuous bone marrow culture. Exp Hematol 1982;10:367 – 372.

Bridges J, Pritchard J. Bone and cartilage induction in the rabbit. J Anat 1958;92:28 – 36.

Brockbank KGM, Van Peer CMJ. Colony-stimulating activity produced by hemopoietic organ fibroblastoid cells in vitro. Acta Hematol 1983;69:369 – 476.

Brockbank KCM, DeJong JP, Piersma AH, Voerman JSA. Hemopoiesis in purified bone-marrow-derived reticular fibroblasts in vitro. Exp Hematol 1986;14:386 – 394.

Brondy VC, Zuckerman KS, Jetmalani S, Fitchen JH, Bagby GC. Monocytes stimulate fibroblastoid bone marrow stromal cells to produce multilineage hemopoietic growth factors. Blood 1986;68:530 – 537.

Castro-Malaspina H, Gay RE, Resnick G, et al. Characterization of human bone marrow fibroblast colony-forming cells (CFUf) and their progeny. Blood 1980;56:289 – 301.

Chamberlin W, Barone J, Kedo A, Fried W. Lack of recovery of murine hemopoietic stromal cells after irradiation-induced damage. Blood 1974;44:385 – 392.

Danis A. Etude de l'ossification dans les greffes de moelle osseuse. Acta Med Belg 1957;3:1 – 120.

Dexter TM, Allen TD, Lajtha LG. Conditions controlling the proliferation of hemopoietic stem cells in vitro. Cellular Physiol 1977;91:335 – 349.

Ebbe S, Phalen E, Ryan MK. The production of megakaryocytic macrocytosis by systemic factors in $Sl/Sl^d$ mice. Proc Soc Exp Biol Med 1977;155:243 – 250.

Epichima SY, Latzinik NV. Proliferative activity of stromal precursor cells with clonogenic properties. Bull Exp Biol Med 1976;1:55 – 59.

Fried W, Chamberlin W, Knospe WH, Trobaugh FE, Jr. Studies on the defective haemopoietic microenvironment of $Sl/Sl^d$ mice. Br J Haematol 1973;24:643 – 650.

Friedenstein AJ. Humoral nature of osteogenic activity of transitional epithelium. Nature 1962;194: 698 – 699.

Friedenstein AJ. Induction of bone tissue by transitional epithelium. Clin Orthop 1968;59:21 – 37.

Friedenstein AJ. Determined and inducible osteogenic precursor cells. In: Hard Tissue Growth Repair and Remineralization. Ciba Foundation Symposium (new series). Amsterdam Elsevier: 1973;170 – 185.

Friedenstein AJ. Precursor cells of mechanocytes. Int Rev Cytol 1976;47:327 – 359.

Friedenstein AJ. Stromal mechanocytes of bone marrow: cloning in vitro and retransplantation in vivo. In: Thierfelder S, Rodt H, Kolb HJ, eds. Immmunology of Bone Marrow Transplantation. Berlin: Springer-Verlag, 1980;19 – 29.

Friedenstein AJ, Kuralesova AJ. Osteogenic precursor cells of bone marrow in radiation chimeras. Transplantation 1971;12:99 – 108.

Friedenstein AJ, Luria EA. Cellular bases of hemopoietic microenvironment. Moscow Med 1980.

Friedenstein AJ, Lalykina KS. Lymphoid cell populations are competent systems for induced osteogenesis. Calcif Tissue Res 1970;4(Suppl):105 – 106.

Friedenstein AJ, Lalykina KS. Thymus cells are inducible to osteogenesis. Eur J Immunol 1972;2: 602 – 603.

Friedenstein AJ, Lalykina KS. Bone induction and osteogenic precursor cells. Moscow:Medicine, 1973.

Friedenstein AJ, Piatetzky-Shapiro JJ, Petrakova KV. Osteogenesis in transplants of bone marrow cells. J Embryol Exp Morph 1966;16:381 – 390.

Friedenstein AJ, Lalykina KS, Tolmacheva AA. Osteogenic activity of peritoneal fluid cells induced by transitional epithelium. Acta Anat 1967;68:532 – 549.

Friedenstein AJ, Petrakova KV, Kuralesova AJ, Frolova GP, Gorskaja UF, Kuralesova AJ, Latzinik NV, Gerasimov JV. Heterotopic transplants of bone marrow. Analysis of precursor cells for osteogenic and hemopoietic tissues. Transplantion 1968;6:230 – 247.

Friedenstein AJ, Chailkhyan RK, Lalykina KS. The development of fibroblasts colonies in monolayer cultures of guinea-pig bone marrow and spleen cells. Cell Tissue Kinet 1970;3:393 – 403.

Friedenstein AJ, Chailkhyan RK, Latzinik NV, Panasyk AF, Keilis-Borok IV. Stromal cells responsible for transferring the microenviroment of hemopoietic tissues. Cloning in vitro and retransplantation in vivo. Transplantation 1974a;17:331 – 340.

Friedenstein AJ, Deriglasova UF, Kulagina NN, Panasyk AF, Rudakowa SF, Luria EA, Rudakow TA. Precursors for fibroblasts in different populations of hematopoietic cells as detected by the in vitro colony assay method. Exp Hematol 1974b;2:83 – 92.

Friedenstein AJ, Gorskaja UF, Kulagina NN. Fibroblast precursors in normal and irradiated mouse hematopoietic organ. Exp Hematol 1976;4:267 – 274.

Friedenstein AJ, Ivanov-Smolenski AA, Chajlakyan RK. Origin of bone marrow stromal mechanocytes in radiochimeras and heterotopic transplants. Exp Hematol 1978;6:440 – 444.

Friedenstein AJ, Latzinik NV, Garskaya UF, Sidorovich SU. Radiosensitivity and postirradiation changes

Friedenstein AJ, Latzinik NV, Grosheva AG, Gorskaya UR. Marrow microenvironment transfer by heterotopic transplantation of freshly isolated and cultured cells in porous sponges. Exp Hematol 1982;10: 217 – 227.

Friedenstein AJ, Chailkhjan RK, Gerasimov UV. Bone marrow osteogenic stem cells: in vitro cultivation and transplantation in diffusion chambers. Cell Tissue Kinet 1987;20:263 – 272.

Friedenstein AJ. Bone marrow osteogenic stem cells. In: Cohn DV, Glorieux FH, Martin TJ, eds. Calcium Regulation and Bone Metabolism. Vol. 10. Amsterdam: Elsevier, 1990;353 – 361.

Gerasimov YV, Chailakhyan RK. Effect of curettage of the medullary cavity on bone marrow stromal precursor cells. Bull Exp Biol Med 1978;86:1243 – 1245.

Golde DW, Hocking WG, Quan SG, Sparkes RS, Gale RP. Origin of human bone marrow fibroblasts. Br J Haematol 1980;44:183 – 187.

Gordon MY, Gordon-Smith EC. Bone marrow fibroblastoid colony-forming cells (FCFU) in aplastic anaemia: colony growth and stimulation of granulocyte-macrophage colony-forming cells (GM-CFC) Br J Haematol 1981;49:465-472.

Gordon MY, Riley GP, Watt SM, Greaves MF. Compartmentization of a haemopoietic growth factor (GM-CFC) by glycosaminoglycans (GAGs) in the bone marrow microenvironment. Nature 1987;326:403 – 405.

Greenberg BR, Wilson FD, Woo L. Granulopoeitic effects of human bone marrow fibroblastic cells and abnormalities in 'granulopoietic microenvironment'. Blood 1981;58:557 – 563.

Gualtieri RJ. Consequences of extremely high doses of irradiation on bone marrow stromal cells and the release of hemopoietic growth factors. Exp Hematol 1987;9:952 – 957.

Gupta V, Rajarman S, Costanzi JJ. Effect of oxygen on the clonal growth of adherent cells (CFUf) from different compartments of mouse bone marrow. Exp Hematol 1987;15:1153 – 1157.

Hauschka PV, Chen TL, Mavarkos AE. Polypeptide growth factors in bone matrix. In: Everad D and Harnett S, eds. Cellular and Molecular Biology of Vertebrate Hard Tissues. Ciba Foundation Symposium 136, Chichester: John Wiley & Sons, 1988;207 – 219.

Hendry JH, Lord BI. The analysis of the early and late response to cytotoxic insults in the haemopoietic cell hierarchy. In: Potten CS, Hendry JH, eds. Cytotoxic Insults to Tissue. Edinburgh: Churchill Livingstone, 1983;1 – 66.

Hirata J, Kaneko S, Nishimura JN, Motamura S, Ibayashi H. Effect of platelet-derived growth factor and bone marrow-conditioned medium on the proliferation of human bone marrow-derived fibroblastoid colony-forming cells. Acta Hematol 1985;74:189 – 194.

Hollings PE, Fitzgerald PH, Heaton DE, Beard MEJ. Host origin of in vitro bone marrow fibroblasts after bone marrow transplantation in man. Int J Cell Cloning 1984;2:348 – 351.

Howlett CR, Cave J, Williamson M, Farmer J, Ali SY, Bab J, Owen ME. Mineralization in vitro of cultures of rabbit marrow stromal cells. Clin Orthop 1986;213:251 – 253.

Huggins C. The formation of bone under the influence of epithelium of the urinary tract. Arch Surg 1931;22:377 – 385.

Kaneko S, Motomura, Ibayashi H. Differentiation of human bone marrow-derived fibroblastoid colony forming cells (CFUf) Br J Haematol 1982;51:217 – 305.

Keating A, Singer JW, Killen PD, et al. Donor origin of the in vitro haemopoietic microenvironment after marrow transplantation in man. Nature 1982;289:280 – 283.

Keilis-Borok IV, Latzinik NV, Epichina SY, Friedenstein AJ. Dynamics of the formation of fibroblast colonies in monolayer cultures of bone marrow, according to $^{3}$H-thymidine incorporation experiments. Cytologia 1971;13:1402 – 1409.

Keilis-Borok IV, Rayevskaya MV, Friedenstein AJ. Properties of the bone tissue induced by the transitional epithelium. Bull Exp Biol Med 1982;94:1725 – 1728.

Knospe WH, Blom J, Crosby WH. Regeneration of locally irradiated bone marrow. I. Dose dependent long-term changes in the rat with particular emphasis upon vascular and stromal reaction. Blood 1966;28:398 – 405.

Knospe WH, Blom J, Crosby WH. Regeneration of locally irradiated bone marrow. II. Induction of regeneration of permanently aplastic medullar cavities. Blood 1968;31:400 – 409.

Kuzmenko GN, Panasyk AF, Friedenstein AJ, Kulagina NN. Radiosensitivity of bone marrow cells forming fibroblast colonies in monolayer cultures. Bull Exp Biol Med 1972;58:94 – 96.

Latzinik NV, Sidorovich SY, Tarchanova IA. Studies of surface receptors of the stromal mechanocytes of hemopoietic organs. Immunology (Moscow) 1980;1:26 – 28.

Latzinik NV, Sidorovich SU, Friedenstein AJ. Effect of bone marrow trypsinization on the efficacy of fibroblast colony formation in monolayer cultures. Bull Exp Biol Med 1981;9:257 – 384.

Latzinik NV, Gorskaya UF, Grosheva AG, et al. The content of stromal colony-forming cells (FCFC) in the mouse bone marrow and the clonal nature of FCFC-derived stromal fibroblast colonies. Ontogenesis 1986;17:27 – 35.

Latzinik NV, Friedenstein AJ, Pavlenko RG. Stimulation of CFUf colony formation by haemopoietic cells (in press).

Le Douarin NM, Houssaint E, Jotereau FV, Belo M. Origin of hemopoietic stem cells in embryonic bursa of Fabricius and bone marrow studied trough interspecific chimeras. Proc Natl Acad Sci 1975;72:2701 – 2705.

Lee M, Segal GM, Bagby GC. Interleukin-1 induces human bone marrow-derived fibroblasts to produce multilinage hemopoietic growth factors. Exp Hematol 1987;15:983 – 988.

Lennon JE, Micklem HS. Stromal cells in long-term murine bone marrow culture: FACS studies and origin of stromal cells in radiation chimeras. Exp Hematol 1986;14:287 – 292.

Lim B, Izagnirre CA, Aye MT, et al. Characterization of reticulofibroblastoid colonies (CFU-RF) derived from bone marrow and long-term marrow culture monolayers. J Cellular Physiol 1986;127:45 – 54.

Lovhang D, Pelus LM, Nordlie EM, Boyum A, Moore MAS. Monocyte-conditioned medium and interleukin induce granulocyte-macrophage colony stimulating factor production in the adherent cell layer of murine bone marrow cultures. Exp Hematol 1986;14:1037 – 1042.

Luria EA. Hematopoietic and Lymphoid Tissue in Culture. New York: Plenum Press, 1977.

Luria EA, Panasyuk AF, Friedenstein AJ. Fibroblast colony formation from monolayer cultures of blood cells. Transfusion 1971;11:345 – 349.

Luria EA, Owen ME, Friedenstein AJ, Morris JF, Kuznetsov SA. Bone formation in organ cultures of bone marrow. Cell Tissue Res 1987;248:449 – 454.

Luria EA, Kuznetsov SA, Genkina EN, Friedenstein AJ. Bone formation by mouse bone marrow cell suspensions in organ cultures. Bull Exp Biol Med 1988;6:720 – 723.

Luria EA, Friedenstein AJ, Groshewa AG, Gleyberman AE. Colony-forming precursors of fibroblast in circulating blood. Bull Exp Biol Med 1989;12:712 – 71.

Maximov AA. Uber experimentelle Erzeugung von Knochenmarks-Gewebe. Vorlaufige Mitteilung Anat Anz 1906;28:24 – 38.

Maximov AA. Cultures of blood leucocytes. From lymphocyte and monocyte to connective tissue. Arch Exp Zellforsch 1928;5:169 – 178.

Marshall MJ, Nisbet NW, Evans S. Donor origin of the in vitro haemopoietic microenvironment after marrow transplantation in mice. Experientia 1984;40:385.

McIntyre AP, Bjornson BH. Human bone marrow stromal cell colonies: response to hydrocortisone and dependence on platelet-derived growth factor. Exp Hematol 1986;14:833 – 839.

Micklein HS, Loutit JF. Tissue Grafting and Radiation. New York: Academic Press, 1966.

Miskarova ED, Lalykina KS, Kokorin JN, Friedenstein AJ. Osteogenic potencies of prolonged diploid cultures of myeloid cells. Bull Exp Med 1970;56:78 – 81.

Munker R, Casson J, Ogawa M, Koeffler HP. Recombinant human TNF induces production of granulocyte-monocyte colony stimulating factor. Nature 1986;323:79 – 87.

Owen M. The origin of bone cells. Intern Rev Cytol 1970;28:213 – 230.

Owen M. Linage of osteogenic cells and their relationship to the stromal system. In: Peck WA, ed. Bone and Mineral Research, Vol. 3. Amsterdam: Elsevier, 1985;1 – 25.

Owen ME, Cave J, Joyner CJ. Clonal analysis in vitro of osteogenic differentiation of marrow CFUf. J Cell Sci 1987;87:731 – 738.

Owen ME, Friedenstein AJ. Stromal stem cells: marrow derived osteogenic precursors. In: Evered D, Harnett S, eds. Cellular and Molecular Biology of Vertebrate Hard Tissues. Ciba Foundation Symposium 136. Chichester: John Wiley & Sons, 1988;42 – 52.

Petrakova KV, Tolmacheva AA, Friedenstein AG. Bone formation occurring in bone marrow transplantation in diffusion chambers. Bull Exp Biol Med 1963;12:87 – 91.

Piersma AH, Ploemacher RE, Brockbank KGM. Transplantation of bone marrow fibroblastoid stromal cells in mice via the intravenous route. Br J Haematol 1983;54:285 – 292.

Pfeilschifter J, D'Souza S, Mundy GR. Transforming growth factor beta is released from resorbing bone and stimulates osteoblast activity. J Bone Miner Res 1986;1:294.

Qusenberry PJ, Ginbrone MA. Vascular endothelium as a regulator of granulopoiesis production of colony-stimulating activity by cultured human endothelial cells. Blood 1980;56:1060.

Roberts R, Gallagher J, Spooncer E, Allen TD, Bloomfield F, Dexter TM. Heparan sulphate bound growth factors: a mechanism for stromal cell mediated haemopoiesis. Nature 1988;332:376 – 378.

Schofield R, Lorimore SA, Wright EG. Ectopic implantation studies using $Sl/Sl^d$ marrow and recipients. Exp Hematol 1987;15:217 – 220.

Sacerdotti C, Frattin G. Ueber die heteroplastische knochenbildung. Arch Path Anat Physiol 1902;168:431 – 446.

Tavassoli M, Crosby WH. Transplantation of marrow to extramedullary sites. Science 1968;161:54 – 56.

Tavassoli M, Friedenstein AJ. Hemopoietic stromal microenvironment. Am J Hematol 1983;15:195 – 203.

Tavassoli M, Maniatis A, Binder RA, Crosby WH. Studies on marrow histogenesis. Proc Soc Exp Biol Med 1971;138:868 – 870.

Termine JD. Non-collagen proteins in bone. In: Evered D, Harnett S, eds. Cellular and Molecular Biology of Vertebrate Hard Tissues. Ciba Foundation Symposium 136. Chichester: John Wiley & Sons, 1988;118 – 202.

Urist MR. Bone formation by autoinduction. Science 1965;150:893 – 899.

Urist MR, Huo YK, Brownell AG. Purification of bovine bone morphogenic protein by hydroxyapatite chromatography. Proc Natl Acad Sci 1984;81:371 – 375.

Wang OR, Wolf NS. The effect of several growth factors on the in vitro growth of bone marrow stromal cells. Exp Hematol 1987;15:610.

Wan-Ming DA, David DF, Biggs JC. Studies of hemopoietic stromal fibroblastic colonies in patients undergoing bone marrow transplantation. Exp Hematol 1986;14:266 – 270.

Willmer N. Morphological problems of cell type, shape and identification. In: Willmer EN, ed. Cell and Tissue in Culture, Vol 1. New York: Academic Press, 1964;143 – 176.

Wilson FD, O'Grady L, McNeill CJ, Munn SL. The formation of bone marrow-derived fibroblastic plaques in vitro. Exp Hematol 1974;2:343 – 349.

Wilson FD, Greenberg GR, Konrad PN, Klein AD, Walling PA. Cytogenetic studies on bone marrow fibroblasts from male-female haemopoietic chimera: evidence that stromal elements in human transplantation recipients are of host type. Transplantation 1978;25:87 – 92.

Zucali JR, Dinarello CA, Oblon DJ, Gross MA, Anderson L, Weiner RS. Interleukin 1 stimulates fibroblasts to produce granulocyte macrophage colony-stimulating activity and prostoglandin $E_2$. J Clin Invest 1986;78:1316 – 1323.

Zucali JR, Broxmeyer HE, Dinarello CA, Gross MA, Weiner RS. Regulation of early human haematopoetic (BFU-E) and CFU-GEMM progenitor cells in vitro by interleukin-1 induced fibroblast conditioned medium. Blood 1987;69:33 – 41.

Zuckerman KS, Prince CW, Rhodes RK, Ribedeneira M. Resistance of the stromal cells in murine long-term bone marrow cultures to damage by ionizing radiation. Exp Hematol 1986;14:1056 – 1062.

*Bone and Mineral Research/7*
*Johan N.M. Heersche and John A. Kanis, editors*



# Estrogens and bone

Erik Fink Eriksen and Leif Mosekilde

*Medical Department III, Division of Endocrinology and Metabolism, Aarhus Amtssygehus, 8000 Aarhus C, Denmark*

## I. Introduction

Estrogen deficiency is recognized as one of the most important causes of osteoporosis and estrogen treatment has been used in the prophylaxis against postmenopausal osteoporosis for more than 15 years (Horsman et al. 1977; Lindsay et al. 1977; Christiansen et al. 1980a, b; Riggs et al. 1986; Munk Jensen et al. 1988). The vast majority of data concerning estrogen action on bone have been derived from bone densitometric studies, and massive evidence for preservation of bone mass during estrogen treatment of postmenopausal women has been obtained.

The effects of estrogen at the level of individual bone cells have, however, remained elusive, mainly because estrogen receptors were thought to be non-existent in bone. Recently, however, two groups independently demonstrated the presence of estrogen receptors as well as postreceptor effects of estradiol in normal human bone cells (Eriksen et al. 1988) and transformed rat bone cells (Komm et al. 1988). These findings in concert with recent advances in cell biology and the understanding of the intermediary organization of bone will probably lead to a mass of new information on the action of estradiol on bone in the coming years. The purpose of this chapter is, therefore, to summarize the current knowledge about estrogens and their action on bone and to point out certain areas that need more attention in the coming years.

## II. Estrogen biosynthesis, secretion and degradation

In women, the ovary is normally the major source of estrogens, although the conversion of androgen precursors to estrone ($E_1$) in other tissues gains clinical importance after the menopause or oophorectomy (Siiteri 1973; Deslypere et al. 1985). During estrogen synthesis cholesterol is converted to pregnenolone. This compound is later converted to androstenedione, the major androgen secreted by the ovary. This conversion takes place either through progesterone and 17-alpha-hydroxyprogesterone or through 17-alpha-hydroxypregnenolone and dehydroepiandrosterone (DHEA) (Fig. 1) (Goldfien and Monroe 1983). Androstenedione is reversibly converted to testosterone, which by the aromatase complex is transformed irreversibly to 17-beta-estradiol ($E_2$), the major estrogen produced by the ovary. $E_2$ is reversibly oxidized to form estrone ($E_1$), which in term is irreversibly hydroxylated at the C-16-alpha position to form 16-alpha-hydroxyestrone and estriol ($E_3$) (Fishman 1960). These metabolites possess some estrogenic potential (Fishman 1980).

During the menstrual cycle, regulation of biosynthesis and release of the hormones is controlled by the gonadotropins as well as by local factors. When $E_2$ is released into the bloodstream it binds to sex hormone binding globulin (SHBG) and with less affinity to albumin. The proportion of free to bound $E_2$ does not vary significantly during the menstrual cycle. However, differences in binding may assume clinical importance after the menopause.

The metabolism of $E_2$ involves a series of oxidative transformations (Goldfien and Monroe 1983) (Table 1). Circulating $E_2$ is rapidly converted in the liver to estrone by 17-beta-hydroxysteroid dehydrogenase. Although some of the estrone re-enters the

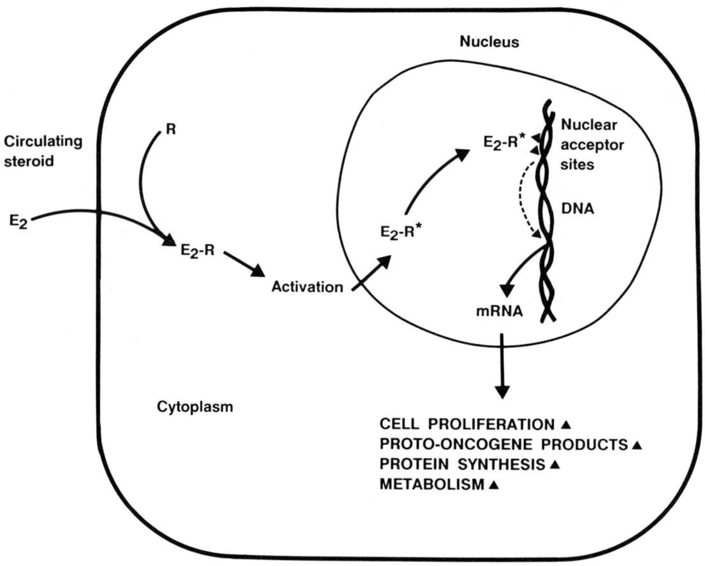


Fig. 1. Schematic drawing showing the current concept of estrogen-receptor interaction with nuclear acceptor sites. Estrogens ($E_2$) enter the cell by diffusion over the cell membrane. In the cytoplasm the steroid ligand interacts with free estrogen receptor (R) and creates a ligand receptor complex ($E_2$-R) which after activation ($E_2$-R*) enters the nuclear compartment and binds to nuclear acceptor sites on the DNA. The binding elicits altered mRNA processing at sites situated some distance away from the acceptor site. In the classical target tissues the final result of faltered mRNA processing is stimulation of proliferation, protein synthesis, cellular metabolism and as recently shown, expression of proto-oncogene mRNA.

TABLE 1. Biosynthesis and degradation of estrogens

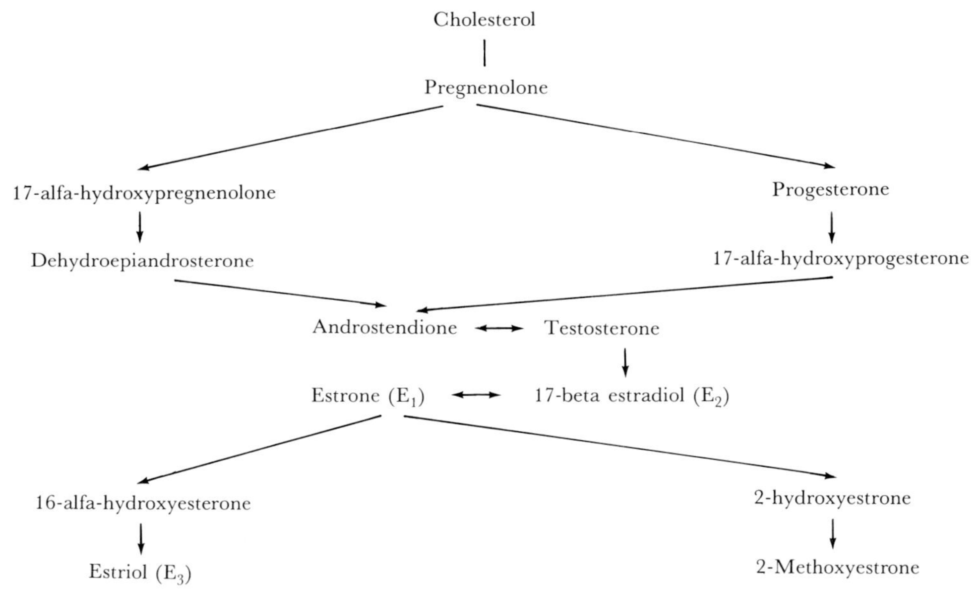


circulation, most of it is irreversibly hydroxylated either in the $C_2$ position to form 2-hydroxyestrone and 2-methoxyestrone, or at the C-16-alpha position to form 16-alpha-hydroxyestrone and estriol ($E_3$). The two pathways are mutually exclusive and lead to products with quite different biological properties. The 16-alpha-hydroxy compounds are biologically active, whereas the 2-hydroxy estrogens are virtually devoid of estrogenic activity (Jellineck 1981). The latter compounds are rapidly cleared from the circulation (Kono 1982) by conjugation processes in the liver to form sulphated and/or glucuronidated metabolites, that are excreted primarily in the urine and to a lesser extent through the bile.

## III. Mechanism of steroid action

The modern concepts of the mechanism of estrogen action are based mainly on studies of breast cancer tissue in the early sixties demonstrating the presence of specific receptor proteins in target cells that recognize and interact with estrogen ligand leading to changes in gene expression in the target cell (Jensen et al. 1969; Korenmann et al. 1970; McGuire et al. 1975). As studies on steroid receptors in bone cells are few, most of the general data on estrogen receptors and mechanisms of estrogen action given below will be based mainly on studies using transformed cell systems or the reproductive system.

The mechanism, whereby estrogen interacts with DNA in order to alter mRNA transscription seems to be the same for all sex steroids and is depicted in Fig. 1. The transport of steroid from blood into the cell across the cell membrane does not seem to involve specific carrier mechanisms, but its thought to take place through passive diffusion. Diffusion over the phospholipid bilayer is facilitated by the general hydrophobic nature of the cholesterol backbone of the steroid molecule. Once the hormone enters the cytoplasm it is bound to a steroid- and tissue-specific receptor macromolecule (Jensen and DeSombre 1973). The ligand is bound with very high affinity ($K_d$ in the range of $10^{-9}$ to $10^{-10}$ M). After binding of ligand the receptor undergoes conformational changes enabling it to bind to nuclear acceptor sites ('activation') (Thrall et al. 1978; Spelsberg et al. 1982; Muller et al. 1983). The binding to nuclear acceptor sites occurs after a few minutes and leads to alteration of gene expression through changes in the processing of mRNA (O'Malley and Means 1974). These changes can be detected after 20 – 30 min and the subsequent processing of these mRNAs into proteins (detectable after 1 – 6 h) affect several aspects of cellular function that will be described in more detail below.

## A. The estrogen receptor (ER): physico-chemical properties

Ultracentrifugation studies have revealed that the occupied nuclear receptor migrates at 4 – 5 S, while the unoccupied receptor migrates at 8 – 9 S. The receptor transformation from 8 to 9 S to 4 – 5 S and the nuclear translocation of the 4 – 5 S species is a temperature-dependent process (Gorski et al. 1968; Jensen and DeSombre 1973). It has been proposed to define receptor transformation in another way, namely as the change in biochemical form of the receptor that results in increased affinity for nuclear components such as DNA or chromatin (Spelsberg et al. 1981b; Muller et al., 1983). The precise mechanism underlying transformation is unknown, but it probably involves a combination of association or dissociation of subunits and conformational changes (Sherman and Stevens 1984). One study has even proposed the existence of an ER transforming factor, which should work as a calcium-dependent protease (Puca et al. 1984).

The fact that the majority of ER reside in the nucleus has further been proven by several other methods: (a) autoradiographic localization based on previous injection with tritiated steroid (Sheridan et al. 1979); (b) subcellular fractionation studies showing the greatest binding to nuclei (Mester and Beaulieu 1972); (c) studies on cytochalasin B enucleated cells (Welshons et al. 1984) and (d) immunocytochemical localization studies employing monoclonal antibodies against the estrogen receptor (Greene et al. 1984).

In the crude cytosol prepared from target tissues ER is present as an 8 – 9 S complex, with a molecular weight of approximately 300 000. If incubated in media of increased ionic strength the receptor transforms into the pure hormone binding 4 – 5 S subunit(s). Two different models of the untransformed 8 – 9 S form have been proposed. One model postulates the participation of two non-steroid binding protein components (apparent $M_r$ 58 000 and 14 000) (Murayama et al. 1980). The alternative model suggests the binding unit being a homo-oligomer (Sica et al. 1976). The most recent study on the untransformed estradiol receptor, however, suggests the presence of two binding subunits arranged as a hetero-oligomer ($M_r$ of 62 000 and 65 000), with two molecules reacting with antibodies against a heat-shock protein ($M_r$ 90 000) attached to the complex (Redeuilh et al. 1987). These authors further suggested that transformation involved the release of this heat-shock protein from the complex leading to nuclear translocation of the pure steroid binding subunit-organized dimers.

In the mouse, similar studies have revealed nuclear ER heterogeneity consisting of a doublet with apparent molecular masses of 66.4 and 65 kDa. ER isolated from the cytoplasmic component revealed only one band of 65 kDa. Binding analysis revealed predominant binding of steroid to the 65 kDa component (Golding and Korach 1988). Analysis of the non-steroid binding component in the calf uterus has revealed a 90 kDa component with close homology to three different heat shock proteins (Ratajcsak et al. 1988).

ER cDNA clones from the transformed breast cancer cell line MCF-7 and the chicken oviduct have been reported. They were found to code for polypeptides of 595 and 589 amino acids, respectively ($M_r$ around 66 000) (Green et al. 1986; Greene et al. 1986) and a certain homology with the proto-oncogene v-erb-a was demonstrable (Green et al. 1986).

Based on observations on tissue specificity and saturability of estrogen binding to nuclei the hypothesis of the existence of nuclear acceptor sites emerged. Spelsberg et al. (1981a, b, 1983, 1987) have performed detailed studies on nuclear acceptor sites. They found that the acceptor sites were confined to a non-histone chromosomal protein fraction. These investigators published evidence for the existence of the association between specific DNA-sequences and acceptor sites, suggesting the existence of a DNA protein complex of non-histone proteins and the DNA backbone (Spelsberg et al. 1987). These findings have further been corroborated by the demonstration of specific DNA sequences that reveal selective binding of purified receptor protein (Jost et al. 1984). According to the hypotheses put forward by these authors steroids bind to acceptor sites distant from the estrogen-regulated structural genes (Spelsberg et al. 1987). Comparison of sequences have shown that all steroid receptors share a common highly conserved cysteine rich region, that functions as the DNA-binding region (Giguere et al. 1988).

## B. Regulation of estrogen receptor concentrations

17-Beta estradiol and several other estrogen analogues are able to increase the concentration of ER in a variety of model systems, while tamoxifen and clomiphene reduces ER concentration (Juriansz et al. 1988). In reproductive tissue, ER concentrations may be altered by concomitant administration of progesterone (Fuentealba et al.

1988), whether this is the case in bone cells too remains to be established. Three different phases may be defined, when dealing with changes in receptor concentrations: (1) rapid changes due to nuclear translocation, (2) an 8 – 12 h recycling phase and (3) changes in receptor concentrations due to alterations in receptor synthesis (Walters 1986). The factors affecting ER concentrations in bone cells are still unknown.

## IV. Receptor assays

### A. Qualitative estrogen receptor assays

*(1) Monoclonal ER antibodies.* Greene et al. (1984) were the first to produce a monoclonal antibody that interacts specifically with the ER. This antibody has mainly been used qualitatively for the demonstration of ER in tissue sections or cell samples. It seems to be less sensitive than assays based on radioligands, but is a good tool for the screening of tissues with high contents of receptor (e.g. breast cancer) (Weiss et al. 1986; Schulze and Barrack 1987).

*(2) [$^3$H]estradiol and [$^{125}$I]estradiol binding.* One study has reported the use of [$^3$H]estradiol as a ligand in binding studies involving frozen sections of prostate and urethra (Thornton 1987). Due to the low specific activity of these isotopes, however, significant problems may arise when using these techniques in tissues with low receptor concentrations.

[$^{125}$I]estradiol possesses a much higher specific activity and has been used for the autoradiographic demonstration of ER in the transformed breast cancer cell line MCF-7, rat and calf uterus (Hochberg 1979; Els et al. 1985; Stumpf et al. 1987). Less data are available on the use in quantitative assays. The ligand has, however, been used for the simultaneous demonstration of estrogen- and progesterone receptor (Thibodeau et al. 1981) and Komm et al. (1988) were able to detect very low levels of ER in rat osteoblasts.

### B. Quantitative estrogen receptor assays

*(1) Methods based on cell lysis and charcoal separation.* The earliest assays for ER were based on quantification of receptors in cell lysates. Lysis of cells was carried out in hypoosmolar environment. Later studies showed that stabilization of the receptor could be obtained by the addition of molybdenum (Sica et al. 1977; Muller et al. 1983). The number of receptors and other characteristics of ligand-receptor interactions were quantitated by the incubation of the lysate with tritiated estrogen ($^3$H-$E_2$) at 4°C. After incubation for 18 – 24 h bound and unbound ligands were separated by addition of either dextran-coated charcoal (DCC) or hydroxyapatite followed by centrifugation (Jensen et al. 1969; Korenman and Dukes 1970; McGuire et al. 1975).

Several problems are associated with this method. First of all, the method relies on the liberation of receptor-material from the nucleus during hypo-osmolar lysis. This liberation may vary, and the stability of the receptor macromolecule may be affected by the assay buffer despite the addition of stabilizers like molybdenum. Moreover, recent studies have demonstrated that the results obtained with the DCC assay lack correlation to the cellular effects of steroid ligand. Studies mainly employing the chick oviduct have demonstrated that estrogen withdrawal-induced alterations in progesterone receptor binding obtained with the DCC assay did not reflect changes in mRNA or avidin production. These findings led to the introduction of the concept of non-functional receptors (i.e. receptors that bind ligand, but do not lead to transcriptional activity; Spelsberg and Boyd Leinen 1980a; Graham et al. 1984).

*(2) The biopsy nuclear binding assay.* The problems with functional and non-functional receptors led to the development of other approaches to steroid receptor quantification, and recently an assay system, the biopsy nuclear binding (BNB) assay, that solves most of the problems associated with conventional DCC assays has been described (Graham et al. 1984; Eriksen et al. 1988). The (BNB) assay involves the addition of tritiated steroid to intact cells either trypsinized from cell cultures or liberated through collagenase treatment of tissue samples. The incubation takes place at physiological temperature and after 1 h the cells are lysed. A nuclear pellet is obtained by centrifuging the lysate through a sucrose gradient and the amount of ligand bound to the nuclei is measured by liquid scintillation together with simultaneous estimation of the DNA content of the pellet. This method has been shown to correlate very well to cellular activity in the chick oviduct system in that it only measures functional receptors. It seems to be more sensitive than the DCC and monoclonal antibody assays (Eriksen et al. 1988), probably because the assay method protects against receptor degradation. Moreover, it requires less tissue or cells than the DCC assay. Nuclear exchange assays have also been shown to correlate well to changes in uterine growth in rats or ovalbumin synthesis in chicks after treatment with estradiol (Anderson et al. 1973).

## V. Estrogen receptors in bone

As the first studies showing clinical effects of estrogens on bone emerged, several authors tried to demonstrate estrogen receptors in bone.

Van Paassen et al. (1978) assayed cytosol preparations from human femoral heads and rat bone, but were unable to demonstrate any receptor binding using sucrose gradient analysis as well as charcoal separation.

Chen and Feldman (1978) investigated cytoplasmic extracts from cultured fetal rat calvarial cells and adult ovariectomized rats for estrogen receptors employing tritiated $E_2$ and Sephadex chromatography for separation of bound and unbound receptor.

None of the prepations exhibited specific binding of estradiol. Corticosteroid receptors were, however, demonstrable. Bone extracts from perinatal rats revealed high levels of estrogen binding, but further analysis of binding characteristics showed that the binding was attributable to the presence of alfa-foetoprotein in the extracts.

Yoshioka et al. (1980) used a whole cell incubation system but were also unable to demonstrate specific binding of estradiol and androgen to cytoplasmatic and nuclear fractions of rat bone cytosol. They were, however, able to demonstrate specific nuclear binding of progesterone analog R5020 and dexamethasone.

In a more recent paper by Morel et al. (1985) monoclonal antibodies against ER were employed in a combined immunocytochemical-electron microscopic analysis of rat bone, but no significant immunoreactivity for estrogen receptor could be demonstrated.

The apparent absence of ER in bone seemed to be further corroborated by studies in rat organ culture systems, showing the absence of direct estrogen effects on bone resorption (Caputo et al. 1976; Stewart and Stern 1987), prostaglandin production (Feyen and Raisz 1987) or osteoblastic collagen synthesis (Canalis et al. 1978).

These studies led to the conclusion that the effects of estrogen on bone were probably indirectly mediated, be it through interaction with the action of PTH or calcitonin on bone or some other mechanism (see Section VIII). The data were, however, confounded by the fact that giant cell tumors, that are mainly of osteoblastic origin, were shown to possess estrogen and progesteron receptors (Malawer et al. 1984). In this study, specific estrogen and progesterone binding was demonstrable by fluorescent histochemical methods. It is worth noting, however, that when the DCC assay was used on two positive cell lines, no binding could be detected.

Lopez et al. (1986) reported estradiol and testosterone binding sites in tibia cytosol from mice, without being able to specifically relate them to bone cells. It is interesting, however, that these authors reported binding sites for estradiol and testosterone only in the epiphyses, but not in the diaphyses.

Gray et al. (1987) reported specific effects of 17-beta estradiol on proliferation and differentiation of the rat osteosarcoma cell line UMR-106, that could not be reproduced if the stereoisomer 17-alfa estradiol was used. This study prompted new attempts to look for estrogen receptors in bone cells, and Eriksen et al. (1988) demonstrated specific nuclear receptors in normal, non transformed human bone cells cultured from trabecular bone. Employing the BNB assay described above it was possible to demonstrate a mean of 1600 receptors per nucleus (Fig. 2). The binding was temperature-dependent, steroid-specific, and saturable. Moreover, the binding was cell type-specific, because human skin fibroblasts and other non-target tissues like colon, spleen and lung revealed much lower binding (less than 500 receptors per nucleus). The number of receptors was in the range of the numbers obtained from freshly isolated endometrium (around 4000 per nucleus). It is worth noting, however, that the number of binding sites calculated for normal human tissue like bone and endometrium is much lower than the number obtained from malignant tissue, e.g. breast

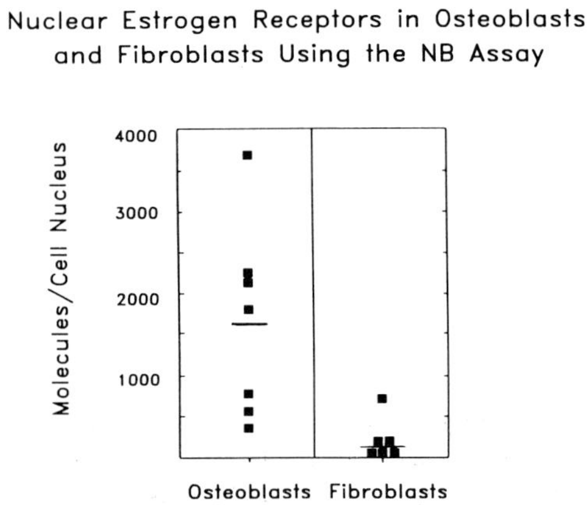


Fig. 2. Estrogen receptor concentrations in seven strains of cultured human osteoblast-like cells obtained from normal women compared to cultured human skin fibroblasts. (From Eriksen et al. 1988, with permission.)

cancer (20 – 30 000 receptors per nucleus). The data were further corroborated by the demonstration of mRNA for the human ER in the same cells using Northern blotting. The full length cDNA probe to human ER hybridized to a band at approximately 6.4 kilobases (kb), which corresponded to the positive band of the strongly ER positive breast cancer cell line MCF-7. The size was furthermore in the range reported in previous papers describing cloning of ER (Greene et al. 1986; Green et al. 1986). Finally, it was possible to induce progesterone receptor, a classical estrogen receptor-mediated response (Sumida et al. 1988), in the majority of cell lines exposed to estrogen for 24 h (Fig. 3).

Simultaneously, Komm et al. (1988) demonstrated specific ER binding in the clonal rat cell line ROS 17/2.8 and the human osteosarcoma cell line HOS TE85 (200 binding sites). They used iodinated 17-beta estradiol and nuclear extracts. Moreover, mRNA coding for ER was demonstrable at 6.0 to 6.2 kb. This group was also able to demonstrate postreceptor responses like increased production of collagen type I and transforming growth factor beta (TGF-beta) mRNA after 17-beta estradiol administration.

Finally, these findings have been further corroborated by a Swiss group (Ernst et al. 1988) demonstrating a dose-dependent and specific 17-beta estradiol-mediated enhancement of proliferation and collagen type I mRNA in normal rat osteoblast-like cells. These responses were abolished after addition of the antiestrogenic analogue tamoxifen.

Thus, evidence indicates that the effects of estradiol on bone could be mainly mediated through binding to a specific nuclear receptor leading to induction of specific responses in the target cell.

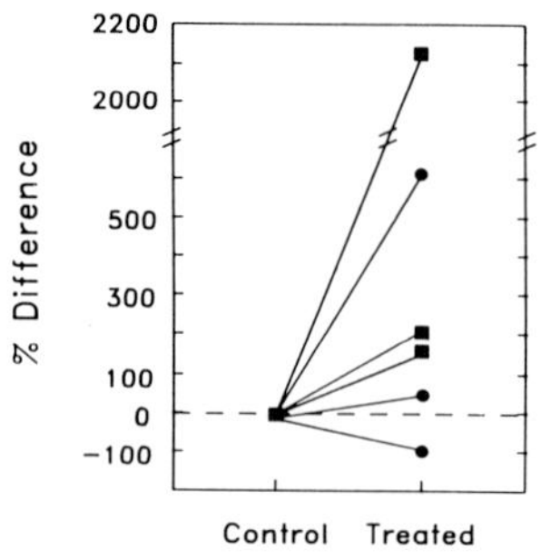


Fig. 3. Induction of progesterone receptor in six strains of cultured human osteoblast-like cells obtained from three normal women (■) and three normal men (●) after a 24-h exposure to 10 nM 17-beta estradiol. The results are expressed as the percentage difference between the specific binding of progesterone analog [$^3$H]R5020 in mean molecules per nucleus in the estrogen-treated cells compared to that of control cells (that is, not estradiol treated) from the same strain. (From Eriksen et al. 1988, with permission.)

## VI. Cellular responses to estrogen receptor binding

The effects of estrogens have been most thoroughly studied in the reproductive system, mainly using the rat uterus or the chick oviduct as models. In these tissues estrogen increases cell proliferation as expressed in increased thymidine incorporation. Messenger RNA polymerase activity is also increased leading to an increase in the total amount of RNA in the tissue. The mRNA codes for several distinct proteins like histones, enzymes and distinct uterine proteins (Hamilton et al. 1953; Jensen and DeSombre 1973; O'Malley 1974). Moreover, the general metabolic activity is increased as reflected in increased glucose utilization, lactate production, amino acid transport and $O_2$ consumption (Szego and Roberts 1953; Coulson and Gorski 1967; Riggs et al. 1968). The mechanism underlying the stimulatory effect of estradiol on cell proliferation is still unknown, but it may be related to the estrogen-mediated effects on *c*-myc and *c*-ras oncogene expression that have been demonstrated in the breast cancer cell line MCF-7 (Katsaros et al. 1988; Wilding et al. 1988). These oncogenes are known to affect cell proliferation. Moreover, estrogen has been shown to regulate the number of receptors for epidermal growth factor in other tissues (Mukku 1986). The estrogen-mediated increases in collagen type I message and other osteoblast-related proteins is probably related to altered mRNA processing as previously described.

In bone cells, $E_2$ increases TGF-beta mRNA (Komm et al. 1988). This finding may explain some of the effects of estradiol on bone cell proliferation *in vitro,* because TGF-beta is a very potent regulator of osteoblast proliferation (Pfeilschifter and Mundy 1987).

## VII. Estrogen effects on bone remodelling

Before reviewing the effects of estrogen on bone remodelling, it is necessary to summarize the current knowledge on the intermediary organization of bone and the mechanisms by which bone is lost from the skeleton.

### A. Remodelling and internal organization of bone

Bone is continuously renewed (remodelled) throughout life (Frost 1969) in order to secure the viability of the cells and the biomechanical competence of the skeleton. Bone remodelling takes place at localized sites in cortical and trabecular bone. In cortical bone following *activation* (i.e. recruitment of osteoclast precursors at the given resorptive site) a group of osteoclasts creates a 'cutting cone', which erodes a canal through existing bone without any notice of the previously formed osteons (Jaworski 1977). When resorption is completed the osteoblasts start forming new concentric layers of lamellar bone, the 'closing cone' (Jaworski 1977). Bone resorption lasts for approximately one month and formation for about 3 months after which a new completed osteon (Bone Structural Unit, BSU) has been formed at the site of previous resorption. The hole created by bone resorption has been refilled and the cells have been renewed. In cortical bone the BSUs form typical patterns of several generations of osteons, which in cross-sections are nearly circular structures with concentric lamellae surrounding a central canal (Jaworski 1977).

During the last few years, it has become obvious that trabecular bone is renewed in the same way as cortical bone. Trabecular bone consists of BSUs (or packets or walls), which in sections present as crescent-shaped structures with parallel lamellae outlined by the trabecular bone surface and the cement line (Kragstrup et al. 1982; Eriksen et al. 1986). These BSUs are, like the osteons of cortical bone, renewed by osteoclastic resorption followed by osteoblastic formation (Eriksen et al. 1986). Following activation, osteoclasts and later mononuclear cells erode from the bone surface to a mean depth of about 65 $\mu$m, the final resorption depth (Eriksen et al. 1984a). The osteoblasts are proceeding to form bone and during this process they gradually become more and more pyknotic and end up as inactively looking flat lining cells or surface osteocytes (Eriksen et al. 1984b).

During remodelling, the *coupling* between bone resorption and bone formation secures the preservation of bone mass in spite of large interindividual variations in bone turnover (Parfitt 1982). Uncoupling, which indicates that resorption is not followed by formation or that formation starts without previous resorption may however, occur at the periosteal and endosteal surfaces. Uncoupling has to be distinguished from *imbalance* between the amount of bone resorbed and formed during one remodelling cycle (Parfitt 1979).

## B. Pathogenetic mechanisms underlying variations in bone mass

In spite of the coupling between resorption and formation changes in bone mass occur, most often in terms of bone loss. Several different mechanisms may be responsible for the loss of bone after menopause (Parfitt 1976, 1984). In order to understand the effects of estrogen on bone loss it is important to distinguish between reversible and irreversible bone loss. Reversible bone loss is induced by enhanced activation of new remodelling cycles followed by a similar gain in bone mass after normalization of bone turnover, in contrast to irreversible bone loss, which denotes permanent loss of bone.

Figure 4b illustrates the effect of increased activation frequency on trabecular bone. Due to the increased number of newly activated remodelling cycles, where bone is resorbed but not yet reformed, the bone will show increased porosity (compare to Fig. 4a). This increased porosity is of course followed by mobilization of bone mineral and temporary reduction of bone mass. Following normalization of the activation frequency (Fig. 4a), resorption will decrease before formation and the holes will be refilled with bone. This is an example of reversible bone loss due an expansion of the remodelling space (i.e. the amount of bone resorbed and yet not reformed during the remodelling process). Such changes occur in hyperparathyroidism (Eriksen et al.

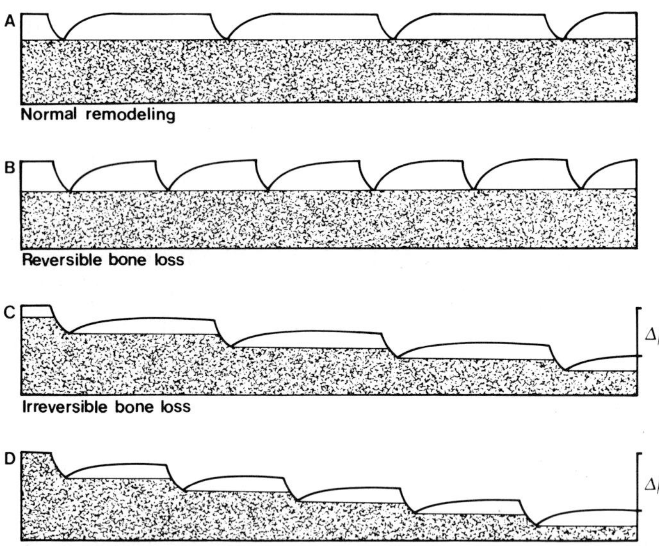


Fig. 4. Different types of bone loss. (A) Remodelling with no imbalance between resorption and formation, resulting in preservation of bone mass; (B) increased activation without a change in balance between resorption and formation leading to an expansion of the remodelling space and reversible bone loss. (C) Bone remodelling with a negative net balance between resorption and formation resulting in an irreversible loss of bone. (D) Net negative balance between resorption and formation associated with an increased activation frequency resulting in an accelerated irreversible bone loss. (From Eriksen 1986, with permission.)

1986) and during antler growth in deer (Parfitt 1976).

A negative balance per remodelling cycle between the amount of bone resorbed and later formed will create an irreversible bone loss (Fig. 4c). This occurs in postmenopausal osteoporosis (Eriksen et al. 1986, 1990). If a simultaneous increase in activation frequency occurs, a mixture of reversible and irreversible bone loss is present and the negative balance at tissue and organ level will be enhanced (Fig. 4d). This type of bone loss is found in hyperthyroidism (Melsen and Mosekilde 1977; Eriksen et al. 1986) and around menopause. In trabecular bone, another mechanism of irreversible bone loss exists, namely trabecular perforation. This process, which by its nature is related to the activation frequency, is probably of major importance for the normal age-related loss of trabecular bone (Parfitt 1984). The average resorption depth in trabecular bone is 60 $\mu$m, but can amount to several hundred $\mu$m in some lacunae (Eriksen et al. 1984a). The average trabecular thickness is around 150 $\mu$m, but shows great scatter from close to zero and up to several hundred $\mu$m. Therefore, the possibility exists that a deep resorption lacuna hits a thin trabeculum or two lacunae meet each other midway through a trabeculum and thus perforates the structure. This will result in the removal of the structural basis for subsequent bone formation (uncoupling), and the final result will be a hole in the trabecular network, irreversible loss of bone and reduced mechanical competence of the bone affected. The risk for perforation increases with increased activation frequency, increased resorption depth and decreased trabecular thickness.

### C. Bone structure and bone strength

Non load-bearing trabecular bone from younger individuals consists of uniform boxes of trabecular plates forming a honeycomb structure, which combines maximum strength with minimal bone mass. The architecture of load-bearing trabecular bone from the same person will be characterized by thick plates and columns oriented in the direction of the compressive forces sustained by thinner trabecular struts in the non load-bearing direction (anisotropy). The trabecular elements of younger individuals are completely connected giving a maximum of support. This trabecular framework changes with age. The thick load-bearing plates are successively perforated during the remodelling processes and converted in columns and the thinner non load-bearing trabeculae are disconnected and often disappear. The biomechanical consequences of this loss of continuity in the three-dimensional lattice are pronounced (Mosekilde and Mosekilde 1986, 1987). As the thinner trabeculae disappear, the slenderness ratio (i.e. the ratio of length between supporting struts to the ratio of the load-bearing columns) of the remaining trabeculae increases. When this ratio reaches a critical level elastic buckling and bending forces will dominate instead of compressive forces (Euler buckling). These processes explain why bone strength decreases with age even after normalization for bone mass (Mosekilde and Mosekilde 1986, 1987).

During adulthood, the skeleton shows a generalized tendency towards slow appositional growth leading to an increased diameter of tubular bones and an expansion of the marrow cavity due to a positive balance at the periosteal envelope and a negative balance at the endosteal envelope. Similar changes have been observed in irregular weightbearing bones where it, to some extent, might reduce the effect on bone strength of the reduction in trabecular bone mass with age (Mosekilde and Mosekilde 1986).

## VIII. Estrogens and other osteotrophic hormones

### A. Estrogens and parathyroid hormone (PTH)

Heaney (1978) put forward the hypothesis that estrogens might act as antiresorptive agents through inhibition of PTH-mediated effects at the cellular level. Estrogen has been shown to decrease the degree of hypercalcemia in primary hyperparathyroid patients (Gallagher and Nordin 1972; Marcus et al. 1984). Recently, two *in vitro* studies have shown 17-beta estradiol-mediated inhibition of PTH-related increases in cAMP and prostaglandin $E_2$ production in bone cells (Fukayama and Tashjian 1988; Pilbeam and Raisz 1988).

At the level of the parathyroid glands, estrogen exerts stimulatory effects. Both estrogen and progesterone increase PTH secretion from bovine parathyroid glands (Duarte et al. 1988), and estrogen administration increases serum PTH in postmenopausal women (Gallagher et al. 1980).

As the most important effect of parathyroid hormone is to increase bone turnover without significantly changing the balance between resorption and formation (Eriksen et al. 1985), the inhibition of PTH action at the cellular level is compatible with the decrease in bone turnover observed after estrogen administration to postmenopausal women. The stimulatory effects at the level of the parathyroid glands would lead to increased serum PTH and increased bone turnover after estrogen administration. Thus, it is possible that the increased serum levels of PTH are offset by reduced cellular responsivity.

### B. Estrogens and calcitonin

Several investigators have reported considerably lower plasma calcitonin levels and secretory reserve in women (Heath and Sizemore 1975; Stevenson et al. 1981). These findings, together with the demonstration of increased immunoreactive calcitonin levels after estrogen treatment (Stevenson et al. 1981), led to the hypothesis that the antiresorptive action of estrogen was mediated by the increase in calcitonin levels (Stevenson et al. 1981). In organ cultures of rat, thyroparathyroid gland estrogens ($10^{-7}$ to $10^{-9}$ M) also increase calcitonin secretion (Greenberg et al. 1986; Williams et al. 1986). The whole concept of estrogen exerting any action via alterations in calcitonin levels is still subject to considerable dispute (Heath et al. 1988; Studd and Baber 1988).

### C. Estrogens and 1,25-dihydroxyvitamin $D_3$ [1,25$(OH)_2D_3$]

Estrogens have been shown to increase serum levels of 1,25$(OH)_2D_3$ (Sørensen et al. 1979). As osteoporotic women have decreased calcium absorption that increases with calcitriol supplementation (Recker et al. 1984; Riggs and Nelson 1985), this effect has been taken as one of the indirect effects of estradiol, that might explain its beneficial role in the prophylaxis against postmenopausal osteoporosis. In a longitudinal study on perimenopausal women (Falch et al. 1987), however, no direct relation between estradiol levels and 1,25-dihydroxyvitamin $D_3$ were demonstrable.

### D. Estrogens and growth hormone

The 24 h integrated growth hormone (GH) concentration is greater in women than in men, and greater in young women than in postmenopausal women, and the differences are highly significantly correlated to endogenous concentrations of estradiol (Ho et al. 1987). Moreover, after correcting for effects of estradiol no significant effects of age or sex were demonstrable (Ho et al. 1987). This would suggest estrogen-mediated amplification of the pulsatile GH release. In another study by Dawson-Hughes et al. (1987), a similar increase in GH secretion after estrogen therapy in postmenopausal women was found, the concentration of somatomedin C was, however, reduced. The latter effect could be due to an estrogen-mediated inhibition of GH-dependent hepatic IGF-1 synthesis (Murphy and Friesen 1988). The inhibition of somatomedin C synthesis may be dose-dependent, however, because lower doses of estrogen increase somatomedin C concentrations (Shulman et al. 1987).

## IX. The menopause

The menopause begins with the last episode of menstrual bleeding induced by cyclic endogenous secretion of steroids. It normally occurs at the age of 51 – 52 years of age (range 42 – 60 years) (Ryan 1979). However, the decrease in serum levels of estrogens and progesterone and a rise in gonadotropin levels starts several years before menopause (Korenman et al. 1976). This premenopausal decrease in estrogen secretion after the age of 35 may be related to some of the premenopausal losses of bone mineral observed in some studies (Johnston et al. 1985; Riggs et al. 1985). In the immediate postmenopausal period, decreases in circulating levels of several sex steroids are observed (Abraham and Maroulis 1975; Manwol and Menan 1977). Estradiol and estrone drop to around 25% and 75% of their premenopausal values, respectively. Minor reductions in circulating levels of testosterone, dihydrotestosterone, and androstenedione are also observed. Most of the estriol still present in the circulation after menopause represents extraglandular conversion of androgen precursors (mainly androstenedione) in muscles and adipose tissues to estrone and then to estriol (Siiteri and MacDonald 1973; Siiteri 1975; Vermuelen and Valdenek 1978). The conversion rate of androstenedione to estrone increases with body weight, years after menopause and age (Hemsell et al. 1974; Vermuelen and Valdenek 1978).

Several different studies have demonstrated an increase in bone turnover after menopause (Fig. 5). The increase in bone remodelling activity has been corroborated using calcium kinetics (Recker et al. 1977) as well as bone markers (Hyldstrup et al. 1984; Eastell et al. 1988) and bone histomorphometry (Eastell et al. 1988). This increase in the number of sites undergoing active remodelling (i.e. increased activation frequency) leads to an increased probability for trabecular perforation (Parfitt 1984). This perforation leads to the removal of whole trabecular plates and reduces trabecular connectivity with serious consequences for the mechanical properties of trabecular bone (Mosekilde et al. 1987). As trabecular thickness stays constant through life

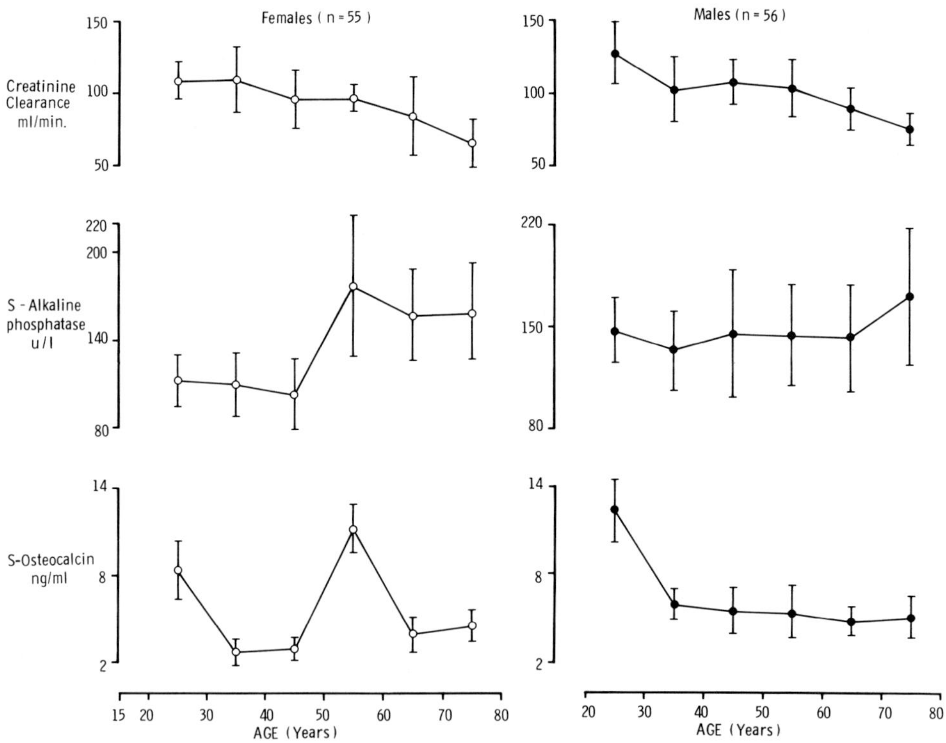


Fig. 5. Variation in creatinine clearance, serum alkaline phosphatase and serum osteocalcin (Bone Gla Protein, BGP) in 55 normal women and 56 normal men. Note the pronounced increase in alkaline phosphatase and osteocalcin in women around menopause. Alkaline phosphatase stays elevated, while osteocalcin decreases to premenopausal values in the sixth decade. Males do not show these abrupt changes in bone turnover with age.

(Birkenhaeger 1985) bone loss due to trabecular perforations seems to be the main mechanism by which bone is lost in the perimenopausal period in women.

## X. Effect of estrogen treatment on bone remodelling and bone mass

In a recent study, we have demonstrated that a one year combined treatment with estrogen and progesterone initiated several years after menopause in patients with spinal osteoporosis reduced the activation frequency in iliac crest trabecular bone to about 50% of the pretreatment value (Fig. 6) (Steiniche et al. 1989). The reduced activation frequency was followed by a marked decrease in the amount of trabecular surface covered by osteoid, mineralizing and erosion surface. The bone formation rate at tissue level was also reduced. These observations are in accordance with previous microradiographic studies on undecalcified bone biopsies demonstrating that estrogen treatment reduced the extent of resorptive surface and later the extent of formative surface (Riggs et al. 1972). Serum alkaline phosphatase and urinary hydroxyproline excretion, which reflect bone formation and resorption rates at the skeletal level (Charles et al. 1985) also decreased during treatment (Fig. 7) (Steiniche et al. 1989). This is in accordance with several other studies which have demonstrated that estrogen treatment to normal and osteoporotic women reduces serum levels of alkaline phosphatase, BGP, urinary hydroxyproline excretion and skeletal uptake of bisphosphonates (Christiansen et al. 1982; Marshall et al. 1984; Thomsen 1987).

In our study (Steiniche et al. 1989) no significant changes were observed in mean wall thickness or in mean final depth of resorption lacunae. Thus, no direct anabolic

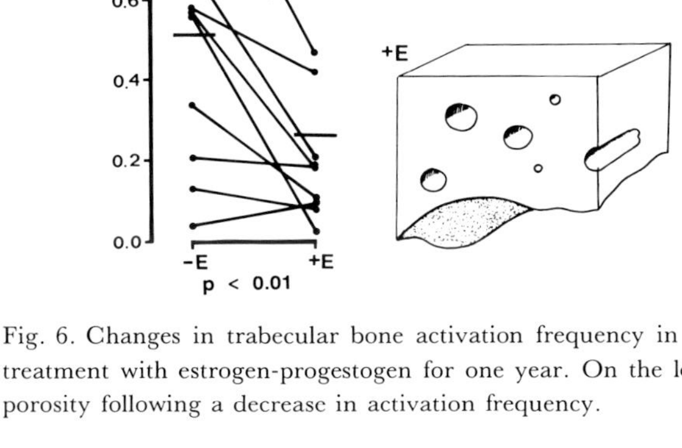


Fig. 6. Changes in trabecular bone activation frequency in spinal crush fracture osteoporosis following treatment with estrogen-progestogen for one year. On the left is shown the striking decrease in cortical porosity following a decrease in activation frequency.

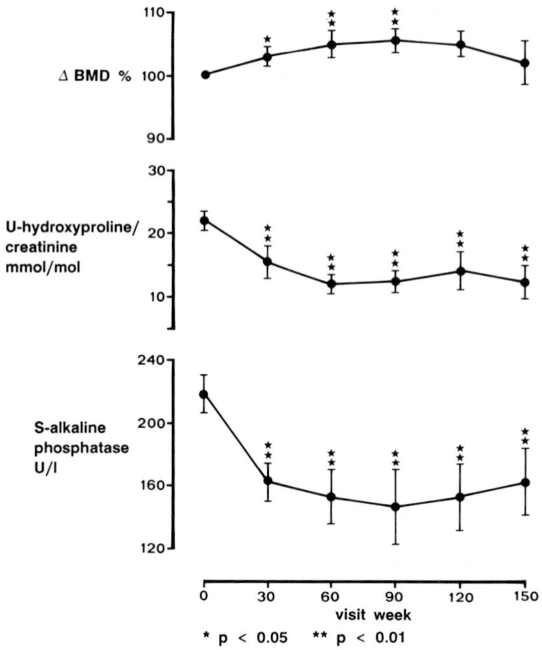


Fig. 7. Changes in lumbar BMD, urinary hydroxyproline/creatinine ratio and S-alkaline phosphatase in spinal crush fracture osteoporosis following treatment with estrogen/progestogen for one year. Bars denote SE.

action of estrogen was demonstrable in this group of patients. Consequently, the balance between thickness of bone resorbed and the thickness of bone formed per remodelling cycle was unchanged (Fig. 8). The lumbar bone mineral density showed a 4 – 5% increase during the first 1 – 2 years of treatment after which a trend towards a decrease was observable (Fig. 7). Identical changes in forearm bone mineral content and lumbar bone mineral density have been reported when estrogen treatment was initiated shortly after the menopause (Christiansen et al. 1980a, b, 1982; Marshall et al. 1984; Munk Jensen et al. 1988). In a double-blind placebo controlled study, Christiansen et al. (1980b) measured forearm BMC in 43 postmenopausal women and observed a 2 – 3% increase over the first 2 years. The increase in BMC was most pronounced during the first year of treatment, after which it started to level off. Munk Jensen et al. (1988) compared the effect of continuous estrogen and progesterone, sequential estrogen and progesterone and placebo on forearm and lumbar bone mineral density in a total of 151 individuals. A net gain in vertebral bone density of 4 – 6% per year was observed with continuous supplementation compared to 4 – 5% per year with sequential supplementation. The net gain in forearm bone mineral density was lower.

The observed changes in bone mineral density can be explained as a direct effect of the reduced activation frequency. Throughout life, lamellar bone forms a renewal

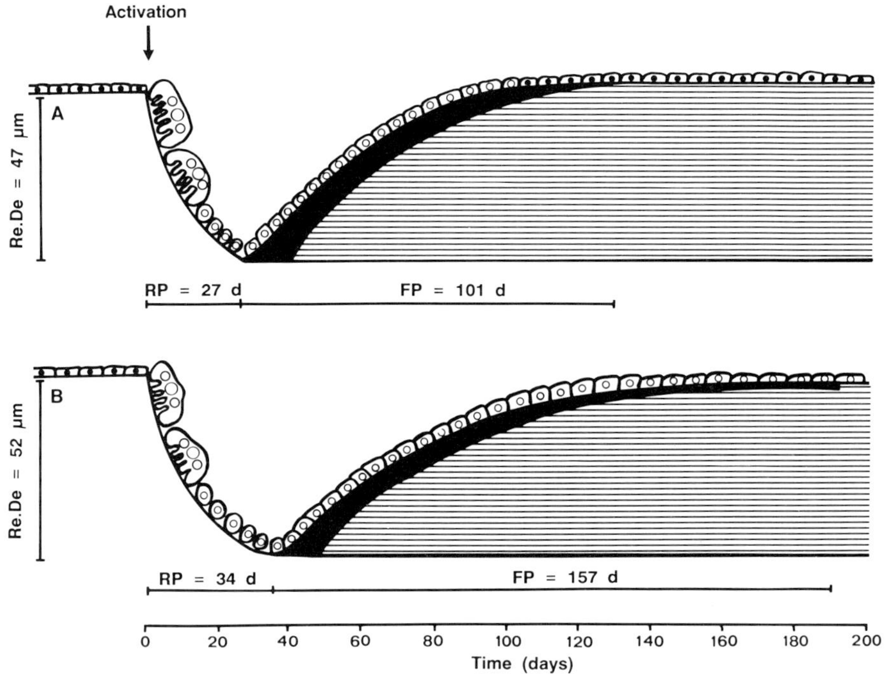


Fig. 8. Reconstruction of trabecular bone remodelling before (A) and after one year of treatment with estrogen/progestogen (B) in postmenopausal crush fracture osteoporosis. Re.De = resorption depth; W.Th = wall thickness; RP = resorption period (days); FP = formative period.

system, where bone is turned over by localized osteoclastic resorption followed by osteoblastic formation (Frost 1966; Eriksen 1986). The amount of bone which has been removed by osteoclasts and not yet reformed by osteoblasts constitutes a transient deficit, the remodelling space (Parfitt 1983). In normal individuals the remodelling space constitutes 6 – 8% of the total skeletal volume (Parfitt 1983). A reduction of the activation frequency to 50% of the pretreatment value reduces the remodelling space by 50% and thus induces a reversible gain in bone volume of 3 – 4%. The reduced bone turnover will furthermore lead to a gradual increase in mean bone age (Frost 1966). As older bone is more heavily mineralized (Amprino and Engstrom 1952) a further increase in bone mineral density will ensue. These mechanisms also explain why the increases in BMC after estrogen treatment are most pronounced during the first year or two of treatment (Christiansen 1980; Steiniche 1988) where the remodelling space is closing down.

The influence of the estrogen-induced increases in bone on biomechanical competence are still unknown. Bone strength depends not only on bone mass but also to a great extent on the integrity of the trabecular network (Parfitt 1984; Mosekilde et al. 1987). During normal remodelling, the trabecular structures are perforated because deep resorption lacunae hit thinner trabecular structures (Parfitt 1984). The probability for perforations depends on the activation frequency, the final resorption depth and trabecular thickness. As shown in the study by Steiniche et al. (1989) the latter two variables were unaffected by estrogen/gestagen treatment, while the activation frequency was reduced. With resorption depth and wall thickness remaining unchanged, this reduction in activation frequency will reduce the probability for perforations by approximately 40%. Thus, despite the balance between resorption and formation remaining unaffected, estrogen/gestagen treatment may protect the trabecular network against fortuitous perforations. This is probably the main mechanism whereby bone mass is maintained, and justifies the use of estrogen as a primary prophylactic in postmenopausal women as well as its use as a secondary prophylactic in osteoporosis.

In postmenopausal spinal osteoporosis the balance per remodelling cycle is typically negative leading to an irreversible bone loss with thinning of trabecular structures (Eriksen et al. 1985, 1988). A reduction in activation frequency should therefore decrease this irreversible bone loss. This theory has been corroborated by the finding of a 19% increase in bone mineral content of the forearm by Ettinger et al. (1985) in postmenopausal women on long-term estrogen/gestagen for at least 5 years (mean 14 years), when compared to age-matched controls. This study also reported an increase in spinal bone mineral density of 54% and an increase in combined cortical thickness of the second metacarp of 16%. Whether the increase in bone thickness can be taken as a mere result of reduced activation at the endosteal surface or constitutes evidence of a direct anabolic action of the steroid remains to be elucidated. The quantitative changes observed in this study are, however, so pronounced that a direct anabolic effect of estrogen cannot be ruled out.

In conclusion, histomorphometrically estrogen/gestagen treatment reduces trabecular bone activation frequency and tissue level bone turnover. Bone markers and the bisphosphonate retention test indicate similar effects on the whole skeleton. The decrease in trabecular activation frequency leads to a reduction in the remodelling space resulting in a reversible increase in bone mass and bone mineral. There is at present no evidence for estrogen creating a positive balance between resorption and formation, but the reduction in activation frequency is sufficient to ensure significant long-term preservation of bone mass due to a reduction of trabecular perforation and preservation of the trabecular lattice. The reduction in bone turnover could theoretically lead to accumulation of older, more heavily mineralized bone and possible accumulation of microdamage.

The effects demonstrated after *in vivo* estrogen administration do not correspond to the general stimulatory role of estradiol in osteoblasts demonstrated with respect to proliferation as well as collagen mRNA production mentioned above. Whether this discrepancy between *in vivo* and *in vitro* effects caused by either local factors or other hormones overriding the stimulatory effect at the cellular level remains to be elucidated.

## XI. Relations between risk factors for osteoporosis and estrogen

The prevalence of symptomatic osteoporosis is positively correlated to estrogen deficiency, low body weight, and smoking. Furthermore, an inverse correlation to obesity has been demonstrated. These risk factors are all associated with altered estrogen production and or degradation, which may be of importance for the accelerated bone loss.

### A. Early menopause and estrogen deficiency

It is generally accepted that an early menopause is associated with osteoporotic fractures. Several case-control studies have, however, given contradictory results. Paganini-Hill et al. (1981) reported that women with hip fractures were younger at the menopause than women without fractures, whereas Hutchinson et al. (1979) reported the opposite trend. In two studies, Krieger et al. (1978) and Kiel et al. (1987) were unable to demonstrate any relation between hip fracture and menopausal age, even if patients with surgical menopause were included.

Oophorectomized women are subject to accelerated bone loss in the first few years after the operation (Lindsay et al. 1977), with biochemical evidence of an increased bone turnover and bone mineral mobilization (Fogelman et al. 1984). After 4 – 6 years, however, the rate of bone loss may show great individual variation (Aitken et al. 1973). In spite of these variations in postoophorectomy bone loss, bone mineral density of the radius, hip and spine is significantly less than that of age-matched controls with intact ovaries in women oophorectomized 20 years before menopause (Richelson et al. 1984). This indicates that early oophorectomy may be of clinical significance for the development of later osteoporosis. Epidemiological studies in women undergoing oophorectomy closer to menopause, however, have been unable to show the same correlation (Krieger et al. 1982; Kiel et al. 1987).

Amenorrhoea affects between 2 and 3% of young females and 25 – 30% of these women have hyperprolactinaemia and reduced serum levels of estrogens (Petterson et al. 1973; Bachman and Kemman 1982). Several studies have demonstrated reduced forearm and spinal bone mineral density in these patients (Klibanski et al. 1980, 1986; Koppelman et al. 1984) with an inverse correlation between the bone mineral content and duration of amenorrhoea (Klibanski et al. 1986). After long-term bromocriptine therapy or curative transsphenoidal hypophysectomy resulting in normalization of periods, cortical bone mineral content increases significantly with the highest rate of increase during the first 6 – 12 months (Klibansky et al. 1986). In patients cured of hyperprolactinaemia without recurrence of periods bone density is still reduced, when compared to age-matched controls (Schlechte et al. 1983; Cann et al. 1984). Prior menstrual history also seems to be important. Drinkwater (1988) demonstrated that women with regular periods throughout their fertile period have higher bone densities than women with irregular periods.

Excessive physical activity in young women may produce hypothalamic amenorrhoea with estrogen deficiency (Schwartz et al. 1981; Loucks and Horvath 1984; Fisher et al. 1986). The prevalence of amenorrhoea among exercising women is around 12% for swimmers, 25% for runners and up to 50% for competitive runners (Shangold and Levine 1982; Shanborne et al. 1982). Several groups have demonstrated reduced bone mineral content in female athletes (Cann et al. 1984; Drinkwater et al. 1984; Fisher et al. 1986) with a positive correlation between serum estradiol and bone mineral content (Fisher et al. 1986). Female athletes who are amenorrhoeic have reduced spinal bone density compared to their counterparts who menstruate (Cann et al., 1984; Drinkwater et al. 1984). It has not been proven, however, whether this reduction in bone mass is irreversible or whether it is associated with increased relative risk for fractures.

Amenorrhoea and estrogen deficiency are some of the physiological sequelae of the self-induced starvation seen in anorexia nervosa (Walsh 1977). Cortical forearm bone mineral content has been reported reduced in these patients when compared to age-matched controls of normal weight (Rigotti et al. 1984). In the study of Rigotti et al. (1984) two of the 18 patients had frank crush fracture spinal osteoporosis. Bone mineral content correlated inversely to age and duration of illness and positively to body weight. No relation to circulating estrogen levels was observed. The exact pathophysiological mechanisms responsible for osteopenia in this disease state are largely unknown. The dietary calcium intake is down in anorexia nervosa (Beaumont et al. 1981; Rigotti et al. 1984), but there are no signs of vitamin D deficiency or secondary hyperparathyroidism (Rigotti et al. 1984). Women with anorexia nervosa have elevated plasma cortisol levels (Casper et al. 1979), which may be a contributing factor to bone loss.

Patients with a reasonable level of physical activity have, however, a higher bone mineral content than patients with less activity (Rigotti et al. 1984) and some studies have demonstrated a direct correlation between $VO_{max}$ and bone density (Pocock et al. 1986).

Osteopenia eventually complicated with low energy fractures is common in Turner's syndrome (Engel and Forbes 1965; Beals et al. 1973). Moreover, metacarpal cortical width has been reported to be reduced among younger patients with Turner's syndrome. The reduction is more pronounced in untreated patients compared to patients on estrogen substitution (Barr et al. 1974) suggesting that the estrogen deficiency is of clinical significance.

Early and late estrogen deficiency probably affect bone mass by different mechanisms. Early estrogen deficiency developed before peak bone mass is obtained around the age of 25 (e.g. Turner's syndrome, most cases of hyperprolactinaemic amenorrhoea and amenorrhoea among athletes), probably affect bone maturation and formation during bone modelling leading to a thinner and more slender skeleton. On the other hand, late estrogen deficiency (e.g. oophorectomy, normal menopause) could induce a state of accelerated bone loss due to increased activation frequency as previously discussed. This mechanism would mainly affect trabecular bone due to increased incidence of trabecular perforations.

### B. Smoking

Daniell (1976) reported a significantly increased risk of osteoporotic vertebral fractures in patients smoking more than 10 cigarettes per day for 5 years versus controls smoking less. Similar but non-significant trends were reported for hip fractures and forearm fractures by Paganini-Hill et al. (1981) and Williams et al. (1982). Daniell (1976) did not consider confounding variables, whereas other studies (Paganini-Hill et al. 1981; Williams et al. 1982) performed proper corrections for age, weight, estrogen use, socioeconomic status, race and menopausal status. Furthermore, several studies have demonstrated that the bones of smokers have thinner cortices and a lower mineral content, than those of non-smokers of the same age and sex (Daniell 1976; Hollo et al. 1979; Lindqvist et al. 1981; Lindsay et al. 1981; Mellstrom et al. 1982).

Cross-sectional and cohort studies strongly support the association between smoking and early menopause even after considering confounding variables (Jick et al. 1977; Kauffman et al. 1980; Adena and Gallagher 1982; Anderson et al. 1982). The studies demonstrated that healthy smokers reach menopause 1.0 – 1.7 years earlier than healthy non-smokers, with a trend towards earlier menopause with increasing amounts smoked. Since an early menopause is a risk factor for postmenopausal osteoporosis (see above), the effect of smoking on fracture incidence could be associated alone with early cessation of menses. However, assuming time since menopause to be the crucial factor for the onset of osteoporotic fractures a 1 – 2 year earlier menopausal age in smokers cannot by itself explain the more than 2-fold increase in fracture rate reported in several studies (Daniell 1976; Paganini-Hill et al. 1981; Williams et al. 1982).

Various suggestions have been made regarding the mechanism of the effect of smoking on menopausal age and osteoporosis. Theoretically, smoking could reduce endogenous estrogen levels through a reduced biosynthesis or an enhanced metabolic clearance, or smoking could impair the binding and effect of estrogen on bone cells and/or exert a direct effect on bone cells. Based on decreased luteal phase urinary excretions of estrone, $E_2$ and $E_3$ in smokers compared to non-smokers, MacMahon et al. (1982) suggested that smoking decreased the biosynthesis of estrogen. However, since the C-2 pathway was not considered and substantial amounts of estrogen are cleared through biliary excretion, estrogen production cannot accurately be estimated from urinary excretion of these metabolites. Furthermore, the proposed reduction in biosynthesis does not explain why serum $E_2$ and serum estrone ($E_3$) are significantly lower in smokers compared to non-smokers on long-term replacement therapy (Jensen et al. 1985). On the other hand, Michnovic et al. (1986) reported a significant increase in the C-2 hydroxylation of estradiol in female smokers compared to non-smokers of the same sex, age and body mass index with a reduction in the competing C-16 pathway leading to a decreased bioavailability of estrogen at the level of target tissues and reduced renal excretion of $E_2$ and $E_3$. The effect was thought to be caused by induction of the hepatic cytochrome P-450 enzyme system by nicotine, 3-methylcholanthrene or benzpyrene.

### C. Body weight

Several studies have reported an inverse relation between body weight (BW) and hip fracture rate (Alffram 1964; Hutchinson et al. 1979; Paganini-Hill et al. 1981; Krieger et al. 1982; Williams et al. 1982; Alderman et al. 1986; Kiel et al. 1987). In the Framingham study (Kiel et al. 1987), the relative risk of fracture was 0.63 in individuals 114 – 123% overweight and 0.33 in individuals with more than 138% overweight. Measurements of bone mass and bone mineral content in obese subjects have shown conflicting results. Without correction for the negative photon absorption coefficient of fat, Danoe et al. (1978) reported reduced forearm bone mineral content (BMC) in 37 obese patients. After correction for this effect, forearm BMC was found to be normal in 23 extremely obese patients (Rickers et al. 1981). In tubular bones, cortical bone area has been reported increased due to a greater outer diameter (Dalen et al. 1975). On the other hand, histomorphometric studies on iliac crest bone biopsies have revealed reduced trabecular bone volume (Compston et al. 1981).

Obesity may protect the skeleton in several ways. In postmenopausal women the small amounts of circulating estrogens are derived from androgen precursors, mainly androstenedione, which are converted to estrone in adipose and muscle tissue (Siiteri and MacDonald 1973; Siiteri 1975; Vermuelen and Valdenek 1978). The extraglandular production of estrogen from circulating androgens in postmenopausal individuals and in oophorectomized patients depend on the amount of adipose tissue (Hemsell 1974; Lindsay et al. 1977; Vermuelen and Valdenek 1978; Frumar et al. 1980). Hence, the postmenopausal obese patients may reduce their risk of fracture by reducing the accelerated bone loss after menopause induced by estrogen deficiency. Alternative explanations would be that obesity may affect PTH (Andersson et al. 1986) or vitamin D endocrine system or that the obese individuals are less likely to fall because of inactivity and are protected against fractures by the cushioning effect of body fat (Kiel et al. 1987). However, based on iliac crest bone biopsies Steiniche et al. (1986) concluded that obese individuals during growth and modelling develop a greater skeleton with larger cortical areas and larger marrow spaces than normal. The absolute amount of trabecular bone was normal but distributed over a larger space resulting in a reduced fractional amount of trabecular bone. These results suggest that the skeleton, in obese patients during growth is adapted to increased weightbearing by an increase in size.

### XII. Effect of estrogen on fracture risk

The aim of the prophylactic treatment in postmenopausal osteoporosis is to prevent the occurrence of low energy fractures in the postmenopausal period and later. As previously discussed, a number of studies have demonstrated beyond any doubt that estrogen replacement therapy (ERT) prevents the postmenopausal loss of bone and bone mineral. There are, however, no corresponding randomized prospective studies which prove a reduction in fracture risk in women on ERT after menopause. Several retrospective and cohort studies, however, support this concept.

In several case-control studies (Hutchinson et al. 1979; Weiss et al. 1980b; Johnson and Specht 1981; Paganini-Hill et al. 1981; Krieger et al. 1982) the occurrence of ERT in patients with osteoporotic fractures were compared to the occurrence in age-matched controls without fractures. Weiss et al. (1980b) evaluated actual and previous ERT in 327 females aged 54 – 73 years with forearm and hip fractures and in 567 randomly selected controls. The fracture risk for women who had used ERT was 50 – 60% lower than in women, who had never received estrogen. The relation between previous ERT and fracture risk was far less convincing. Hutchinson et al. (1979) investigated 157 pairs and found that the relative risk for forearm fracture or hip fracture was 0.69 in the postmenopausal women on previous ERT for more than 6 months. In a similar case-control study involving 95 postmenopausal women with hip fractures and 190 matched controls, Paganini-Hill et al. (1981) found a relative fracture risk of 0.42 in women who had taken estrogen for more than 60 months. The effect was most pronounced in oophorectomized women who had a relative risk of 0.14 after more than 60 months of ERT. These case-control studies are limited by imprecise recall of past estrogen use, lack of precise information on previous fractures in the control group, inclusion of only survivors of hip fractures (about 25% of hip fracture patients die within one year) and the use of short-term ERT as discriminator (Hutchinson et al. 1979).

Retrospective cohort studies can to some extent compensate for these limitations. Hammond et al. (1979a, b) compared 301 postmenopausal women on ERT with a corresponding number of controls. The observation period was 13 years. The prevalence of all fractures was 15.9% in the control group compared to 8.6% in the ERT group. However, the mean age at the end of the study period was only 56 years and there was no information on the different fracture types. Furthermore, the two groups differed in race, height and body stature. Ettinger et al. (1985) compared the occurrence of fractures in different parts of the skeleton in 245 postmenopausal caucasian females on long-term ERT (more than 5 years, average 14 years) with matched controls. The two groups were comparable with respect to menopausal age, height, body weight, parity, smoking, education and occupation. The observation period was 17.6 years and the mean age at the end of the study was 69 years. The investigation showed a marked reduction in overall fracture rate in the ERT group. The reduction was only related to the occurrence of osteoporotic fractures which was reduced to 54%

in controls. The number of vertebral compression fractures was 34 in the control group compared to 11 in the estrogen group ($p < 0.001$). For the other osteopenic fractures the difference was not significant. Kiel et al. (1987) performed a retrospective cohort study of 2873 women in the Framingham Heart Study in order to assess the effect of ERT on the subsequent risk of hip fracture. There were 191 hip fractures in 179 postmenopausal women. The mean age at the first fracture was 75 years or around 30 years after the menopause. The relative risk of hip fracture in individuals who had taken estrogen at any time was 0.65 after adjustment for age and weight. The adjusted relative risk in women who had taken estrogen within the last 2 years was further reduced to 0.34.

In a 10-year prospective study, Lindsay et al. (1980) reported a reduced fracture rate in oophorectomized women on ERT compared to untreated women. In the ERT group 4% of the women had infractions in the vertebral bodies compared to 38% in the untreated group. After 10 years crush fractures were observed in 1.7% of the estrogen-treated compared to 8.5% in the controls. The patients were, however, not randomized to the two groups.

It should be emphasized that retrospective and prospective non-randomized studies are unable to confirm causality due to the study design. The seemingly protective effect of ERT on fracture risk may result from selection bias due to, for instance, life style factors which protect against bone loss or fractures, and at the same time influences the chance of ERT. The final proof, based on a randomized prospective study, that ERT after natural menopause reduces fracture risk is still awaited.

## XIII. Side effects to long-term estrogen replacement therapy

The potential serious side effects to long-term ERT are endometrial cancer, breast cancer and acute myocardial infarction (thromboembolic disease and possibly gall stones). The risks of these side effects seem to depend on whether the estrogen treatment is given with or without concomitant gestagen administration.

### A. Endometrial cancer

A number of studies have clearly demonstrated that unopposed continuous estrogen treatment increases the risk of endometrial cancer (Ziel et al. 1975; Gray et al. 1977; Macdonald et al. 1977; Horwitz and Feinstein 1978; Hammond et al. 1979a, b; Jick et al. 1979; Weiss et al. 1979a; Hulka et al. 1980). The relative risk is related to the dose and duration of treatment and varies between 2 and 15 (Ziel et al. 1982). The most important risk factor is the duration of treatment. The risk is significantly increased after 2 – 4 years of continuous treatment. A steep rise in relative risk is observed up to a 10 – 15-fold increase in relative risk after 10 years (Cramer et al. 1979). The risk is further increased in obese patients with late menopause (Davies et al.

1981). It is possible that the relative risk is slightly overestimated due to detection bias (Macrae et al. 1981). Furthermore, it has been claimed that the endometrial cancer induced by ERT is less malignant (Collins et al. 1980). It is now generally accepted, however, that a cause relationship exists between unopposed estrogen exposure after the menopause and endometrial carcinoma (Hulka et al. 1980).

Progesterone given for 7 – 10 days in combination with cyclic estrogen seems to reduce the risk of endometrial carcinoma — some studies even propose that the relative risk is below 1 (Hammond et al. 1979a, b; Nachtigall et al. 1979a, b; Thom et al. 1979; Gambrell et al. 1980; Whitehead et al. 1981; Judd et al. 1983). However, the combined estrogen/gestagen treatment has not been used on a larger scale for a sufficient period of time in relation to the development of malignancies in order to give a precise estimate of relative risks.

### B. Breast carcinoma

The incidence of breast cancer is around 4 times that of endometrial carcinoma and the mortality is higher. Even a small increase in the relative risk of breast carcinoma induced by ERT would therefore carry potential serious consequences. It has been difficult, however, to demonstrate any significant association between ERT and breast carcinoma. In a prospective cohort study, Hoover et al. (1976) reported a 2-fold increase in relative risk after 15 years exposure to estrogen. This is in accordance with an ongoing prospective cohort study which after an average observation period of 5.7 years found a 20% increase in the risk of breast cancer (Persson et al. 1987). The study gave no evidence for a protective effect of concomitant progesterone administration. Other studies have been unable to show this increase in relative risk (Nomura et al. 1986) or even reported decreased relative risk especially among those taking opposed estrogen (Gambrell et al. 1983). Ross et al. (1980) and Jick et al. (1980), however, reported an increased relative risk in subgroups of patients depending on whether hysterectomy and/or oophorectomy had been performed. Patients around the menopause and on a high estrogen dose, were found to be particularly prone to develop breast carcinoma.

Thus, from the data available it cannot be excluded that opposed or unopposed estrogen treatment given after menopause may be associated with an increased risk of breast cancer.

### C. Cardiovascular disorders

Menopause is associated with increased risk of cardiovascular diseases (Gordon et al. 1978). Before 60 years of age, the incidence of acute myocardial infarction (AMI) is lower among females than males (Gordon et al. 1978). After menopause this trend reverses. These findings suggest that estrogen protects against cardiovascular disorders. A significant reduction in the overall mortality has been demonstrated after long-term estrogen use (Burch 1975; Bush 1983). Moreover, a number of case control studies have shown unchanged (Rosenberg et al. 1976, 1980; Pfeffer et al. 1978, 1979) or reduced (Bain et al. 1981; Ross et al. 1981; Szklo et al. 1984) risk of AMI after postmenopausal estrogen therapy. Based on questionnaires distributed among 58 000 nurses in the U.S.A., Stampfer et al. (1985) found a reduced risk of cardiovascular disorders in those taking estrogen. However, in a prospective study including 1200 women, Wilson et al. (1985) found a 50% increase in risk of cardiovascular morbidity and a 2-fold increased risk of cerebrovascular disease among estrogen users.

Administration of unopposed estrogen to postmenopausal women is followed by a decrease in serum total cholesterol with an increase in serum high-density lipoprotein (HDL) cholesterol and a reduction in serum low-density-lipoprotein (LDL) cholesterol (Wallentin and Larsson Cohn 1977; Wallace et al. 1979; Wahl et al. 1983). These changes protect against ischaemic heart disease. Serum triglyceride levels, however, increased slightly during treatment (Wahl et al. 1983). Opposed estrogen reduced serum total LDL cholesterol without changes in serum HDL cholesterol and triglyceride (Christiansen et al. 1981, 1984). Hence, in some studies, cyclic progesterone does not compromise the beneficial effects of estrogen on blood lipids.

In a single case-control study a positive relation between the use of conjugated estrogen and hypertension, in younger women was reported. In the elderly the association even extended to non-fatal stroke (Pfeffer et al. 1976). During treatment with opposed estrogen, however, unchanged systolic pressure and a small drop in diastolic blood pressure has been reported (Christiansen et al. 1981).

Thus, most available data suggest a reduction of the risk of cardiovascular disease after unopposed estrogen treatment. It is, however, worth noting that the results from the Framingham study show an increased risk (Wilson et al. 1985). Progestagen given in a cyclic fashion together with estrogen probably modifies the effects of estrogen on cardiovascular risk factors but there is at present no epidemiological data on the effects of opposed estrogen treatment on cardiovascular risk.

### D. Deep venous thrombosis

It is well known that administration of oral contraceptives increases the risk of deep venous trombosis (Sagar et al. 1975; Vessey et al. 1980). Estrogen exerts several effects on the clotting system including increased concentrations of the clotting factors VII, IX and X complex (Von Kaulla et al. 1975; Bonner et al. 1976) and reduced concentrations of the anticoagulant component Antithrombin III, which inactivates thrombin and enzymes engaged in thrombin formation (Bonner et al. 1976; Wessler et al. 1976). Some studies have reported reduced platelet counts after estrogen (Beller et al. 1972). The fibrinolytic system is also affected by estrogens. ERT increases circulating fibrin degradation products and reduces circulating plasminogen and the endothelial content of plasminogen activator (Bonner et al. 1976; Davies et al. 1976; Mendel et al. 1982).

Some of the effects on the clotting system seem to be dose-dependent (Conrad et al. 1972) and the doses used in ERT are usually lower than the doses used in oral contraceptives. This may explain why case-control studies as well as two smaller prospective studies have failed to demonstrate an increased relative risk of venous thrombosis in postmenopausal women on ERT (Report 1974; Hart et al. 1978; Nachtigall et al. 1979; Petitti et al. 1979).

### E. Gall stones

A single case-control study demonstrated a 2.5-fold increase in relative risk for surgically proven gall stone in postmenopausal women receiving estrogen replacement (Report 1974).

## XIV. Conclusion

Despite the widespread use of estrogen as a prophylactic agent against osteoporosis the exact mechanisms whereby the hormone exerts its action on bone cell remain to be elucidated. Most of the positive effects on bone mass reported in bone densitometric studies can be explained through changes in the remodelling space. *In vitro* studies have shown effects similar to the effects of estrogen on the classical target tissue, the reproductive system, that is stimulation of cell proliferation and protein synthesis. The few *in vivo* studies conducted so far have, however, shown effects that must be interpreted as being the opposite of the *in vitro* effects. This could be due to the antiresorptive effect of estrogen overriding a general stimulatory effect on the osteoblasts. Another reason might be that the *in vivo* studies have been performed in osteoporotics. Osteoporotic women are characterized by decreased bone formative potential (Eriksen et al. 1990) and it is possible that anabolic effects could be demonstrated in perimenopausal women. In order to address these questions, longitudinal prospective *in vivo* studies on estrogen effects in the pre-, peri- and postmenopausal period are urgently needed. Such studies should furthermore focus on (a) anti-fracture efficacy of estrogen, (b) identification of individuals at risk for osteoporosis, (c) identification of individuals that may benefit from ERT and (d) safety of ERT.

## References*

Abraham GE, Maroulis GB. Effect of exogenous estrogens on serum pregnenolone, cortisol and androgens in postmenopausal women. Obstet Gynecol 1975;45:271 – 274.

Adena MA, Gallagher HG. Cigarette smoking and the age at menopause. Ann Hum Biol 1982;9: 121 – 130.

---

**Author's note:* List completed October 1988.

Aitken JM, Hart DM, Anderson JB, Lindsay R, Smith DA. Osteoporosis after oophorectomy for non malignant disease. Br Med J 1973;1:325 – 328.

Alderman BW, Weiss NS, Daling JR, Ure CL, Ballard JH. Reproductive history and postmenopausal risk of hip and forearm fracture. Am J Epidemiol 1986;124:262 – 267.

Alffram PA. An epidemiological study of cervical and trochanteric fractures in the femur in an urban population: analysis of 1,664 cases with special reference to etiological factors. Acta Orthop Scand 1964;(Suppl):65.

Amprino R, Engstrom A. Studies of x-ray absorption and diffraction of bone tissue. Acta Anat (Basel) 1952;75:1 – 22.

Anderson JN, Peck EJ, Clark JH. Complex relationship between concentration of estrogen receptor and uterotrophic responses. Endocrinology 1973;92:1488 – 1495.

Anderson FS, Transboel I, Christiansen C. Is cigarette smoking a promotor of the menopause. Acta Med Scand 1982;212:137 – 139.

Anderson T, McNair P, Fogh Andersen N, Nielsen TT, Hyldstrup L, Transboel I. Increased parathyroid hormone as a consequence of changed complex binding of plasma calcium in morbid obesity. Metabolism 1986;35:147 – 151.

Bachman GA, Kemman E. Prevalence of oligomenorrhoea and amenorrhoea in a college population. Am J Obstet Gynecol 1982;144:98 – 102.

Bain C, Willett W, Hennekens CH, Rosner M, Belanger C, Speizer FE. Use of postmenopausal hormones and risk of myocardial infarction. Circulation 1981;64:42 – 46.

Barr DG. Bone deficiency in Turners syndrome measured by metacarpal dimensions. Arch Dis Child 1974;49:821 – 822.

Beals RK. Orthopedic aspects of the XO (Turners) syndrome. Clin Orthop Rel Res 1973;97:19 – 30.

Beller FK, Nachtigall L, Rosenberg M. Coagulation studies of menopausal women taking oestrogen replacement. Obstet Gynecol 1975;39:775 – 778.

Beumont PJV, Chambers TL, Rouse L, Abraham SF. The diet composition and nutritional knowledge of patients with anorexia nervosa. J Hum Nutr 1981;35:265 – 273.

Birkenhaeger-Frenkel DH, Courpron P, Clermont E, Huepscher E, Coutinho MF, Meunier PJ. Trabecular thickness, intertrabecular distance and age related bone loss. Bone 1985;6:402.

Bonner J, Haddon M, Hunter DH, Richards DH, Thornton C. Coagulation postmenopausal women receiving oestrogen preparations. Postgradr Med J 1976;52(Suppl 6):30 – 34.

Bursch JC, Byrd BF, Vaughn WK. Effect of long term estrogen administration to women following hysterectomy. Front Horm Res 1975;3:208 – 214.

Bush TL, Cowan LD, Barret-Connor E, Criqui Mh, Kason JM, Wallace RB, Tyroler A, Rifkind BM. Estrogen use and all-cause mortality. J Am Med Assoc 1983;249:903 – 906.

Canalis E, Raisz LG. Effect of sex steroids on bone collagen synthesis in vitro. Calcif Tissue Res 1978;25:105 – 110.

Cann CE, Martin MC, Genant HK, Jaffe RB. Decreased spinal mineral content in amenorrheic women. J Am Med Assoc 1984;251:626 – 629.

Caputo CB, Meadows D, Raisz LG. Failure of estrogens and androgens to inhibit bone resorption in tissue culture. Endocrinology 1976;98:1065 – 1068.

Casper RC, Chatterton R, Davis JM. Alterations in serum cortisol binding characteristics in anorexia nervosa. Am J Psychiatry 1979;49:406 – 411.

Charles P, Poser JW, Mosekilde L, Jensen FT. Estimation of bone turnover evaluated by $^{47}$Ca kinetics: Efficiency of serum bone carboxyglutamic acid containing protein, serum alkaline phosphatase and urinary hydroxyproline. J Clin Invest 1985;76:2254 – 2258.

Chen TL, Feldman D. Distinction between alpha-foetoprotein and intracellular estrogen receptors: evidence against the presence of estradiol receptors in rat bone. Endocrinology 1978;102:236 – 244.

Christiansen C, Christensen MS, McNair P, Hagen C, Stocklund KE, Transboel I. Prevention of early postmenopausal bone loss: a controlled 2-year study in 315 normal females. Eur J Clin Invest

1980a;10:273 – 277.

Christiansen C, Christensen MS, Larsen NE, Transboel I. Bone mass in postmenopausal women after withdrawal of estrogen/gestagen replacement therapy. Lancet 1980b;1:459 – 461.

Christiansen C, Christensen MS, Hagen C, Stocklund KE, Transboel I. Effects of natural oestrogen/gestagen and thiazide on coronary risk factors in normal postmenopausal women. Acta Obstet Gynecol 1981;60:407 – 412.

Christiansen C, Christensen MS, Grande F, Transboel I. Low-risk lipoprotein pattern in postmenopausal women on sequential estrogen/progestogen treatment. Maturitas 1984;5:193 – 199.

Collins J, Donner A, Allen LH, Adams O. Oestrogen use and survival in endometrial cancer. Lancet 1980;ii:961 – 964.

Compston JE, Vedi S, Ledger JE, Webb A, Gazed JC, Pelkington TRE. Vitamin D status and bone histomorphometry in gross obesity. Am J Clin Nutr 1981;34:2359 – 2363.

Conrad J, Samama M, Salomon Y. Antithrombin III and the oestrogen content of combined oestrogen-progestagen cotraceptives. Lancet 1972;ii:1148 – 1149.

Coulson P, Gorski J. Effect of estrogen on cycloleucine $^{14}C$ an putrescine $^{3}H$-uptake by the rat uterus. Endocrinology 1967;80:357 – 361.

Cramer DW, Knapp RC. Review of epidemiologic studies of endometrial cancer and exogenous estrogen. Obstet Gynecol 1979;54:521 – 526.

Dalen N, Halberg D, Lamke B. Bone mass in obese subjects. Acta Med Scand 1975;197:353 – 355.

Daniell HW. Osteoporosis of the slender smoker: vertebral compression fractures and loss of metacarpal cortex in relation to postmenopausal cigarette smoking and lack of obesity. Arch Intern Med 1976;136:298 – 304.

Danoe P, Christiansen P. Bone decalcification following intestinal by pass operation for obesity and absence of calcium malabsorption: A comparison of two types of operation. Scand J Gastroenterol 1978;13:81 – 75.

Davies JL, Rosenstein NB, Antunes CMF, Stolley PD. A review of the risk factors for endometrial carcinoma. Obstet Gynecol Surv 1981;36:107 – 116.

Davies T, Fieldhouse G, McNichol GP. The effects of therapy with oestriol succinate and ethinylestradiol on the hemostatic mechanism in postmenopausal women. Thrombo Haemosts (Stuttgart) 1976;35:403 – 414.

Dawson-Hughes B, Stern D, Goldman J, Reichlin S. Regulation of growth hormone and somatomedin C secretion in postmenopausal women: effect of physiological estrogen replacement. J Clin Endocrinol Metab 1986;63:424 – 432.

Deslypere JP, Verdonck L, Vermuelen A. Fat tissue: a steroid reservoir and site of steroid metabolism. J Clin Endocrinol Metab 1985;61:564 – 570.

Drinkwater BL, Nilson K, Chestnut CH, Brenner WJ, Shainholtz S, Southworth MB. Bone mineral content of amenorrheic and eumenorrheic athletes. N Engl J Med 1984;311:277 – 279.

Drinkwater BL. Maximizing bone mass in the premenstrual years: positive and negative factors. In: Christiansen CC, Johansen JS, Riis BJ, eds. Proceedings of the Second International Symposium on Osteoporosis. Aalborg, Denmark: Aalborg Stiftsbogtrykkeri 1987;484 – 488.

Duarte B, Hargis GK, Krukreja SC. Effects of estradiol and progesterone on parathyroid secretion from human parathyroid tissue. J Clin Endocrinol Metab 1988;66:584 – 587.

Eastell R, Delmas PD, Hodgson SF, Eriksen EF, Mann KG, Riggs BL. Bone formation in older women: concurrent assessment with bone histomorphometry, calcium kinetics and biochemical markers. J Clin Endocrinol Metab 1988;67:741 – 748.

Els M, Berns JJ, Focko FGR, Mulder E. Rapid and sensitive detection of oestrogen receptors in cells and tissue sections by autoradiography with $^{125}I$-oestradiol. Histochemical J 1985;17:1185 – 1196.

Engel E, Forbes AP. Cytogenetic and clinical findings in 48 patients with congenitally defective or absent ovaries. Medicine 1965;44:135 – 164.

Eriksen EF, Melsen F, Mosekilde L. Reconstruction of the resorptive site in iliac trabecular bone: a kinetic model for bone resorption in 20 normal individuals. Metab Bone Dis Rel Res 1984a;5:235 – 242.

Eriksen EF, Gundersen HJG, Melsen F, Mosekilde L. Reconstruction of the formative site in iliac trabecular bone in 20 normal individuals employing a kinetic model for matrix and mineral apposition. Metab Bone Dis Rel Res 1984b;5:243 – 252.

Eriksen EF, Mosekilde L, Melsen F. Effect of sodium fluoride, calcium phosphate and vitamin $D_2$ on bone balance and remodelling in osteoporotics. Bone 1985;6:381 – 389.

Eriksen EF, Mosekilde L, Melsen F. Trabecular bone remodelling and balance in primary hyperparathyroidism. Bone 1986;7:213 – 222.

Eriksen EF. Normal and pathological remodelling of human trabecular bone: Three dimensional reconstruction of the remodelling sequence in normals and in metabolic bone disease. Endocr Rev 1986;7:379 – 408.

Eriksen EF, Colvard DS, Berg NJ, Graham ML, Mann KG, Spelsberg TC, Riggs BL. Evidence of estrogen receptors in normal human osteoblast cells. Science 1988a;241:84 – 86.

Eriksen EF, Hodgson SF, Eastell R, O'Fallon WM, Riggs BL. Trabecular bone formation and resorption rates in type I (postmenopausal) osteoporosis. J Bone Min Res 1990;5:311 – 319.

Ernst M, Schmid CH, Froesch ER. Enhanced osteoblast proliferation and collagen gene expression by estradiol. Proc Natl Acad Sci USA 1988;85:2307 – 2310.

Ettinger B, Genant HK, Cann CE. Long term estrogen replacement therapy prevents bone loss and fractures. Ann Intern Med 1985;102:319 – 325.

Falch JA, Oftebro H, Haug E. Postmenopausal osteoporosis: no effect of 3 years treatment with $1,25(OH)_2D_3$. J Clin Endocrinol Metab 1987;64:836 – 840.

Feyen JHM, Raisz LG. Prostaglandin production by calvariae from sham operated and oophorectomized rats: effect of 17-beta estradiol in vivo. Endocrinology 1987;121:819 – 821.

Fishman J, Martucci C. Biological properties of 16-alpha hydroxyestrone: implications in estrogen physiology and pathophysiology. J Clin Endocrinol Metab 1980;51:611 – 615.

Fishman J, Bradlow HL, Gallagher TF. Oxidative metabolism of estradiol. J Biol Chem 1960;235:3104 – 3107.

Fisher EC, Nelson ME, Frontera WR, Turksov RN, Evans WJ. Bone mineral content and levels of gonadotropins and estrogens in amenorrheic women. J Clin Endocrinol Metab 1986;62:1232 – 1236.

Fogelman I, Poser JW, Smith ML, Hart DM, Bevan JA. Alterations in skeletal metabolism following oophorectomy. In: Christiansen C, Arnaud CD, Nordin BEC, Parfitt AM, Peck WA, Riggs BL, eds. Osteoporosis. Aalborg, Denmark: Aalborg Stiftsbogtrykkeri, 1984;519 – 522.

Frost HM. The Bone Dynamics in Osteoporosis and Osteomalcia. Springfield, IL: Charles C Thomas, 1966.

Frost HM. Tetracycline based histological analysis of bone remodelling. Calcif Tissue Res 1969;3:211 – 237.

Frumar A, Moldsin D, Geola F, Shamamki I, Talaryh I, Deftos L, Judd H. Relationship of fasting urinary calcium to circulating estrogen and body weight in postmenopausal women. J Clin Endocrinol 1980;50:70 – 75.

Fuentealba B, Nieto M, Croxatto HB. Progesterone abbreviated the nuclear retention of estrogen receptor in the rat oviduct and counteracts estrogen action on egg transport. Biol Reprod 1988;38:63 – 69.

Fuakayama S, Tashjian Jr. A. Acute actions of estradiol on human bone cells in culture. J Bone Miner Res 1988;3(Suppl. 1):S219.

Gallagher JC, Nordin BEC. Treatment with estrogen of primary hyperparathyroidism in postmenopausal women. Lancet 1972;i:503 – 505.

Gallagher JC, Riggs BL, Jerpbak CM, Arnaud CD. The effect of age on serum immunoreactive parathyroid hormone in normal and osteoporotic women. J Lab Clin Med 1980;95:373 – 378.

Gambrell Jr. RD. The role of hormones in the etiology of breast and endometrial cancer. Acta Obstet Gynecol (Suppl) 1979;88:73 – 81.

Gambrell Jr. RD, Massey FM, Castenada TA, Ugenas AJ, Ricci CA, Wright FH. The use of progesterone challenge test to reduce the risk of endometrial cancer. Obstet Gynecol 1980;55:732 – 738.

Gambrell Jr. RD, Maier RC, Sanders BI. Decreased incidence of breast cancer in postmenopausal estrogen-progestagen users. Obstet Gynecol 1983;62:435 – 443.

Giguere V, Yang N, Segui P, Evans RM. Identification of a new class of steroid hormone receptors. Nature 1988;331:91 – 94.

Goldfien A, Monroe SE. The ovaries. In: Greenspan FS and Forsham PH, eds. Basic and Clinical Endocrinology. Los Altos, California: Lange Medical Publications, 1983;368 – 413.

Golding TS, Korach KS. Nuclear receptor molecular heterogeneity in the mouse uterus. Proc Natl Acad Sci USA 1988;85:69 – 73.

Gordon T, Kannel WB, Hjortland MC, McNamara PN. Menopause and coronary heart disease: The Framingham study. Ann Intern Med 1978;89:157 – 161.

Gorski J, Todt D, Shyamala G, Smith D, Notides A. Hormone receptors: studies on the interaction of estrogen with the uterus. Recent Prog Horm Res 1968;24:45 – 50.

Graham ML, Spelsberg TC, Dines DE, Spencer Payne W, Bjornsson J, Lie JT. Pulmonary lymphangiomyomatosis: with particular reference to steroid receptor assay studies and pathologic correlation. Mayo Clinic Proc 1984;59:3 – 11.

Gray LA, Christopherson WM, Hoover RN. Estrogens and endometrial carcinoma. Obstet Gynecol Surg 1977;32:619 – 621.

Gray TK, Flynn TC, Gray KM, Nabell. Specific effects of 17-beta estradiol on osteoblast proliferation and differentiation. Proc Natl Acad Sci USA 1987;84:6267 – 6281.

Greenberg C, Kukreja SC, Bowser EN, Hargis GK, Henderson WJ, Williams GA. Effects of estradiol and progesterone on calcitonin secretion. Endocrinology 1986;118:2594 – 2598.

Green S, Walter P, Kumar V, Bornest JM, Argos P, Chambon P. Human estrogen receptor cDNA sequence, expression and homology to v-erb-a. Nature 1986;320:134 – 139.

Greene GL, Sobel NB, King WJ, Jensen EV. Immunocytochemical studies of estrogen receptors. J Steroid Biochem 1984;20:51 – 56.

Greene GL, Gilna P, Waterfield M, Baker A, Hort Y, Shine J. Sequence and expression of human estrogen receptor complementary DNA. Science 1986;231:1150 – 1159.

Hamilton TH. Control by estrogen of genetic transcription and translation. Science 1968;161:649 – 651.

Hammond CB, Jelovsek FR, Lee KL, Creasman WT, Parker RT. Effects of long term estrogen replacement therapy. I. Metabolic effects. Am J Obstet Gynecol 1979a;133:525 – 529.

Hammond CB, Jalovsek FR, Lee KL, Creasman WT, Parker RT. Effects of long term estrogen replacement therapy. II. Neoplasia. Am J Obstet Gynecol 1979b;133:537 – 547.

Hart DM, Lindsay R, Purdie D. Vascular complications of long term oestrogen therapy. Hormon Res 1978;242:1150 – 1154.

Heaney RP, Recker RR, Saville PD. Menopausal changes in bone remodelling. J Lab Clin Med 1978;92:964 – 969.

Heath H III, Sizemore GW. Plasma calcitonin in normal man: difference between men and women. J Clin Invest 1977;60:1135 – 1140.

Heath H III, Tiegs RD, Hurley DL. Is inhibition of bone resorption by estrogen or calcium mediated by increased calcitonin secretion. In: Christiansen C, Johansen J, Riis BJ, eds. Osteoporosis. Copenhagen: Osteopress, 1987;840 – 843.

Hemsell DL, Spodin JM, Brenner PF, Siiteri PK, MacDonald PC. Plasma precursors of estrogen II. Correlation of the extent of conversion of plasma androstendione to estrone with age. J Clin Endocrinol Metab 1974;38:476 – 479.

Ho Ky, Evans WS, Blizzard RM, et al. Effects of sex and age on the 24-hour profile of growth hormone secretion in man: importance of endogenous estradiol concentrations. J Clin Endocrinol Metab 1987;64:51 – 58.

Hochberg RB. Iodine-125-labeled estradiol: a gamma-emitting analog of estradiol that binds to the estrogen receptor. Science 1979;205:1138 – 1140.

Hollo I, Gergely I, Boross M. Influence of heavy smoking upon the bone mineral content of the radius of the aged and effect of tobacco smoke on the sensitivity to calcitonin of the rats. Aktuel Gerontol 1979;9:365 – 368.

Horsman A, Gallagher JC, Simpson M, Nordin BEC. Prospective trial of estrogen and calcium in postmenopausal women. Br Med J 1977;2:789 – 792.

Hoover R, Gray LA, Cole P, Macmahon B. Menopausal estrogens and breast cancer. N Engl J Med 1976;295:402 – 405.

Horwitz RI, Feinstein MD. Alternative analytic methods for case-control studies of estrogen and endometrial cancer. N Engl J Med 1978;299:1089 – 2004.

Hulka BS, Fowler WC, Kaufman DG, Grimson RC, Greenberg BG, Houge CJR, Berger GS, Fulliam CC. Estrogen and endometrial cancer: Cases and two control groups from North Carolina. Am J Obstet Gynecol 1980;137:92 – 101.

Hutchinson TA, Polansky SM, Feinstein AR. Postmenopausal oestrogen protects against fractures of hip and distal radius: a case control study. Lancet 1979;2:705 – 709.

Hyldstrup L, McNair P, Mogensen NB, Jensen GF, Transboel I. Measurement of whole body retention of diphosphonate and other indices of bone metabolism in 125 normals: dependence on age, sex and glomerular filtration. Scand J Clin Lab Invest 1984;44:373 – 378.

Jaworsky ZF. Some morphologic and dynamic aspects of remodelling on the endosteal-cortical and trabecular surfaces. In: Menczel J, Harell A, eds. Calcified Tissue, Structural, Functional and Metabolic Aspects. New York: Academic Press, 1971;159 – 160.

Jellineck PH, Krey I, Davis PG, et al. Central and peripheral action of estradiol and catecholestrogens administered at low concentrations by constant infusion. Endocrinology 1981;108:1848 – 1854.

Jensen EV, Suzuki T, Numata M, Smith S, DeSombre ER. Estrogen binding substances of target tissues. Steroids 1969;13:417 – 420.

Jensen EV, DeSombre ER. Estrogen receptor interaction. Science 1973;182:126 – 128.

Jensen J, Christiansen C, Roedbro P. Cigarette smoking, serum estrogens and bone mineral loss during hormone replacement therapy early after menopause. N Engl J Med 1985;313:973 – 975.

Jick H, Porter J, Morrison AS. Relation between smoking and age at natural menopause. Lancet 1977;1:1354 – 1355.

Jick H, Watkins RN, Hunter JR, Dinan BJ, Madsen S, Rothman KJ, Walker AM. Replacement estrogens and endometrial cancer. N Engl J Med 1979;300:218 – 222.

Jick H, Walker AM, Watkins RN, D'Ewart DC, Hunter JR, Danford A, Madsen S, Dinan BJ, Rothman KJ. Replacement estrogens and breast cancer. Am J Epidemiol 1980;112:586 – 594.

Johnson RE, Specht EE. The risk of hip fracture in postmenopausal females with and without estrogen exposure. Am J Public Health 1981;71:139 – 144.

Johnston CC, Hui SL, Witt RM, Appledorn R, Baker RS, Longcope C. Early menopausal changes in bone mass and sex steroids. J Clin Endocrinol Metab 1985;61:905 – 911.

Jost JP, Seldran M, Gieser M. Preferential binding of estrogen-receptor complex to a region containing the estrogen dependent hypomethylation site preceding the chicken vitellogenin II gene. Proc Natl Acad Sci USA 1984;81:429 – 433.

Judd HL, Meldrum DR, Deftos LJ, Henderson BE. Estrogen replacement therapy: indications and complications (UCLA conference). Ann Intern Med 1983;98:195 – 205.

Jurianz RL, Huseby RA, Wilcox RB. Interactions of putative estrogens with the intracellular receptor complex in mouse Leydig cells: relationship to preneoplastic hyperplasia. Cancer Res 1988;48:14 – 18.

Katsaros D, Ally S, Cho-Chung YS. Site-selective cyclic AMP analogues are antagonistic to estrogen stimulation of growth and proto-oncogene expression in human breast cancer cells. Int J Cancer 1988;41:863 – 867.

Kauffman DW, Slone D, Rosenberg L, et al. Cigarette smoking and age at natural menopause. Am J Public Health 1980;70:420 – 422.

Kiel DF, Felson DT, Anderson JJ, Wilson FWF, Moskowitz MA. Hip fracture and the use of estrogens in postmenopausal women: The Framingham Study. N Engl J Med 1987;317:1169 – 1174.

Klibanski A, Neer RM, Beitins IZ, Ridgway EC, Zervas NT, McArthur JW. Decreased bone density in hyperprolactinaemic women. N Engl J Med 1980;303:1511 – 1514.

Klibanski A, Greenspan SL. Increase in bone mass after treatment of hyperprolactinaemic amenorrhoea. N Engl J Med 1986;315:542 – 546.

Komm BS, Terpening CM, Benz DJ, et al. Estrogen binding, receptor mRNA and biologic response in osteoblast osteosarcoma cells. Science 1988;241:81 – 84.

Kono S, Merriam GR, Brandon DD, Loriaux DL, Lipsett MB. Radioimmunoassay and metabolism of the catechol estrogen 2-hydrocyestradiol. J Clin Endocrinol Metab 1982;54:150 – 154.

Korenmann SG, Dukes BA. Specific estrogen binding to the cytoplasm of human breast carcinoma. J Clin Endocrinol Metab 1970;30:639 – 645.

Korenmann SG, Sherman BM, Korenmann JC. Reproductive hormone function: the perimenopausal period and beyond. Clin Endocrinol Metab 1976;42:629 – 636.

Koppelman MCS, Kurtz DW, Morrish KA, et al. Vertebral body bone mineral content in hyperprolactinaemic women. J Clin Endocrinol Metab 1984;59:1050 – 1053.

Kragstrup J, Gundersen HJG, Melsen F, Mosekilde L. Estimation of the three dimensional wall thickness of completed remodelling sites in iliac trabecular bone. Metab Bone Dis Rel Res 1982;4:113 – 119.

Krieger N, Kelsey JL, Holford TR, O'Connor T. An epidemiologic study of hip fracture in postmenopausal women. Am J Epidemiol 1978;116:141 – 148.

Lindqvist O, Bengtsson C, Hansson T, et al. Bone mineral content in relation to age and menopause in middle aged women. Scand J Clin Lab Invest 1981;41:215 – 223.

Lindsay R, Coutts JRT, Sweeney A, Hart DM. Endogenous oestrogen and bone loss following oophorectomy. Calcif Tissue Res 1977;22:213 – 216.

Lindsay R, Hart DM, MacLean A, Clark AC, Kraszowski A, Garwood J. Bone response to termination of oestrogen treatment. Lancet 1978;1:1325 – 1327.

Lindsay R, Hart DM, Forrest C, Baird C. Prevention of spinal osteoporosis in oophorectomized women. Lancet 1980;2:1151 – 1154.

Lindsay R. The influence of cigarette smoking on bone mass and bone loss. In: DeLuca HF, Frost H, Jee WSS et al, eds. Osteoporosis: Recent Advances in Pathogenesis and Treatment. Baltimore: University Park Press, 1981;481.

Lopez A, Ventanas J, Burgos J. Oestradiol and testosterone binding sites in mice tibiae and their relationship to bone growth. Exp Clin Endocrinol 1986;88:31 – 38.

Loucks AB, Horvath SM. Exercise induced stress responses of amenorrheic and eumenorrheic runners. J Clin Endocrinol Metab 1984;59:1100 – 1112.

MacDonald TW, Annegers JF, O'Fallon WM, Dockerty MB, Malkasian GD, Kurland LT. Exogenous estrogen and endometrial carcinoma: case-control and incidence study. Am J Obstet Gynecol 1977;127:572 – 580.

MacMahon B, Trichoupoulos D, Cole P, et al. Cigarette smoking, relative weight and menopause. Am J Epidemiol 1983;117:651 – 658.

MacRae KD. Health risks of estrogen therapy. J Endocrinol 1981;89:145P – 148P.

Malawer M, Bray M, Kass M. Fluorescent histochemical demonstration of estrogen and progesterone binding in giant cell tumors of bone: preliminary observations. J Surg Oncol 1984;25:148 – 152.

Manwol SE, Menan KMJ. Changes in reproductive hormone secretion during the climacteric and postmenopausal periods. Clin Obstet Gynecol 1977;20:113 – 122.

Marshall RW, Selby PL, Chivers DC, Hodgkinson A. The effect of ethinylestradiol on calcium and bone metabolism in peri- and postmenopausal women. Horm Metab Res 1984;16:97 – 103.

McGuire WL, Carbone PP, Sears ME, Escher GC. Estrogen receptors in human breast cancer: an overview. In: McGuire WL, Carbone PP, Vollmer EP, eds. Estrogen Receptors in Human Breast Cancer. New York: Raven Press, 1975;1 – 7.

Melsen F, Mosekilde L. Morphometric and dynamic studies of bone changes in hyperthyroidism. Acta Pathol Scand Sect A 1977;85:141 – 150.

Mellstrom D, Rundgren A, Jagenburg R, et al. Tobacco smoking, ageing and health among the elderly:

a longitudinal population study of 70 year old men and an age cohort comparison. Age Ageing 1982;11:45 – 58.

Mendel FP, Geola FL, Lu JKH, et al. Biological effects of various doses of ethinyl estradiol on postmenopausal women. Obstet Gynecol 1982;59:673 – 679.

Mester J, Baulieu EE. Nuclear estrogen receptor of chick liver. Biochim Biophys Acta 1972;261:236 – 241.

Michnovicz JJ, Hershcopf H, Naganuma H, Bradlow HL, Fishman J. Increased 2-hydroxylation of estradiol as a possible mechanism to the anti-estrogenic effect of cigarette smoking. N Engl J Med 1986;315:1305 – 1309.

Morel G, Boivin G, David L, Dubois PM, Meunier PJ. Immunocytochemical evidence for endogenous calcitonin and parathyroid hormone in osteoblasts from the calvaria from neonatal mice. Absence of endogenous estradiol and estradiol receptors. Cell Tissue Res 1985;240:89 – 93.

Mosekilde L, Mosekilde L. Normal vertebral body size and compressive strength: relations to age and to vertebral and iliac trabecular bone compressive strength. Bone 1986;7:207 – 212.

Mosekilde L, Mosekilde Li, Danielsen CC. Biomechanical competence of vertebral trabecular bone in relation to ash density and age in normal individuals. Bone 1987;8:79 – 85.

Mukku VR, Stancel GM. Regulation of epidermal growth factor receptor by estrogen. J Biol Chem 1986;260:9820 – 9824.

Muller RE, Traish AM, Wotiz HH. Estrogen receptor activation precedes transformation: effects of ionic strength, temperature and molybdate. J Biol Chem 1983;258:9227 – 9236.

Munk Jensen N, Pors Nielsen S, Obel EB, Bonne Eriksen P. Reversal of postmenopausal vertebral bone loss by oestrogen and progestagen: a double blind placebo controlled study. Br Med J 1988;296:1150 – 1152.

Murayama A, Fukai F, Haroto T, Yamamoto T. Estrogen receptor of cow uterus. 3. Molecular constitution of estrogen receptor binding factors. J Biochem 1980;88:969 – 976.

Murphy LJ, Friesen HG. Differential effects of estrogen and growth hormone on uterine and hepatic insulin like growth factor I gene expression in the ovariectomized hypophysectomized rats. Endocrinology 1988;122:325 – 332.

Nachtigall LE, Nachtigall RH, Nachtigall RD. Estrogen replacement therapy II: a prospective study on the relationship to carcinoma and cardiovascular and metabolic problems. J Obstet Gynecol 1979a;54:74 – 79.

Nachtigall LE, Nachtigall RH, Nachtigall RD, Beckman EM. Estrogen replacement therapy II: a prospective study in relationship to carcinoma and cardiovascular and metabolic problems. Obstet Gynecol 1979b;54:74 – 79.

Nomura AMY, Kolonel LN, Hirohata T, Lee J. The association of replacement estrogens with breast cancer. Int J Cancer 1986;37:49 – 53.

O'Malley BW, Means AR. Female steroid hormones and target cell nuclei: the effects of steroid hormones on target cell functions. Science 1974;183:610 – 620.

Paganini-Hill A, Ross RK, Gerkins VR, Henderson BE, Arthur M, Marci TM. Menopausal estrogen therapy and hip fractures. Ann Intern Med 1981;95:28 – 31.

Parfitt AM. The actions of parathyroid hormone on bone: relation to bone remodelling and turnover, calcium homeostasis and metabolic bone disease. Part III of IV parts: PTH and osteoblasts, the relationship between bone turnover and bone loss, and the state of bone in primary hyperparathyroidism. Metabolism 1976;25:1033 – 1087.

Parfitt AM. Quantum concept of bone remodelling and turnover: implications for the pathogenesis of osteoporosis. Calcif Tissue Int 1979;28:1 – 5.

Parfitt AM. The coupling of bone formation and bone resorption: a critical analysis of the concept and its relevance to the pathogenesis of osteoporosis. Metab Bone Dis Rel Res 1982;4:1 – 6.

Parfitt AM. The physiologic and clinical significance of bone histomorphometric data. In: Recker RR, ed. Bone histomorphometry, techniques and interpretation. Boca Raton, Florida: CRC Press Inc., 1983;143 – 224.

Parfitt AM. Age related structural changes in trabecular and cortical bone: cellular mechanisms and biomechanical consequences. Calcif Tissue Int 1984;36:123 – 128.

Petitti DB, Wingerd ZJ, Pellerin G, Ramcharan S. Risk of vascular disease in women: smoking, oral contraceptives, noncontraceptive estrogens and other factors. J Am Med Assoc 1979;242:1150 – 1154.

Pfeffer RI, Van den Noort S. Estrogen use and stroke risk in postmenopausal women. Am J Epidemiol 1976;103:445 – 456.

Pfeffer RI, Whipple GH, Kuorsaki TT, Chapman JM. Coronary risk and estrogen use in postmenopausal women. Am J Epidemiol 1978;107:479 – 487.

Persson I. Cancerrisker efter langtidsbehandling med oestrogen-gestagen. Laekartidningen 1987;84:4256 – 4257.

Petterson F, Fries H, Nillius SJ. Epidemiology of secondary amenorrhoea I. Incidence and prevalence rates. Am J Obstet Gynecol 1973;117:80 – 86.

Pfeilschifter J, Mundy GR. Modulation of type-beta transforming growth factor activity in bone cultures by osteotropic hormones. Proc Natl Acad Sci USA 1987;84:2024 – 2028.

Pilbeam CC, Raisz LG. In vitro inhibition of PTH-stimulated prostaglandin ($PGE_2$) production by 17-beta estradiol. J Bone Miner Res 1988;3(Suppl. 1):S219.

Pocock NA, Eisman JA, Yeates MG, Sambrook PN, Eberl S. Physical fitness is a major determinant of femoral neck and lumbar spine bone mineral density. J Clin Invest 1986;78:618 – 622.

Puca GA, Nola E, Sica V, Bresciani F. Estrogen binding proteins of calf uterus. Molecular and functional characterization of the receptor transforming factor: a $Ca^{++}$ activated protease. J Biol Chem 1977;252:1358 – 1366.

Ratajczak T, Brockway MJ, Hahnel R, Moritz RL, Simpson RJ. Sequence analysis of the nonsteroid binding component of the calf uterine estrogen receptor. Biochem Biophys Res Commun 1988;151:1156 – 1163.

Recker RR, Saville PD, Heaney RP. Effect of estrogens and calcium carbonate on bone loss in postmenopausal women. Ann Intern Med 1977;87:549 – 555.

Recker RR, Gallagher JC, Heaney RP. The metabolic effects of treatment with calcitriol in patients with postmenopausal osteoporosis. Clin Res 1984;32:406A.

Redeuilh G, Moncharmont B, Secco C, Baulieu EE. Subunit composition of the molybdate stabilized '8-9S' nontransformed estradiol receptor purified from calf uterus. J Biol Chem 1988;262:6969 – 6975.

Report from Boston Collaborative Drug Surveillance Program. Surgically confirmed gall bladder disease, venous thromboembolism and breast tumors in relation to postmenopausal estrogen therapy. N Engl J Med 1974;290:15 – 19.

Richelson LS, Wahner HW, Melton LJ III, Riggs BL. Relative contributions of aging and estrogen deficiency to postmenopausal bone loss. N Engl J Med 1984;311:1273 – 1275.

Rickers H, Balslev I, Foltved H, Roedbro P. Bone mineral content before and after intestinal bypass operation in obese patients. Acta Med Scand 1981;209:203 – 207.

Riggs BL, Jowsey J, Goldsmith RS, Kelly PJ, Hoffman DL, Arnaud CD. Short and long term effects of estrogens and synthetic anabolic steroids in postmenopausal osteoporosis. J Clin Invest 1972;51:1959 – 1964.

Riggs BL, Nelson KI. Effects of long term treatment with calcitriol on calcium absorption and mineral metabolism in postmenopausal osteoporosis. J Clin Endocrinol Metab 1985;61:457 – 461.

Riggs BL, Wahner HW, Melton LJ III, Richelson LS, Judd HL, Offord KP. Rates of bone loss in the appendicular and axial skeletons of women: evidence of substantial vertebral bone loss prior to menopause. J Clin Invest 1985;77:1487 – 1491.

Riggs BL, Melton LJ, III. Involutional osteoporosis. N Engl J Med 1986;314:1676 – 1686.

Riggs TR, Pan MW, Feng HW. Transport of amino acids into the estrogen primed uterus I. General characteristics of the effect in vitro. Biochim Biophys Acta 1968;150:92 – 96.

Rigotti NA, Nussbaum SR, Herzog DB, Neer RM. Osteoporosis in women with anorexia nervosa. N Engl J Med 1984;311:1601 – 1606.

Rosenberg L, Armstrong B, Jick H. Myocardial infarction and estrogen therapy in postmenopausal women. N Engl J Med 1976;294:1256 – 1259.

Rosenberg L, Sloane D, Shapiro S, Kaufman D, Stolley PD, Miettenen OS. Noncontraceptive estrogens and myocardial infarction in young women. J Am Med Assoc 1980;244:339 – 342.

Ross RK, Paganini-Hill A, Gerkins NR, Mack TM, Pfeffer R, Arthur M, Henderson BE. A case-control study of menopausal estrogen therapy and breast cancer. J Am Med Assoc 1980;243:1635 – 1639.

Ross RK, Paganini-Hill A, Mack TM, Arthur M, Henderson BE. Menopausal oestrogen therapy and protection from death from ischaemic heart disease. Lancet 1981;1:858 – 860.

Ryan KJ. Estrogen use and postmenopausal women: a National Institute of Health Consensus Development Conference. Ann Intern Med 1979;91:921 – 922.

Sagar S, Stamatakis JD, Thomas DP, Kakkar VV. Oral contraceptive, antithrombin III activity and postoperative deep vein thrombosis. Lancet 1976;1:509 – 511.

Schlechte JA, Sherman B, Martin R. Bone density in amenorrheic women with and without hyperprolactinaemia. J Clin Endocrinol Metab 1983;56:1120 – 1123.

Schwartz B, Cummings DC, Riordan E, Selye M, Yen S, Rebar R. Exercise associated amenorrhoea: a distinct entity? Am J Obstet Gynecol 1981;141:662 – 665.

Schulze H, Barrack ER. Immunocytochemical localization of estrogen receptors in the normal acanine urinary tract and prostate. Endocrinology 1987;121:1773 – 1783.

Shanborne CF, Martin BJ, Wagner WW. Is athletic amenorrhoea specific to runners. Am J Obstet Gynecol 1982;143:859 – 860.

Shangold MM, Levine HS. The effect of marathon training upon menstrual function. Am J Obstet Gynecol 1982;143:882 – 885.

Sheridan PJ, Buchanan JM, Anselmo VC, Martin PM. Equilibrium: the intracellular distribution of steroid receptors. Nature 1979;282:579 – 582.

Sherman MR, Stevens J. Structure of mammalian steroid receptors: evolving concepts and methodological developments. Annu Rev Physiol 1984;46:83 – 105.

Shulman DI, Sweetland M, Duckett G, Root AW. Effect of estrogen on the growth hormone (GH) secretory response to GH-releasing factor in the castrate female rat in vivo. Endocrinology 1987;120:1047 – 1051.

Sica V, Puca GA, Nola E, Bresciani F. Use of chaotropic salts to prevent aggregation of estrogen receptors. Fed Proc 1977;R10.

Siiteri PK. Postmenopausal estrogen production. Front Horm Res 1973;3:40 – 44.

Siiteri PK, MacDonald PC. Role of extraglandular estrogen in human endocrinology. In: Greep RD, Astwood EB, eds. Handbook of Physiology, Sect 7: Endocrinology. Washington DC: American Physiological Society, 1973;603 – 613.

Sørensen OH, Lund B, Lund B, Andersen RB, Danneskjold Samsoe B, Mosekilde L, Melsen F, Saltin B, Friis T, Selnes A. Effects of 1-alpha vitamin D on bone and muscle in senile osteopenia. Proceedings from 'Endocrinology 79'. In: McIntyre I, Szelke J, eds. Molecular Endocrinology. Amsterdam: Elsevier/North-Holland Biomedical Press, 1979;309 – 318.

Spelsberg TC, Boyd-Leinen PA. Identification of biologically active and inactive steroid receptors. Clin Biochem 1980;13:198 – 203.

Spelsberg TC, Boyd-Leinen PA, Martin-Dani G, Kon OL. Novel regulations in steroid action: Role of receptor subunits and chromosomal proteins in nuclear bindings. In: Birdsell NJM, ed. Drug Receptors and Their Effectors. London: Macmillan Press Limited, 1981;133 – 154.

Spelsberg TC, Littlefield BA, Seelke R, Dani GM. Toyoda H, Boyd-Leinen P, Thrall C, Kon OL. Role of specific chromosomal proteins and DNA sequences in the nuclear binding sites for steroid receptors. Rec Prog Horm Res 1983;39:463 – 517.

Spelsberg TC, Goldberger A, Horton M, Hora J. Nuclear acceptor sites for sex steroid hormone receptors in chromatin. J Steroid Biochem 1987;27:133 – 147.

Stampfer MJ, Willet WC, Colditz GA, Rosner B, Spizer FE, Hennekens CH. A prospective study of postmenopausal estrogen therapy and heart disease. N Engl J Med 1985;313:1044 – 1049.

Steiniche T, Vesterby A, Eriksen EF, Mosekilde L, Melsen F. A histomorphometric determination of iliac bone structure and remodelling in obese subjects. Bone 1986;7:77 – 82.

Steiniche T, Hasling C, Charles P, Eriksen EF, Mosekilde L, Melsen F. A randomized study on the effects of estrogen/gestagen or high dose oral calcium on trabecular bone remodelling in postmenopausal osteoporosis. Bone 1989;10:313 – 320.

Stewart PJ, Stern PH. Vertebral bone resorption in vitro: effects of parathyroid hormone, calcitonin, 1,25-dihydroxyvitamin $D_3$, epidermal growth factor, prostaglandin $E_2$ and estrogen. Calcif Tissue Int 1987;40:21 – 26.

Stevenson JC, Abeyasekera G, Hillyard CJ, Phang KG, MacIntyre I, Campbell S, Townsent PT, Young O, Whitehead MI. Calcitonin and the calcium regulating hormones in postmenopausal osteoporosis: Effect of estrogens. Lancet 1981;i:693 – 695.

Stumpf WE, Morin JK, Ennis BW, Zielinksi JE, Hochberg RB. Utility of [$^{16}$alfa-$^{125}$I] Iodoestradiol for autoradiography for the study of cellular and regional distribution of receptors. J Histochem Cytochem 1987;33:87 – 92.

Sumida C, Lecerf F, Pasqualini JR. Control of progesterone receptors in fetal uterine cells in culture: effects of estradiol, progestins, antiestrogens, and growth factors. Endocrinology 1988;122:3 – 11.

Szego CM, Roberts S. Steroid action and interaction in uterine metabolism. Rec Prog Horm Res 1953;8:149.

Szklo M, Tonascia J, Gordis L. Estrogen use and myocardial infarction risk: a case control study. Prev Med 1984;13:510 – 516.

Thibodeau SN, Freeman L, Jiang NS. Simultaneous measurement of estrogen and progesterone receptors in tumor cytosols with use of $^{125}$I-labelled estradiol and of $^{3}$H-R5020. Clin Chem 1980;27:687 – 691.

Thom MH, White PJ, Williams RM. Prevention and treatment of endometrial disease in climacteric women receiving oestrogen therapy. Lancet 1979;2:455 – 457.

Thomsen K, Roedbro P, Christiansen C. Bone turnover determined by urinary excretion of $^{99m}$Tc-diphosphonate in the prediction of postmenopausal bone loss. Bone Miner 1987;2:125 – 131.

Thornton JG, Wells M. Oestrogen receptor in glands and stroma of normal and neoplastic human endometrium: a combined histochemical, immunocytochemical and morphometric study. J Clin Pathol 1987;40:1437 – 1442.

Thrall C, Webster R, Spelsberg TC. Steroid receptor interaction with chromatin. In: Busch H, ed. The Cell Nucleus, Vol VI, Part I. New York: Academic Press 1978;461 – 529.

Van Paassen HC, Poortman J, Bogart-Creutzburg IHC, Thijssen JHH, Duursma SA. Oestrogen binding in bone cell cytosol. Calcif Tissue Res 1978;25:249 – 254.

Vermuelen A, Valdenek L. Sex hormone concentrations in postmenopausal women: relation to obesity, fat mass age and years post menopause. Clin Endocrinol 1978;9:59 – 66.

Vessey MP. Female hormones and vascular disease: epidemiologic overview. Br J Fam Plann 1980;6:1 – 12.

Von Kaulla E, Drogmueller W, Von Kaulla KN. Conjugated oestrogen and hypercoagulability. Am J Obstet Gynecol 1975;122:775 – 778.

Wahl P, Walden C, Knopp R, Wallace R, Hiess G, Rifkind B. Effect of estrogen/progestin potency on lipid/lipoprotein cholesterol. N Engl J Med 1983;308:862 – 867.

Wallace RB, Hoover J, Barret-Cono E, et al. Altered plasma lipid and lipoprotein levels associated with oral contraceptive and estrogen use. Lancet 1979;2:111 – 115.

Wallentin L, Larsson Cohn U. Metabolic and hormonal effects of postmenopausal oestrogen replacement treatment: II Plasma lipids. Acta Endocrinol (Kbh) 1977;86:597 – 607.

Walsh BT. The endocrinology of anorexia nervosa. Adv Psychoneuroendocrinol 1977;3:597 – 607.

Walters MR. Steroid hormone receptors and the nucleus. Endocr Rev 1985;6:512 – 543.

Weiss NS, Szekely DR, Dallas R, English MS, Abraham I, Schweid AI. Endometrial cancer in relations to patterns of perimenopausal estrogen use. J Am Med Assoc 1980a;242:299 – 312.

Weiss NS, Ure CL, Ballard JH, Williams AR, Daling JF. Decreased risk of fractures of the hip and lower forearm with postmenopausal use of estrogen. N Engl J Med 1980b;303:1195 – 1197.

Weiss SW, Langloss JM, Shmookler BM, Malawer MM, D'Avis J, Enzinger FM, Stanton R. Estrogen receptor protein in bone and soft tissue tumors. Lab Invest 1986;54:689 – 693.

Welshons WV, Lieberman ME, Gorski J. Nuclear localization of unoccupied oestrogen receptors. Nature 1984;307:747 – 749.

Wessler SS, Gitel SN, Wan LS, Pasternack BS. Estrogen-containing oral contraceptive agents: a basis for their thrombogenicity. J Am Med Assoc 1976;236:2197 – 2182.

Whitehead MI, Townsend PT, Pryse-Davies J, Ryder TA, King JB. Effects of estrogen and progestins on the biochemistry and morphology of the postmenopausal endometrium. N Engl J Med 1981;305:1599 – 1605.

Wilding G, Lippman ME, Gelmann EP. Effects of steroid hormones and peptide growth factors on proto-oncogene c-fos expression in human breast cancer cells. Cancer Res 1988;48:802 – 805.

Williams AR, Weiss NS, Ure CL, Balladr J, Daling JR. Effect of weight, smoking and estrogen use on the risk of hip and forearm fractures in postmenopausal women. Obstet Gynecol 1982;60:695 – 699.

Williams GA, Kukreja SC, Bowser EN, Hargis GK, Greenberg CP, Henderson WJ. Prolonged effect of estradiol on calcitonin secretion. Bone Miner 1986;1:415 – 420.

Wilson FWF, Garrison RJ, Castelli WP. Postmenopausal estrogen use, cigarette smoking and cardiovascular morbidity in women over 50. N Engl J Med 1985;313:1038 – 1043.

Yoshioka T, Sato B, Matsumoto K, Ono K. Steroid receptors in osteoblasts. Clin Orthop Rel Res 1980;148:297 – 303.

Ziel KH. Estrogen's role in endometrial cancer. Obstet Gynecol 1982;60:509 – 515.

Ziel HK, Finkle WK. Increased risk of endometrial carcinoma among users of conjugated estrogens. N Engl J Med 1975;293:1167 – 1170.

*Bone and Mineral Research/7*
*Johan N.M. Heersche and John A. Kanis, editors*



# Vitamin D and the skin: photobiology, physiology and therapeutic efficacy for psoriasis

Michael F. Holick

*Boston University School of Medicine, 80 East Concord St., M-1013 Boston, MA 02118, U.S.A.*

## I. Introduction

Vitamin D is a unique vitamin/hormone whose origin dates back at least 500 million years when it was produced in ocean-dwelling photoplankton while they were being exposed to sunlight (Holick 1989a). There is mounting evidence that most plants and animals exposed to sunlight have the capacity to produce this seco-sterol (Holick 1989a). Although the biologic function of vitamin D in plants and invertebrates is unknown it appears that the intimate relationship between sunlight and vitamin D became essential in the evolution of terrestrial vertebrates. The major physiologic function of vitamin D is to maintain extracellular fluid concentrations of calcium and phosphorus within the normal range. This seco-sterol accomplishes this by regulating the efficiency of intestinal calcium and phosphorus transport and by stimulating the mobilization of calcium and phosphorus stores from the bone (DeLuca 1984; Holick 1987; Reichel et al. 1989).

During the past two decades, intensive research on vitamin D has revealed that vitamin D is a hormone and not a vitamin. Once vitamin D is formed in the skin it requires obligate hydroxylations in the liver and kidney to form 1,25-dihydroxyvitamin D ($1,25(OH)_2D$) (DeLuca 1988; Holick 1989b; Reichel et al. 1989). It is $1,25(OH)_2D$ that is responsible for enhancing the efficiency of intestinal absorption of dietary calcium and phosphorus and the mobilization of calcium and phosphorus stores from bone.

During the past decade, it has been recognized that high affinity, low capacity receptors for $1,25(OH)_2D$ are present not only in expected target tissues such as the intestine bone and kidney but also in a diversity of other tissues and cells including the brain, gonads, stomach, pancreas, mononuclear cells, lymphocytes, and skin (Stumpf et al. 1979; Bhalla et al. 1983; Tsoukas et al. 1984; Holick et al. 1987). The hormonal form of vitamin D can inhibit the proliferation and induce maturation of both normal and tumor cells that possess its receptor (Eisman 1984; Suda et al. 1984).

Of special interest to our research group was that the skin was not only the site for the synthesis of vitamin $D_3$ but it also was a potential target tissue for its activated form. One practical application for this phenomenon was the possible use of 1,25-$(OH)_2D_3$ and its analogs for the treatment of the hyperproliferative skin disorder psoriasis. This chapter focuses on advances in our understanding of the photobiology of vitamin $D_3$ and the potential therapeutic use of 1,25 $(OH)_2D_3$ and its analogs for psoriasis.

## II. Historical perspective of rickets

### A. Epidemiology

Archaeological records show that humans have worshipped the sun for its life-giving powers from almost the beginning of time. Although the relationship of sunshine to health began to be appreciated at the turn of the 20th century, its roots began over 300 years ago. As people began to migrate to city-centers in Northern Europe and live in an environment that was devoid of direct exposure to sunlight (Fig. 1), a disease identified by deformities of the skeleton (Fig. 2), including enlargement of the joints of the long bones and rib cage, curvature of the spine and thighs, enlargement of the head, and generalized muscular weakness was recognized. Glisson and Whistler in 1650 identified this bone-deforming disease as a major health problem for the young children in the industrialized cities of Great Britain (Fraser and Scriver 1979; Holick 1987). The incidence of the disease commonly known as rickets or 'English disease', continued to increase during the industrial revolution and by the turn of the 20th century this disease was epidemic in industrialized cities of Northern Europe and in northeastern United States. One study conducted in Leiden, the Netherlands, reported that more than 80% of young children dying of various causes had clinical manifestations of this bone-deforming disease (Schmorl 1909). The consequences of this disease were quite profound, especially for children who often had deformities of their legs making it difficult for them to walk and work. For women, a deformed pelvis often caused difficulty in child birth and resulted in a high incidence of infant and maternal morbidity and mortality.

The first insight into the potential cause of this devastating bone disease was made by Sniadecki in 1822 (Sniadecki 1939). He reported that children in Warsaw, Poland had a very high incidence of rickets while children living in the nearby rural areas were essentially free of the disease. He advocated that 'if parents financial status permits it is best to take children out into the country and keep them as much as possible in the dry, open and pure air. If not, they should be carried out in the open air especially in the sun, the direct action of which on their bodies must be regarded as one of the most efficient methods for the prevention and cure of this disease . . . thus strong and obvious is the influence of the sun on the cure of 'English disease' [i.e. rickets], and the frequent occurrence of the disease in densely populated towns, where the streets are narrow and the dwellings of the working class low and poorly lit.'

Unfortunately, these brilliant insights were not appreciated by the medical and scientific communities at the time and little attention was focused on the environment

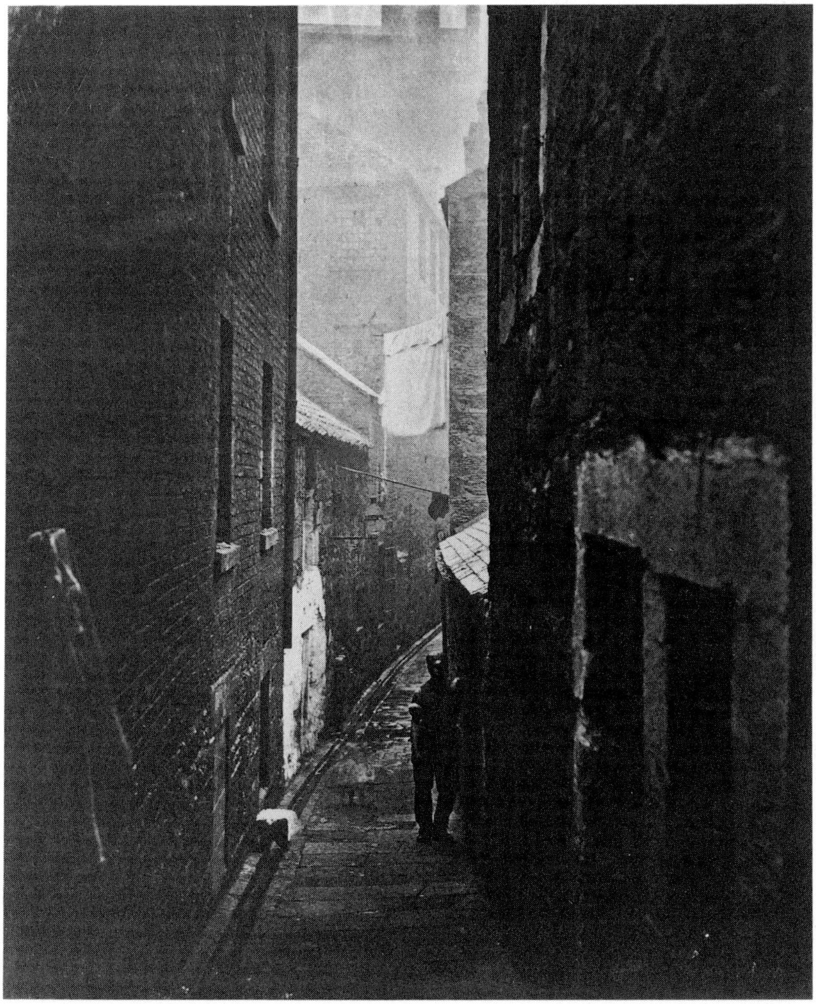

Fig. 1. A typical scene in Glasgow in the mid-1800s as captured by this photograph taken by Thomas Annan. (Reproduced with permission, Thomas Annan's Photographs of the Old Closes and Streets of Glasgow 1868/1877, Dover Publications, Inc., New York, 1977.)

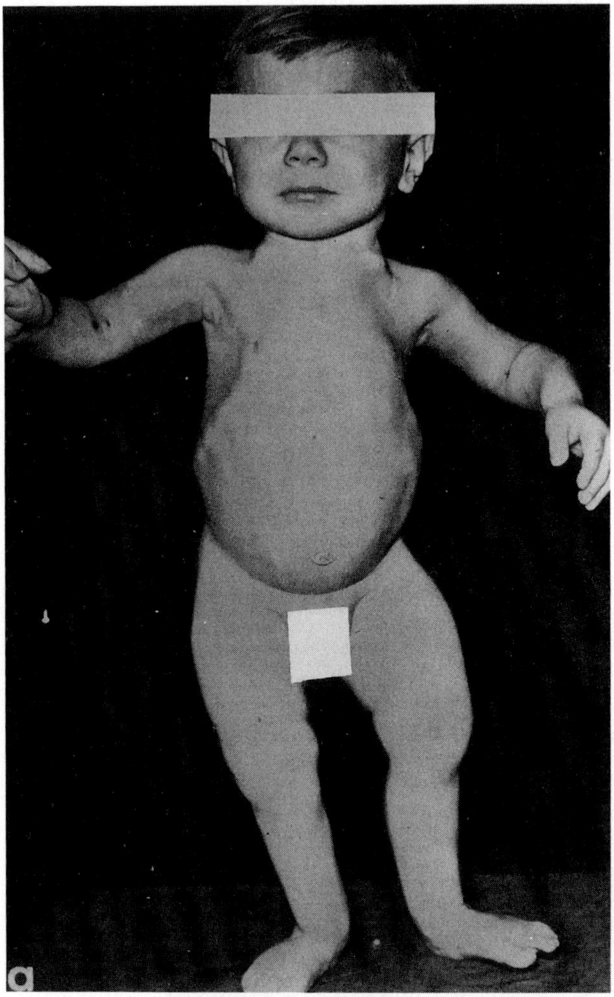

Fig. 2. Child with rickets showing rachitic rosary of the rib cage, bowed legs, deformity of the long bones, and muscle weakness. (From Fraser and Scriver 1979, with permission.)

as a cause for this disease until 1889 when an investigative committee of the British Medical Association reported that rickets was unknown in rural districts of the British Islands but that it was prevalent in the large industrialized towns (Owen 1889). A year later, Palm (1890) reported an epidemiologic survey regarding potential factors that cause rickets. He evaluated the prevalence of rickets around the world and found that children who had poor nutrition and lived in squalor in many of the cities in China, Japan, and India were not afflicted with this dreaded disease. Therefore, ruling out nutrition and infection as likely causes of rickets, he concentrated his efforts on other potential causes. He reasoned the only difference between children who were living in rural areas in Britain and the underdeveloped countries from middle-class British children living in the inner cities was the latter were not exposed to sunlight. Palm concluded that the common denominator for rickets in children was the lack of sunlight exposure. He encouraged systematic sunbathing as a means for preventing and curing rickets and encouraged the scientific community to appreciate the healthful effects of sunlight. However, the response of the medical and scientific community to these insightful observations went unheeded just as were Sniadecki's. Indeed it was inconceivable for the medical and scientific communities to believe that exposure to sunlight could have any significant impact on bone disease (Holick 1989b).

By the turn of the 20th century rickets continued to be a major health problem in the industrialized cities of Europe and North America. Numerous investigators from almost every field of science began a major effort to define the cause and find a cure for this disease. Because of its prevalence many investigators thought that rickets was caused by a heritable disorder. Koch (1911) was convinced that rickets was caused by a bacteria. At the time syphilitic bone disease was rampant as was rickets and Koch as well as other prominent physicians believed that the two were related. To prove that rickets was caused by a bacteria he inoculated dogs with *Streptococcus longus* and found that 10% of the dogs developed rickets. Findlay (1908) suggested that it was lack of activity that was most responsible for causing this disease.

### B. Nutritional factor

The concept that rickets was caused by a nutritional deficiency was first suggested by the common folklore practice of giving children cod liver oil to prevent and cure this disease. As early as 1827, Bretonneau treated a 15-month-old child with acute rickets with cod liver oil and noted the incredible speed at which the patient was cured. His student, Trousseau, used the liver oils from a variety of fish including rays, herring as well as whale and seal liver oils for the treatment of rickets and osteomalacia. In his treatise on therapeutics in 1858 he advocated the use of fish liver oil preferably accompanied by exposure to sunlight to rapidly cure both rickets and osteomalacia (Mayer 1957). Unfortunately, by 1900 these insightful observations were disregarded. It was not until 1918 when Mellanby (1918) fed rachitic beagle puppies cod liver oil and found their rickets was cured that the scientific community began to consider rickets as a nutritional deficiency disease. He concluded that cod liver oil possessed a fat soluble nutritional factor that he called the antirachitic factor. Originally it was thought the antirachitic factor was vitamin A. However, when cod liver oil was heated and exposed to oxygen to destroy the vitamin A activity, the resulting oil continued to have antirachitic activity (McCollum et al. 1922). Thus, a new fat soluble compound in cod liver oil was recognized and called vitamin D.

### C. Ultraviolet and solar radiation

Almost simultaneous with Mellanby's observations, Huldschinsky (1919) exposed four rachitic children to radiation from a mercury vapor arc lamp and demonstrated by X-ray analysis that the rickets was cured after 4 months of therapy. He cleverly showed that the effect of this phototherapy was not a local effect on the bone by demonstrating that exposure of one arm to this radiation had an equal and dramatic curative effect on both arms. In 1921, Hess and Unger (1921) exposed seven rachitic children in New York City to sunshine and reported that X-ray examination showed marked improvement in rickets of each child. Thus, one century after Sniadecki had first suggested the importance of sunlight exposure for prevention of rickets it was unequivocally shown that exposure to sunlight alone could prevent and cure this crippling bone disease.

### D. Vitamin D fortification of foods

Initially, it was believed that exposure to radiation from a mercury arc lamp enhanced the mobilization of the fat soluble antirachitic factor from the skin rather than causing its photosynthesis (Goldblatt and Soames 1923). However, this theory was proven to be incorrect when it was shown that irradiation of muscle and liver imparted these tissues with antirachitic activity. The appreciation that exposure to sunlight could cure rickets in children prompted Hess and Weinstock (1924) and Steenbock and Black (1924) to expose a variety of foods and other substances including human and rat plasma, wheat, lettuce, cotton, olive and linseed oils, and rat chow to ultraviolet radiation. They found that the ultraviolet irradiation imparted antirachitic activity to the substances. These observations led Steenbock (1924) to conclude that there may be great utility in irradiating food substances for the prevention and cure of rickets in children. This concept led to the addition of provitamin D to milk and its subsequent irradiation to impart antirachitic activity. This simple concept led to the eradication of rickets as a significant health problem in the United States and other countries that use this practice. Once the structure of vitamin D was characterized, it was chemically synthesized and directly added to milk, making the irradiation of milk obsolete.

Today each quart of milk in the United States is fortified with 400 I.U. (10 $\mu$g, twice the recommended daily allowance of adults) of either vitamin $D_2$ or vitamin $D_3$ (Fig. 3). This process has eradicated rickets as a significant health problem for children living in the industrialized cities of the United States and Canada. However, in the 1940s the amount of vitamin D added to milk was not well regulated in Europe and many infants became intoxicated with vitamin D which caused hypercalcemia and irreversible brain damage. In response, vitamin D fortification was severely restricted in Europe and other countries. As a result, childhood rickets continues to be a health problem in Europe (Stamp et al. 1980; Ala-Houhala et al. 1984; Markestad et al. 1984). Recently, many European countries have begun adding vitamin D to various food stuffs including margarine and cereals.

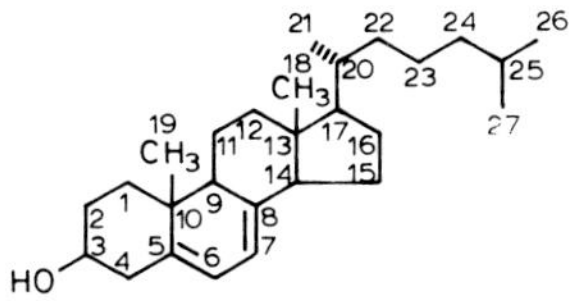

7-Dehydrocholesterol
(provitamin D3)

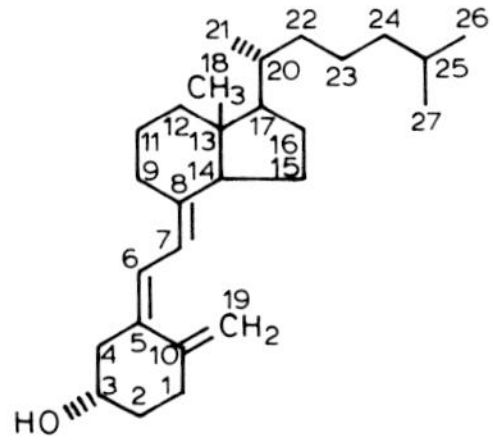

Vitamin D3

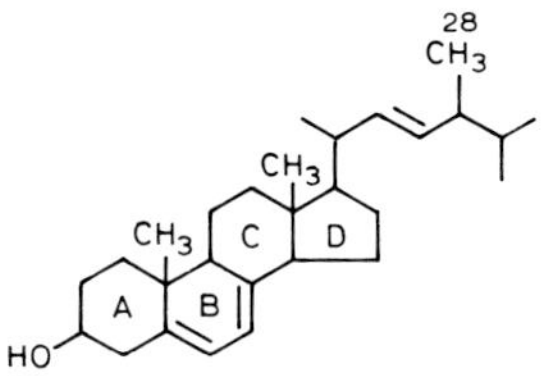

Ergosterol
(provitamin D2)

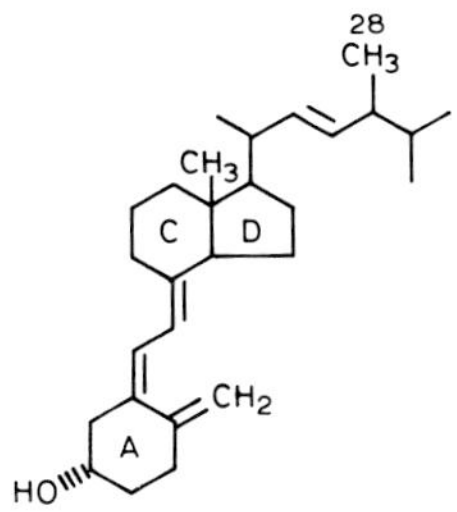

Vitamin D2

Fig. 3. Structure of vitamins $D_3$ and $D_2$ and their respective precursors, 7-dehydrocholesterol and ergosterol. The only structural difference between vitamins $D_2$ and $D_3$ is their side chains; the side chain for vitamin $D_2$ contains a double bond between $C_{22}$, $C_{23}$, and a $C_{24}$ methyl group. (From MacLaughlin and Holick 1983, with permission.)

## E. Identification of vitamin $D_2$ and vitamin $D_3$

Once it was appreciated that exposure of skin to ultraviolet radiation produced antirachitic activity it was of great interest to identify the precursor of vitamin D in the skin. The first precursor of vitamin D was isolated from yeast and identified as ergosterol (Fig. 3) (Fieser and Fieser 1959). Ergosterol, a major sterol in the fungal and plant kingdoms contains a four member ring system with double bonds between carbons 5 and 6 and 7 and 8. When ergosterol was first irradiated the resulting product was called vitamin $D_1$. However, it was quickly appreciated that this vitamin D preparation was a mixture of several compounds and the term vitamin $D_1$ was dropped (Fieser and Fieser 1959). The vitamin D that was isolated in pure form from irradiated ergosterol was called vitamin $D_2$ or ergocalciferol.

Originally it was believed that the vitamin D produced in the skin during exposure to sunlight was vitamin $D_2$. However, in the 1930s investigators (Massengale and Nussmeier 1930; Steenbock and Kletzien 1932; Waddell 1934) found that vitamin $D_2$ was ineffective as an antirachitic factor in chickens when compared to the vitamin D obtained from mammalian skin. These observations suggested that vitamin $D_2$ was not the vitamin D that was produced in mammalian skin. At the same time Windaus and colleagues were synthesizing analogs of vitamin $D_2$, one of which had a side chain for cholesterol. It was found that the vitamin D originating from 7-dehydrocholesterol had the same antirachitic potency in chickens as the vitamin D isolated from mammalian skin (Fieser and Fieser 1959; MacLaughlin and Holick 1983). Finally in 1937, Windaus and Boch (1937) isolated 7-dehydrocholesterol from pig skin. Irradiation of 7-dehydrocholesterol gave rise to a vitamin D called vitamin $D_3$ or cholecalciferol. Vitamin $D_3$ has since been isolated from abdominal human cadaver skin (Rauschkolb et al. 1969) and rat skin (Okano et al. 1977; Esvelt et al. 1978).

## III. Photobiology of vitamin $D_3$

### A. Photosynthesis of previtamin $D_3$ in human skin

At first it was believed that direct exposure of 7-dehydrocholesterol in the skin to sunlight resulted in its conversion to vitamin $D_3$. However, in 1948, Velluz et al. (1948) exposed 7-dehydrocholesterol in an organic solvent to ultraviolet radiation at 0°C and were unable to recover vitamin $D_3$ from the irradiated solution. Instead they isolated a compound that they called previtamin $D_3$. They noted that previtamin $D_3$ was unstable at room temperature and that it slowly isomerized to vitamin $D_3$ (Velluz et al. 1949).

When humans are exposed to sunlight the high energy photons (that are not absorbed by the thin ozone layer that envelops the earth) with energies above 290 nm strike the surface of the skin. Some of this solar energy is reflected, refracted, and absorbed. In whites, 20 – 30% of the radiation at 295 nm is transmitted through the epidermis; the majority of the ultraviolet B (UVB) photons (UVB; 290 – 320 nm) are absorbed by the stratum spinosium of the epidermis. Whereas in blacks only 2 – 5% of the UVB photons penetrate through the epidermis (Anderson and Parrish 1982; MacLaughlin

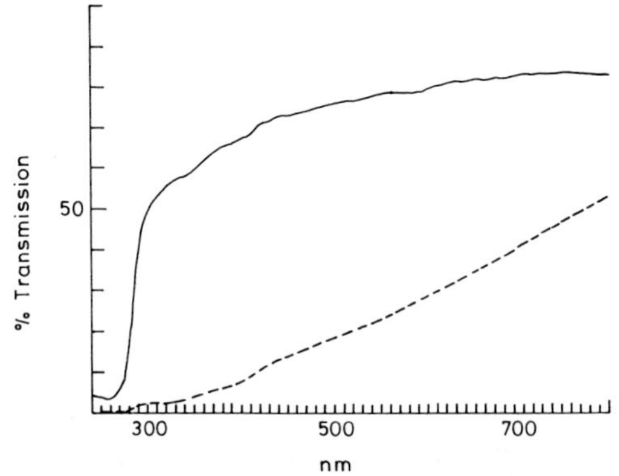


Fig. 4. Percentage transmission of 250 – 800 nm radiation through Caucasoid (——) and Black ( – – – ) epidermis. (From MacLaughlin and Holick 1983, with permission.)

and Holick 1983) (Fig. 4). As the ultraviolet radiation penetrates the epidermis on its journey to the dermis it is absorbed by a variety of molecules including DNA, RNA, proteins, urocanic acid, as well as 7-dehydrocholesterol. The 5,7-diene of 7-dehydrocholesterol absorbs solar radiation between 290 and 315 nm (Fig. 5) causing it to isomerize resulting in a bond cleavage between carbons 9 and 10 to form a 9, 10-seco-sterol (seco from the Greek term to split) previtamin $D_3$ (Fig. 6) (Holick et al. 1980; MacLaughlin et al. 1982). Approximately 65% of the provitamin $D_3$ per unit area is found in the epidermis and the remaining 35% is in the dermis. Because most of the radiation responsible for producing previtamin $D_3$ is absorbed in the epidermis greater than 95% of the previtamin $D_3$ that is produced is in the epidermis (Holick et al. 1980). Once previtamin $D_3$ is synthesized in the skin its conversion to vitamin $D_3$ is controlled by the temperature of its environment. At body temperature (37°C) this conversion takes approximately two days to reach conpletion (Fig. 7). Because the temperature of the viable layers of the epidermis are relatively constant the thermal isomerization of previtamin $D_3$ to vitamin $D_3$ is not affected by the surface temperature of the skin.

Once vitamin $D_3$ is formed in the cytoplasm of the epidermal cells it must be translocated into the extracellular space for transport into the dermal capillary bed. Although the mechanism by which vitamin $D_3$ exits the epidermis is not well understood, it is recognized that the vitamin-D binding protein, an $\alpha_1$-globulin commonly known as the group-specific protein (Cooke and David, 1985) has a relatively high specificity for vitamin $D_3$ when compared to previtamin $D_3$ and provitamin $D_3$ (Fig. 8) (Holick et al. 1981). Therefore, although the vitamin-D binding protein in the dermal capillary circulation does not enter into the epidermis it probably acts like a sponge and helps to selectively direct vitamin $D_3$ from the epidermis into the circulation (Fig. 6).

There are several physiological advantages for producing previtamin $D_3$ in the

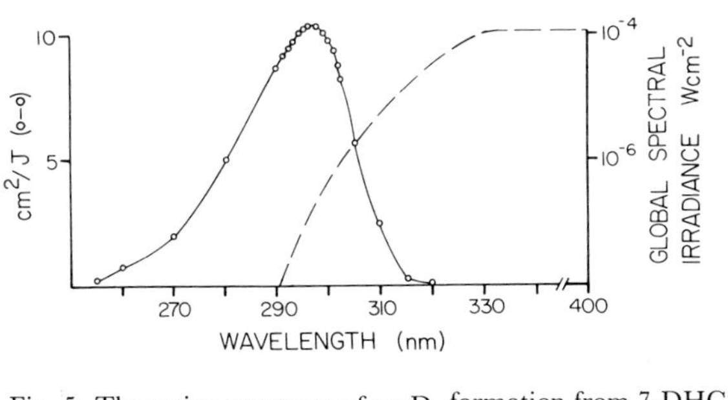


Fig. 5. The action spectrum of pre$D_3$ formation from 7-DHC in human epidermis (○) and the spectral irradiance curve for sunlight ( – – – ). The action spectrum was obtained by plotting the reciprocal of the dose as a function of wavelength. At any wavelength, no more than 5% of product was made. The overlay of the curve of the action spectrum with that of the solar spectrum demonstrates the small portion of the solar UV spectrum that is involved with the production of pre$D_3$ from 7-DHC. (From MacLaughlin et al. with permission. Copyright 1982 by the American Association for the Advancement of Science.)

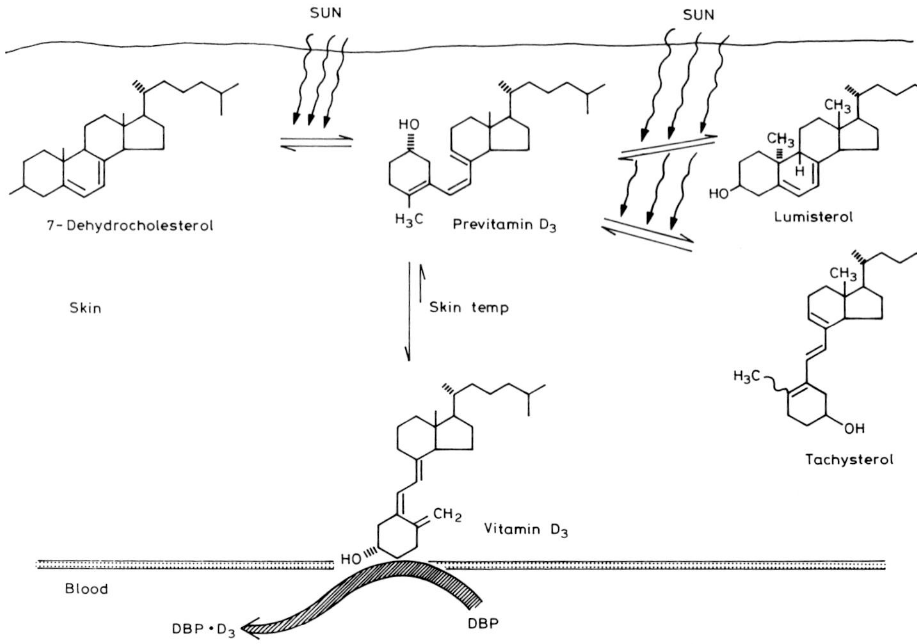


Fig. 6. Schematic representation of the formation of previtamin $D_3$ (pre$D_3$) in the skin during exposure to the sun and the thermal isomerization of pre$D_3$ to vitamin $D_3$, which is specifically translocated by the vitamin-D-binding protein (DBP) into the circulation. During the continual exposure to the sun, pre$D_3$ also photoisomerizes to lumisterol$_3$ and tachysterol$_3$, which are photoproducts that are biologically inert (i.e. they do not stimulate intestinal calcium absorption). Because the DBP has no affinity for lumisterol$_3$ but has minimal affinity for tachysterol$_3$, the translocation of these photoisomers into the circulation is negligible, and these photoproducts are sloughed off during the natural turnover of the skin. Because these photoisomers are in a state of quasiphotoequilibrium, as soon as pre$D_3$ stores are depleted (owing to thermal isomerization to vitamin $D_3$), exposure of lumisterol and tachysterol to UV radiation will provoke these isomers to photoisomerize to pre$D_3$. (From Holick et al. with permission. Copyright 1981 by the American Association for the Advancement of Science.)

skin. Since previtamin $D_3$ is biologically inert and not well recognized by the vitamin-D binding protein, it remains in the epidermis and slowly converts over a period of several days to vitamin $D_3$. The effect of the highly selective translocation of vitamin $D_3$ from the epidermis into the circulation permits removal of vitamin $D_3$ from the epidermis and shifts the previtamin $D_3 \rightleftarrows$ vitamin $D_3$ equilibrium to the right thus ensuring that small quantities of previtamin $D_3$ that are produced in the skin are efficiently converted to vitamin $D_3$ (Fig. 7). In addition, the epidermis retains previtamin $D_3$ for it to continue isomerizing to vitamin $D_3$ thereby limiting its exit into the circulation for metabolic destruction.

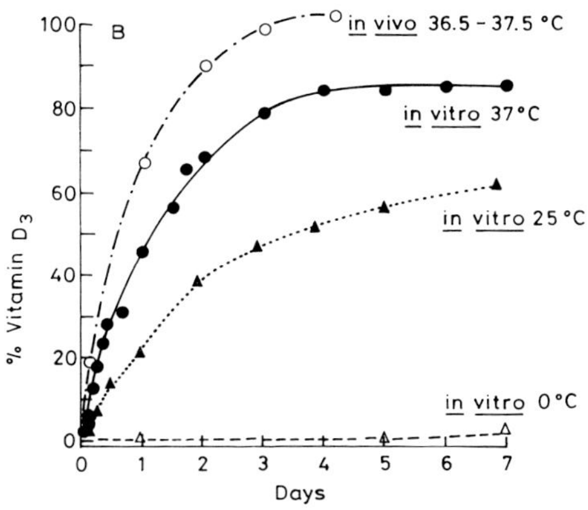


Fig. 7. Thermal conversion of pre$D_3$ to $D_3$ as a function of time *in vitro* at 0°C (- - - △ - - -), 25°C (· · · ▲ · · ·), 37°C (—— ● ——), and *in vivo* at 36.5 – 37.5°C (- ○ -). Each time point represents two experiments, each determined in triplicate. There was excellent agreement for each of the data points, with less than 2% variation. (From Holick et al. with permission. Copyright 1980 by the American Association for the Advancement of Science.)

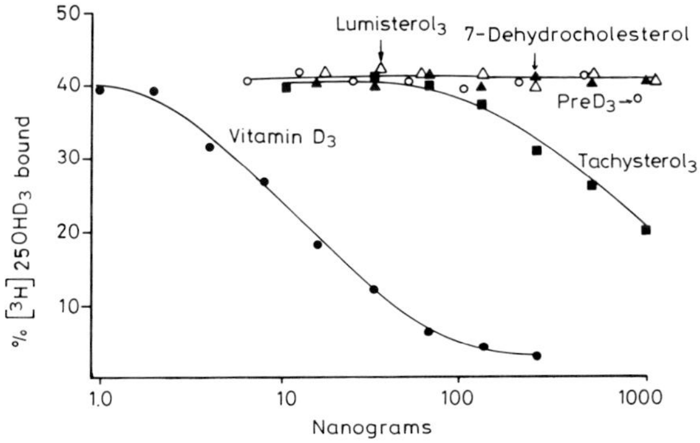


Fig. 8. Displacement of $^3$H-labelled 25-OH-$D_3$ from rat vitamin-D binding protein by vitamin $D_3$, previtamin $D_3$ (pre$D_3$), lumisterol$_3$, tachysterol$_3$, and 7-dehydrocholesterol. Each point represents an average of three determinations. (From Holick et al. with permission. Copyright 1981 by the American Association for the Advancement of Science.)

## B. Factors that affect the cutaneous synthesis of previtamin $D_3$

*1. Effect of hair and feathers.* The concentration of provitamin $D_3$ as well as the quantity and quality of solar radiation reaching the provitamin $D_3$ in the skin are the major factors governing the amount of previtamin $D_3$ that is produced. Hair and feathers on the surface of the skin can absorb most of this radiation and decrease the production of previtamin $D_3$ (Holick et al. 1982). Originally it was believed that 7-

dehydrocholesterol was deposited on the surface of the skin, hair, or feathers to permit its efficient conversion to vitamin $D_3$ during the daytime before being absorbed through the skin or licked off and ingested (Hou 1931). However, there is mounting evidence that his hypothesis is incorrect. For example, in the chicken, Koch and Koch (1941) showed that very little, if any, 7-dehydrocholesterol could be detected in the lipid extracts from feathers and preen glands of chickens compared to relatively high concentrations of the provitamin $D_3$ content in the skin of the legs and feet. Recently, it was found that the skin on the comb of the chicken also had high concentrations of provitamin $D_3$ and when exposed to sunlight the 7-dehydrocholesterol in the comb efficiently converted to previtamin $D_3$ (Young Soo Yoeh and M. F. Holick, unpublished results). Similarly, an analysis of rat hair revealed very little provitamin $D_3$. However, exposure of rats to simulated sunlight demonstrated the production of previtamin $D_3$ in their skin.

*2. Effect of melanin.* It has long been believed that melanin pigmentation evolved for the prevention of vitamin D intoxication due to excessive exposure to sunlight (Loomis 1967). Although melanin is an effective neutral filter that efficiently absorbs UVB-radiation thus diminishing the production of previtamin $D_3$ in the skin, it appears that sunlight itself is the most important factor for regulating the total production of vitamin $D_3$ in the skin (Holick et al. 1981). As can be seen in Fig. 9, when caucasian skin was exposed to simulated equatorial sunlight for 10 min, approximately 15% of provitamin $D_3$ in the stratum basale was converted to previtamin $D_3$. Continued exposure of caucasian skin to simulated equatorial sunlight, however, did not increase the amount of previtamin $D_3$. After one hour of exposure 40% of provitamin $D_3$ had been photolyzed; however, only 15% of the photolyzed provitamin $D_3$ was accounted for as previtamin $D_3$ (Fig. 9). The majority of photolyzed provitamin $D_3$ was accounted for by the presence of two photoproducts identified as lumisterol and tachysterol (Holick et al. 1981) (Fig. 6). The concentrations of lumisterol increased with increasing exposure times. When black skin was subjected to the same conditions, longer exposure times were needed to maximize previtamin $D_3$ formation (Holick et al. 1981). Therefore, it is the photochemical degradation of previtamin $D_3$ rather that melanin pigmentation that is most responsible for limiting the production of previtamin $D_3$ in human skin.

*3. Effect of season, latitude and time of the day.* It is well known that vitamin D deficiency is more prevalent during the winter months. In 1897, Kassowitz (1897) reported on the increased incidence of rickets during the winter months and its decline during the summer and autumn. Similarly, Schmorl (1909) demonstrated from his autopsy studies that the highest percentage of rickets was found between November and May while Hansemann (1906) noted that almost all children who were born in the autumn and died in the spring showed marked manifestation of rickets while those born in the spring and dying in the fall were essentially free of the disease.

It has always been assumed that during the winter people were outdoors less and they wore more clothing, thereby decreasing the surface area of the skin exposed to sunlight. Furthermore, the zenith angle of the sun increased in the autumn and

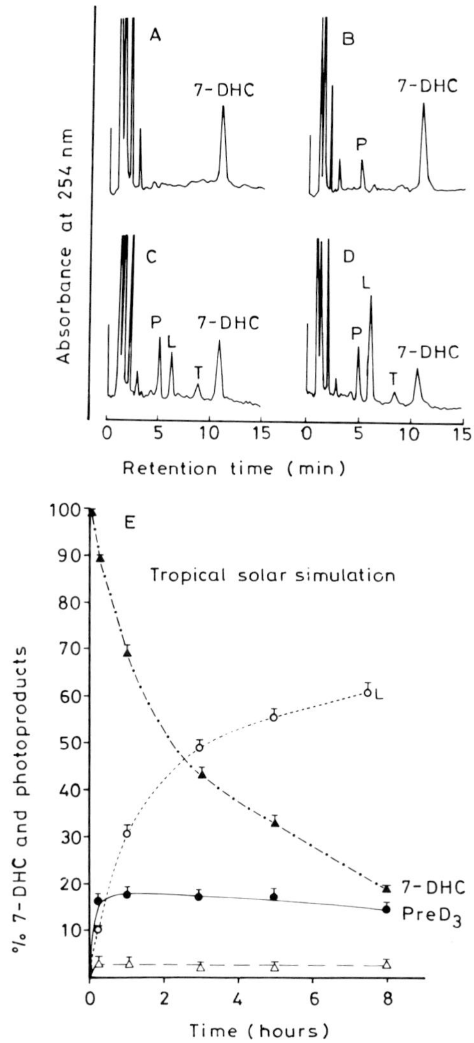


Fig. 9. High-performance liquid-chromatographic profiles of a lipid extract from the basal cells of surgically obtained hypopigmented skin that was previously shielded from (A) or exposed to equatorial simulated solar ultraviolet radiation that reaches the Earth at sea level at noon for (B) 10 min; (C) 1 h; and (D) 8 h. (E) represents an analysis of the photolysis of 7-dehydrocholesterol (7-DHC) (– – ▲ – –) in the basal cell layer and the appearance of the photoproducts previtamin $D_3$ (pre$D_3$) (—— ● ——), lumisterol$_3$ (L) (– – – ○ – – –), and tachysterol (T) (– – – △ – – –) with increasing exposure time. $\bar{\Delta}$ represents the S.E.M. from three determinations. (From Holick et al. with permission. Copyright 1981 by the American Association for the Advancement of Science.)

winter, and the amount of solar UVB radiation that reached the earth's surface was diminished.

The quantity of ultraviolet photons that penetrate to the earth's surface is dependent on many factors including the pathlength through which sunlight penetrates through the stratospheric ozone layer; the distance that solar radiation must travel through the atmosphere is a function of the solar zenith angle and depends on latitude, season, and time of day (Webb et al. 1988). To determine the effects of latitude, season and time of day on the cutaneous production of previtamin $D_3$, we developed a model that consisted of quartz tubes containing $^3$H-7-dehydrocholesterol in methanol. This model and human skin were exposed to sunlight on the roof of our laboratory on cloudless days throughout the year (Webb et al. 1988). In Boston (42°N) the conversion of 7-dehydrocholesterol to previtamin $D_3$ was greatest in June and July (Fig. 10) (Webb et al. 1988). There was a gradual decline in the efficiency of conversion of 7-dehydrocholesterol to previtamin $D_3$ after August and by October less than 4% of 7-dehydrocholesterol was photolyzed to previtamin $D_3$ between the hours of 11:30 and 14:30 EST. By November, however, there was no detectable production of the previtamin $D_3$.

To determine the impact of latitude on the cutaneous synthesis of previtamin $D_3$ a similar study was conducted in Edmonton, Canada (52°N). As can be seen in Fig.

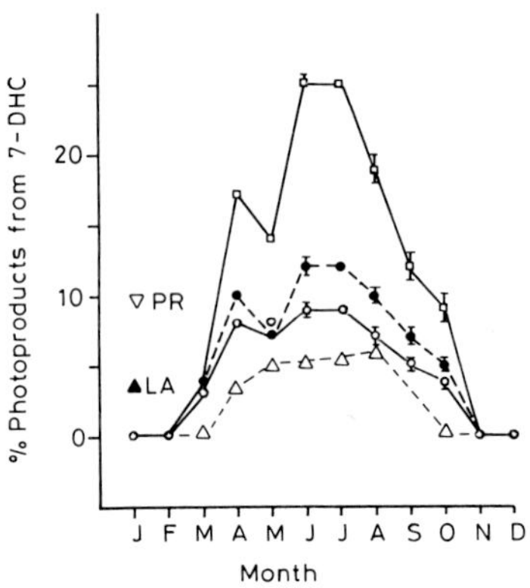


Fig. 10. [3α-$^3$H] 7-DHC in methanol was exposed to sunlight at different seasons and latitudes. Shown are the mean ± 2 S.D. ($n = 3$) annual change in percent conversion of 7-DHC to previtamin $D_3$ after sunlight exposure for 1 h (○ – – ○) and 3 h (● – – ●), and total photoproducts (previtamin $D_3$, lumisterol, and tachysterol) after 3 h (□——□) in Boston. The data were collected from November 1985 through 1986 to May 1987, and the figure shows compiled data for the 12 calendar months. For months where data was available for more than 1 year, the results were the same within the uncertainty of a single point measurement except for the photosynthesis of previtamin $D_3$ in May when exposure for 1 and 3 h gave the same result in 1986 (●), and only a 1 h value is available for 1987 (○). Also shown is the conversion of 7-DHC to previtamin $D_3$ throughout the year after exposure to 1 h of sunlight in Edmonton (△ – – △) and in January in Los Angeles (LA) and Peurto Rico (PR; single samples accurate to ± 1% photoproduct). (From Webb et al. 1988, with permission.)

10, the photosynthesis of previtamin $D_3$ began in the middle of April and ceased after the middle of October. However, in Los Angeles (34°N) and in San Juan (18°N) previtamin $D_3$ production occurred throughout the year (Fig. 10).

Recently, we have evaluated the effect of the time of day on the cutaneous production of previtamin $D_3$. Preliminary results have revealed that during the summer months the photolysis of 7-dehydrocholesterol to previtamin $D_3$ can occur as early as 7:00 EST and as late as 17:00 EST. However, in the spring and autumn previtamin $D_3$ synthesis begins at around 10:00 EST and ceases around 15:00 EST (Z. Liu and M.F. Holick, unpublished results).

*4. Photodegradation of vitamin $D_3$.* Once vitamin $D_3$ is formed in the skin from previtamin $D_3$ it escapes into the circulation by diffusing from the epidermis into the dermal capillary bed prompted by its attraction to the vitamin D-binding protein. However, if vitamin $D_3$ does not escape into the circulation before it is exposed to sunlight the triene-system of vitamin $D_3$ absorbs solar ultraviolet radiation and photolyzes to three principal products identified as 5,6-*trans*-vitamin $D_3$, supersterol 1 and supersterol 2 (Webb et al. 1989) (Fig. 11). To determine the sensitivity of the photodegradation of vitamin $D_3$ by season, samples of radiolabelled vitamin $D_3$ in an organic solvent were exposed to sunlight on cloudless days between the hours of 10:30 and 14:30 EST in the middle month throughout the year. As revealed in Fig. 12, exposure for as little as 10 min in Boston in the summer resulted in the photodegradation

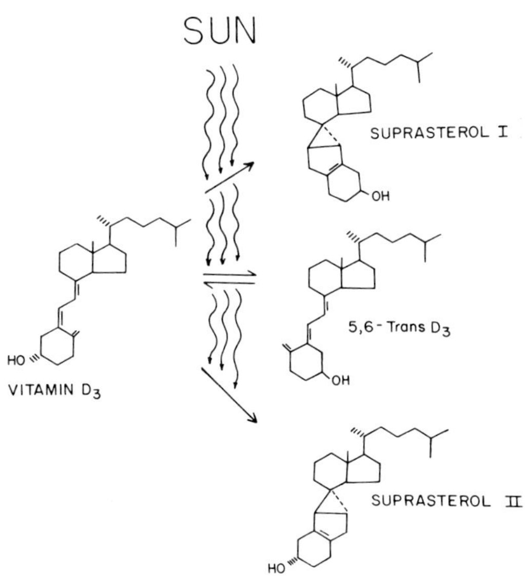


Fig. 11. Photolysis of vitamin $D_3$ to 5, 6-*trans*-vitamin $D_3$, suprasterol 1, and suprasterol 2. (From Holick et al. 1987 with permission.)

of 30% of vitamin $D_3$; after 0.5, 1 and 3 h greater than 50, 75 and 95% was destroyed. Although exposure to sunlight in Boston during the winter does not promote the cutaneous synthesis of previtamin $D_3$ it was found that solar radiation that reached Boston can photolyze vitamin $D_3$ (Fig. 12) (Webb et al. 1989). The reason that vitamin $D_3$ is photolyzed at a time when previtamin $D_3$ cannot be formed is due to the fact that lower energy ultraviolet radiation (316 – 335 nm) that reach Boston during the winter can photodegrade vitamin $D_3$ (Fig. 12). Thus, 7-dehydrocholesterol cannot be photolyzed in late fall and winter in Boston because there are few solar photons reaching the earth's surface with sufficient energy below 315 nm. However, vitamin $D_3$ can absorb the relatively large number of low energy ultraviolet

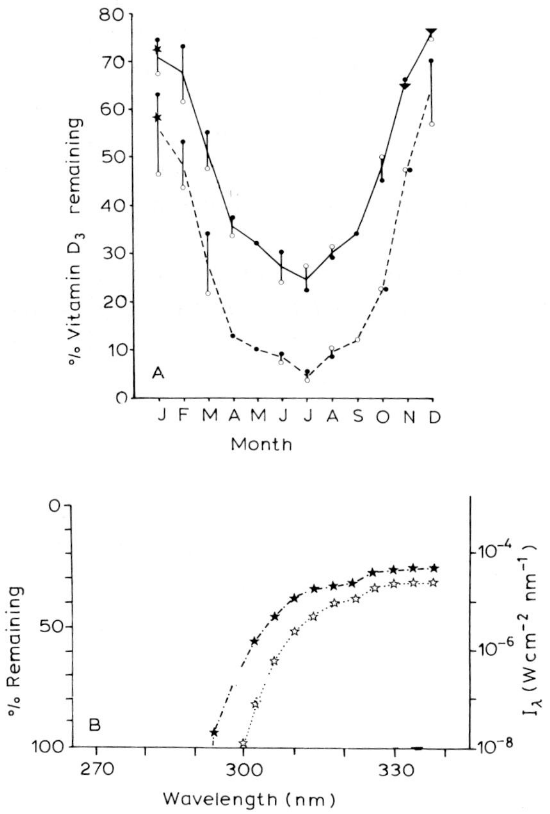


Fig. 12. (A) The percentage of [$^3$H]vitamin $D_3$ remaining after exposure to 1 and 3 h of sunlight in each month of the year. Each point represents the mean ± S.E. of three determinations. (B) Solar spectra measured in Boston at noon on clear days: June ( ★ – . – ★ ) and January ( ☆. . . ☆). Note that in January 300 nm was the shortest detectable wavelength, whereas in June the intensity at 300 nm was 2 orders of magnitude greater than that in January, and the shortest detectable wavelength was 294 nm. (From Webb et al. 1989, with permission.)

photons between 316 and 335 nm that are present in winter sunlight resulting in the photoisomerization of vitamin $D_3$ throughout the year (Fig. 12). Since this low energy ultraviolet radiation can penetrate through the epidermis into the dermal capillary bed (Anderson and Parrish 1982) it is possible that throughout the year vitamin $D_3$ in the circulation is photoisomerized upon exposure to solar ultraviolet radiation. Thus, although winter sunlight cannot produce vitamin $D_3$ in the skin it may, however, promote the photodestruction of nutritionally obtained vitamin D that is present in the bloodstream (Webb et al. 1989).

*5. Effect of aging.* Vitamin D deficiency and its associated metabolic bone disease, osteomalacia is an unrecognized epidemic (Chalmers et al. 1967; Jenkins et al. 1973; Sokoloff 1978; Doppelt et al. 1983). It has been estimated both in the United States and in Great Britain that about 30 – 40% of elderly persons with hip fractures are vitamin D-deficient. There are a variety of causes for vitamin D deficiency in the aged. Although aging does not decrease the efficiency of the intestine to absorb dietary vitamin D (Holick 1986) the aged do not obtain sufficient vitamin D in their diet to meet their body's requirement (Omdahl et al. 1982). In the United States and Canada, the principal food source for vitamin D is milk. One of the primary causes of poor vitamin D nutrition in the elderly in the United States and Canada is due to a decrease of or complete abstinence from the consumption of milk. This decrease is related to the misconception among the elderly that they no longer need to drink milk because milk is important only for maintaining a healthy skeleton in growing children, and the gastrointestinal discomfort caused by the lack of the enzyme lactase which is responsible for digesting the lactose in milk. If an elderly adult does not consume milk or fish liver oils that contain vitamin D or take a vitamin D supplement, it then becomes essential for that person to sunbathe to generate enough vitamin $D_3$ for the maintenance of a healthy skeleton (Holick 1986). Indeed there are two studies in the elderly that clearly demonstrate the importance of vitamin D supplementation along with exposure to sunlight as a means of maintaining calcium homeostasis. Lamberg-Allart (1984) evaluated circulating concentrations of 25-OH-D in three groups of elderly people during one year. They found low circulating concentrations of 25-OH-D in long-stay geriatric patients and in residents at the old people's home was a consequence of both a low dietary vitamin D intake and low exposure to sunlight. Similarly, Webb et al. (1990) monitored 25-OH-D concentrations in free-living elderly people at a nursing home throughout the year. The elderly, who were taking a vitamin D supplement of 400 I.U. a day or had milk as a component of their diet providing them with approximately 200 – 350 I.U. of vitamin D had normal circulating concentrations of 25-OH-D throughout the year. However, residents who did not drink milk and who had low exposure to sunlight had low-normal 25-OH-D levels in their circulation and during the winter months approximately 60% of the group were found to be vitamin D-deficient.

Therfore, based on these studies the elderly depend on exposure to sunlight for their vitamin D requirement. However, Lester et al. (1977) were among the first to investigate the effect of aging on cutaneous vitamin D production. They reported that during the summer months the circulating concentrations of 25-OH-D were lower in non house-bound elderly subjects than in healthy young British ones.

Indeed aging has a dramatic impact on the skin. After the age of 20 years, skin thickness decreases linearly with age (Tan et al. 1982). An analysis of the concentrations of 7-dehydrocholesterol in the epidermis and dermis from skin samples of people of varying ages revealed that there was a marked age-dependent decrease in the epidermal concentrations of this vitamin $D_3$ precursor while the concentrations of 7-dehydrocholesterol did not change in the dermis (Fig. 13) (MacLaughlin and Holick 1985). When human skin samples from various ages were exposed to simulated sunlight it was found that the skin from an 8- and 18-year-old subject was 2 to 3 times greater that the amount produced in the skin from a 77- and 82-year-old subject. To be certain that these *in vitro* data were relevant, healthy young and older adults were exposed to a whole body dose of the same amount of ultraviolet radiation that was comparable to being at Cape Cod on a sunny afernoon in the summer for about 15 min. Circulating concentrations of vitamin $D_3$ were determined before and at various times after the exposure. Whereas the young volunteers (age range 22 – 30 years) raised their circulating concentrations of vitamin D to a maximum of 30 ng/ml within 24 h after their exposure the elderly subjects (62 – 80 years) were only able to achieve a maximum concentration of about 8 ng/ml (Fig. 14) (Holick et al. 1989a).

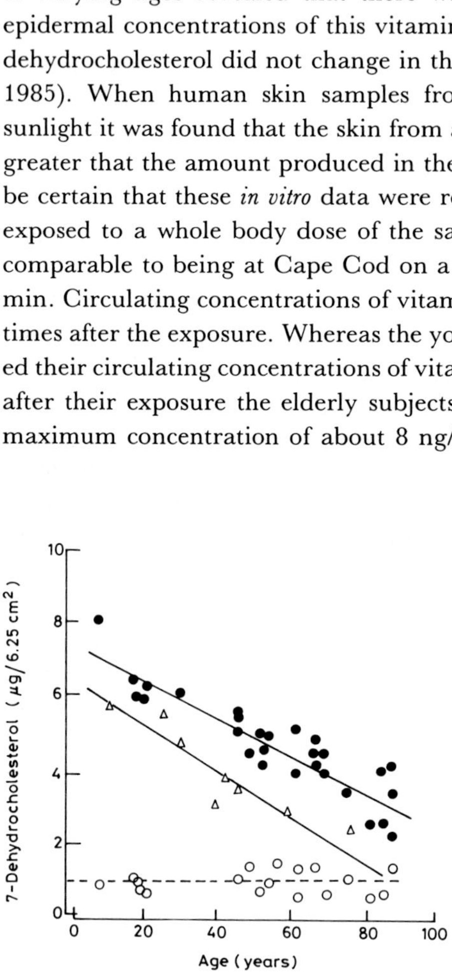


Fig. 13. Effect of aging on 7-dehydrocholesterol concentrations in human epidermis and dermis. Concentrations of 7-dehydrocholesterol (provitamin $D_3$) per unit area of human epidermis (●), stratum basale (△), and dermis (○) were obtained from surgical specimens from donors of various ages. Linear regression analysis gave slopes of $-0.05$, $-0.06$, and $-0.0005$ for epidermis ($r = -0.89$), stratum basale ($r = -0.92$), and dermis ($r = -0.04$), respectively. Slopes of epidermis and stratum basale are significantly different from slope of dermis ($P < 0.001$). (From MacLaughlin and Holick 1985, with permission.)

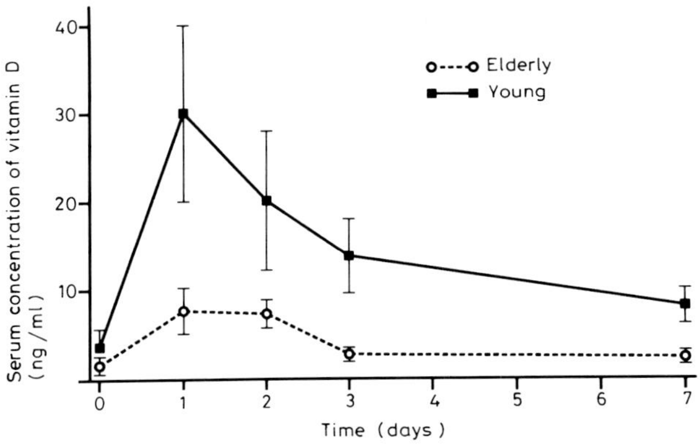


Fig. 14. Circulating concentrations of vitamin D in healthy young and elderly volunteers exposed to ultraviolet radiation. (From Holick et al. 1989a, with permission.)

*6. Effect of sunscreen use.* There is great concern today about the damaging effects of chronic exposure to sunlight (Parrish et al. 1979). Long-term exposure to sunlight can cause significant damage to the structural integrity of the skin, causing dry wrinkled skin as well as increased risk of the skin cancer (Montagna and Carlisle 1979). As a result of this heightened awareness of the damaging effects of sunlight there has been a major effort to encourage all caucasians to wear sunscreens before going outdoors. Although there is no question of the benefit of sunscreen use for the prevention of sunburn, skin cancer and skin damage, it has been shown that sunscreens can also prevent the beneficial effect of sunlight, the production of previtamin $D_3$ (Matsuoka et al. 1987). This is not surprising because the radiation that is responsible for causing sunburn and skin damage is the same radiation that is responsible for producing previtamin $D_3$ (Fig. 15). It was shown when young white adults were covered with either a sunscreen preparation containing para-aminobenzoic acid (PABA) which had a sun protection factor of 8 or a baby oil that did not contain PABA the sunscreen prevented any increase in the circulating concentrations of vitamin $D_3$, after exposure to simulated sunlight that would have caused a mild sunburn (Matsuoka et al. 1987) (Fig. 16). Therefore, any UVB blocking agent that prevents the damaging effects of sunlight will also prevent the cutaneous production of previtamin $D_3$.

The use of sunscreens by children and young adults should not affect their vitamin D status because it is unlikely that they will always wear a sunscreen before going outdoors. However, the elderly often follow the advice of their physician and will put a sunscreen on their skin before going outdoors in order to prevent skin wrinkles. There is evidence that the chronic use of sunscreens by the elderly can decrease circulating concentrations of 25-OH-D and cause vitamin D deficiency (Matsuoka et al. 1988) (Fig.17) which could increase the risk of hip fracture (Chalmers et al. 1967; Doppelt et al. 1983; Kavookjian et al. 1990).

## C. Recommendations for the safe use of sunlight for producing vitamin $D_3$

It should be appreciated that it is casual exposure to sunlight that provides all humans with their vitamin D requirement. It is important to provide some perspective about all of the negative publicity regarding exposure to sunlight. It is known that if a young adult receives a whole body exposure to sunlight that causes a slight sunburn the

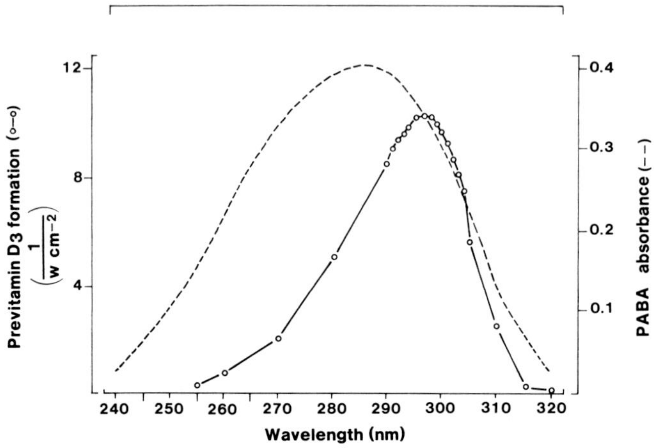


Fig. 15. Absorption spectrum of PABA superimposed on the action spectrum of previtamin $D_3$ formation spectrum was obtained by plotting the reciprocal of photoenergy as a function of wavelength. At any wavelength, no more than 5% of the 7-dehydrocholesterol was converted to previtamin $D_3$. (From Matsuoka et al. 1987, with permission.)

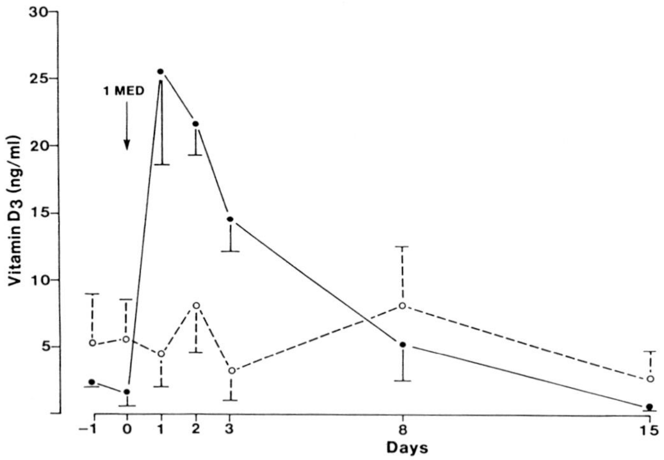


Fig. 16. Mean (± S.E.M.) serum vitamin $D_3$ concentrations in eight normal subjects. Four subjects (○ – – ○) applied PABA and four applied vehicle (●——●) to the entire skin before exposure to UVB. On day 0, all subjects underwent total body exposure to 1 MED UVR. To convert nanograms of vitamin D per milliliter to nanomoles per liter, multiply by 2.599. (From Matsuoka et al. 1987, with permission.)

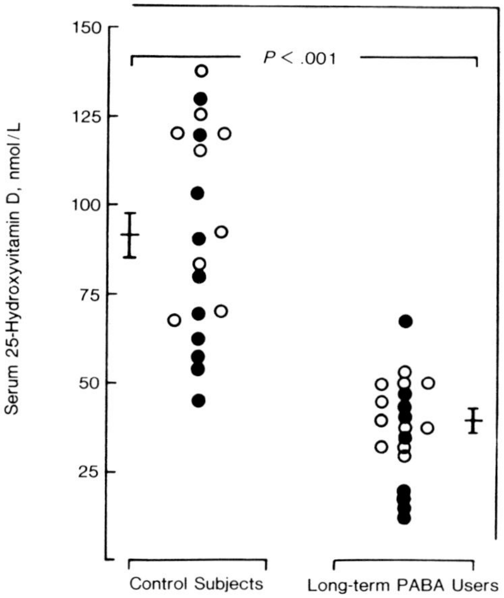


Fig. 17. Serum concentration of 25-hydroxyvitamin D in long-term sunscreen users and in age- and sex-matched controls from same geographical area. Blood samples were obtained simultaneously from patients and controls. Mean serum 25-hydroxyvitamin D level was significantly lower in long-term sunscreen users ($p < 0.001$). Two long-term sunscreen users had absolute vitamin-D deficiency, 25-hydroxyvitamin D level below 20 nmol/l. PABA indicates *p*-aminobenzoic acid; ○, subjects from Philadelphia; ●, subjects from Springfield, IL. (From Matsuoka et al. 1988, with permission.)

amount of vitamin $D_3$ that enters the circulation is comparable to taking 10 000 I.U. of vitamin $D_3$ (250 $\mu$g) orally (Holick 1986). Therefore, because the skin has a very large capacity to produce vitamin $D_3$ and since aging will decrease this capacity I recommend for elderly Caucasian men and women in Boston that exposure of hands, arms, and face to suberythemal amounts of sunlight in the spring, summer, and fall, which is equal to about 10 – 15 min between the hours of 9:00 and 16:00 EST, is more than adequate to provide them with their vitamin D requirement. If they wish to stay outdoors for longer periods I encourage them to apply a sunscreen with a sun protection factor of 15. This sensible advice permits the elderly who are prone to developing vitamin D deficiency to acquire their vitamin D requirement while preventing the damaging effects that are caused by chronic long-term exposure to sunlight. Needless to say, the consumption of two 8 oz glasses of milk or a multivitamin containing 400 I.U. of vitamin D can replace sunlight.

### D. Effects of exposure to sunlight and artificial ultraviolet radiation on circulating concentrations of vitamin D and its metabolites

It is known that circulating concentrations of 25-OH-D fluctuate with season of the year and are usually higher in the summer and lower in the winter (Fig. 18) (Poskitt et al. 1979; Chesney et al. 1981; Tjellesen et al. 1982; Clemens and Holick 1983; Audran et al. 1984). Because of its long circulating half life, 25-OH-D has become a valuable indicator for determining the cumulative effect of sunlight and diet on the vitamin D status in the body. However, because of the tight regulation of the renal synthesis of $1,25(OH)_2D$ the circulating concentrations of $1,25(OH)_2D$ are not affected by season (Chesney et al. 1981; Tjellesen et al. 1982; Clemens and Holick 1983; Audran et al. 1984).

To quantitatively determine the effects of a single exposure of simulated solar ultraviolet radiation on circulating concentrations of vitamin D and its metabolites, young healthy volunteers exposed their entire bodies to various doses of ultraviolet radiation. Circulating concentrations of vitamin D increased in proportion to the exposure dose (Adams et al. 1982) (Fig. 19). In response to a single whole body exposure to a dose of ultraviolet radiation that caused a minimal sunburn (one minimal erythema dose; MED) circulating concentrations of vitamin D increased approximately 5 to 10-fold within the first 24 – 48 h before declining towards the baseline by 7 days. Increases in exposure from 1 – 1.5, 3 and 4 MEDs resulted in proportionally higher peak concentrations of vitamin $D_3$ at 24 h. It was estimated that the apparent half-life of vitamin D in the circulation was approximately 48 h and that at least 30 $\mu$g of vitamin $D_3$ was made in the skin and released into the circulation from each square meter of body surface after exposure to 1 MED of ultraviolet radiation (Adams et al. 1981).

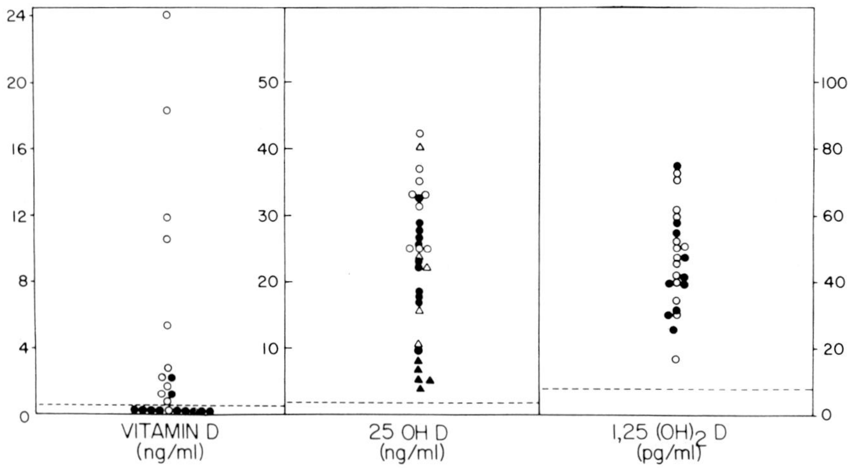


Fig. 18. Distribution of circulating concentrations of vitamin D, 25-OH-D, and $1,25(OH)_2D$ in healthy subjects determined in the authors' laboratory. Vitamin D and 25-OH-D values determined in subjects during summer months (○,△) were higher than those determined during winter months (●,▲), whereas no seasonal variation was apparent for $1,25(OH)_2D$ concentration. Elderly adults (△,▲) (age 50 – 80) had significantly lower 25-OH-D concentrations than did younger adults (○,●).

To determine the effect of skin pigmentation on the cutaneous production of vitamin $D_3$, healthy young adult black, asian, and white subjects were exposed to identical amounts of ultraviolet radiation. The circulating concentration of vitamin D increased 30-fold in the white subjects exposed to a 1.5 MED dose of ultraviolet radiation. When black and asian subjects were exposed to exactly the same amount of radiation there was no significant change in the circulating concentrations of vitamin D. However, when black and asian subjects were exposed to increasing doses of ultraviolet radiation they were able to increase their circulating concentrations of vitamin D to comparable levels of the white subjects (Figs. 20 and 21) (Clemens et al. 1982; Lo et al. 1984). Therefore, black, asian, and white people all have the same capacity to produce vitamin $D_3$ in their skin, however, blacks and asians require longer exposure times because of increased melanin pigmentation in their skin.

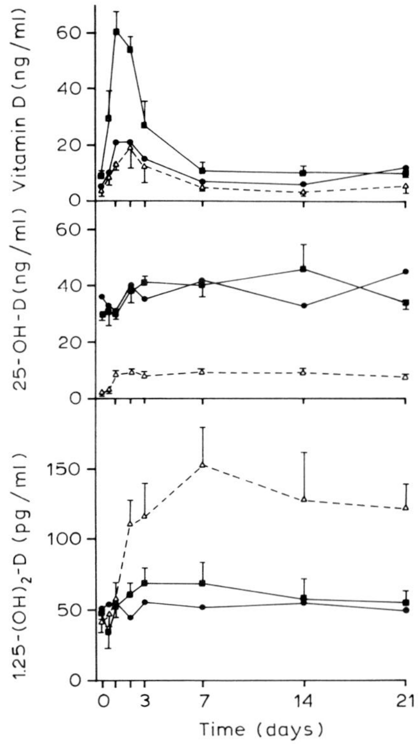


Fig. 19. Changes in serum concentrations of vitamin D and its metabolites after exposure to ultraviolet radiation. Concentrations of vitamin D, 25-OH-D, and $1,25(OH)_2D$ were measured in three normal subjects exposed to three minimal erythemal doses of ultraviolet radiation (UVR) (——■——), in a representative normal subject exposed to one minimal erythemal dose of UVR (——●——), and in three vitamin-D-deficient patients exposed to one minimal erythemal dose of UVR (- - - △ - - -). To convert nanograms of vitamin D per milliliter to nanomoles per liter, nanograms of 25-OH-D per milliliter to nanomoles per liter, and picograms of $1,25(OH)_2D$ per milliliter to picomoles per liter, multiply by 2.58, 2.50, and 2.40, respectively. Bars denote S.E.M. (From Adams et al. 1982, with permission.)

To determine the effect of a single exposure of ultraviolet radiation on circulating concentrations of 25-OH-D and $1,25(OH)_2D$, young white healthy subjects were exposed to a whole body dose 1 MED of radiation. Whereas the circulating concentrations of vitamin D-increased 10-fold within 24 h after a whole body exposure to 3 MEDs of ultraviolet radiation, the circulating concentrations of 25-OH-D increased

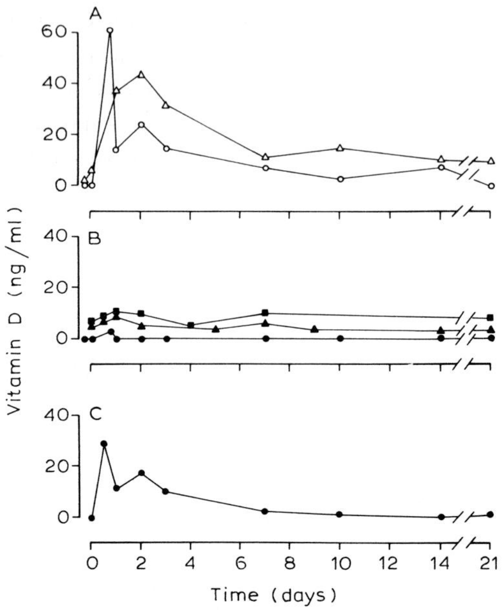


Fig. 20. In two lightly pigmented caucasian (A) and three heavily pigmented black subjects (B) after total-body exposure to 0.054 J/cm$^2$ of UVR. (C) Serial change in circulating vitamin D after re-exposure of one black subject (° in panel B) to a 0.32 J/cm$^2$ dose of UVR. (From Clemens et al. 1982, with permission.)

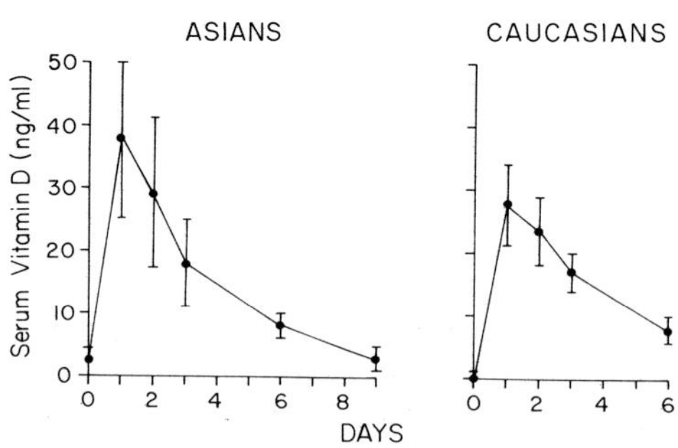


Fig. 21. Serum vitamin D concentrations in Asians and Caucasians after 1.5 MED whole-body ultraviolet irradiation. Means ± standard deviations are shown at 0, 1, 2, 3, 6, and 9 days. There are no significant differences in serum vitamin-D concentrations between Asians and Caucasians at any time point. (From Lo et al. 1986, with permission.)

by no more than 30 – 50% over a period of one week and the circulating concentrations of $1,25(OH)_2D$ did not increase significantly above baseline (Fig. 19). To determine whether vitamin D deficiency influenced the capacity to the skin to produce vitamin $D_3$, three patients with vitamin D deficiency were exposed to a whole body dose equivalent to 1 MED. The circulating concentrations of vitamin D and 25-OH-D in these vitamin D deficient subjects increased in a pattern comparable to that of the young, healthy volunteers. However, the circulating concentrations of $1,25(OH)_2D$ in vitamin D-deficient patients markedly increased from about 50 to 160 pg/ml within one week after exposure and persisted at this concentration throughout the next 2 weeks (Fig. 19). The marked increase in the $1,25(OH)_2D$ concentration was most likely due to the positive feedback effect of parathyroid hormone on the renal 25-OH-D-1-hydroxylase (Holick 1989b).

## E. Cutaneous production of 24-dehydrovitamin $D_3$

It has been assumed for the past 60 years that exposure to sunlight results in the cutaneous production of only one vitamin D, vitamin $D_3$. However, our evolutionary

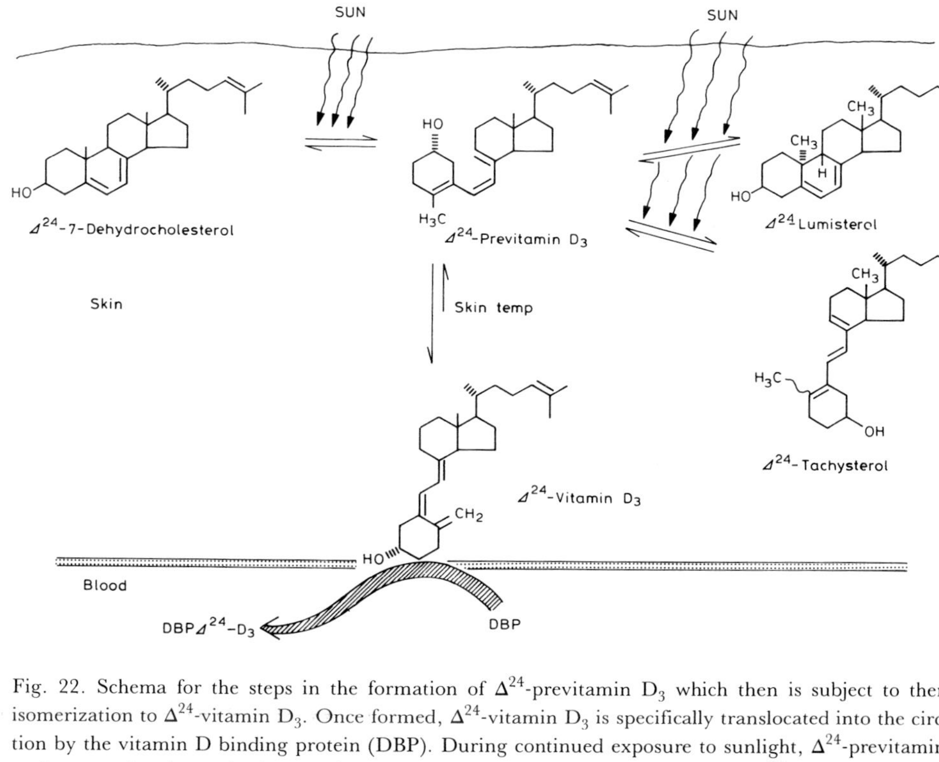


Fig. 22. Schema for the steps in the formation of $\Delta^{24}$-previtamin $D_3$ which then is subject to thermal isomerization to $\Delta^{24}$-vitamin $D_3$. Once formed, $\Delta^{24}$-vitamin $D_3$ is specifically translocated into the circulation by the vitamin D binding protein (DBP). During continued exposure to sunlight, $\Delta^{24}$-previtamin $D_3$ undergoes photoisomerication to form the biologically inert photoproducts, $\Delta^{24}$-lumisterol and $\Delta^{24}$-tachysterol. (From Holick SA, 1985, with permission.)

studies on the photosynthesis of vitamin D has revealed that plants and animals have the capacity to produce several vitamin Ds when exposed to sunlight (Holick 1989a). Amphibians and reptiles have up to six different provitamin Ds in their skin (Table 1) that are susceptible to photolysis to their previtamin D counterparts. An analysis of rat and human skin has revealed the presence of another provitamin D that was

TABLE 1. Provitamin D content in the skin from amphibians, reptiles and mammals

| Species | Provitamin D | | | | |
|---|---|---|---|---|---|
| | RT (min) | Type | ng/cm$^2$ | ng/mg Lipid | % Total |
| Northern Grass Frog | 6.10 | U[a] | 18.0 | 90.0 | 0.3 |
| | 6.39 | U | 71.0 | 360.0 | 1.2 |
| | 6.90 | U | 165.0 | 840.0 | 2.8 |
| | 7.25 | 7-DHC[b] | 5240.0 | 26700.0 | 89.3 |
| | 8.07 | U | 277.0 | 1400 | 4.7 |
| | 8.83 | U | 88.0 | 450 | 1.5 |
| Bullfrog | 8.42 | U | 6.9 | 14.0 | 1.6 |
| | 8.89 | U | 4.7 | 9.6 | 1.1 |
| | 9.87 | 7-DHC | 365.0 | 739.0 | 85 |
| | 18.82 | U | 25.0 | 50.0 | 5.8 |
| | 11.75 | U | 25.0 | 50.0 | 5.8 |
| Anolis Lizard | 8.66 | U | 548 | 152 | 3.7 |
| | 10.15 | 7-DHC | 13340 | 3700 | 90.0 |
| | 11.08 | U | 608 | 169 | 4.1 |
| | 12.01 | U | 356 | 99 | 2.4 |
| Chicken | 9.82 | 7-DHC | | | 99 |
| | 11.64 | U | | | < 1 |
| Rat (14 days) | 8.42 | $\Delta^{24}$-7-DHC[c] | 905 | 135 | 31 |
| | 9.82 | 7-DHC | 2014 | 300 | 69 |
| Rat (14 weeks) | 8.30 | $\Delta^{24}$-7-DHC | 15 | 2.3 | 16 |
| | 9.68 | 7-DHC | 77 | 12.0 | 84 |
| Seal | 8.47 | U | 288 | 280 | 39 |
| | 9.90 | 7-DHC | 4500 | 438 | 61 |
| Common Dolphin | | 7-DHC | 1165 | 28 | 100 |
| White-Sided Dolphin | | 7-DHC | 5060 | 321 | 100 |
| Harbor Porpoise | | 7-DHC | 1815 | 119 | 100 |
| Human (65 years) | 8.6 | $\Delta^{24}$-7-DHC | 2.5 | 0.7 | 0.5 |
| | 10.3 | 7-DHC | 490 | 130 | 99.5 |

[a] U = Unknown.
[b] 7-DHC = 7-dehydrocholesterol.
[c] $\Delta^{24}$-7-DHC = 24-dehydroprovitamin $D_3$.

identified as 24-dehydroprovitamin $D_3$ (cholesta-5, 7, 24-trien-3β-ol). During exposure to simulated sunlight this provitamin is efficiently converted to 24-dehydroprevitamin $D_3$ (Fig. 22). Although the physiologic function of this new vitamin D is unknown, *in vitro* studies have revealed that 24-dehydrovitamin $D_3$ is an effective competitive inhibitor of the hepatic vitamin D-25-hydroxylase (Bolt et al.

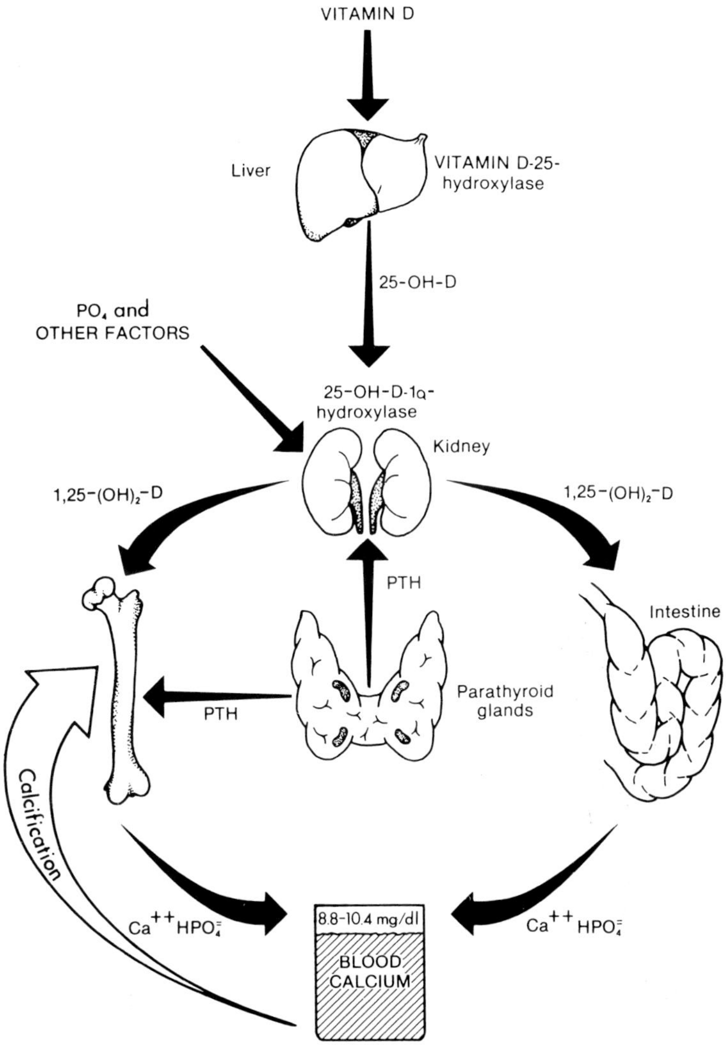


Fig. 23. Schematic representation of the hormonal control loop for vitamin D metabolism and function. A reduction in the serum calcium below approximately 8.8 mg/ml prompts a proportional increase in the secretion of parathyroid hormone, which enhances the mobilization of calcium stores from bone. Parathyroid hormone also promotes the synthesis of $1,25(OH)_2D$ in the kidney, which, in turn, stimulates the mobilization of calcium from the bone and intestine. (From Holick 1987, with permission.)

1988). Therefore, during excessive exposure to sunlight, 24-dehydrovitamin $D_3$ that is produced in the skin could potentially inhibit the hepatic production of 25-OH-D.

## IV. Biologic function of 1,25-dihydroxyvitamin $D_3$ in the skin

### A. Vitamin D metabolism and physiology

Vitamin D (the term vitamin D refers to either vitamin $D_2$ or $D_3$) whether coming from the skin or the diet is biologically inert and enters into the circulation where it is transported to the liver and metabolized in hepatocytes to 25-OH-D (Fig. 23) (DeLuca 1984, 1988; Holick 1989b; Reichel et al. 1989). Although 25-OH-D is the major circulating form of vitamin D it is not biologically active. 25-OH-D is transported to kidney where it is hydroxylated on carbon 1 to form $1,25(OH)_2D$ (Fig. 23). $1,25(OH)_2D$ carries out its physiologic actions on calcium and phosphorus metabolism by interacting with specific nuclear receptors in the intestine. This interaction results in the phosphorylation of the receptor complex that, in turn, activates transcription of specific genes (Fig. 24) (Haussler et al. 1985; Pike 1985). Originally it was believed that $1,25(OH)_2D$ enhanced the mobilization of calcium and phosphorus from the bone by directly interacting with mature osteoclasts to increase their activity. However, there is mounting evidence that mature osteoclasts do not

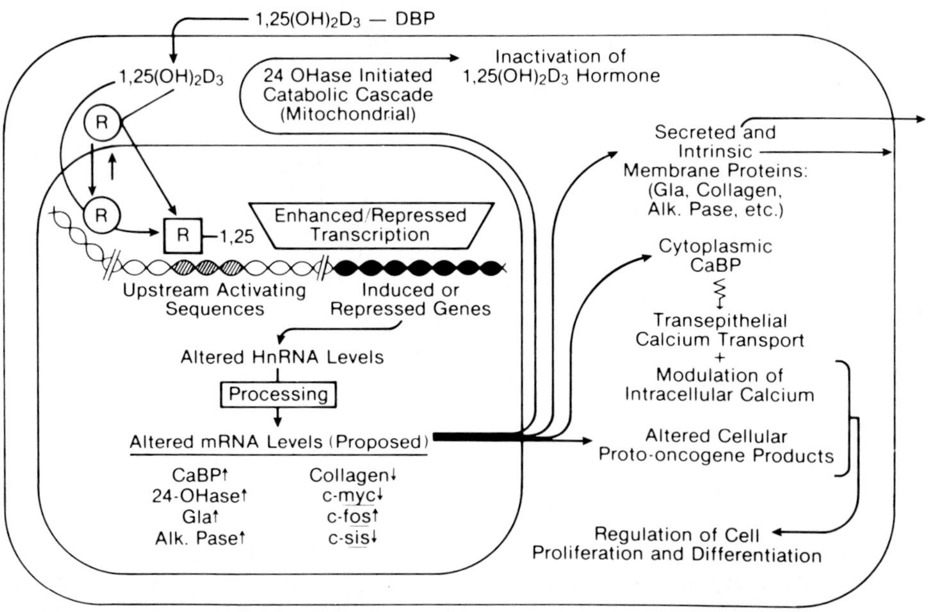


Fig. 24. Proposed mechanism of action of $1,25(OH)_2D_3$ in target cells resulting in a variety of biological responses. (From Haussler et al. 1985, with permission.)

possess nuclear receptors for 1,25$(OH)_2D_3$ (Merke et al. 1986). It is now believed that 1,25$(OH)_2D_3$ acts on bone indirectly by mobilizing mononuclear stem cells to become osteoclasts. Once the osteoclasts have matured, they lose their nuclear receptor for the hormone and are no longer responsive to it (Holick 1989b).

During the past decade, a new appreciation has developed regarding the vast potential biologic actions of 1,25$(OH)_2D$. There are a variety of tissues and cells that are not related to calcium or phorphous metabolism but possess high affinity, low capacity nuclear receptors for 1,25$(OH)_2D_3$ (Stumpf et al. 1979; Colston et al. 1981a). These include brain, stomach, skeletal muscle, parathyroid glands, gonads, cardiac muscle, pancreas, activated T and B lymphocytes, monocytes, dermal fibroblasts, keratinocytes, and cells in the outer root sheath of hair. In addition, a variety of cultured tumor cell lines including malignant melanoma, breast cancer, and leukemia possess receptors for this hormone (Tanaka et al. 1982; Eisman 1984; Mason 1985; Smith and Holick 1987).

Although the physiologic function of 1,25$(OH)_2D$ in these tissues and cells is not well understood, under experimental conditions 1,25$(OH)_2D$ has such diverse actions as stimulating calcium binding protein activity in certain specific regions of the brain, inhibiting interleukin-2 production, enhancing interleukin-1 production, inhibiting gamma-globulin synthesis, inhibiting parathyroid hormone synthesis and enhancing thyrothropin secretion (DeLuca 1984; Holick 1989b; Reichel 1989). When tumor cells are exposed to 1,25$(OH)_2D_3$ in culture, at low concentrations this hormone can enhance their proliferation (Eisman 1984). However, at physiologic and pharmacologic concentrations, 1,25$(OH)_2D_3$ often inhibits proliferation and induces maturation of these cells. For example, when 1,25$(OH)_2D_3$ receptor positive malignant melanocytes are exposed to 1,25$(OH)_2D_3$ the proliferative activity of these cells is decreased and melanin synthesis is enhanced (Colston et al. 1981b). Receptor positive malignant human promyleocytic cells respond to 1,25$(OH)_2D_3$ by decreasing their proliferative activity and inducing cell maturation as defined by an induction of cell surface antigens including Fc and $C_3$ receptors, lysozyme and phagocytic activity (Tanaka et al. 1982; Suda et al. 1984). In addition, these mononuclear cells are transformed within days to biochemically functioning multinucleated giant cells. The effect of 1,25$(OH)_2D_3$ on these cells is reversible (Bar Shavit et al. 1986). Furthermore, when clones of HL-60 cells that possessed less than 10% of the nuclear binding activity for the hormone were incubated with 1,25$(OH)_2D_3$, there was little difference in their proliferative activity.

These observations have important clinical implications. Although it is exciting to consider the use of 1,25$(OH)_2D_3$ for the treatment of a variety of malignancies including certain leukemias, it is likely that tumor cells become resistant to the antiproliferative effect of 1,25$(OH)_2D_3$ by decreasing their nuclear binding activity to the hormone. This may be the explanation for why patients with preleukemia who were treated with 1,25$(OH)_2D_3$ initially responded to the hormone but eventually reverted into blastic phase (Koeffler et al. 1985).

## B. Effect of $1,25(OH)_2D_3$ on cultured fibroblasts and keratinocytes

Of great interest to us was the observation that $1,25(OH)_2D_3$ specifically localized in the nuclei of the germative layer of the epidermis (Stumpf et al. 1979). In the mouse, the $1,25(OH)_2D_3$ receptors were first apparent in the skin during the third trimester and its binding activity increased throughout the neonatal development (Horiuchi et al. 1985; Merke et al. 1985) (Fig. 25). Incubation of receptor positive cultured murine (Hosomi et al. 1983) and human (Smith et al. 1986) keratinocytes with $1,25(OH)_2D_3$ resulted in an inhibition of proliferation (Fig. 26) and stimulation of differentiation (Fig. 27) as evidenced by a shift in the distribution of cellular density and size, and an increase in the percentage of attached and desquamated cells and of cells with cornified envelopes (Fig. 28). $1,25(OH)_2D_3$ also increased the activity of the epidermal transglutaminase, the enzyme that is responsible for cross-linking proteins for the development of the cornified envelope (Holick et al. 1987; Smith and Holick 1987). To determine whether the effect of $1,25(OH)_2D_3$ on keratinocyte growth and differentiation was similar to the biologic action of retinoic acid on these cells, we compared their biologic activities. Whereas cultured human keratinocytes exposed to $1,25(OH)_2D_3$ showed morphologic evidence of differentiation the keratinocytes exposed to retinoic acid ($10^{-6}$ M) revealed a stratification of the keratinocytes. Furthermore, retinoic acid ($10^{-6}$ M) stimulated soluble transglutaminase activity and in-

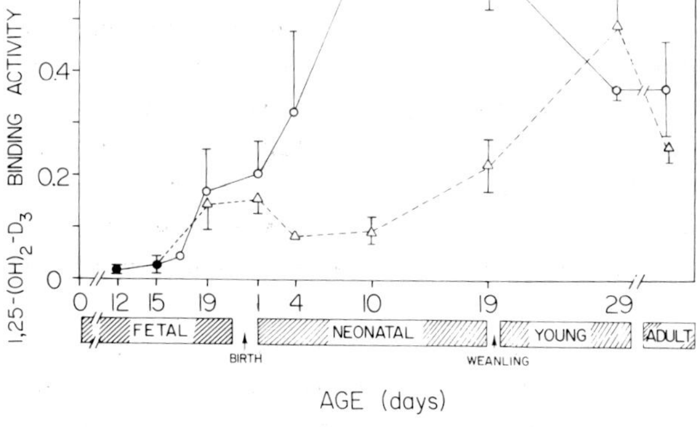


Fig. 25. Developmental changes of $1,25(OH)_2D_3$ receptor in the entire small intestine and skin. Crude chromatin was prepared from whole 12- and 15-day-old fetuses (●), whereas the receptor concentration in whole small intestine (△ – – △) and skin (○ – – – ○) was quantitatively measured by chromatin binding assay. Each point represents up to 5 determinations + S.E.M. (From Horiuchi et al. 1985, with permission.)

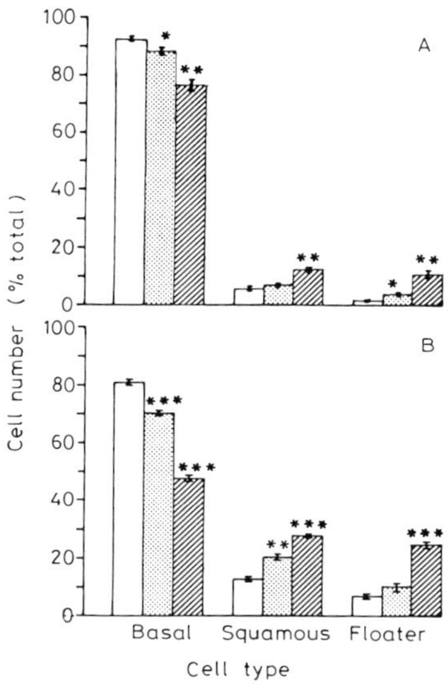


Fig. 26. Effect of $1\alpha,25\text{-}(OH)_2D_3$ on the morphological differentiation of cultured human keratinocytes. The proportion of different keratinocyte cell types after one week (A) or 2 weeks (B) of incubation with vehicle alone (open bar); $1\alpha,25\text{-}(OH)_2D_3$ at $10^{-10}$ M (dotted bar); or $1\alpha,25(OH)_2D_3$ at $10^{-8}$ M (striped bar). Each bar represents the mean of triplicate determinations ± S.E.M. Student's $\tau$-test was used to assess level of significance ($^*p < 0.05$; $^{**}p < 0.01$; $^{***}p < 0.001$). (From Smith et al. 1986, with permission. Copyright 1986 by the Society for Investigative Dermatology, Inc.)

hibited particulate enzyme activity (Holick et al. 1987; Smith and Holick 1987). $1,25(OH)_2D_3$ in a dose-dependent manner enhanced both the soluble and particulate forms of the enzyme. Since the particulate form of the transglutaminase is thought to be responsible for cornified envelope development, these observations are consistent with our finding that $1,25(OH)_2D_3$ enhanced the development of cornified envelopes whereas retinoic did not have any effect on this process.

### C. Biologic activity of $1,25(OH)_2D_3$ on melanogenesis and hair growth

The concept that vitamin D and its metabolites may play a role in melanogenesis is not new. As early as 1974, Oikawa and Nakayasu (1974) reported that pharmacologic concentrations of vitamin D stimulated melanogenesis and tyrosinase activity in cultured melanotic mouse melanoma cells. Since this initial observation, several melanoma cell lines that possess nuclear receptors for $1,25(OH)_2D_3$ have been shown to increase melanin synthesis in a dose-dependent manner when exposed to $1,25(OH)_2D_3$ (Colston et al. 1981b; Hosoi et al. 1985; Mason 1985; Smith and Holick 1987). Ranson et al. (1988) reported that cultured neonatal foreskin melanocytes internalized $^3H\text{-}1,25(OH)_2D_3$ and that incubation of those cells for 48 h with $1,25(OH)_2D_3$ ($10^{-9}$ M) resulted in a 50 and 100% increase in tyrosinase and

25-OH-D-24R-hydroxylase activity, respectively. One *in vivo* study has also made a direct link between melanogenesis and tyrosinase activity. Pavlovitch et al. (1982) found that the ultraviolet stimulation of tyrosinase was markedly diminished in vitamin D-deficient rats.

Although these data suggest that $1,25(OH)_2D_3$ may regulate melanogenesis in nor-

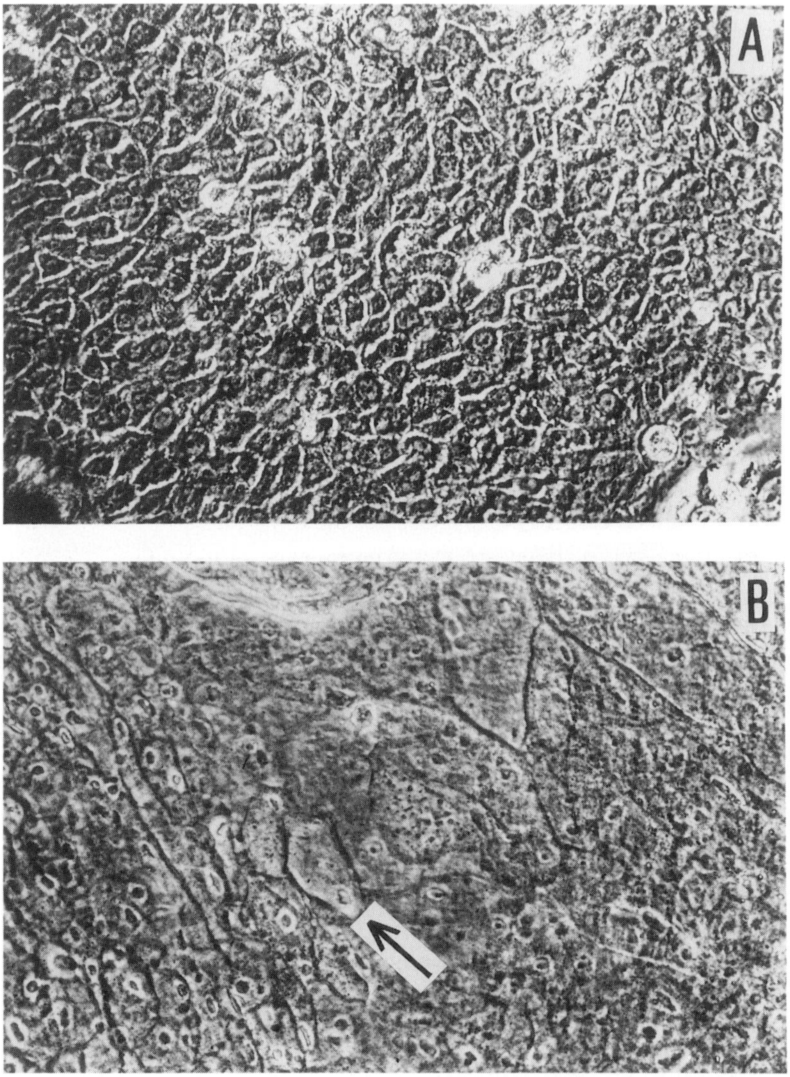


Fig. 27. Phase-contrast micrographs of cultured human keratinocytes grown in the absence (A) or presence (B) of $1\alpha,25$-$(OH)_2D_3$ for 2 weeks ($\times$ 100). Note the formation of enlarged squamous cells in the $1\alpha,25$-$(OH)_2D_3$-dosed culture (arrow) (From Smith et al. 1986, with permission. Copyright 1986 by the Society for Investigative Dermatology, Inc.)

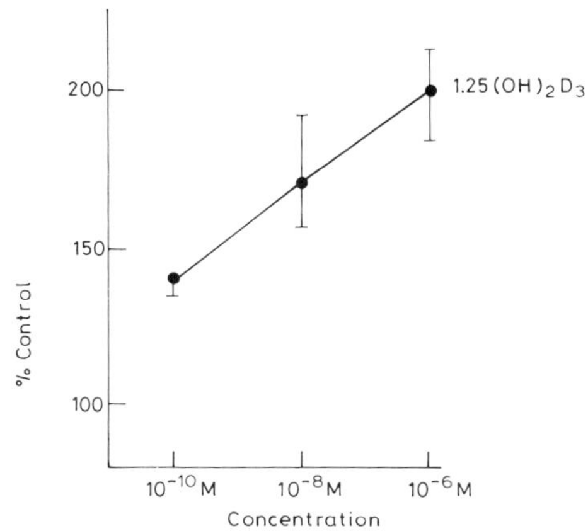


Fig. 28. Dose-dependent effect of $1,25(OH)_2D_3$ on the development of cornified envelopes in cultured human keratinocytes when compared to cornified envelopes that develop in similar cultured human keratinocytes that were exposed to vehicle.

mal melanocytes there are several lines of evidence against $1,25(OH)_2D_3$ being a direct mediator of melanogenesis. Mansur et al. (1988) reported that normal neonatal melanocytes do not have nuclear receptors for $1,25(OH)_2D_3$. Furthermore, $1,25(OH)_2D_3$ did not affect tyrosinase activity in these cultured cells confirming Tomita et al. (1986). It is curious, however, that Tomita et al. (1986) found that while $1,25(OH)_2D_3$ had no effect on melanogenesis, vitamin $D_3$ itself increased tyrosinase activity and altered morphologic characteristics of the cells.

To put these observations into physiologic perspective it should be recognized that there are several clinical observations that also mitigate against $1,25(OH)_2D_3$ having a direct role in melanogenesis. There is no evidence that blacks with vitamin D deficiency and who have undetectable circulating concentrations of $1,25(OH)_2D_3$ have any defect in melanogenesis. Similarly, anephic patients and patients with chronic renal failure who are incapable of making $1,25(OH)_2D_3$ are capable of producing melanin when exposed to sunlight. Furthermore, patients with chronic granulomatous disorders who have an extrarenal unregulated synthesis of $1,25(OH)_2D_3$ do not show an increase in skin melanin synthesis (Holick et al. 1987). Finally, what I believe is most compelling, is that the topical application of $1,25(OH)_2D_3$ for the treatment of psoriasis has not shown any increase in melanogenesis locally (Holick 1989c).

Stumpf et al. (1984) called attention to the possibility that the outer root sheath of the hair follicle was a target tissue for $1,25(OH)_2D_3$ when they showed that $^3H$-$1,25(OH)_2D_3$ localized in the nuclei of the cells in the outer root sheath of hair follicles in the rat. In addition, it has been argued that patients with vitamin D-dependent rickets type II [these patients lack or have defective receptor for $1,25(OH)_2D_3$] also have alopecia totalis (Fig. 29) (Feldman et al. 1982; Lieberman et

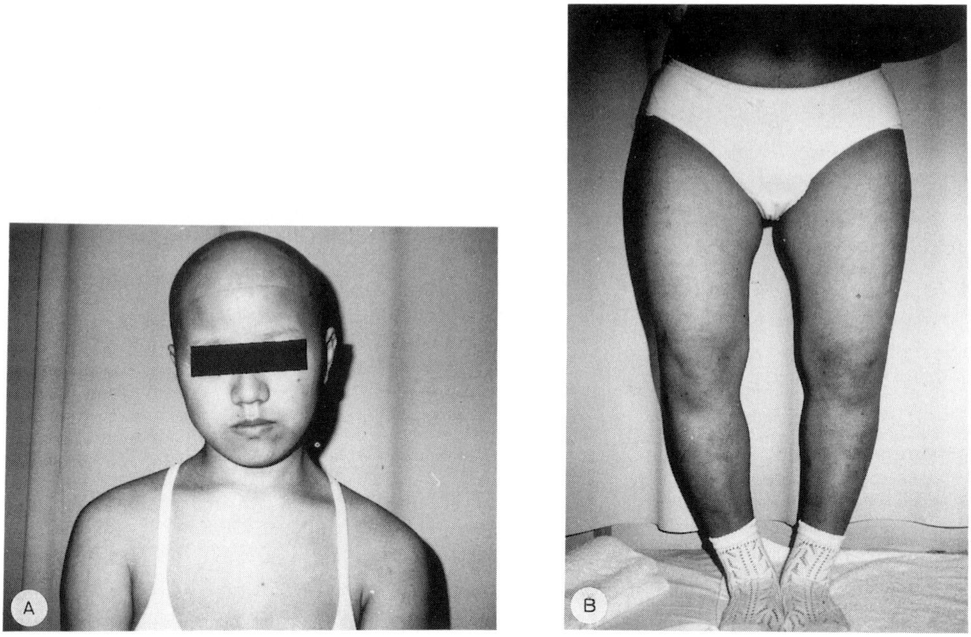

Fig. 29. Fifteen-year-old girl with vitamin D-dependent rickets type II, showing total alopecia (A) and rickets (B). (From Holick 1985, with permission.)

al. 1983; Marx et al. 1984; Hirst et al. 1985; Holick 1985). Marx et al.(1984) have argued that patients with the most severe defect in $1,25(OH)_2$ $D_3$ nuclear binding activity also have the most significant alopecia. Although it would appear that there is a direct relationship between $1,25(OH)_2D_3$ nuclear binding activity and hair growth, there is other evidence that suggests that the resistance to $1,25(OH)_2D_3$ and alopecia is a casual rather than causal relationship (Holick 1985). In addition, there are several lines of clinical evidence that also mitigate against the role of $1,25(OH)_2D_3$ in the promotion of hair growth. There is no evidence that children or adults who suffer from vitamin D-deficiency have excessive hair loss. Furthermore, patients with chronic renal failure and who cannot make $1,25(OH)_2D$ do not suffer from alopecia. From our experience with the topical application of $1,25(OH)_2D_3$ to patients suffering with psoriasis, we have not seen any increase in hair growth over the areas that receive $1,25(OH)_2D_3$ compared to the control side. Therefore, it may be that $1,25(OH)_2D_3$ plays a role in the embryogenesis of the hair follicle during gestation or it may have some indirect effect on hair follicle development and maturation. There is no evidence that $1,25(OH)_2D_3$ is absolutely essential for hair growth (Holick 1985).

## D. Metabolism of 25-hydroxyvitamin $D_3$ in the skin

It is now recognized that most target tissues and cells that possess receptors for $1,25(OH)_2D_3$ also have the capacity to metabolize 25-OH-$D_3$ to 24,25-dihydroxyvitamin $D_3$ [$24,25(OH)_2D_3$] (DeLuca 1984; Napoli and Horst 1984; Holick 1989b). When cultured normal human fibroblasts that possess nuclear receptors for $1,25(OH)_2D_3$ are exposed to $1,25(OH)_2D_3$, this hormone in a dose-dependent manner increases 25-OH-D-24R-hydroxylase activity (Feldman et al. 1982; DeLuca 1984; Hirst et al. 1985; Smith and Holick 1987). This appears to be a specific nuclear effect since cultured human fibroblasts from patients with vitamin D-dependent rickets type II, who either lack or have a defective receptor for $1,25(OH)_2D_3$, do not increase 25-OH-D-24R-hydroxylase activity when exposed to $1,25(OH)_2D_3$ (Fig. 30).

Similar to cultured human fibroblasts when cultured human keratinocytes are exposed to $1,25(OH)_2D_3$ this hormone induced in a dose-dependent manner 25-OH-D-24R-hydroxylase activity (Smith and Holick 1987). In addition, Bikle et al. (1986) demonstrated that cultured human keratinocytes metabolized 25-OH-D not only to $24,25(OH)_2D_3$ but also to a more polar metabolite that was unequivocally identified as $1,25(OH)_2D_3$. This observation is quite interesting although its physiologic relevance remains to be determined. The skin is the largest organ in the body; and therefore, it would be expected that if the epidermis produced $1,25(OH)_2D_3$ it would ultimately enter the circulation. However, anephric patients have undetectable circulating concentrations of $1,25(OH)_2D$ and develop severe abnormalities in calcium and bone metabolism because of this acquired disorder in vitamin D metabolism (Horst 1984; Holick 1987). It has been argued, however, that $1,25(OH)_2D_3$ is made and used by the epidermis in an autocrine/paracrine manner. Further experiments

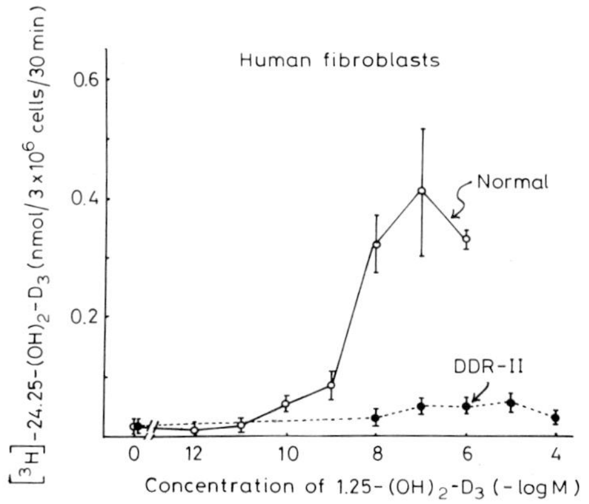


Fig. 30. Measurement of 25-OH-D-24-hydroxylase activity in cultured human fibroblasts from a normal volunteer and a patient with D-dependent rickets type II (DDR-II) in response to varying doses of $1,25(OH)_2D_3$. (Horiuchi and Holick, unpublished results.)

will be required to determine the role of the epidermis in synthesizing $1,25(OH)_2D_3$.

The study by Hollis et al. (1989) that showed that the *in vitro* metabolism of 25-OH-$D_3$ by human trophoblastic homogenates may be due to a nonspecific autooxidation rather than a specific mitochondrial hydroxylation also raises the question as to whether the *in vitro* production of $1,25(OH)_2D_3$ by keratinocytes is caused by an enzymatic rather than an autooxidative mechanism. Clearly, the identification of a mitochondrial enzyme system that produces $1,25(OH)_2D_3$ in keratinocytes would be of great value.

## V. Therapeutic efficacy of $1,25(OH)_2D_3$ for the treatment of psoriasis

### A. Rationale for using $1,25(OH)_2D$ for psoriasis

Psoriasis is a perplexing disease that afflicts approximately 1 to 3% of the population. Worldwide it is estimated that 50 million people suffer from this psychologically debilitating and disfiguring disease. The etiology of psoriasis is unknown although the proximate event is a hyperproliferation of the epidermis. As a result, many of the therapies have been designed to in some way inhibit the proliferative activity of the epidermis. Unfortunately, most of these attempts also injure the epidermis. Thus, the variety of treatments available for this disease including UVB exposure, exposure to UVA plus psoralen, retinoids, methotrexate, and steroids, all have significant side effects (Champion 1981; Baughman 1987; Potten et al. 1987; Smith et al. 1988). Therefore, to date, there is no safe and effective treatment for this skin disorder.

Since psoriasis is a hyperproliferative disorder of the epidermis and $1,25(OH)_2D_3$ inhibits the proliferation of epidermal cells, it seemed reasonable to consider the possible use of $1,25(OH)_2D_3$ for the treatment of this disease. However, before launching into a clinical trial we wondered whether psoriatic epidermal cells would respond to the antiproliferative activity of $1,25(OH)_2D_3$ like normal cultured keratinocytes did. We obtained skin biopsies from patients with psoriasis. Because it was difficult to obtain enough cultured psoriatic keratinocytes from the biopsies, it was reasoned that since skin fibroblasts also respond to the antiproliferative effect of $1,25(OH)_2D_3$ the psoriatic fibroblasts could be used as a measure of whether the psoriatic keratinocytes could respond to $1,25(OH)_2D_3$. Psoriatic and normal cultured fibroblasts were exposed to $1,25(OH)_2D_3$ in increasing concentrations and the antiproliferative activity of the hormone was monitored. Initially it was found that cultured fibroblasts from six psoriatic patients had a partial resistance to the antiproliferative activity of $1,25(OH)_2D_3$ (Fig. 31) (MacLaughlin et al. 1985). Upon further examination of cultured fibroblasts from 20 psoriatic patients, it was concluded that about 25% of the patients had fibroblasts that had a partial resistance to the antiproliferative activity of $1,25(OH)_2D_3$ while the other 75% of the patients had fibroblasts that responded normally to $1,25(OH)_2D_3$ (Fig. 32) (Smith et al. 1988). Cultured fibroblasts and

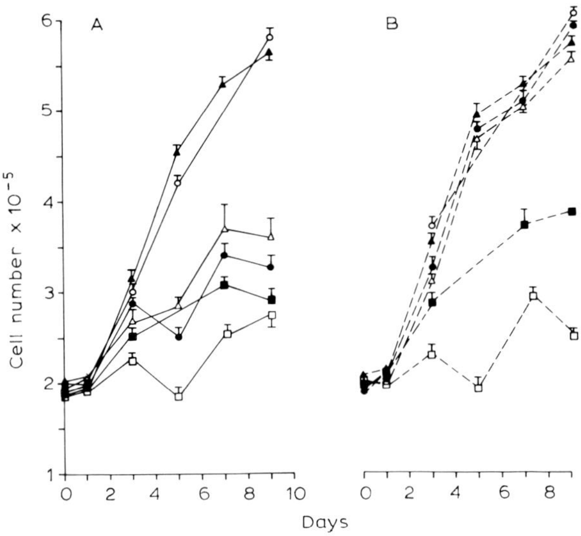


Fig. 31. Human dermal fibroblasts cultured from a skin biopsy from a normal age-matched volunteer (A) or an uninvolved area from a psoriatic patient (B) were incubated at day 0 with either EtOH (○) or $1{,}25(OH)_2D_3$ at one of the following concentrations: 0.0001 (▲), 0.01 (△), 1 (●), 10 (■), or 100 (□) $\mu$M. Each point represents the mean ± S.E.M. of fibroblasts, plated in triplicate. (From MacLaughlin et al. 1985, with permission.)

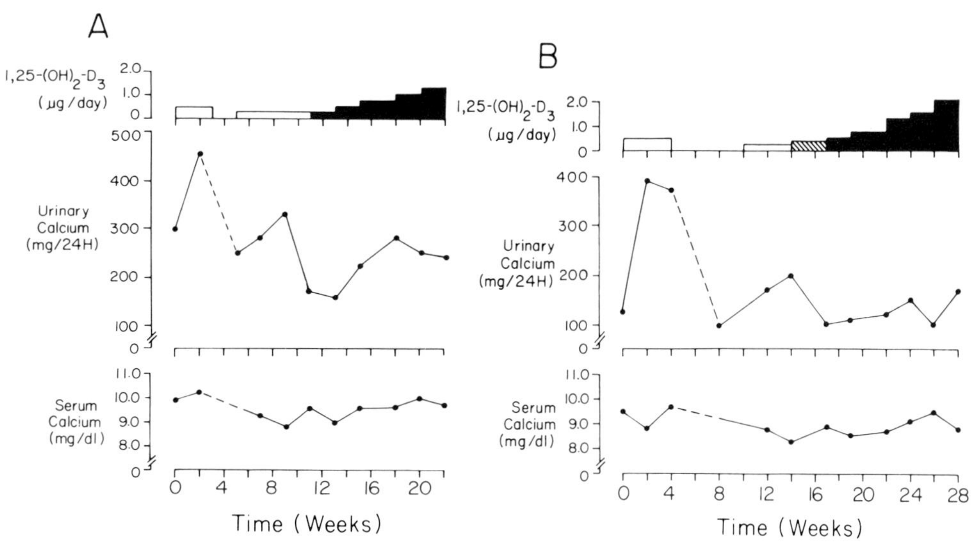


Fig. 32. Effect of $1{,}25(OH)_2D_3$ on the growth of cultured dermal fibroblasts obtained from a normal adult or from four different patients with psoriasis. Fibroblasts were incubated in medium containing vehicle alone or with $1{,}25(OH)_2D_3$ at $10^{-8}$, $10^{-6}$, or $10^{-5}$ mol/l. After 7 days the cells were harvested and counted. Each bar represents the mean ± S.E.M. cell number of triplicate cultures. (From Smith et al. 1988, with permission.)

keratinocytes from skin biopsies of psoriatic patients were analyzed for their $1,25(OH)_2D_3$ receptor. Both cell types had qualitatively and quantitatively the same $1,25(OH)_2D_3$ receptor as normal aged-matched controls (Fig. 33) (MacLaughlin et al. 1985; Smith et al. 1988). We successfully cultured psoriatic keratinocytes from three patients and exposed them to $1,25(OH)_2D_3$. The hormone inhibited their proliferation and induced terminal differentiation in a dose-dependent manner (Fig. 34). However, when Abe et al. (1989) cultured keratinocytes from three patients they found that they had a partial resistance to $1,25(OH)_2D_3$.

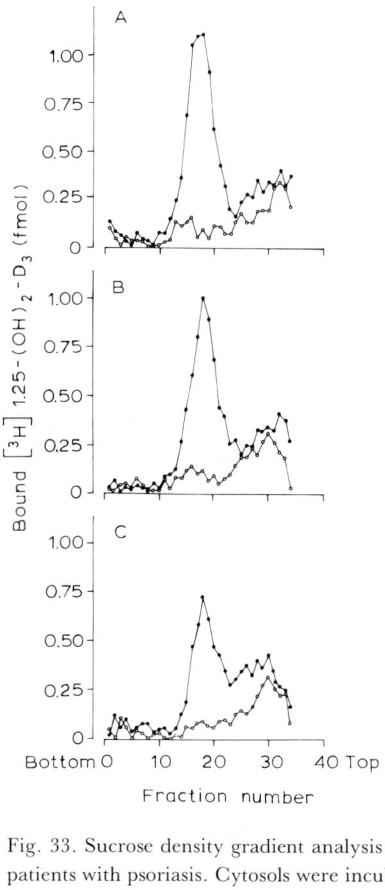


Fig. 33. Sucrose density gradient analysis of cultured keratinocyte cytosol from (A) normal subject, (B,C) patients with psoriasis. Cytosols were incubated with $1,25(OH)_2$-$[^3H]D_3$ alone (●) or in the presence of excess radioinert $1,25(OH)_2D_3$ (○). After incubation the unbound $1,25(OH)_2D_3$ was removed and the cytosols were centrifuged through sucrose gradients. For comparison a radiolabelled standard with a known sedimentation coefficient (ovalbumin, 3.7 S) was run through a separate gradient. (From Smith et al. 1988, with permission.)

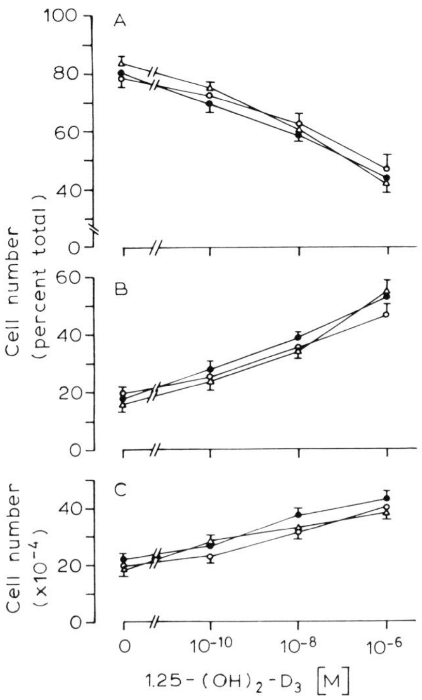


Fig. 34. Dose-dependent effect of $1{,}25(OH)_2D_3$ on the growth and differentiation of cultured epidermal keratinocytes obtained from a normal subject (●) and two patients with psoriasis, patient 1 (○) and patient 2 (△). Triplicate cultures were incubated for 7 days in serum-free medium containing $1{,}25(OH)_2D_3$ at $10^{-10}$, $10^{-8}$, or $10^{-6}$ mol/l or in medium with vehicle alone. After incubation the cultures were harvested and the numbers of attached proliferative basal cells (A), attached differentiated squamous cells (B), and cells with cornified envelopes (C) were counted. Each point represents the mean ± S.E.M. cell number of triplicate cultures. (From Smith et al. 1988, with permission.)

### B. Clinical experience with topical $1{,}25(OH)_2D_3$ for psoriasis

Thus, with the knowledge that cultured psoriatic skin cells responded to the antiproliferative activity of $1{,}25(OH)_2D_3$ (MacLaughlin et al. 1985), a clinical trial was initiated to evaluate the therapeutic efficacy of oral and topical $1{,}25(OH)_2D_3$ for patients with either plaque or erythrodermal psoriasis. Initially three patients with plaque psoriasis on their extensor surfaces applied once a day either 0.1 mg of petrolatum to a 30 $cm^2$ area on one side or 0.1 g of petrolatum containing 0.3 $\mu$g of $1{,}25(OH)_2D_3$ on a comparable lesion on the contralateral side in a double-blind study. The treated side could readily be distinguished at 2 weeks in all three patients as evidenced by a marked thinning of the plaque and decreased erythema when compared to the thickness and erythema of the control side. Complete resolution was noted after 6 weeks of therapy. The concentration of $1{,}25(OH)_2D_3$ was increased 5-fold to 15 $\mu$g/g of petrolatum to see if the response time could be shortened. The patients were instructed to apply 0.1 g of either petrolatum or petrolatum plus $1,25(OH)_2D_3$ (15 $\mu g/g$) on a 20 – 30 $cm^2$ lesion in a right/left double-blind control study. The patients noted that within 2 to 4 days there was a significant decrease in their plaque thickness and erythema on the lesion that received $1,25(OH)_2D_3$. By 4 weeks, there was often complete resolution of their lesions on the treated side (Fig. 35). Of the 60 patients we have treated, approximately 60% had complete clearing and an additional 30% showed marked thinning of their plaque, resolution in the scaling, and decreased erythema (Holick et al. 1989b).

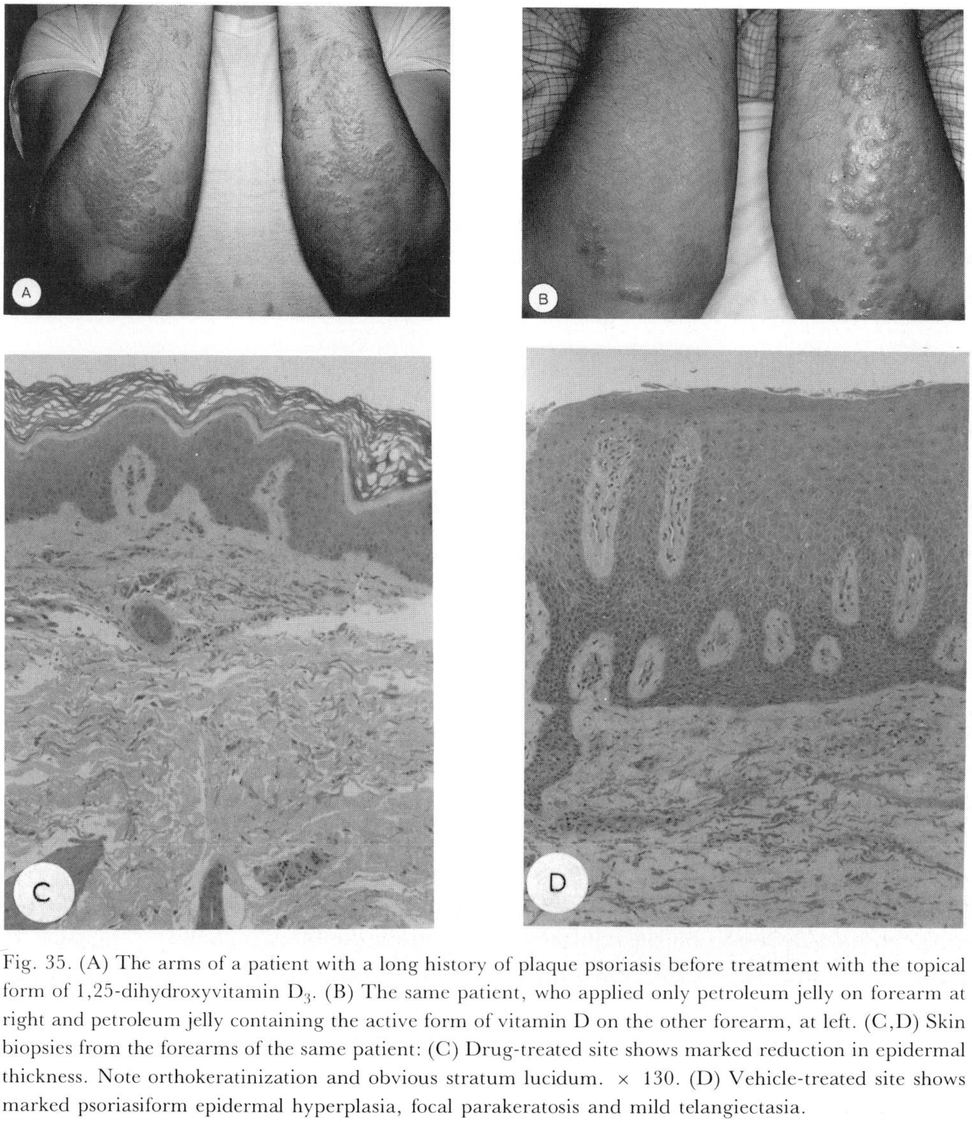


Fig. 35. (A) The arms of a patient with a long history of plaque psoriasis before treatment with the topical form of 1,25-dihydroxyvitamin $D_3$. (B) The same patient, who applied only petroleum jelly on forearm at right and petroleum jelly containing the active form of vitamin D on the other forearm, at left. (C,D) Skin biopsies from the forearms of the same patient: (C) Drug-treated site shows marked reduction in epidermal thickness. Note orthokeratinization and obvious stratum lucidum. × 130. (D) Vehicle-treated site shows marked psoriasiform epidermal hyperplasia, focal parakeratosis and mild telangiectasia.

When patients topically applied $1,25(OH)_2D_3$ over a relatively small area there was no change in either their 24 urinary calcium concentrations, circulation concentrations of calcium, phosphate, alkaline phosphatase, or $1,25(OH)_2D$. As a result larger areas were treated. Figure 36 shows a patient's abdomen before and after applying petrolatum containing 15 $\mu$g of $1,25(OH)_2D_3$/g. Considering the amount of ointment used which was 2 to 3 g each day, she was applying between 30 and 45 $\mu$g of $1,25(OH)_2D_3$ on her skin each day. After 8 weeks of therapy there was dramatic improvement in her psoriasis (Fig. 36B) and her 24 h urinary calcium and circulating concentrations of calcium, phosphate, alkaline phosphatase, and $1,25(OH)_2D$ did not increase above normal levels (Holick 1989c, d). To put the amount of $1,25(OH)_2D_3$ that was used in this and other patients into perspective, it has been estimated that the kidney produces about 1 to 2 $\mu$g of $1,25(OH)_2D$ a day (Grey et al. 1978) and the amount of $1,25(OH)_2D_3$ that can be given orally without toxicity is no more than 2 $\mu$g/day (Koeffler et al. 1985). Thus, because of the large amounts of $1,25(OH)_2D_3$ that can be potentially topically applied to patients with extensive psoriasis, there remains understandable concern about the potential of storing $1,25(OH)_2D_3$ in the skin and its eventual entrance into the circulation to cause severe hypercalciuria and hypercalcemia (Holick 1989d). However, our experience to date, using up to 60 $\mu$g of $1,25(OH)_2D_3$ topically each night on the skin of psoriatic patients, has not shown this to be true. There are several possible reasons for why such a large amount of $1,25(OH)_2D_3$ can be applied to the skin without causing toxicity. Firstly, both the keratinocytes in the epidermis and dermal fibroblasts possess receptors for $1,25(OH)_2D_3$. As the topically applied $1,25(OH)_2D_3$ works its way through the skin it could be sequestered by nuclear receptors in the cells throughout the entire epidermis and dermis. Therefore, the skin could act as a buffering zone preventing significant quantities of $1,25(OH)_2D_3$ from entering the circulation. Secondly, $1,25(OH)_2D_3$ enhances its own destruction once it enters its target cell (DeLuca 1984;

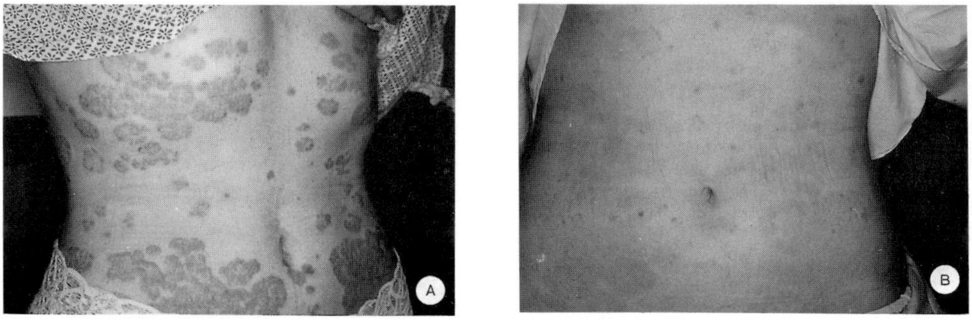


Fig. 36. Psoriatic plaques on the abdomen of this 22-year-old female with psoriasis for 11 years (A). She topically applied 2 to 3 g of Vaseline containing 15 $\mu$g of $1,25(OH)_2D_3$/g on her abdominal lesions for 6 weeks. She showed a remarkable improvement in her psoriasis and an evaluation of circulating concentrations of calcium, phosphorus, and $1,25(OH)_2D$ showed no change from her pretreatment values.

Horst 1984; Napoli and Horst 1984). The chronic application of 1,25(OH)$_2$D$_3$ could also enhance the catabolic activity of the skin cells to prevent significant quantities of 1,25(OH)$_2$D$_3$ from exiting the skin into the circulation (Holick 1989d). Thus, it appears that the topical use of 1,25(OH)$_2$D$_3$ over large areas does not present a health hazard for psoriatic patients who have a barrier break in their epidermis that could potentially enhance the absorption of this drug into their circulation.

### C. Clinical experience with the oral use of 1,25-dihydroxyvitamin D$_3$ for the treatment of psoriasis

It is now well documented that topical 1,25(OH)$_2$D$_3$ is a safe and effective therapy for the treatment of psoriasis. However, ideally patients who have extensive disease would benefit by taking 1,25(OH)$_2$D$_3$ orally for the treatment of their disease rather than having to apply 1,25(OH)$_2$D$_3$ in vaseline over most of their skin each night.

However, the treatment of psoriasis with oral 1,25(OH)$_2$D$_3$ is potentially complicated by the risk of developing hypercalciuria and hypercalcemia. It has been previously shown that 50% of preleukemic patients treated with 1,25(OH)$_2$D$_3$ developed hypercalcemia and this side effect prevented the administration of greater amounts of this drug (Koeffler et al. 1985). When we gave psoriatic patients 0.5 $\mu$g of 1,25(OH)$_2$D$_3$ orally once a day, a majority of patients developed hypercalciuria (Fig. 37) (Smith et al. 1988). Because we were interested in the antiproliferative activity of 1,25(OH)$_2$D$_3$ rather than its effect on enhancing intestinal absorption of calcium, it was reasoned that providing the hormone at night would minimize the calcemic effect of this drug thereby permitting the use of larger doses to achieve a higher circulating concentration of 1,25(OH)$_2$D$_3$ without the risk of toxicity (Smith et al. 1988). As can be seen in Fig. 37, two patients that were begun on 0.5 $\mu$g in the

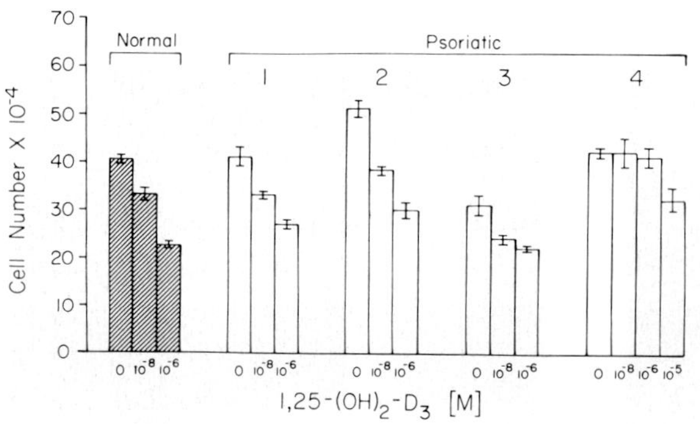


Fig. 37. Effect of 1,25(OH)$_2$-D$_3$ on the growth of cultured dermal fibroblasts obtained from a normal adult or from four different patients with psoriasis (nos. 1 – 4). Fibroblasts were incubated in medium containing vehicle alone or with 1,25(OH)$_2$-D$_3$ at $10^{-8}$, $10^{-6}$, or $10^{-5}$ mol/l. After 7 days the cells were harvested and counted. Each bar represents the mean ± S.E.M. cell number of triplicate cultures.

daytime quickly developed hypercalciuria. The drug was stopped and reinstated at bedtime. The patients were monitored for 24 h urinary calcium and serum calcium bi-monthly. When there was no increase above normal in both urine and serum calcium values, the dose of $1,25(OH)_2D_3$ was increased by 0.25 $\mu$g every 2 weeks up to a therapeutic dose of between 1.5 and 2.5 $\mu$g. Although oral $1,25(OH)_2D_3$ at 1 $\mu$g or less is ineffective for relieving the manifestations of psorasis (Morimoto and Yoshikawa 1989), it is effective at between 1.5 and 2.0 $\mu$g each night (Fig. 38). Our experience of 50 patients on oral therapy is that 26% received complete clearing of their disease while another 40% noted marked decrease in the amount of scale and thickness of plaque (Fig. 39) (Holick et al. 1989c). By giving $1,25(OH)_2D_3$ at night in a step-wise fashion, it is likely that (1) there is little or no calcium in the intestine during the ensuing 6 to 8 h and therefore there is minimum effect on the enhancement of intestinal calcium absorption; (2) exogenous $1,25(OH)_2D_3$ decreased the endogenous production of $1,25(OH)_2D_3$; (3) exogenous $1,25(OH)_2D_3$ increased the catabolism of $1,25(OH)_2D_3$ in target tissues thereby decreasing its biologic and circulating half-life; (4) $1,25(OH)_2D_3$ metabolites inhibited the association of $1,25(OH)_2D_3$ with its nuclear receptor (Lohnes and Jones 1989).

## VI. Design and therapeutic efficacy of analogs of 1,25-dihydroxyvitamin $D_3$ for the treatment of psoriasis

Although $1,25(OH)_2D_3$ is an extremely safe and effective therapy when used topically, the oral use of $1,25(OH)_2D_3$, if not monitored properly, can potentially cause significant hypercalciuria and hypercalcemia. An ideal drug for the treatment of psoriasis would be an analog of $1,25(OH)_2D_3$ that is effective in inhibiting the proliferation of epidermal cells while having little effect on calcium metabolism. Indeed there are a variety of analogs that have been synthesized and evaluated *in vitro* for their

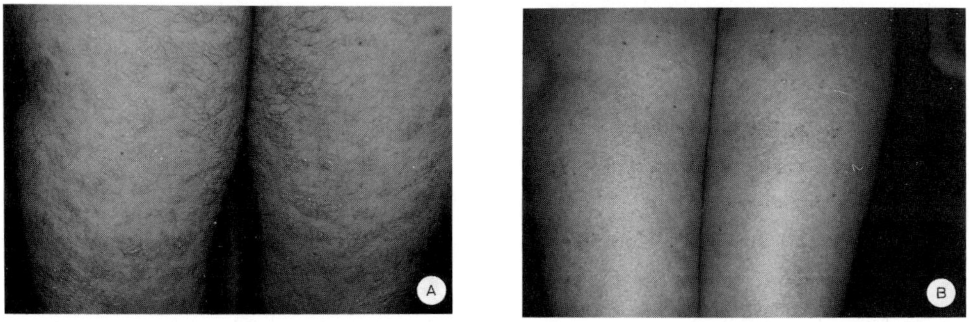


Fig. 38. Psoriatic plaques on the back of the legs of a 21-year-old female with psoriasis for 18 years (A). She was begun on oral $1,25(OH)_2D_3$ (0.5 $\mu$g) and the dose was increased in a stepwise manner. After 3 months, while taking 2.0 $\mu$g of $1,25(OH)_2D_3$ there was complete resolution of her scale and plaques (B).

antiproliferative activity in cultured human keratinocytes and HL-60 promyelocytic leukemic cells as well as *in vivo* for their effect on intestinal calcium transport and bone calcium mobilization. Several analogs in Table 2 show minimal effect on intestinal calcium absorption *in vivo* while maintaining a very high antiproliferative activity *in vitro* (Holick et al. 1988; Holick 1989c). A novel analog, 22-oxa-1,25-dihydroxyvitamin $D_3$ has also been shown *in vivo* to have little effect on intestinal calcium transport while *in vitro* maintaining its potent antiproliferative activity for both tumor cells and cultured human and murine keratinocytes (Brown et al. 1989).

However, caution is needed when designing analogs of $1,25(OH)_2D_3$ that have little effect on calcium metabolism while having potent antiproliferative activity. When judging a $1,25(OH)_2D_3$ analog for its calcemic versus antiproliferative activity, it will be important to evaluate the analogs parenterally in order to evaluate both effects *in vivo*. An example of this can be seen with the analog MC-903 (Binderup and Bramm 1988; Stagberg et al. 1989). This analog is 100 times less active on calcium metabolism when provided *in vivo* when compared to $1,25(OH)_2D_3$. However, *in vitro* it is equally as active as $1,25(OH)_2D_3$ in inhibiting the proliferation of cultured human keratinocytes. Although it is possible that there are specific $1,25(OH)_2D_3$ receptors in

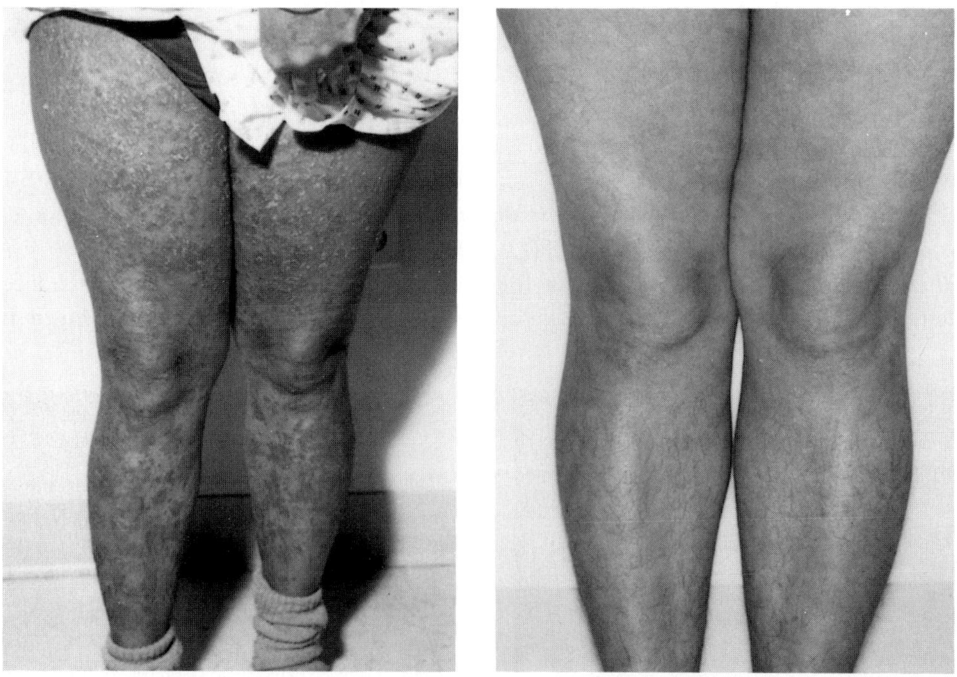

A B

Fig. 39. Views of legs of a patient with erythrodermal psoriasis before treatment (A) and after 3 months of treatment with oral $1,25(OH)_2D_3$ (B). (From Smith et al. 1988, with permission.)

TABLE 2

| Differentiation human HL-60 leukemia cells line $ED_{50}$ at $10^{-9}$ M | 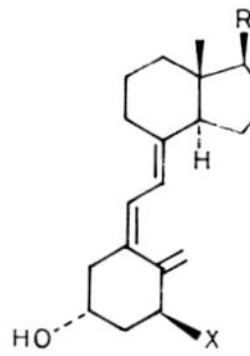 | Human keratinocytes in culture relative to the effect of $1.25\text{-}(OH)_2D_3$ as 1: Inhibition of proliferation | Human keratinocytes in culture relative to the effect of $1.25\text{-}(OH)_2D_3$ as 1: Induction of cornified envelopes | % of $1.25\text{-}(OH)_2D_3$ effect at 12.5 NG in rat: Intestinal calcium absorption | % of $1.25\text{-}(OH)_2D_3$ effect at 12.5 NG in rat: Bone calcium mobilization | Competitive binding to $1.25\text{-}(OH)_2D_3$ rat intestine receptors: % of $1.25\text{-}(OH)_2D_3$ effect |
|---|---|---|---|---|---|---|
| 10 | Ro 21-5535 X = OH<br>R = 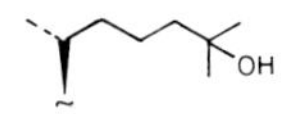 | 1 | 1 | 100 | 100 | 100 |
| 10 | Ro 21-5535/2 X = OH<br>R = 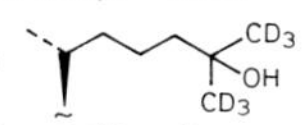 | 1 | 1 | 92 | 64 | 100 |
| 10 | Ro 21-5535/3 X = OH<br>R = 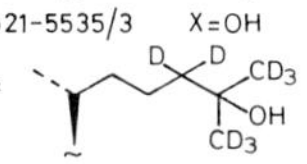 | 1 | 1 | 106 | 147 | 104 |
| 30 | Ro 23-0233 X = OH<br>R = 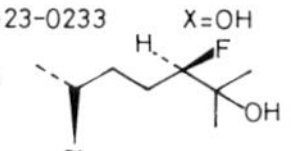 | 1 | 1 | 65 | 40 | 115 |
| 1 | Ro 22-9343 X = OH<br>R = 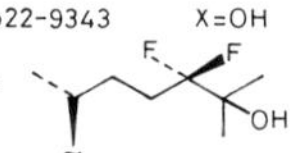 | 1 – 10 | 1 | 235 | 58 | 229 |
| 3 | Ro 23-6889 X = OH<br>R = 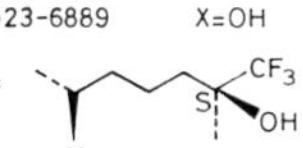 | 1 | 1 | 197 | 163 | 199 |
| 0.5 | Ro 23-4194 X = OH<br>R = 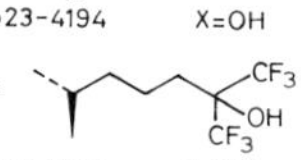 | 0.5 | 0.5 | 229 | 137 | 82 |
| 8 | Ro 23-6710 X = OH<br>R = 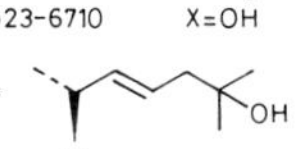 | $10^{-2}$ | $10^{-3}$ | 92 | 133 | 122 |
| 0.3 | Ro 23-6536 X = OH<br>R = 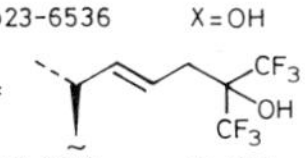 | 1 | $10^{-3}$ | 221 | 110 | 62 |
| 10 | Ro 17-6218 X = OH<br>R = 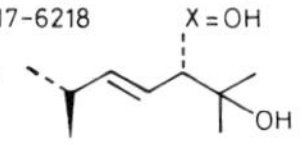 | 1 | $10^{-4}$ | 111 | 39 | |
| 10 | Ro 23-6709 X = OH<br>R = 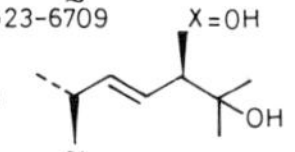 | 100 | $10^{-4}$ | 27 | 22 | |
| 3 | Ro 23-7498 X = OH<br>R = 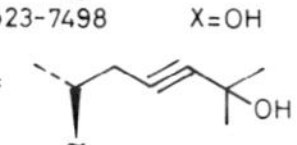 | 1 | 1 – 10 | 95 | 15 | 39 |
| 1000 | Ro 23-9375 X = H<br>R = 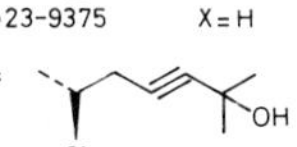 | 1 | 1 | 71 | 0 | |
| 10 | Ro 23-4319 X = OH<br>R = 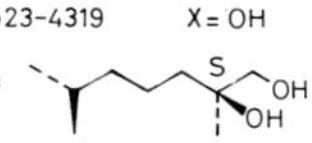 | 0.1 | 1 | 51 | 10 | 6 |
| 10 | Ro 23-6005 X = OH<br>R = 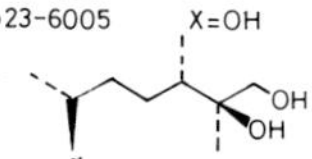 | 0.1 | 1 | 47 | 0 | |
| 70 | Ro 23-6474 X = OH<br>R = 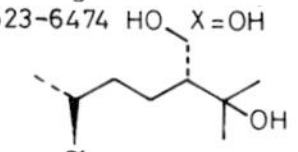 | 1 | 1 | 0 | 0 | 1 |

the skin that are different from the intestine so that analogs such as MC-903 can be designed to function in the skin while having little or no effect on intestinal calcium transport, this does not appear to be likely. There is strong evidence that the nuclear receptor for 1,25$(OH)_2D_3$ in keratinocytes, fibroblasts, and intestinal cells are one and the same (Clemens et al. 1983; Pike 1985). The most likely explanation is that MC-903 is rapidly degraded and therefore has minimum biologic action *in vivo*.

There is an alternative explanation for why analogs of 1,25$(OH)_2D_3$ can be developed to have little calcemic action while having potent antiproliferative activity. There is mounting evidence that 1,25$(OH)_2D_3$ not only interacts with a specific nuclear receptor, but it also can interact with the plasma membrane to alter intracellular calcium (Fig. 40) and phosphoinositol metabolism (Baran et al. 1986; Smith and Holick 1987; MacLaughlin et al. 1990). It may be possible to develop synthetic analogs of 1,25$(OH)_2D_3$ that enhance intracellular calcium movement and phosphoinositol metabolism while having little effect on the 1,25$(OH)_2D_3$ nuclear receptor. It is well known that intracellular calcium concentrations have a dramatic influence on inhibiting keratinocyte proliferation and inducing differentiation (Hennings et al. 1980); it may be possible to direct 1,25$(OH)_2D_3$ analogs for this purpose (Holick 1989d).

Three analogs of 1,25$(OH)_2D_3$ have been tested for their clinical therapeutic efficacy in psoriasis. 1-OH-$D_3$ was found to be effective when given orally (Morimoto and Kumahara 1985; Morimoto et al. 1986). However, since this analog is metabolized to 1,25$(OH)_2D_3$ in humans it is unlikely that 1-OH-$D_3$ will have any selective biologic actions. In addition, the half-life of 1-OH-$D_3$ is much longer than 1,25$(OH)_2D_3$ and therefore if toxicity was to occur it would take a much longer time to reverse it (Paterson 1981). 1,24-dihydroxyvitamin $D_3$ (1,24$(OH)_2D_3$) is recognized by the 1,25$(OH)_2D_3$ receptor with almost equal affinity as the natural hormone. This analog appears to be as effective as 1,25$(OH)_2D_3$ for psoriasis when used topically

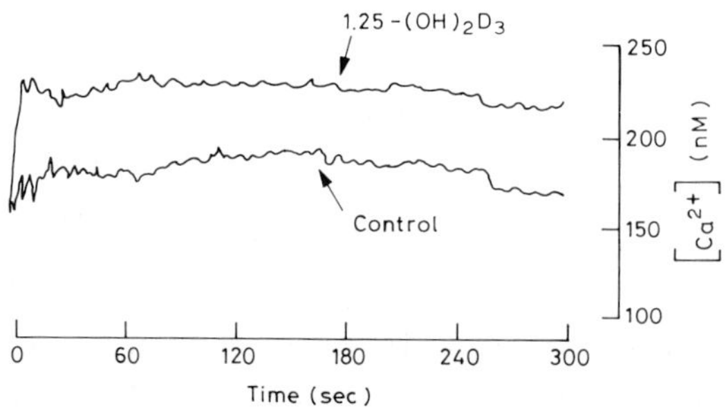


Fig. 40. Effect of 1,25$(OH)_2D_3$ on free cytosolic calcium concentration of cultured human keratinocytes. Cells were loaded with Quin2/AM and then treated with vehicle alone (control) or 1,25$(OH)_2D_3$ ($10^{-8}$ M). The fluorescence (F) was measured at 495 nm over the 5-min time course. The calcium concentration was calculated according to the equation: $[Ca^{+2}]i = 115\ \text{nM}\ (F - F_{min})/(F_{max} - F)$. (From Smith and Holick 1987, with permission.)

(Kato et al. 1986). Although it was suggested that this analog is less toxic than $1,25(OH)_2D_3$ there is little evidence for this in humans.

MC-903 when used in concentrations of 50 and 100 μg/g ointment or cream is as effective as $1,25(OH)_2D_3$ at a concentration of 15 μg/g (Kragballe et al. 1988; Holick 1989d; Kragballe et al. 1989) in resolving psoriatic lesions. However, unlike $1,25(OH)_2D_3$, approximately 10% of the patients using MC-903 develop a dermatitis similar to that induced by steroids (Kragballe et al. 1989).

Caution will be required when designing analogs of $1,25(OH)_2D_3$ that have little effect on calcium metabolism while having potent antiproliferative activity. For example, it is possible that the oral or topical administration of an analog that has no calcemic effect could enter into the bloodstream and travel to the kidney and liver to interact with nuclear receptors to inhibit $1,25(OH)_2D$ production and enhance the catabolism of endogenously produced $1,25(OH)_2D$, respectively. This could result in an acquired disorder in the metabolism and catabolism of 25-OH-D and $1,25(OH)_2D$, respectively, that could ultimately lead to hypocalcemia and metabolic bone disease. Alternatively, a $1,25(OH)_2D_3$ analog could interact with the nuclear receptor for $1,25(OH)_2D_3$ in the intestine and prevent the natural hormone from expressing its biologic activity. This could lead to an acquired defect in the target tissue recognition and utilization for the natural hormone and could also result in hypocalcemia and metabolic bone disease (Holick 1989d).

## VII. Conclusion

The sun has been responsible for providing all humans with some or all of their vitamin D requirement. There needs be a reawakening of the fact that it is casual exposure to sunlight that provides all of us with our vitamin D requirement. Since there are a variety of factors that can limit the cutaneous production of vitamin $D_3$, sensible guidelines need to be developed to provide us with a more even-handed appreciation of both the beneficial effects of short-term exposure to sunlight as well as the damaging effects due to chronic exposure to this wonderful natural resource (Holick 1990).

Based on the clinical trials to date, one of the major pharmacologic uses of $1,25(OH)_2D_3$ and its analogs in the future will be for the treatment the hyperproliferative skin disease psoriasis. Although Staberg et al. (1987) have reported a significant decrease in serum $1,25(OH)_2D_3$ in 17 psoriatic patients compared to age-matched controls, there is little reason to believe that psoriasis is in any way due to an acquired or inborn error in the metabolism or recognition of $1,25(OH)_2D_3$. Our extensive experience with psoriatic patients has not revealed any alteration in the metabolism of 25-OH-D to $1,25(OH)_2D$ (Smith et al. 1988; Holick et al. 1989c, d). Furthermore, although there is some evidence for a partial resistance to $1,25(OH)_2D_3$ in cultured fibroblast and keratinocytes from psoriatic patients it is unlikely that this is the etiologic factor for psoriasis.

## Acknowledgements

This work was supported by AM-32324, AG-02918, AG-04390 and M01 RR 00533.


## References


Abe J, Kondo S, Nishii Y, Kuroki, T. Resistance to 1,25-dihydroxyvitamin D3 of cultured psoriatic epidermal keratinocytes isolated from involved and uninvolved skin. J Clin Endocrinol 1989;68:851 – 854.

Adams JA, Clemens TL, Parrish JA, Holick, MF. Vitamin D synthesis and metabolism after ultraviolet radiation of normal and vitamin D deficient subjects. N Engl J Med 1981;306:722 – 725.

Ala-Houhala M, Parvianen MT, Pyykko K, Visakorpi, JK. Serum 25-hydroxyvitamin D levels in Finnish children. Acta Paediatr Scand 1984;73:232 – 236.

Anderson I, Campbell AER, Dunn A, Runciman, JBM. Osteomalacia in elderly women. Scot Med J 1966;11:429 – 435.

Anderson RR, Parrish, JA. Optical properties of human skin. In: Regan JD, Parrish JA, (eds.) The Science of Photomedicine. New York: Plenum Press, 1982;147 – 194.

Aubran M, Jallet P, Avenel M, Bidet M, Galland R, Renier JC. Vaiations saisonnieres des metabolites de la vitamin D chez l'homme. Presse Med 1984;13:661 – 663.

Bar-Shavit Z, Kahn AJ, Stone KR, Trial J, Hilliard T, Reitsma PH, Teitlelbaum L. Reversibility of vitamin D-induced human leukemia cell-line maturation. Endocrinology 1986;118:679 – 686.

Baran DT, Moira L, Mine L. 1,25-Dihydroxyvitamin D increases hepatocyte cytosolic calcium levels: A potential regulator of vitamin D-25-hydroxylase. J Clin Invest 1986;77:1622 – 1626.

Baughman RD. Psoriasis practices. (Editorial) Arch Dermatol 1987;123:1299 – 1300.

Bhalla AK, Clemens T, Amento E, Holick MF, Krane SM. Specific high-affinity receptors for 1,25-dihydroxyvitamin D3 in human peripheral blood mononuclear cells: Presence in monocytes and induction in T lymphocytes following activation. J Clin Endrocrinol Metab 1983;57:1308 – 1310.

Bikle DD, Nemanic MD, Whitney JO, Elias PO. Neonatal human foreskin keratinocytes produce 1,25-dihydroxyvitamin D3. Biochemistry 1986;25:1545 – 1548.

Binderup L, Bramm E. Effect of a novel vitamin D analogue MC 903 on cell proliferation and differentiation in vitro and on calcium metabolism in vivo. Biochem Pharmacol 1988;37:889 – 895.

Bolt MJG, Holick SA, Holick MF, MacLaughlin J, Rosenberg IH. 24-Dehydrovitamin D3 is a potent inhibitor of rat liver microsomal vitamin D-25-hydroxylase. Arch Biochem Biophys 1988;266:532 – 538.

Brown AJ, Ritter CR, Finch JL, Morrissey J, Martin KJ, Murayama E, Nishii Y. The noncalcemic analogue of vitamin D, 22-oxacalcitriol, suppresses parathyroid hormone synthesis and secretion. J Clin Invest 1989;84:728 – 732.

Chalmers J, Conacher DH, Gardner DL, Scott PJ. Osteomalacia — a common disease in elderly women. J Bone Jt Surg (Br) 1967;403 – 423.

Champion RH. Psoriasis and its treatment. Br Med J 1981;282:343 – 346.

Chesney RW, Rosen JF, Hamstra AJ, Smith C Mahaffey K, DeLuca HF. Absence of seasonal variation in serum concentrations of 1,25-dihydroxyvitamin D despite a rise in 25-hydroxyvitamin D in summer. J Clin Endocrinol Metab 1981;53:139 – 142.

Clemens TL, Holick MF. Recent advances in the hormonal regulation of calcium and phosphorus in adult animals and humans. In: Holick MF, Anast CS, Gray TK, eds. Perinatal Calcium and Phosphorus Metabolism. New York: Elsevier, 1983;1 – 18.

Clemens TL, Henderson SL, Adams JS, Holick MF. Increased skin pigment reduces the capacity of skin to synthesise vitamin D3. Lancet 1982;74 – 76.

Clemens TL, Adams JS, Horiuchi N, et al. Interaction of 1,25-dihydroxyvitamin D3 with keratinocytes and fibroblasts from skin of normal subjects and a subject with vitamin D-dependent rickets, type II. J Clin

Endocrinol Metab 1983;56:824 – 830.

Colston K, Colston MJ, Feldman, D. 1,25-Dihydroxyvitamin D3 and malignant melanoma: the presence of receptors and inhibition of cell growth in culture. Endocrinology 1981a;108:1083 – 1086.

Colston K, Horst M, Feldman D. Organ distribution of the cytoplasmic 1,25-dihydroxycholecalciferol receptor in various mouse tissues. Endocrinology 1981b;107:1916.

Cooke NE, David EV. Serum vitamin D-binding protein is a third member of the albumin and alpha fetoprotein gene family. J Clin Invest 1985;76:2420 – 2424.

Czarnetzki BM. Vitamin D3 in dermatology: a critical appraisal. Dermatologica 1989;178:184 – 188.

DeLuca, H. The vitamin D story: A collaborative effort of basic science and clinical medicine. Fed Proc Am Soc Exp Biol 1988;2: 224 – 236.

DeLuca, HF. The metabolism, physiology, and function of vitamin D. In: Kumar R, ed. Vitamin D: Basic and Clinical Aspects. Boston, The Hague: Martinus Nijhoff, 1984;1 – 68.

Doppelt SH, Neer RM, Daly M, Bourret L, Schiller A, Holick MF. Vitamin D deficiency and osteomalacia in patients with hip fractures. Orthop Trans 1983;7:512 – 513.

Eisman JA. 1,25-Dihydroxyvitamin D3 receptor and role of 1,25-dihydroxyvitamin D3 in human cancer cells in vitamin D. In: Kumar R, ed. Vitamin D: Basic and Clinical Aspects. Boston, Martinus Nijhoff, The Hague: 1984;365 – 382.

Esvelt RP, Schnoes HK, DeLuca HF. Vitamin D3 from rat skins irradiated in vitro with ultraviolet light. Arch Biochem Bioshys 1978;188:282 – 286.

Feldman D, Chen T, Cone C, Hirst M, Shani S, Benderli A, Hochberg Z. Vitamin-D resistant rickets with alopecia: cultured skin fibroblasts exhibit defective cytoplasmic receptors and unresponsiveness to 1,25(OH)2D3. J Clin Endocrinol Metab 1982;55:1020 – 1022.

Fieser LD, Fieser M. Vitamin D. In: Steroids. New York: Reinhold, 1959;90 – 168.

Findlay, L. The etiology of rickets: a clinical and experimental study. Br Med J 1980;ii:13.

Fraser D, Scriver CR. Hereditary disorders associated with vitamin-D resistance or defective phosphate metabolism. In: DeGroot L, Besser G, Cahill G, Marshall J, Nelson D, Odell W, Potts JT, Rubenstein A, Steinberger E, eds. Endocrinology, Vol.2. New York: Grune and Stratton, 1979;797 – 807.

Goldblatt H, Soames KM. Studies on the fat soluble growth-promoting factor. Biochem J 1923;17:446 – 453.

Gray RW, Caldas AE, Wilz DR, Lemann J, Smith GA. Execretion of 3H-1,25-dihydroxyvitamin D3 in healthy adults. J Clin Endocrinol Metab 1978;46:756 – 765.

Hanesmann D. Veber den einfluss der domestikation auf die entstehung der krankheiten. Berl Klin Wochenschr Xliii, 1906;629:670.

Haussler MR, Donaldson CA, Kelly MA, Mangelsdorf DJ, Marion SL, Pike JW. Functions and mechanism of action of the 1,25-dihydroxyvitamin D3 receptor. In: Norman AW, Schaefer K, Grigoleit HG, Herrath Dv, eds. Vitamin D: A Chemical, Biochemical and Clinical Update. New York: Walter de Gruyter, 1985;83 – 92.

Hennings H, Michael D, Cheng C, Steinert P, Holbrook K, Yuspa SH. Calcium regulation of growth and differentiation of mouse epidermal cells in culture. Cell 1980;19:245 – 254.

Hess AF, Unger LF. Cure of infantile rickets by sunlight. J Am Med Assoc 1921;77:39.

Hess AF, Weinstock M. Antirachitic properties imparted to inert fluids and green vegetables by ultraviolet irradiation. J Biol Chem 1924;62:301 – 313.

Hirst MA, Hochmann HI, Feldman, D. Vitamin D resistance and alopecia: a kindred with normal 1,25-dihydroxyvitamin D binding, but decreased receptor affinity for deoxyribonucleic acid. J Clin Endocrinol Metab 1985;60:490 – 495.

Holick MF. Vitamin D resistance and alopecia: A causal or casual relationship? Arch Dermatol 1985;121:601 – 603.

Holick MF. Vitamin D requirements for the elderly. Clin Nutr 1986;5:121 – 129.

Holick MF. Vitamin D and the kidney. Kidney Int 1987;32:912 – 929.

Holick MF. Phylogenetic and evolutionary aspects of vitamin D from phytoplankton to humans. In: Pang

PKT, Schreibman MP, eds. Vertebrate Endocrinology: Fundamentals and Biomedical Implications, Vol 3. Orlando: Academic Press, 1989a;7 – 43.

Holick MF. Vitamin D: biosynthesis, metabolism, and mode of action. In: DeGroot LJ, Besser G, Cahill G, Marshall J, Nelson D, Odell W, Potts JT, Rubenstein A, Steinberger E, eds. Endocrinology, Vol. 2. New York: Grune and Stratton, 1989b;902 – 926.

Holick MF. 1,25-Dihydroxyvitamin D3 and the skin: a unique application for the treatment of psoriasis. In: Proceedings, Society for Experimental Biology and Medicine, 1989c;19:246 – 257.

Holick MF. Will 1,25-dihydroxyvitamin D3, MC 903 and their analogs herald a new pharmacologic era for the treatment of psoriasis? Arch Dermatol 1989d;125:1692 – 1697.

Holick MF. An intimate relationship between the sun, skin, and vitamin D: A new perspective. Bone 1990;7:66 – 69.

Holick MF, MacLaughlin JA, Doppelt. Factors that influence the cutaneous photosynthesis of previtamin D3. Science 1981;211:590 – 593.

Holick MF, MacLaughlin JA, Parrish JA, Anderson RR. The photochemistry and photobiology of vitamin D3. In: Regan JD, Parrish JA, eds. The Science of Photomedicine. New York: Plenum Press, 1982;195 – 218.

Holick MF, Smith EL, Pincus S. Skin as the site of vitamin D3 synthesis and target tissue for 1,25-dihydroxycholecalciferol. Use of calcitriol (1,25-dihydroxycholecalciferol) for treatment of psoriasis. Arch Dermatol 1987;123:1677a – 1683a.

Holick MF, Uskokovic M, Persons KS. An evaluation of a variety of analogs of 1,25-dihydroxyvitamin D3 on the inhibition of proliferation and induction of terminal differentiation in cultured human normal keratinocytes. In: Norman AW, Schaefer K, Grigoleit HG, Herrath DV eds. Vitamin D. Berlin: Walter de Gruyter, 1988;362 – 363.

Holick MF, Matsuoka, LY, Wortsman J. Age, vitamin D, and solar ultraviolet radiation. Lancet 1989a;ii:1104 – 1105.

Holick MF, McCarthy E, Joyce-Otis D, Pochi P, Bhawan J. Long-term effects of orally and topically administered 1,25-dihydroxyvitamin D3 on calcium and bone metabolism in healthy young and middle-aged male and female adults who suffer from psoriasis. 10th Int Confer Calcium Regulating Hormones. ASBMR 1989b;4:723a,s298.

Holick SA, St Lezin M, Young D, Malaikal S, Holick MF. Isolation and identification of 24-dehydroprovitamin D3 and its photolysis to 24-dehydroprevitamin D3 in mammalian skin. J Biol Chem 1985;260:12181 – 12184.

Hollis BW, Iskersky VN, Chang MK. In vitro metabolism of 25-hydroxyvitamin D3 by human trophoblastic homogenates, mitochondria, and microsomes: lack of evidence for the presence of 25-hydroxyvitamin D3-1$\alpha$-and 24R-hydroxylases. Endocrinology 1989;125:1224 – 1230.

Horiuchi N, Clemens TL, Schiller AL, Holick, MF. Detection and developmental changes of the 1,25(OH)2D3 receptor concentration in mouse skin and intestine. J Invest Dermatol 1985;84:461 – 464.

**Horst R. Recent advances in the quantitation of vitamin D and vitamin D metabolists. In: Kumar R, ed. Vitamin D: Basic and Clinical Aspects. Boston, The Hague: Martinus Nijhoff 1984;423–478.**

Hosoi J, Abe E, Suda T, Kuroki T. Regulation of melanin synthesis of B16 mouse melanoma cells by 1,25-dihydroxyvitamin D3 and retinoic acid. Cancer Res 1985;45:1474 – 1478.

Hosomi J, Hosoi J, Abe E, Suda T Kuroki T. Regulation of terminal differentiation of cultured mouse epidermal cells by 1,25-dihydroxyvitamin D3. Endocrinology 1983;113:1950 – 1957.

Hou H. Relation of preen gland of birds to rickets. III. Site of activation during irradiation. Chin J Physiol 1931;5:11 – 18.

Huldschinsky K. Heilung von Rachitis durch Kunstliche Hohensonne. Dtsch Med Wochenschr 1919;45:712 – 713.

Jenkins DH, Roberts JG, Webster D, Williams EO. Osteomalacia in elderly patients with fracture of the femoral neck. J Bone Jt Surg (Br) 1973;55B:575 – 580.

Kassowitz M. Tetanie and autointoxication in kindersalter. Wien Med Presse XXXViii, 1897;97:139.

Kato T, Rokugo M, Terui T, Tagami H. Successful treatment of psoriasis with topical application of active vitamin D3 analogue, 1$\alpha$,24-dihydroxycholecalciferol. Br J Dermatol 1986;115:431 – 433.

Kavookjian H, Whitelaw G, Lin S, Holick MF. Role of vitamin D deficiency in the level of age-associated fractures in patients treated at an inner city hospital. Orthopediac Trans (1990).

Koch EM, Koch FC. The provitamin D of the covering tissues of chickens. J Poult Sci 1941;20:33.

Koch J. Untersuchungen uber die localixation der bakterian das verhalten des knochenmarkes und die veranderungen der knochen, insbesondere der epiphysen, bei infektionskranheiten. Mit bemerkungen zur theorie der rachitis. Z Hyg Infektionskr IXIX, 1911;436.

Koeffler HP, Hirjik J, Iti L and the Southern California Leukemia Group. 1,25-Dihydroxyvitamin D3: in vivo and in vitro effects on human preleukemic and leukemic cells. Cancer Treat Rep 1985;69:1399 – 1407.

Kragballe K. Treatment of psoriasis by the topical application of the novel vitamin D3 analogue MC 903. Arch Dermatol 1989;125:1647 – 1652.

Kragballe K, Beck HI, Sogaard H. Improvement of psoriasis by a topical vitamin D3 analogue (MC903) in a double-blind study. Br J Dermatol 1988;119:223 – 230.

Lamberg-Allard T. Vitamin D intake, sunlight exposure, and 25-hydroxyvitamin D levels in elderly during on year. Ann Nutr Met 1984;28:144 – 150.

Lester E, Skinner RK, Wills, MR. Seasonal variation in serum 25-hydroxyvitamin D in the elderly in Britain. Lancet 1977;1:979 – 980.

Lieberman UA, Eil C, Marx SJ. Resistance to 1,25-dihydroxyvitamin D: Association with heterogeneous defects in cultured skin fibroblasts. J Clin Invest 1983;71:192 – 200.

Lo C, Paris PW, Holick, MF. Indian and Pakistani immigrants have the same capacity as Caucasians to produce vitamin D in response to ultraviolet irradiation. Am J Clin Nutr 1986;44:683 – 685.

Lohnes D, Jones G. Calcitroic acid production limits vitamin D receptor occupation in osteoblast derived cells. 10th Int Conf Calcium Regulating Hormone. ASBMR 1989;4:576a, S261.

Loomis F. Skin-pigment regulation of vitamin D biosynthesis in man. Science 1967;157:501 – 506.

MacLaughlin JA, Holick MF. Mediation of cutaneous vitamin D3 synthesis by UV radiation. In: Goldsmith LA, ed. Biochemistry and Physiology of the Skin, Vol. 1. North Carolina: Oxford University Press, 1983;734 – 754.

MacLaughlin JA, Anderson RR, Holick MF. Spectral character of sunlight modulates photosynthesis of previtamin D3 and its photoisomers in human skin. Science 1982;216:1001 – 1004.

MacLaughlin JA, Gange W, Taylor D, Smith E, Holick MF. Cultured psoriatic fibroblasts from involved and uninvolved sites have a partial but not absolute resistance to the proliferation-inhibition activity of 1,25-dihydroxyvitamin D3. Proc Natl Acad Sci 1985;82:5409 – 5412.

MacLaughlin JA, Cantley LC, Holick MF. 1,25(OH)2D3 Increases calcium and phosphatidylinositol metabolism in differentiating cultured human keratinocytes. J Nutr Biochem (1990).

Mansur CP, Gorden PR, Ray S, Holick MF, Gilchrest BA. Vitamin D, its precursors, and metabolites do not affect melanization of cultured human melanocytes. J Invest Dermatol 1988;91:16 – 21.

Marksted T, Halvorsen S, Halvorsen KS, et al. Plasma concentrations of vitamin D metabolites before and during treatment of vitamin D deficiency rickets in children. Acta Padiatr Scand 1984;73:225 – 231.

Marx SJ. Resistance to vitamin D. In: Kumar R, ed. Vitamin D: Basic and Clinical Aspects. Boston, The Hague: Martinus Nijhoff, 1984;721 – 745.

Mason RS. Extra-renal production of 1,25(OH)2D3, the metabolism of vitamin D by non-traditional tissues. In: Norman AW, Schaefer K, Grigoleit HG, Herrath DV, eds. Vitamin D: A Chemical, Biochemical and Clinical Update. New York: Walter de Gruyter & Co., 1985;23 – 32.

Massengale ON, Nussmeier M. The action of activated ergosterol in the chicken. J Biol Chem 1930;87:423 – 425.

Matsuoka LY, Ide L, Wortsman J, MacLaughlin J, Holick MF. Sunscreens suppress cutaneous vitamin D3 synthesis. J Clin Endocrinol Metab 1987;64:1165 – 1168.

Matsuoka LY, Wortsman J, Hanifan N, Holick MF. Chronic sunscreen use decreases circulating concentrations of 25-hydroxyvitamin D: a preliminary study. Arch Dermatol 1988;124:1802 – 1804.

Mayer J. Armand Trousseau and the arrow of time. Nutr Rev 1957;15:321 – 323.

McCollum EF, Simmonds N, Becker JE, Shipley PG. Studies on experimental rickets; and experimental demonstration of the existence of a vitamin which promotes calcium deposition. J Biol Chem 1922;53:293 – 312.

Mellanby T. The part played by an 'accessory factor' in the production of experimental rickets. J Physiol 1918;52:11 – 14.

Merke J, Schwittay D, Furstenberger G, Gross M, Marks F, Ritz E. Demonstration and characterization of 1,25-dihydroxyvitamin D3 receptors in basal cells of epidermis of neonatal and adult mice. Calcif Tissue Int 1985;37:257 – 267.

Merke J, Klaus G, Hugel U, et al. No 1,25-dihydroxyvitamin D3 receptors on osteoclasts of calcium-deficient chicken despite demonstrable receptors on circulating monocytes. J Clin Invest 1986;77:312 – 314.

Montagna W, Carlisle MS. Structural changes in aging human skin. J Invest Dermatol 1979;73:47 – 53.

Morimoto S, Kumahara Y. A patient with psoriasis cured by 1a-hydroxyvitamin D3. Med J Oska Univ 1985;35:51.

Morimoto S, Yoshikawa K. Psoriasis and vitamin D3 (Editorial). Arch Dermatol 1989;125:231 – 234.

Morimoto S, Yochikawa K, Kozuka T, et al. An open study of vitamin D3 treatment in psoriasis. Br J Dermatol 1986;115:421 – 429.

Napoli J, Horst, R. Vitamin D metabolism. In: Kumar R. ed. Vitamin D: Basic and Clinical Aspects. Boston, The Hague: Martinus Nijhoff, 1984;91 – 124.

Oikawa A, Nakayasu M. Stimulation of melanogenesis in cultured melanoma cells by calciferols. FEBS Lett 1974;42:32 – 35.

Okano T, Yasumura M, Mizuno K, Kobayashi T. Photochemical conversion of 7-dehydrocholesterol into vitamin D3 in rat skins. J Nutr Sci Vitaminol (Tokyo) 1977;23:165 – 168.

Omdahl JL, Garry PJ, Hunsaker LA, et al. Nutritional status in a healthy elderly population: vitamin D. Am J Clin Nutr 1982;36:1225 – 1233.

Owen I. Geographical distribution of rickets, acute and subacute rheumatism, chorea, cancer and urinary calculus in the British Islands. Br Med J 1889;1:113 – 116.

Palm TA. The geographic distribution and etiology of rickets. Practioner 1980;45:270 – 279, 321 – 342.

Parrish JA, White HAD, Pathak MA. Photomedicine. In: Fitzpatrick TB, et al. eds. Dermatology in General Medicine. New York: McGraw-Hill, 1979;942.

Paterson CR. Hypercalcemia and alphacalcidiol therapy. Postgradr Med J 1981;57:431 – 432.

Pavlovitch JH, Rizk M, Balsan S. Vitamin D nutrition increases skin tyrosinase response to exposure to ultraviolet radiation. Molecular Cell Endocrinol 1982;25:295 – 302.

Pike JW. Intracellular receptors mediate the biologic action of 1,25-dihydroxyvitamin D3. Nutr Rev 1985;43:161 – 168.

Poskitt EME, Cole TJ, Lawson DEM. Diet, sunlight and 25-hydroxyvitamin D in healthy children and adults. Br Med J 1979;1:221 – 223.

Potten CS. Possible defects in the proliferative organization and control mechanismin psoriasis. In: Farber EM, Nall L, Mohenn V, Jacobs PH, eds. Psoriasis: Proceedings of the Fourth International Symposium. New York: Elsevier, 1987;15 – 35.

Powers GF, Park EA, Shipley PG, McCollum EV, Simmonds N. The prevention of rickets in the rat by means of radiation with the mercury vapor quartz lamp. Proc Soc Exp Biol Med 1921;19:120 – 121.

Ranson M, Posen S, Mason, R. Human melanocytes as a target tissue for hormones: in vitro studies with 1$\alpha$,25, dihydroxyvitamin D3, $\alpha$-melanocyte stimulating hormone, and beta-estradiol. J Invest Dermatol 1988;91:593 – 602.

Rauschkolb EW, Winston D, Fenimore DC, Black HS, Fabre LF. Identification of vitamin D3 in human skin. J Invest Dermatol 1969;53:289 – 293.

Reichel H, Koeffler HP, Norman AW. The role of the vitamin D endocrine system in health and disease.

N Engl J Med 1989;320:981 – 991.

Schmorl G. Die pathologigische anatomie de rachitischen knochenerkrankung mit besonderer ber ucksichtigung imer histologie und pathogenese. Ergeb d. Inn Med Kinderheilkd IV, 1909;403.

Smith EL, Holick MF. The skin: The site of vitamin D3 synthesis and a target tissue for its metabolite 1,25-dihydroxyvitamin D3. Steroids 1987;49:103 – 131.

Smith EL, Walworth ND, Holick MF. Effect of 1,25-dihydroxyvitamin D3 on the morphologic and biochemical differentiation of cultured human epidermal keratinocytes grown in serum-free conditions. J Invest Dermatol 1986;86:709 – 714.

Smith EL, Pincus SH, Donovan L, Holick MF. A novel approach for the evaluation and treatment of psoriasis. J Am Acad Dermatol 1988;19:516 – 528.

Sniadecki J (1940) Cited by W Mozolowski. Jerdrzej Sniadecki (1768 – 1883) on the cure of rickets. Nature 1939;143:121.

Sokoloff L. Occult osteomalacia in American patients with fracture of the hip. Am J Surg Pathol 1978;2:21 – 30.

Staberg B, Oxholm A, Klemp P, Christiansen C. Abnormal vitamin D metabolism in patients with psoriasis. Acta Derm Venereol (Stockh) 1987;67:65 – 68.

Staberg B, Roed-Petersen J, Meene T. Efficacy of topical treatment in psoriasis with MC903, a new vitamin D analogue. Acta Dermatol Venereol 1989;69:147 – 150.

Stamp TC, Walker PG, Perry W, Jenkins, MV. Nutritional osteomalacia and late rickets in greater London, 1974 – 1979: clinical and metabolic studies in 45 patients. Clin Endocrinol Metab 1980;9:81 – 105.

Steenbock H. The induction of growth-prompting and calcifying properties in a ration exposed to light. Science 1924;60:224 – 225.

Steenbock H, Black A. The reduction of growth-promoting and calcifying properties in a ration by exposure to ultraviolet light. J Biol Chem 1924;61:408 – 422.

Steenbock H, Kletzien SWF. The reaction of chicken to irradiated ergosterol and irradiated yeast as contrasted with the natural vitamin D in fish liver oil. J Biol Chem 1932;97:249 – 264.

Stumpf WE, Sar M, Reid FA, et al. Target cells for 1,25-dihydroxyvitamin D3 in intestinal tract, stomach, kidney, skin, pituitary, and parathyroid. Science 1979;206:1188 – 1190.

Stumpf WE, Clark SA, Sar M, DeLuca HF. Topographical and developmental studies on target sites of 1,25(OH)2 vitamin D3 in skin. Cell Tissue Res 1984;238:489 – 496.

Suda T, Abe E, Miyaura C, Tanak H, Shiina Y, Kuribayashi T. Vitamin D and its effects on myeloid leukemia cells. In: Kumar R, ed. Vitamin D: Basic and Clinical Aspects. Boston, The Hague: Martinus Nijhoff, 1984;365 – 382.

Tan CY, Strathum B, Marks R. Skin thickness measurement by pulsed ultrasound: its reproducibility, validation and variability. Br J Dermatol 1982;106:657 – 667.

Tanaka H, Abe E, Miyaura C. 1,25-Dihydroxycholeciferol and human myeloid leukemia cell line (HL-60): The presence of cytosol receptor and induction of differentiation. Biochem J 1982;204:713 – 719.

Tjellesen L, Nielsen B, Christiansen C. Seasonal fluctuations in serum concentrations of vitamin D metabolites. Br Med J 1982;284:196.

Tomita Y, Fukushima M, Hachiro T. Stimulation of melanogenesis by cholecalciferol in cultured human melanocytes: A possible mechanism underlying pigmentation after ultraviolet irradiation. Tokyo J Exp Med 1986;149:451 – 452.

Tsoukas CD, Provvedine DM, Manolagas SC. 1,25-Dihydroxyvitamin D3, a novel immuno-regulatory hormone. Science 1984;221:1438 – 1440.

Velluz L, Petit A, Amiard G. Sur un stage non photochimique dans la formation des calciferols: essais d'interpretation. Bull Soc Chim Fr 1948;15:1115 – 1120.

Velluz L, Amiard G, Petit A. Le precalciferol—ses relations d'equilibre avec le calciferol. Bull Soc Chim Fr 1949;16:501 – 508.

Waddell J. The provitamin D of cholesterol. I. The antirachitic efficacy of irradiated cholesterol. J Biol Chem 1934;105:711 – 739.

Webb AR, Kline L, Holick MF. Influence of season and latitude on the cutaneous synthesis of vitamin D3: Exposure to winter sunlight in Boston and Edmonton will not promote vitamin D3 synthesis in human skin. J Clin Endocrinol Metab 1988;67:373 – 378.

Webb AR, deCosta BR, Holick MF. Sunlight regulates the cutaneous production of vitamin D3 by causing its photodegradation. J Clin Endocrinol Metab 1989;68:882 – 887.

Webb AR, Pilbeam C, Hanafin N, Holick MF. An evaluation of the relative contributions of exposure to sunlight and diet on the circulating concentrations of 25-hydroxyvitamin D in an elderly nursing home population in Boston. J Clin Nutr 1990;51:1075 – 1081.

Windaus A, Bock F. Uber das provitamin aus dem sterin der schweineschwarte. Hoppe-Seyler's Z Physiol Chem 1937;245:168.

# Subject Index

Prepared by J.C. Netelenbos, University Hospital, Free University, Amsterdam